PROGRESS IN BRAIN RESEARCH

VOLUME 39

DRUG EFFECTS ON NEUROENDOCRINE REGULATION

PROGRESS IN BRAIN RESEARCH

PROGRESS IN BRAIN RESEARCH

VOLUME 39

DRUG EFFECTS ON NEUROENDOCRINE REGULATION

EDITED BY

E. ZIMMERMANN

Department of Anatomy
University of California, School of Medicine
Los Angeles, Calif. 90024, U.S.A.

W. H. GISPEN

Rudolf Magnus Institute for Pharmacology
University of Utrecht, Medical Faculty
Vondellaan 6, Utrecht, The Netherlands

B. H. MARKS

Department of Pharmacology
The Ohio State University
Columbus, Ohio 43210, U.S.A.

D. DE WIED

Rudolf Magnus Institute for Pharmacology
University of Utrecht, Medical Faculty
Vondellaan 6, Utrecht, The Netherlands

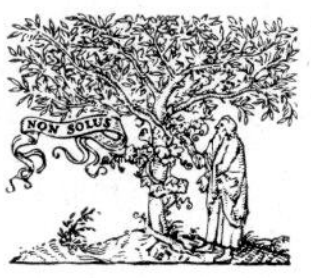

ELSEVIER SCIENTIFIC PUBLISHING COMPANY

AMSTERDAM / LONDON / NEW YORK

1973

ELSEVIER SCIENTIFIC PUBLISHING COMPANY
335 JAN VAN GALENSTRAAT
P.O. BOX 1270, AMSTERDAM, THE NETHERLANDS

AMERICAN ELSEVIER PUBLISHING COMPANY, INC.
52 VANDERBILT AVENUE
NEW YORK, NEW YORK 10017

LIBRARY OF CONGRESS CARD NUMBER: 73-77069

ISBN 0-444-41129-1

WITH 197 ILLUSTRATIONS AND 50 TABLES

PRINTED IN THE NETHERLANDS

This volume contains the Proceedings of an International Symposium on

DRUG EFFECTS ON NEUROENDOCRINE REGULATION

The Symposium was sponsored by the National Institute of Mental Health and National Aeronautics and Space Administration, and held at Snowmass-at-Aspen, Colorado, U.S.A., 17–19 July 1972

List of Contributors

R. Ader, Department of Psychiatry, University of Rochester School of Medicine and Dentistry, Rochester, N.Y. 14642, U.S.A.

M. Amoss, The Salk Institute, 10010 North Torrey Pines Road, La Jolla, Calif. 92037, U.S.A.

J. D. Barchas, Department of Psychiatry, Stanford University Medical School, Stanford, Calif., U.S.A.

H. Barry, III, University of Pittsburgh School of Pharmacy, Pittsburgh, Pa. 15261, U.S.A.

P. Berger, Department of Psychiatry, Stanford University Medical School, Stanford, Calif., U.S.A.

B. Bohus, Rudolf Magnus Institute for Pharmacology, Medical Faculty, University of Utrecht, Vondellaan 6, Utrecht, The Netherlands

R. A. Browning, Department of Pharmacology, The University of Chicago, Chicago, Ill. 60637, U.S.A.

R. Burgus, The Salk Institute, 10010 North Torrey Pines Road, La Jolla, Calif. 92037, U.S.A.

K. D. Cairncross, School of Biological Sciences, Macquarie University, North Ryde, N.S.W. 2113, Australia

R. D. Ciaranello, Section on Pharmacology, Laboratory of Clinical Science, National Institute of Mental Health, Bethesda, Md., U.S.A.

R. Collu, Department of Pediatrics, University of Montreal, Canada

O. M. Cramer, Department of Physiology, The University of Texas Southwestern Medical School, Dallas, Tex. 75235, U.S.A.

D. de Wied, Rudolf Magnus Institute for Pharmacology, Medical Faculty, University of Utrecht, Vondellaan 6, Utrecht, The Netherlands

W. W. Douglas, Department of Pharmacology, Yale University Medical School, 333 Cedar Street, New Haven, Conn. 06510, U.S.A.

H. W. Elliott, Department of Medical Pharmacology and Therapeutics, California College of Medicine, University of California, Irvine, Calif., U.S.A.

A. G. Frantz, Department of Medicine, Columbia University College of Physicians and Surgeons, 630 West 168th Street, New York, N.Y. 10032, U.S.A.

F. Fraschini, Department of Pharmacology, University of Milan, Milan, Italy

J. F. Garcia, Lawrence Radiation Laboratory, University of California, Berkeley, Calif., U.S.A.

R. George, Department of Pharmacology and Brain Research Institute, Center for the Health Sciences, University of California, Los Angeles, Calif. 90024, U.S.A.

W. H. Gispen, Rudolf Magnus Institute for Pharmacology and Laboratory for Physiological Chemistry, University of Utrecht, Medical Faculty, Utrecht, The Netherlands

R. A. Gorski, Department of Anatomy and Brain Research Institute, UCLA School of Medicine, Los Angeles, Calif. 90024, U.S.A.

G. Grant, The Salk Institute, 10010 North Torrey Pines Road, La Jolla, Calif. 92037, U.S.A.

P. Gray, Rockefeller University, New York, N.Y., U.S.A.

H. M. Greven, Research Laboratories, Organon, Oss, The Netherlands

L. J. Grota, Department of Psychiatry, University of Rochester School of Medicine and Dentistry, Rochester, N.Y. 14642, U.S.A.

R. Guillemin, The Salk Institute, 10010 North Torrey Pines Road, La Jolla, Calif. 92037, U.S.A.

A. Heller, Department of Pharmacology, The University of Chicago, Chicago, Ill. 60637, U.S.A.

T. Higuchi, Second Department of Physiology, Yokohama City University School of Medicine, Yokohama, Japan

L. E. Hollister, Veterans Administration Hospital and Stanford University School of Medicine, Palo Alto, Calif. 94304, U.S.A.

M. Hyyppä, Laboratory of Neuroendocrine Regulation, Department of Nutrition and Food Science, Massachusetts Institute of Technology, Cambridge, Mass., U.S.A.

D. M. Jacobowitz, Laboratory of Clinical Science, National Institute of Mental Health, Bethesda, Md. 20014, U.S.A.

S. A. Joseph, Department of Anatomy, The University of Rochester School of Medicine and Dentistry, Rochester, N.Y. 14642, U.S.A.

P. S. Kalra, Department of Physiology, University of Texas Southwestern Medical School, Dallas, Tex., U.S.A.

I. A. KAMBERI, Department of Obstetrics and Gynecology, UCLA School of Medicine, Harbor General Hospital Campus, Division of Reproductive Biology, Torrance, Calif. 90509, U.S.A.
A. J. KASTIN, VA Hospital, Tulane University School of Medicine and Louisiana State University at New Orleans and Medical Center, New Orleans, La., U.S.A.
M. KAWAKAMI, Second Department of Physiology, Yokohama City University School of Medicine, Yokohama, Japan
F. KIMURA, Second Department of Physiology, Yokohama City University School of Medicine, Yokohama, Japan
H. G. KING, School of Biological Sciences, Macquarie University North Ryde, N.S.W. 2113, Australia
K. M. KNIGGE, Department of Anatomy, The University of Rochester School of Medicine and Dentistry, Rochester, N.Y. 14642, U.S.A.
N. KOKKA, Department of Medical Pharmacology and Therapeutics, California College of Medicine, University of California, Irvine, Calif. U.S.A.
N. KONDA, Second Department of Physiology, Yokohama City University School of Medicine, Yokohama, Japan
L. KORANYI, Institute of Physiology, University Medical School, Pécs, Hungary
W. KRIVOY, National Institute of Mental Health, Addiction Research Center, Lexington, Ky., U.S.A.
R. K. KUBENA, ICI America, Inc., Wilmington, Del. 19899, U.S.A.
S. LANDE, Yale University School of Medicine, Department of Dermatology, New Haven, Conn., U.S.A.
N. A. LEOPOLD, Department of Neurology, Boston University School of Medicine, Boston, Mass., U.S.A.
N. LING, The Salk Institute, 10010 North Torrey Pines Road, La Jolla, Calif. 92037, U.S.A.
B. H. MARKS, Department of Pharmacology, The Ohio State University Columbus, O. 43210, U.S.A.
L. MARTINI, Department of Pharmacology, University of Milan, Milan, Italy
S. M. MCCANN, Department of Physiology, University of Texas Southwestern Medical School, Dallas, Tex., U.S.A.
B. S. MCEWEN, Rockefeller University, New York, N.Y., U.S.A.
B. MESS, Department of Anatomy, University Medical School, Szigeti ut 12, Pécs, Hungary
B. J. MEYERSON, Department of Pharmacology, Biomedicum, Box 573, 75123 Uppsala, Sweden
L. H. MILLER, VA Hospital, Tulane University School of Medicine and Louisiana State University at New Orleans and Medical Center, New Orleans, La., U.S.A.
M. MONAHAN, The Salk Institute, 10010 North Torrey Pines Road, La Jolla, Calif. 92037, U.S.A.
P. L. MUNSON, Department of Pharmacology, School of Medicine, University of North Carolina, Chapel Hill, N.C. 27514, U.S.A.
R. NOCKTON, VA Hospital, Tulane University School of Medicine and Louisiana State University at New Orleans and Medical Center, New Orleans, La., U.S.A.
E. PAPAIKONOMOU, Department of Pharmacology, Free University Medical Faculty, Amsterdam, The Netherlands
J. L. PERHACH, Jr., Mead Johnson Research Center, Evansville, Ind. 47721, U.S.A.
S. PODOLSKY, Boston University School of Medicine; Intermediate Care Service and Clinical Metabolic Research Unit, Veterans Administration Hospital, Boston, Mass., U.S.A.
J. C. PORTER, Department of Physiology, The University of Texas Southwestern Medical School, Dallas, Tex. 75235, U.S.A.
P. PREZIOSI, Institute of Pharmacology, University of Naples, Via Pansini 5, 80131 Naples, Italy
R. L. REITER, Department of Anatomy, The University of Texas Medical School at San Antonio, San Antonio, Tex. 78229, U.S.A.
J. RIVIER, The Salk Institute, 10010 North Torrey Pines Road, La Jolla, Calif. 92037, U.S.A.
C. A. SANDMAN, VA Hospital, Tulane University School of Medicine and Louisiana State University at New Orleans and Medical Center, New Orleans, La., U.S.A.
M. SAR, Departments of Anatomy and Pharmacology, Laboratories for Reproductive Biology, University of North Carolina, Chapel Hill, N.C. 27514, U.S.A.
U. SCAPAGNINI, Institute of Pharmacology, University of Naples, Via Pansini 5, 80131, Naples, Italy
A. V. SCHALLY, VA Hospital, Tulane University School of Medicine and Louisiana State University at New Orleans and Medical Center, New Orleans, La., U.S.A.
S. SCHOFIELD, School of Biological Sciences, Macquarie University, North Ryde, N.S.W. 2113, Australia

P. Schotman, Rudolf Magnus Institute for Pharmacology and Laboratory for Physiological Chemistry, University of Utrecht, Medical Faculty, Utrecht, The Netherlands

A. J. Silverman, Department of Anatomy, The University of Rochester School of Medicine and Dentistry, Rochester, N.Y. 14642, U.S.A.

P. G. Smelik, Department of Pharmacology, Free University Medical Faculty, Amsterdam, The Netherlands

L. O. Stratton, VA Hospital, Tulane University School of Medicine and Louisiana State University at New Orleans and Medical Center, New Orleans, La., U.S.A.

W. E. Stumpf, Departments of Anatomy and Pharmacology Laboratories for Reproductive Biology, University of North Carolina, Chapel Hill, N.C. 27514, U.S.A.

E. Terasawa, Second Department of Physiology, Yokohama City University School of Medicine, Yokohama, Japan

L. Tima, Department of Anatomy, University Medical School, Szigeti ut 12, Pécs, Hungary

G. P. Trentini, Department of Pathology, University of Modena, Via Berengario 4, 41100 Modena, Italy

S. Vaala, Department of Anatomy, The University of Rochester School of Medicine and Dentistry, Rochester, N.Y. 14642, U.S.A.

W. Vale, The Salk Institute, 10010 North Torrey Pines Road, La Jolla, Calif. 92037, U.S.A.

J. Vernikos-Danellis, Biomedical Research Division, Ames Research Center, NASA, Moffett Field, California, U.S.A.

P. H. Volkman, Department of Pharmacology, The University of Chicago, Chicago, Ill. 60637, U.S.A.

R. I. Weiner, Department of Anatomy, University of Southern California, School of Medicine, Los Angeles, Calif. 90033, U.S.A.

J. M. Weiss, Rockefeller University, New York, N.Y., U.S.A.

A. Witter, Rudolf Magnus Institute for Pharmacology, Medical Faculty, University of Utrecht, Vondellaan 6, Utrecht, The Netherlands

R. J. Wurtman, Laboratory of Neuroendocrine Regulation, Department of Nutrition and Food Science, Massachusetts Institute of Technology, Cambridge, Mass., U.S.A.

E. Zimmermann, National Institute of Mental Health, Addiction Research Center, Lexington, Ky., U.S.A.

The proceedings of the International Symposium "Drug Effects on Neuroendocrine Regulation" are dedicated to the late Professor GEOFFREY W. HARRIS, whose outstanding work has been a major impetus in the development of Neuroendocrinology.

Preface

Several years ago, a group representing the scientific disciplines of pharmacology, psychology, neuro-anatomy and endocrinology met in conference in Vierhouten, The Netherlands, to evaluate the state of our knowledge concerning the mutual interaction between the pituitary–adrenal system and the brain. The proceedings of that conference were published in 1970 as *Pituitary, Adrenal, and The Brain,* in Progress in Brain Research, Vol. 32 (Elsevier, Amsterdam). It was clear from that meeting that we were on the threshold of exciting new developments in relationship to the interactions between the endocrine and nervous systems. The second discovery which many of us made was that the special combination of disciplines represented at that meeting provided for particularly interesting and enthusiastic discussions and that the group dynamics generated were rather special.

It was with the background of that experience at Vierhouten that a group of us felt impelled to organize a meeting in the U.S.A. several years later in order to measure the advances that had taken place in the understanding of the regulation of the neuro-endocrine system. So it was, therefore, that scientists representing the same combination of disciplines gathered at Snowmass-At-Aspen, Colorado, in the splendid isolation of the Rocky Mountains, to exchange ideas about mechanisms that regulate neuro-endocrine function. There were 90 participants present, including both senior professors and young postdoctoral men and women just entering their careers in neuro-endocrinology. It was apparent from the beginning that the spirit of free exchange, of friendship and of the search for real understanding was with us at this meeting. This spirit was evident from the first morning session, devoted to neuro-anatomical and neuro-chemical aspects of neurosecretion. The vigorous and critical exchange continued through intervening sessions which considered various steroid, biogenic amine and drug effects on neuro-endocrine mechanisms, and great interest and enthusiasm were generated by the discussion of pituitary–adrenal effects upon learning and behavior, the final scientific session.

For all of the good fellowship and invaluable intellectual stimulation, we express sincere gratitude to all of the speakers and to the conference participants in general for their excellent discussion. All of this was made possible by the effort of the various session chairmen, who were instrumental in arranging the program and in insuring the prompt publication of these proceedings—John Porter, Charles Sawyer, Joan Vernikos-Danellis, Luciano Martini, Samuel McCann, William Krivoy, Emery Zimmermann, Robert Ader, Willem Gispen—thank you all!

On a more personal note, our thanks and admiration to our conference secretaries Daria Cverna and Carol Jones, and the graduate students Kenneth Kellar, Paul

McCauley and David Schneider, who made impossible tasks look easy. We also like to thank Greet Hoekstra and Victor Wiegant for their assistance in editing the manuscripts. Finally, the cooperation of the organizing committee, including Willem Gispen, Harold Goldman, William Krivoy and Emery Zimmermann, made it possible for the initial plans for the conference to be fulfilled.

BERNARD H. MARKS
Professor of Pharmacology
Chairman of the Department of Pharmacology
Ohio State University
Columbus, Ohio, U.S.A.

DAVID DE WIED
Professor of Pharmacology
Chairman of the Rudolf Magnus
Institute for Pharmacology
State University of Utrecht
Utrecht, The Netherlands

Acknowledgements

We gratefully acknowledge the

National Institute of Mental Health (U.S.A.)

and the

National Aeronautics and Space Administration (U.S.A.)

for sponsoring this International Symposium.

We also like to express our gratitude to the following organizations:

Abbott Laboratories
Carter-Wallace, Incorporated
CIBA Pharmaceutical Company
Organon Company
Schering Corporation
G. D. Searle and Company
Smith Kline and French Laboratories
Dr. Saal van Zwanenberg Stichting
Wyeth Laboratories

for their generous additional financial support.

Contents

Neuroendocrine Systems: the Need for Precise Identification and Rigorous Description of their Operations*

JOHN C. PORTER

Department of Physiology, The University of Texas Southwestern Medical School, Dallas, Tex. 75235 (U.S.A.)

Neuroendocrinology is a heady science, but it guards its truths with care. It sometimes seems to follow unusual rules which appear to change from time to time and which make it difficult to distinguish fact from fancy. The prober of the secrets of neuroendocrinology often feels like a traveler in *Wonderland* who is not quite sure whether he is seeing the Cat or only its grin. I can imagine that when the historian looks back on these days of neuroendocrinology, he will be sometimes amused and sometimes aghast at our attempts to bring understanding and precision to this fledgling science. As he reviews the accounts detailing our successes and our failures, our insights and our naiveties, he may see a similarity between our plight and that described in *A Tale of Two Cities* by Dickens: "It was the best of times, it was the worst of times, it was the age of wisdom, it was the age of foolishness, it was the epoch of belief, it was the epoch of incredulity, it was the season of Light, ..."

Still, neuroendocrinology has come far in our day, and it is satisfying to participate in a symposium dedicated to the advanced and optimistic topic of "Drug Effects on Neuroendocrine Regulation". Such a symposium may stand as a landmark, signifying the demarcation between two successive phases in the development of neuroendocrinology. The first phase was a period filled with intuitive concepts and characterized by efforts directed toward the establishment of a firm base for the science. The second phase deals with attempts to control and manipulate neuroendocrine systems. This Symposium is a formal recognition of the beginning of this phase.

By way of introduction into the factual portion of the program, let us review the brief past of neuroendocrinology, summarize its present status, and consider where we may be going. In doing so, perhaps we can restate some old questions which are in need of answers. For example, if neuroendocrinology is the science dealing with neuroendocrine systems, what precisely is a neuroendocrine system? Do neuroendocrine systems possess properties and characteristics that are unique and distinguishable from those of other endocrine systems? We begin our search for answers to these

* This investigation has been supported by research grant No. AM 01237 from the National Institutes of Health, Bethesda, Maryland, and by a research grant from the Population Council, New York, N.Y.

References p. 5

questions by reviewing some of the well-known, general characteristics of endocrine systems.

Neither endocrinology nor its subdivision, neuroendocrinology, can be said to have begun at a sharply defined point in time. Instead, both had diffuse beginnings and both acquired many adherents long before either science was recognized; and each arose from advances attributable to experiments emanating solely from research of curiosity. For example, Berthold observed in 1849 that the consequences of castration in the rooster were either prevented or ameliorated by testicular transplantation. Some years later, Brown-Séquard (1889a, 1889b) wrote that the injection into himself of aqueous extracts of animal testes improved his personal well-being, a conclusion that is believed today to be somewhat inflated. Yet, in Brown-Séquard's case, as in others, experiments which were done incorrectly, which yielded erroneous results, and which led to fallacious conclusions are still sometimes useful. Brown-Séquard introduced the valuable experimental technique of hormone replacement.

However, the era of modern endocrinology began when Starling (1905) formalized a concept by use of the word *hormone* in reference to a product secreted into blood by the intestinal mucosa. Today, several sets of cellular systems are known to secrete hormones; and blood is held to be an essential transference vehicle for hormones since they are transported as solutes of plasma. The plasma of blood is, of course, a sub-compartment of the extracellular fluid (ECF), *i.e.*, plasma is the intravascular compartment of the ECF. Before a hormone passes from the secretory cells to plasma, the hormone first enters the ECF adjacent to the secretory cells and thence into plasma. In passage to effector cells, the hormone follows a reverse course. The movement of a hormone within the extracellular fluid appears to be a function of two processes, of which one is diffusion of the hormone along a concentration gradient and the other is movement within the vasculature resulting from the flow of blood.

Neuroendocrinology probably began in 1895 when Oliver and Schäffer found that extracts of adrenomedullary tissue possessed pronounced pressor activity and when Dale (1909) demonstrated that extracts of posterior pituitary tissue stimulated the contractile activity of muscle. Still, the concepts of neurosecretion did not take form until it was shown that certain intraneuronal inclusions were in fact secretory granules, a view which owes much to Scharrer (1933).

Neurosecretory products are often placed into one of two classes. One class consists of those cellular secretions which are known to be involved in such neuronal functions as synaptic transmission and neuronal conduction. The other class consists of substances which are involved in somatic cell function such as renal reabsorption of water, myometrial contraction, and anterior pituitary regulation.

However, the tendency in contemporary usage has been to employ less restrictive constraints as revealed by Green (1966). In a review, he wrote, "a neurosecretory cell will be defined as a neuron which liberates an active substance into the blood stream or tissue fluids, thereby influencing the behavior of somatic cells not necessarily in immediate contact with it". I believe that even this liberal definition is too restrictive and suggest a more general view: *A neuroendocrine system consists of a neural cell or cells which secrete into the extracellular fluid a substance which upon reaching other cells modify their behavior*. This definition does not exclude the possibility that non-neuronal cells may also be neurosecretory cells; it does not require that the secretory product be transported through blood; and the effector cells may be neural cells and/or somatic cells.

One might argue that this view is too inclusive, encompassing as it does such well-known neurotransmitters as acetylcholine and noradrenaline. Indeed, neurotransmitters should be considered as neurohormones. I suggest that the interaction of a neuron with another cell through the intermediacy of a neurotransmitter which passes through the extracellular fluid separating the two cells merely represents the ultimate reduction of an endocrine system. An advantage of this view is that it permits one to consider the entire brain as a collection of heterogeneous neuroendocrine systems, which may not only influence the behavior of somatic cells but also influence the behavior of other neural cells, including other neurosecretory cells.

Now we come to the question: How does a neuroendocrine system differ from a typical endocrine system? First, an essential characteristic of a neuroendocrine system is that the secretory cells are neural cells. Vasopressin, oxytocin, and adrenaline are examples of hormones which are synthesized, stored, and released by neural cells. These hormones, which are secreted by well-defined neuroendocrine systems, *viz*., the neurohypophysial system and adrenomedullary system, are transported *via* plasma of blood to effector cells. These particular neuroendocrine systems differ little from such well-recognized endocrine systems as the adrenocortical system, thyroidal system, parathyroidal system, *etc*.

However, other brain hormones, *viz*., hypophysiotrophic hormones, which stimulate or inhibit the release of anterior pituitary hormones are also present in hypothalamic tissue (*cf*. McCann and Porter, 1969). The molecular structures of two of these hypophysiotrophic hormones have already been determined (Burgus *et al*., 1969; Matsuo *et al*., 1971). Since the activities of several hypophysiotrophic hormones have been demonstrated in hypophysial stalk blood (Porter and Jones, 1956; Kamberi *et al*., 1969, 1970a, 1970b; Wilber and Porter, 1970), it seems probable that these hormones enter portal blood *via* the primary capillary plexus in the median eminence of the hypothalamus. However, the secretory cells elaborating the hypophysiotrophic hormones have not been identified; and consequently the precise location of the secretory cells is not known. It is also not known whether the secretory elements are neuronal cells or non-neuronal cells, but the possible involvement of non-neuronal cells should not be totally discounted. Recently, Zimmerman *et al*. (1972), using a histochemical procedure involving a specific antiserum to neurophysin I, found that neurophysin not only was present in cell bodies and axons of neurons in the supraoptic and paraventricular nuclei but also was present in ependymal cells of the third ventricle. The presence of neurophysin in ependymal cells raises several questions. Do the ependymal cells secrete neurophysin? Or, are the ependymal cells involved in the transference of substances from the cerebrospinal fluid (CSF) of the third ventricle to the capillaries of the portal vessels? Although there is no direct evidence showing that hypophysiotrophic substances are present in CSF, it is noteworthy that Ondo

References p. 5

et al. (1972) found that luteinizing hormone and other substances could pass from CSF into hypophysial portal blood.

It is interesting to speculate that passage of hormonally active products from secretory cells to CSF and from CSF to effector cells represents a general phenomenon and that the movement of CSF through the ventricular system enables substances secreted by the anterior portions of the brain to reach certain posterior regions of the brain that could not be attained by diffusion alone. For example, substances secreted into the CSF by brain tissue surrounding the lateral ventricles could be extracted by the hypothalamus from the CSF as the CSF flowed through the third ventricle.

The findings of Carr and Moore (1969) would seem to support this thesis. They injected tritiated noradrenaline into a lateral ventricle and allowed the radio-labeled compound to equilibrate with the brain stores of this catecholamine. Then, when *d*-amphetamine was infused into the ventricular system to release noradrenaline, they found that the newly released tritiated noradrenaline diffused into the CSF. This finding shows that noradrenaline can pass back and forth between ventricular CSF and brain cells, and it seems probable that other substances can move similarly within the brain.

The flow of CSF in the ventricles would seem to make it possible for neurohormones to be exposed to a larger volume of brain tissue than would be possible if diffusion alone were the sole vehicle for hormonal transfer. Although in comparison to the flow of blood, the flow of CSF is slow (Davson, 1967), but it is not insignificant. In our laboratory, we have seen repeatedly by direct observation that a liquid bolus, placed in the third ventricle or in the cisterna magna, disappears from view within 10 to 30 min (unpublished observations). Our colleague, Dr. J. G. Ondo, has found that synthetic luteinizing hormone-releasing factor placed as a bolus in the cisterna magna initiates the release of luteinizing hormone after a few min lag period (unpublished observations). This observation indicates that solutes in the CSF can enter with modest rapidity the general circulation, presumably by way of the subdural sinuses.

If subsequent investigations confirm the validity of this hypothesis, then many aspects of neural activity should become amenable to experimental as well as therapeutic manipulation. For example, it is conceivable that certain forms of aberrant mentation may be found to be consequences of inappropriate neuroendocrine function. If so, perhaps some problems can be brought to taw by manipulation of certain neuroendocrine systems. Many other opportunities also suggest themselves. Thus, our mission is clear. We must localize precisely the neurosecretory cells of the brain, identify the cells responding to the neurohormones, elucidate the nature of the neurohormones, and determine the functional characteristics of each neuroendocrine system. The task will be difficult, but the reward should be great; and if along the way the mission should seem too much, let us be encouraged by the timeless words of Robert Browning: "A man's reach should exceed his grasp, or what's a heaven for?"

ACKNOWLEDGMENT

The author thanks Mrs. Betty Bechtel for assistance in the preparation of the manuscript.

REFERENCES

BERTHOLD, A. A. (1849) Transplantation der Hoden. *Arch. Anat. Physiol. wiss. Med.*, 42–46.

BROWN-SÉQUARD, C. E. (1889a) Expérience démontrant la puissance dynamogénique chez l'homme d'un liquide extrait de testicules d'animaux. *Arch. Physiol. norm. et path.*, **21**, 651–658.

BROWN-SÉQUARD, C. E. (1889b) The effects produced on man by subcutaneous injections of a liquid obtained from the testicles of animals. *Lancet*, **2**, 105–107.

BURGUS, R., DUNN, T. F., DESIDERIO, D. AND GUILLEMIN, R. (1969) Structure moléculaire du facteur hypothalamique hypophysiotrope TRF d'origine ovine: mise en évidence par spectrométrie de masse de la séquence PCA–His–Pro–NH_2. *C. R. Acad. Sci. [D] (Paris)*, **269**, 1870–1873.

CARR, L. A. AND MOORE, K. E. (1969) Norepinephrine: Release from brain by d-amphetamine in vivo. *Science*, **164**, 322–323.

DALE, H. H. (1909) The action of extracts of the pituitary body. *Biochem. J.*, **4**, 427–447.

DAVSON, H. (1967) *Physiology of The Cerebrospinal Fluid.* Churchill, London, p. 131.

GREEN, J. D. (1966) Microanatomical aspects of the formation of neurohypophysial hormones and neurosecretion, In *The Pituitary Gland, vol. 3.* G. W. HARRIS AND B. T. DONOVAN (Eds.), University of California Press, Berkeley, pp. 240–268.

KAMBERI, I. A., MICAL, R. S. AND PORTER, J. C. (1969) Luteinizing hormone-releasing activity in hypophysial stalk blood and elevation by dopamine. *Science*, **166**, 388–390.

KAMBERI, I. A., MICAL, R. S. AND PORTER, J. C. (1970a) Follicle stimulating hormone releasing activity in hypophysial portal blood and elevation by dopamine. *Nature (London)*, **227**, 714–715.

KAMBERI, I. A., MICAL, R. S. AND PORTER, J. C. (1970b) Prolactin-inhibiting activity in hypophysial stalk blood and elevation by dopamine. *Experientia*, **26**, 1150–1151.

MATSUO, H., BABA, Y., NAIR, R. M. G., ARIMURA, A. AND SCHALLY, A. V. (1971) Structure of the porcine LH- and FSH-releasing hormone. I. The proposed amino acid sequence. *Biochem. biophys. Res. Commun.*, **43**, 1334–1339.

MCCANN, S. M. AND PORTER, J. C. (1969) Hypothalamic pituitary stimulating and inhibiting hormones. *Physiol. Rev.*, **49**, 240–284.

OLIVER, G. AND SCHÄFER, E. A. (1895) The physiological effects of extracts of the suprarenal capsules. *J. Physiol.*, **18**, 230–276.

ONDO, J. C., MICAL, R. S. AND PORTER, J. C. (1972) Passage of radioactive substances from CSF to hypophysial portal blood. *Endocrinology*, **91**, 1239–1246.

PORTER, J. C. AND JONES, J. C. (1956) Effect of plasma from hypophyseal-portal vessel blood on adrenal ascorbic acid. *Endocrinology*, **58**, 62–67.

SCHARRER, E. (1933) Histopathologische Befunde im Zentralnervensystem bei Thalliumvergiftung. *Z. Ges. Neurol. Psychiat.*, **145**, 454–461.

STARLING, E. H. (1905) The chemical correlation of the functions of the body. *Lancet*, **II**, 339–341.

WILBER, J. F. AND PORTER, J. C. (1970) Thyrotropin and growth hormone releasing activity in hypophysial portal blood. *Endocrinology*, **87**, 807–811.

ZIMMERMAN, E. A., HSU, K. C., ROBINSON, A. G., TANNENBAUM, M. AND FRANTZ, A. G. (1972) Distribution of intraneuronal neurophysin I in hypothalamic-posterior pituitary neurosecretory material revealed by immunoenzyme techniques. *IV International Congress of Endocrinology*, Excerpta Medica, Amsterdam, p. 45.

DISCUSSION

GOLDMAN: I'd like to add a modification and perhaps an expansion of your definition of neuroendocrinology, that is, the idea that the subject matter of neuroendocrinology really is the organized interaction between secretory and conductile systems and that this interaction involves a transfer of information by means of specific chemical substances.

PORTER: I think that one thing is certain by our definitions and that is that neuroendocrinologists are going to take over.

Further Observations on the Structure and Function of Median Eminence, With Reference to the Organization of RF-producing Elements in the Endocrine Hypothalamus*

K. M. KNIGGE, S. A. JOSEPH, A. J. SILVERMAN** AND S. VAALA

Department of Anatomy, The University of Rochester, School of Medicine and Dentistry, Rochester, N.Y. 14642 (U.S.A.)

INTRODUCTION

The integration of brain and peripheral endocrine function is accomplished by (*a*) neurohormonal activity of a specialized pool of neurons in the "endocrine hypothalamus" whose secretions are concerned with anterior and posterior lobe function, and (*b*) reciprocal neural connections between this endocrine hypothalamus and higher centers, particularly with the central limbic forebrain–mesencephalic reticular formation circuits. Hormones of the peripheral endocrine organs (including the anterior pituitary) complete closed-loop feedback circuits by participating in the secretory and neural processes at the levels of the pituitary, hypothalamus and higher centers. We have recently reviewed some of the anatomical aspects of this brain-endocrine complex (Knigge and Silverman, 1972b). A major unresolved problem is the identity and location of those specialized parvicellular neurones in the central nervous system (CNS) responsible for secretion of the releasing factors.

An important component of this complex upon which we have focused investigative attention is the median eminence. This tissue, according to our present understanding, represents the final point of convergence of the CNS upon the peripheral endocrine system; its structure and function are therefore of singular importance. Fibers of the tuberoinfundibular tract, ascending noradrenergic systems and possibly others, terminate in the palisade or external layer of median eminence. On the assumption that the parvicellular, releasing factor (RF)-producing neurosecretory system projects directly to the median eminence, much work has been done to identify morphological correlates of their neuroendocrine activity in terminals and axonal inclusions of the palisade layer. Based upon the traditional model of neurosecretion, the magnocellular supraopticohypophyseal axis, it is generally held that parvicellular neurones of the tuberoinfundibular tract are the source of releasing factors and that these hormones are axonally transported to the median eminence and stored in nerve endings in the palisade zone. A further unresolved problem is the validity of this concept, namely

* Supported by U.S.P.H.S. Grant AM-10002 and N.S.F. Grant GB3113.

** U.S.P.H.S. Post Doctoral Fellow 2-FO2NS43754.

References p. 18–19

that releasing factors are axonally delivered to and stored in nerve terminals of the median eminence.

In 1959, Löfgren (1959a and b) called attention to the possibility of a role of the ventricular system in regulation of the secretion of pituitary hormones. In 1968, Knigge *et al.* (Knigge *et al.*, 1971) postulated that "RF-producing elements can ... deliver their product into the ventricle from which it is recovered and delivered to the portal vessels by ependymal cells in the lower wall and floor of the third ventricle". Several other laboratories (Kendall *et al.*, 1969; Kendall *et al.*, 1971; Kendall *et al.*, 1972; Porter *et al.*, 1970; Porter *et al.*, 1972) have explored such a possibility.

This chapter offers additional morphological and functional data suggesting that ependyma of the median eminence are capable of recovering thyrotrophin-releasing factor (TRF) from cerebrospinal fluid (CSF) and delivering it to the portal vessels; this capability is necessarily a fundamental requisite to an hypothesis in which the CSF is a part of the route of delivery of releasing factors from brain to the anterior pituitary.

MATERIALS AND METHODS

The concentration of rat plasma thyrotrophin (TSH) was measured with minor modifications by radioimmunoassay according to Reichlin *et al.* (1970); all samples were assayed in duplicate and at two plasma dilutions. Standard curves of our own rat pituitary extract paralleled those of beef TSH (Pierce, 20 U./mg); results are expressed as mU. TSH/100 ml plasma against the bovine standard.

The methods used in our *in vitro* studies of the transport capacity of median eminence have been described in several previous communications (Silverman *et al.*, 1972; Silverman and Knigge, 1972a; Knigge and Silverman, 1972a). In the present work, we have used essentially similar techniques to examine *in vitro* uptake and binding of TRF. Radioactive preparations included a tritiated TRF, [^{14}C]TRF and a high specific activity (40 Ci/mmole) [^{3}H]proline-labeled TRF. Other releasing factors used in competition studies included luteinizing hormone-releasing factor (LRF) (Burgus), growth hormone-releasing factor (GRF) (Schally) and melanocyte-stimulating hormone-inhibiting factor (MIF) (Kastin).

Tissues for light microscopic autoradiography were processed according to a modified method of Anderson and Greenwald (1969). The unfixed tissue was mounted in minced liver, rapidly quenched in liquid propane, and stored in liquid nitrogen until sectioned. Frozen sections 2 μ thick were cut in a cryostat at $-35°$ in a humidity-controlled room. Under safelight, individual sections were picked up from the knife with glass slides which were previously coated with Kodak NTB-3 liquid emulsion and stored over drierite. The autoradiograms were exposed from 11 to 21 days at $-15°$ in sealed, black light-tight boxes containing ample drierite. Following the exposure period, autoradiograms were developed for 1 min in Kodak D-19 at 19°, rinsed in tap water and treated in fixer for 5 min. Slides were stained with toluidine blue. Appropriate controls were processed for positive and negative chemography.

OBSERVATIONS

Intraventricular infusion of TRF

Large (400 g) male Sprague–Dawley rats were used in all these experiments. The time courses of plasma TSH response to single intravenous injections of TRF are shown in Fig. 1. In these animals, 5 ng of TRF results in a detectable but not significant rise of plasma TSH in 5 min. Following injections of 25 or 100 ng of TRF, plasma TSH levels reach a maximum of 4.5 and 6.9 mU./100 ml respectively at 10 min; in both cases, plasma hormone levels are still elevated approximately four-fold 20 min after injection of the TRF.

A comparison of the response and time course of plasma TSH following intravenous injection or infusion of TRF is depicted in Fig. 2. A constant rate infusion pump delivered total amounts of TRF ranging from 5 to 100 ng of TRF in 1 ml saline at a

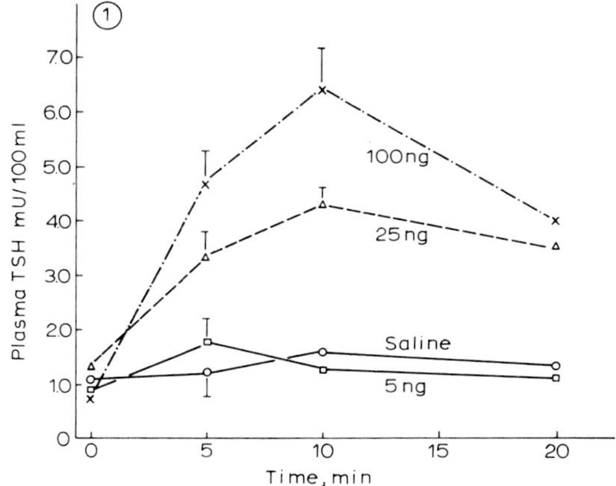

Fig. 1. Time course of plasma TSH response to single intravenous injections of TRF in male (400 g), Sprague–Dawley rats.

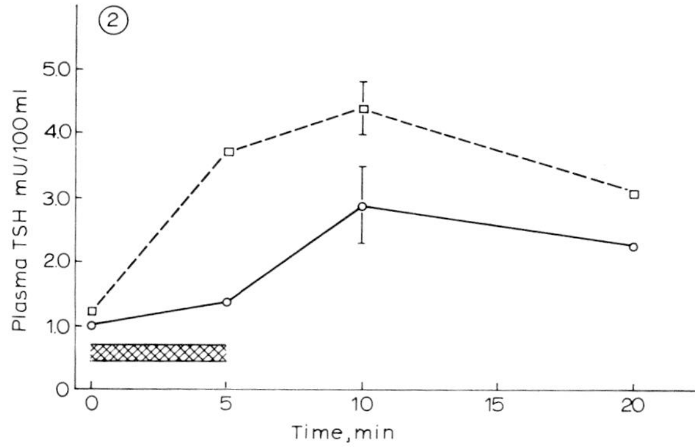

Fig. 2. Comparison of the time course and response of plasma TSH to a single intravenous injection of 25 ng TRF (□– – – –□) *vs.* the same dose (○———○) infused intravenously over a 5-min period.

References p. 18–19

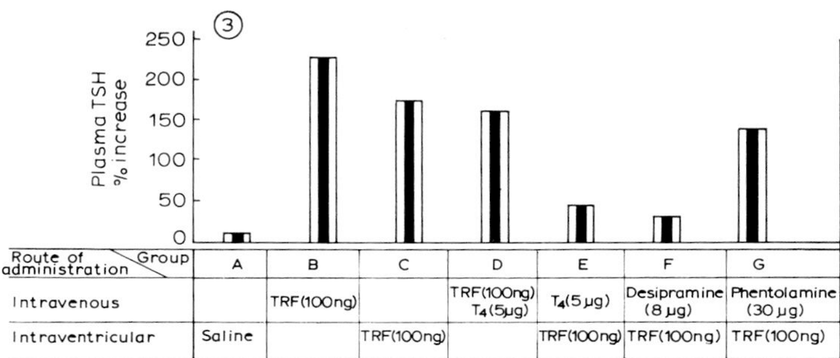

Fig. 3. Plasma TSH response to TRF (100 ng) infused into the lateral ventricle. In all cases of intraventricular administration of TRF, the hormone was infused over a period of 5 min; plasma TSH values represent those measured 5 min after cessation of infusion. In Group D, TRF and thyroxine (T_4) were infused simultaneously into the jugular vein. In groups E, F and G, thyroxine, desipramine or phentolamine were injected intravenously approx. 7 min before infusion of TRF into the lateral ventricle.

rate of approximately 0.2 ml/min. Within this dose range, we have consistently observed a maximal plasma TSH response at 10 min after the beginning of infusion and a significantly smaller rise in plasma TSH compared to an equal dose of TRF given as a single injection.

Fig. 3 summarizes several experiments in which TRF was administered intraventricularly. In all cases, TRF was introduced stereotaxically into the lateral ventricle (De Groot coordinates: AP: + 5.9; L: 1.5). The cannula and tubing used for intraventricular infusion contained an initial 2–3 μl of saline as an "advance fluid"; this was followed by a small "separator" air bubble and finally the TRF solution. These were delivered by positive pressure from an infusion pump and monitored *via* strain gauge and oscilloscope while the cannula was being inserted into the brain. The strain gauge recorded increasing pressure while the cannula and emerging saline traversed tissue; an abrupt fall in pressure was indicated upon entering the ventricle. Solutions were infused at rates of 1–1.5 μl/min and concentrations were adjusted so that a total desired dose was delivered in 5 min. The beginning of infusion of TRF solutions was recorded as zero-time for the purpose of blood sampling and describing the time course of plasma TSH response. This response was recorded as percent difference from that of animals subjected to identical procedures of anesthesia, stereotaxy and cannula insertion but without infusion of any fluid except the 2–3 μl of advance saline. Infusion of TRF into the lateral ventricle results in a plasma TSH response whose time course between zero and 20 min, with maximal hormone levels at 10 min, was similar to that produced by intravenous infusion. At 10 min, maximal response to 100 ng of intraventricularly infused TRF is less (Group C, Fig. 3), but not significantly lower, than the response to 100 ng of intravenously infused TRF (Group B). When 100 ng of TRF and 5 μg of thyroxine (T_4) are infused intravenously at the same time (Group D), plasma TSH response is not modified by the presence of thyroxine. In the animals of Group E, 5 μg of thyroxine was injected intravenously immediately prior to stereotaxy and intraventricular infusion of 100 ng of TRF. An average of 7 min elapsed between the intravenous thyroxine injection and beginning of the intraventricular infusion of TRF; in this group, the plasma TSH response was significantly diminished. The effects of drugs known to alter catecholaminergic transmitter activity were examined using the same protocol as in Group E. 8 μg of desipramine administered intravenously immediately before intraventricular infusion of 100 ng of TRF resulted also in a marked abatement of plasma TSH response (Group F); 30 μg of intravenous phentolamine did not prevent the action of intraventricular TRF (Group G).

In vitro uptake and binding of [^{3}H]TRF by median eminence

Fig. 4 illustrates the *in vitro* uptake of TRF by normal rat median eminence from a solution containing 10 ng/ml [^{3}H]TRF. Uptake is extremely rapid, with saturation at 0.48 ng/mg dry wt. being achieved in approximately 5 min and maintained at this level for the duration (30 min) of these experiments. With longer periods of incubation, a second uptake phase appears, leading to an approximate doubling of the amount of TRF in the tissue (Silverman and Knigge, 1973). The initial uptake of TRF by median eminence as illustrated in Fig. 4 is unaffected by temperature; similar binding is achieved at 4°. Binding of TRF by median eminence is also independent of K^+ and Ca^{++}; incubation in media free of these ions leads to TRF uptake equivalent to that achieved in normal Krebs–Ringer media. A slow turnover of the receptor protein is suggested by the observation that preincubation of median eminence in actinomycin (1–10 μg/ml) for 1–2 h did not influence TRF binding. In competition studies, concentrations of 10–20 ng/ml of LRF, GRF or MIF were incubated together with TRF. None of these factors competed for TRF binding sites in median eminence; increasing the concentration of unlabeled TRF led to a decrease in binding of the labeled hormone. Fig. 4 illustrates also the dissociation of bound [^{3}H]TRF from median eminence. In these experiments, tissues were preincubated for 30 min with

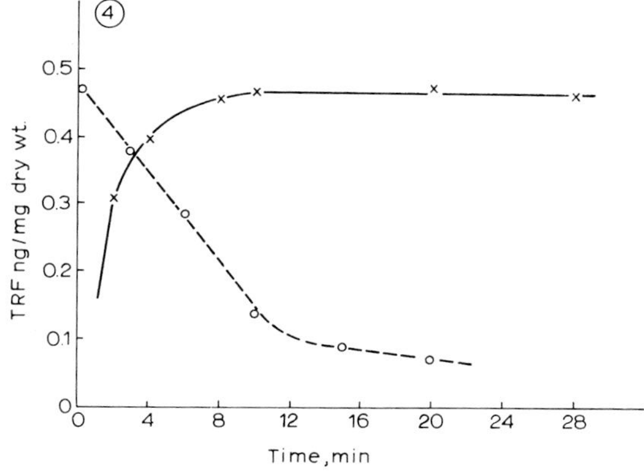

Fig. 4. *In vitro* uptake (x———x) of [^{3}H]TRF by rat median eminence. Also illustrated is the dissociation (○– – – –○) of bound [^{3}H]TRF; median eminence was first incubated for 30 min with 10 ng/ml [^{3}H]TRF and then transferred to fresh medium containing unlabeled hormone.

References p. 18–19

10 ng/ml [^{3}H]TRF and then transferred to fresh media containing unlabeled TRF at a concentration of 1000 ng/ml. The dissociation of [^{3}H]TRF from its binding sites is initially linear with a half-life of approximately 7 min; the overall dissociation process does not appear to follow simple first-order kinetics. Some 20% of the [^{3}H]-TRF initially bound during the 30 min preincubation period may have entered a compartment from which it can less readily exchange.

Autoradiographic localization of thyroxine and TRF

Our previous studies have indicated that median eminence has a considerable capacity to concentrate thyroxine by a mechanism which is in part an active, energy-requiring, Na^+-dependent transport process. We have suggested that the ependymal component of median eminence is the compartment responsible for this activity. Additional support has been provided by the demonstration that thyroxine transport capacity is retained, and even possibly increased, in tissue which has been organ-cultured a sufficient period of time to allow degeneration of virtually all neuronal elements (Silverman *et al.*, 1972). We provide here further evidence for the cellular localization of thyroxine in median eminence. Figs. 5 and 6 are photomicrographs of median eminence from animals in which radiolabeled thyroxine was presented to the ventricular surface of the median eminence by infusion into the lateral ventricle. At 10 min after infusion, autoradiographically demonstrable grains are clearly localized within ependyma. At the apical pole of the cell, cytoplasmic, rather than nuclear, localization of thyroxine, is apparent. The linear arrays of autoradiographic grains (Fig. 6) are clearly associated with the initial, unbranched shafts of ependyma characteristic in this zone of the median eminence. The identification of these autoradiographic grains as thyroxine is considerably strengthened by the knowledge that 70–80% of the thyroxine which enters median eminence is present in a free-pool of unaltered hormone. It is of interest that there is little if any autoradiographic evidence of thyroxine in pars tuberalis.

Figs. 7 and 8 are autoradiographic preparations of median eminence from animals in which [^{3}H]TRF together with 100 ng of unlabeled hormone were infused into the lateral ventricle. A 200% increase in plasma TSH resulted from this dose of infused hormone. The presence of TRF in median eminence, as represented by autoradiographic grains, is apparent. In our preparations thus far, the major grain concentration is in the apical cytoplasm of ependyma (Fig. 8); significant grain concentrations are consistently present also in the portal capillaries and their ansae (Fig. 7). This suggests a localization of TRF in the apical portions of the cell with rapid movement through median eminence. Fig. 9 is an autoradiograph preparation of anterior pituitary from the same group of animals described above. TRF, as represented by autoradiographic grains, is present in both sinusoids as well as in adenohypophyseal cells. The distribution of autoradiographic grains is apparently not restricted to a specific morphological compartment, *i.e.*, membrane, cytoplasm or nucleus. The staining procedure for unfixed tissue causes difficulty in exact identification of the specific cell types with which the grains are associated.

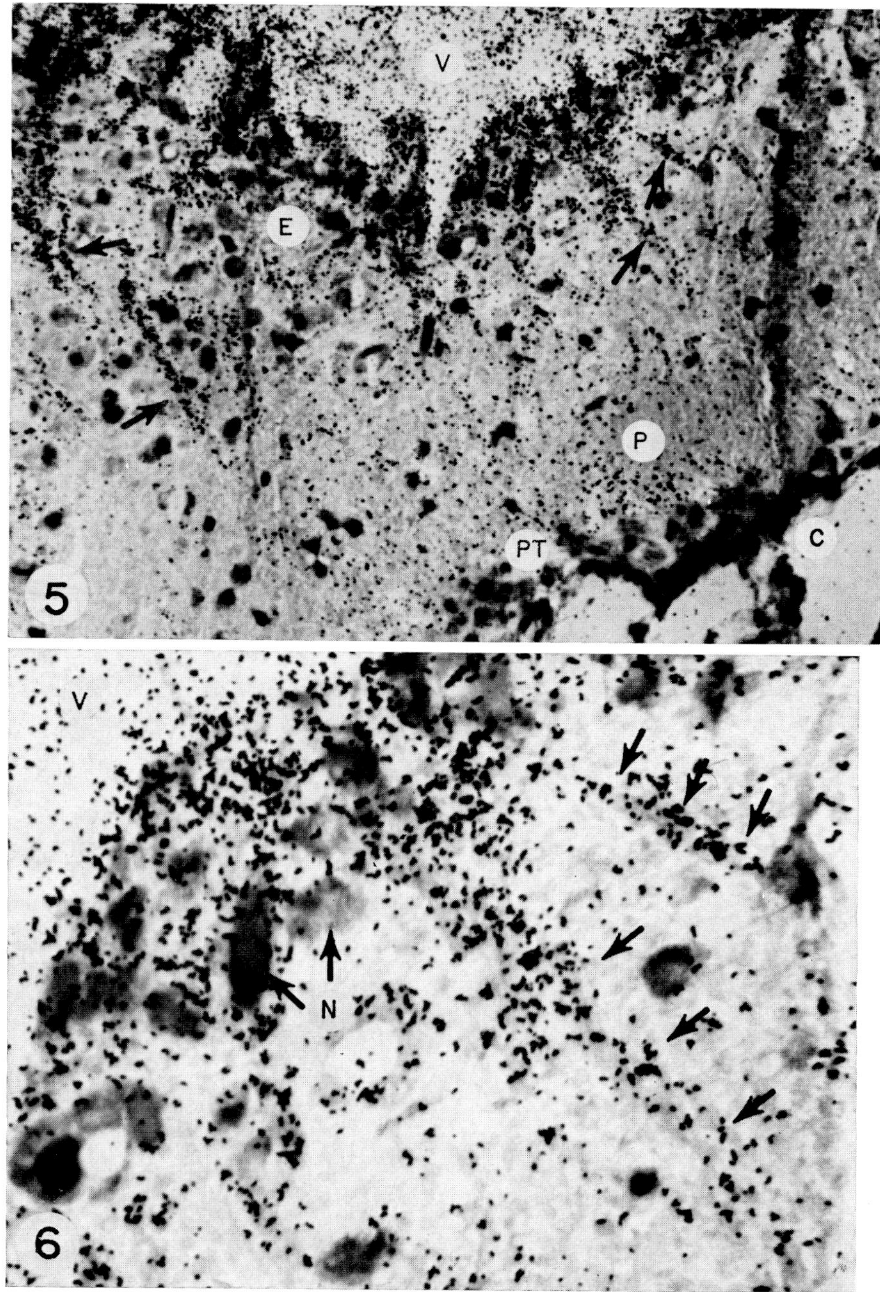

Fig. 5. Low power micrograph (× 533) of an autoradiogram of median eminence from an animal in which radiolabeled thyroxine was infused into the lateral ventricle. Even at low power, grain localization is apparent in the apical ependymal region (E) and palisade zone (P). A linear organization of "grain columns" (→) is evident. The ventricle (V) exhibits intense activity. Pars tuberalis (PT) is relatively devoid of activity, while the portal capillaries (C) contain grain concentrations above background. Exposure time was 11 days.

Fig. 6. Higher magnification (× 1120) of the ependymal surface of median eminence. The columns of autoradiographic grains (→) are superimposed upon the thick shafts of ependyma in this portion of their traverse through the median eminence. The nuclear regions (N) of the ependyma are notably devoid of significant grain concentrations.

References p. 18–19

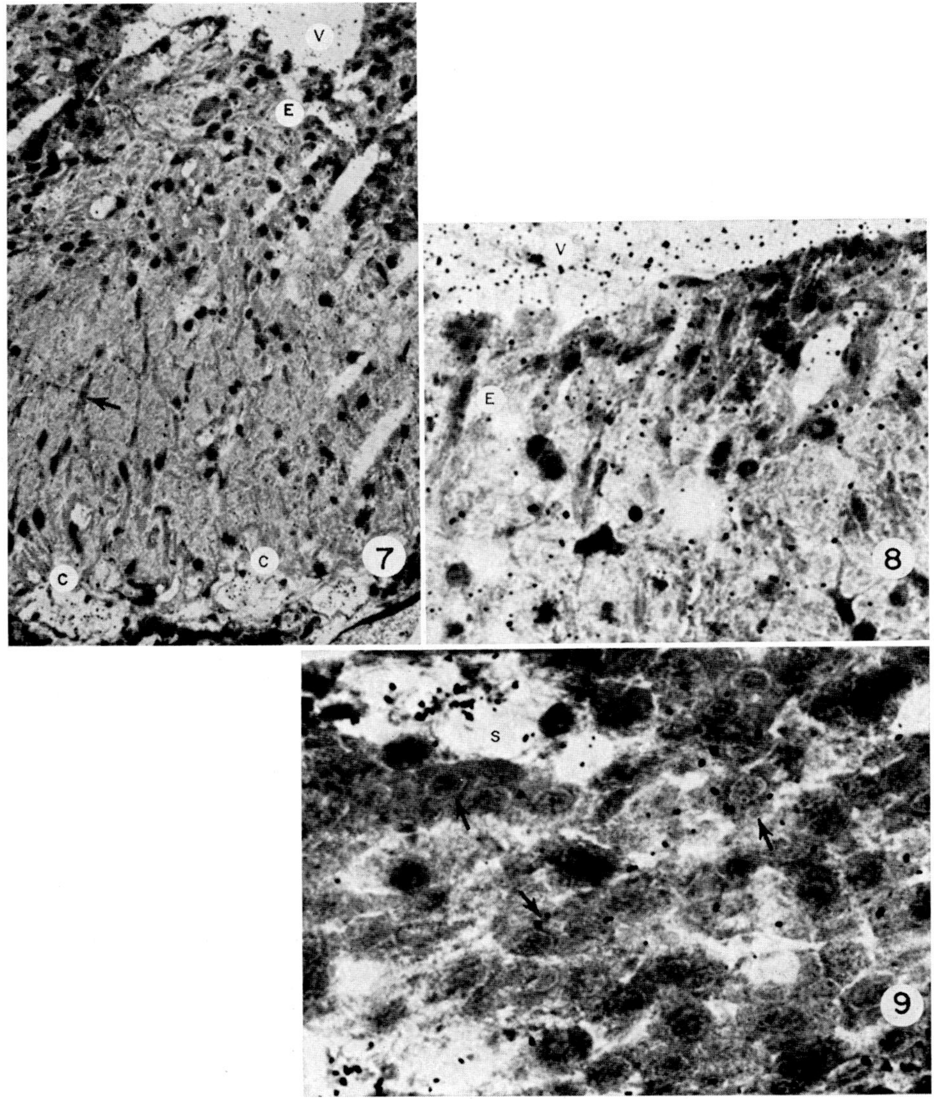

Fig. 7. Low power micrographs (× 334) of an autoradiogram of median eminence from an animal in which [^{3}H]TRF was infused into the lateral ventricle. Grain concentrations are apparent in the ventricular lumen (v), over the apical portions of ependyma (E) and in the portal capillaries (c). Grain concentrations are notably absent from the shafts of ependymal cells (→) in the middle region of the median eminence. Exposure time was 21 days.

Fig. 8. Higher magnification (× 750) of the ependymal (ventricular) surface of the median eminence. Grain concentrations equivalent to that seen in the ventricle (v) are present in the apical portions of the ependyma (E). Exposure time was 21 days.

Fig. 9. Micrograph (K1400) of an autoradiogram of anterior pituitary from an animal in which [^{3}H]TRF was infused into the lateral ventricle. The TRF was infused over a 5-min period and the animal sacrificed 5 min after cessation of infusion. Grain concentrations are apparent in the sinusoids (s) and in the parenchyma (→), although detailed cellular localization as well as cell-type identification is difficult in this preparation. Exposure time was 21 days.

DISCUSSION

A number of laboratories have examined the effect of intraventricularly administered releasing factors upon discharge of pituitary hormones. Most investigators thus far have noted that when administered *via* this route, releasing factors *can* discharge pituitary hormones, but for a variety of considerations, have concluded that the delivery of RF's to median eminence *via* the cerebrospinal fluid is probably not a normal physiological process. It has been observed, for example, that the intraventricular route of administration is generally less effective than when a releasing factor is given intravenously; it is argued that an amount of releasing factor delivered *via* the CSF should be *more* effective than an equivalent dose given intravenously because of the smaller dilution of the hormone when placed in the ventricle. The present authors favor the opinion that such arguments are too simplistic in view of the many unknown factors involved in the movement of substances in the CSF and their transport across the median eminence; this tissue cannot be viewed as a passive membrane separating CSF from portal blood and subject only to simple rules of diffusion. Our studies to date on median eminence indicate clearly the dynamic nature and considerable metabolic capability of this tissue. An example of the regulatory capability of median eminence is seen in our present study in which intravenously administered thyroxine was capable of notably diminishing the effect of TRF infused into the lateral ventricle. Our analysis of this experiment is that thyroxine accumulation by median eminence during the 7–12 min interval between its intravenous administration and intraventricular TRF infusion was sufficiently great to influence the transfer of TRF from the cerebrospinal fluid to the portal capillaries. The initial phase of both *in vitro* and *in vivo* thyroxine uptake by median eminence suggests that nearly half-saturation of the transport process is achieved in less than 10 min. The absence of any effect of thyroxine when it and TRF were administered intravenously at the same time reflects the time course of thyroxine (20–30 min) necessary *at the level of the pituitary* to prevent TRF stimulation of TSH secretion (Vale *et al.*, 1968).

A description of the entire mechanism by which TRF is transported from CSF to pituitary portal blood is not possible at the present time. Our studies to date, however, suggest strongly that a TRF-receptor complex at the ventricular surface of median eminence may be an initial step. The *in vitro* binding properties of [^{3}H]TRF to some element in median eminence parallel strongly the behavior of [^{3}H]TRF with a specific receptor in adenohypophyseal plasma membranes (Grant *et al.*, 1972; Labrie *et al.*, 1972). Our autoradiographic data support the suggestion that the cellular localization of this TRF-receptor complex is in the apical portions of ependyma which line the recess of the third ventricle.

The *in vivo* and *in vitro* capacity of the median eminence with respect to thyroxine transport has led us to suggest that this tissue possesses a mechanism for regulating the level of free thyroxine reaching the anterior pituitary (Knigge and Silverman, 1972a). Previous morphological studies (Knigge and Scott, 1970; Scott and Knigge, 1970), the present autoradiographic localization of thyroxine in ependyma, as well

References p. 18–19

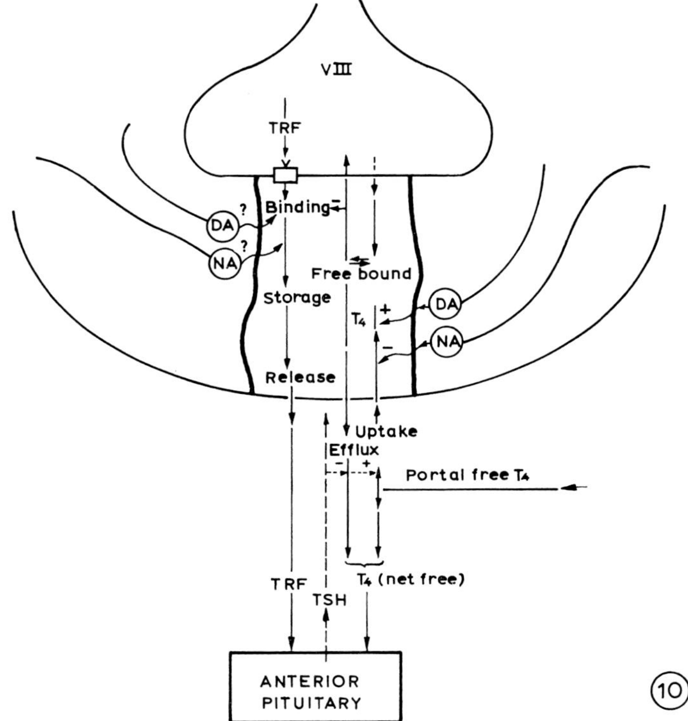

Fig. 10. Schema of thyroxine and TRF transport by median eminence. V III, third ventricle; T4, thyroxine; DA, dopamine; NA, noradrenaline.

as our *in vitro* studies on the transport capacity of the organ-cultured median eminence, point to this cellular element as the one responsible for thyroxine transport and the one which constitutes the physiological compartment linking the cerebrospinal fluid and pituitary portal blood.

Our present studies indicate, furthermore, that in addition to its role in thyroxine transport, the ependyma are also the most likely element of median eminence responsible for transport of TRF from the cerebrospinal fluid to pituitary portal blood. Fig. 10 incorporates our previous conceptualizations of the thyroxine transport compartment of median eminence and our present information that TRF may be transported by the same compartment. The dynamics of this TRF transport process, including binding, storage, intracellular transport and release at the portal face remain to be further explored. Our current studies suggest the presence of a TRF-receptor complex, most likely located in the apical membranes of ependyma at their ventricular face. We have previously suggested that the presence of a large, mobile pool of free thyroxine in this compartment offers a potential regulatory influence; some documentation of this possibility is seen in the present data that an increase of thyroxine in this compartment diminishes the rate of delivery of TRF to portal blood. The site of action of thyroxine in the TRF-transport process requires further study.

TSH has a feedback effect at the level of the median eminence. Its action upon thyroxine transport is to stimulate uptake and diminish efflux. The result of an elevated TSH level is thus to decrease the net amount of free thyroxine reaching the anterior pituitary and to increase the thyroxine level in median eminence. According to our present data, this elevated intracellular thyroxine will depress the transport of TRF. A negative feedback of TSH upon TRF delivery to the anterior pituitary is thus accomplished indirectly by its influence on thyroxine transport.

The precise function of neuronal systems, particularly the catecholaminergic afferents, which terminate in the median eminence has not been entirely resolved. With our initial observations presented here regarding the effect of desipramine and phentolamine on TRF delivery across the median eminence, together with previous evidence that dopamine and noradrenaline influence thyroxine transport, it may be tentatively suggested that these aminergic afferents are organized in a functional (synaptic) relationship to the ependyma. Their neuro-transmitter activity may influence transport or other activities of the ependyma and thus provide a neural input into the regulatory process which controls delivery of releasing factors to the anterior pituitary.

SUMMARY

The hypothesis of ventricular route of delivery of releasing factors to anterior pituitary is further examined. Infusion of TRF into the lateral ventricle of the rat results in plasma TSH responses whose time course is similar to that following intravenous infusion of TRF. The effect of intraventricularly infused TRF upon plasma TSH can be diminished by prior intravenous administration of thyroxine; desipramine produced a similar effect, while phentolamine was without action. Evidence is presented also suggesting the existence of a specific receptor for TRF in median eminence. Following intraventricular infusion of radiolabeled thyroxine or TRF, autoradiographic evidence was obtained for their localization in ependyma. It is suggested that the ependyma of median eminence are capable of transporting TRF from cerebrospinal fluid to the pituitary portal capillaries; thyroxine, and possibly catecholamines, influence the rate of this transport.

ACKNOWLEDGEMENTS

The authors express their sincere appreciation to Dr. Seymour Reichlin for his generosity in providing ABTSH-GP antiserum, Dr. John Pierce (bovine TSH), Dr. Roger Guillemin ([^{3}H]TRF), Dr. Michael Anderson of Abbot Laboratories ([^{14}C]TRF), Dr. Ralph Hirschman of Merck, Sharp and Dohme (GRF), Dr. Abba Kastin (MIF) and Dr. Roger Burgus (LRF). We acknowledge the excellent technical assistance of Dolores Schock, Gail Adams, Marianne Swift and Susan Wischhusen.

References p. 18–19

REFERENCES

ANDERSON, C. H. AND GREENWALD, G. S. (1969) Autoradiographic analysis of estradiol uptake in the brain and pituitary of the female rat. *Endocrinology*, **85**, 1160–1165.

GRANT, G., VALE, W. AND GUILLEMIN, R. (1972) Interaction of thyrotropin releasing factor with membrane receptors of pituitary cells. *Biochem. biophys. res. Commun.*, **46**, 28–34.

KENDALL, J. W., GRIMM, Y. AND SHIMSHAK, G. (1969) Relation of cerebrospinal fluid transport to the ACTH-suppressing effects of corticosteroid implants in the rat brain. *Endocrinology*, **85**, 200–208.

KENDALL, J. W., REES, L. H. AND KRAMER, R. (1971) Thyrotropin-releasing hormone (TRH) stimulation of thyroidal radioiodine release in the rat: comparison between intravenous and intraventricular administration. *Endocrinology*, **88**, 1503–1506.

KENDALL, J. W., JACOBS, J. J. AND KRAMER, R. M. (1972) Studies on the transport of hormones from the cerebrospinal fluid to hypothalamus and pituitary. In *Brain-Endocrine Interaction. Median Eminence: Structure and Function.* Symp. Munich, 1971, K. M. KNIGGE, D. E. SCOTT AND A. WEINDL (Eds.), Karger, Basel, pp. 343–349.

KNIGGE, K. M. AND SCOTT, D. E. (1970) Structure and function of the median eminence. *Amer. J. Anat.*, **129**, 223–244.

KNIGGE, K. M. AND SILVERMAN, A. J. (1972a) Transport capacity of the median eminence. In *Brain-Endocrine Interaction. Median Eminence: Structure and Function.* Symp. Munich, 1971, K. M. KNIGGE, D. E. SCOTT AND A. WEINDL (Eds.), Karger, Basel, pp. 350–363.

KNIGGE, K. M. AND SILVERMAN, A. J. (1972b) The anatomy of the endocrine hypothalamus. In *Handbook of Physiology, Section 7: Endocrinology*, R. O. GREEP AND E. B. ASTWOOD (Eds.), Amer. physiol. Soc., in press.

KNIGGE, K. M., JOSEPH, S. A., SCOTT, D. E. AND JACOBS, J. J. (1971) Observations on the architecture of the arcuate-median eminence region after deafferentation, with reference to the organization of hypothalamic RF-producing elements. In *The Neuroendocrinology of Human Reproduction.* Symp. Detroit, 1968, H. C. MACK AND A. I. SHERMAN (Eds.), Thomas, Springfield, pp. 6–22.

KNIGGE, K. M., SILVERMAN, A. J. AND SCOTT, D. E. (1972) Neurohumoral influences on cellular metabolism in median eminence of the hypothalamus. In *Proc. Int. Symp. Environ. Physiol.*, R. EM. SMITH (Ed.), FASEB, Washington, pp. 51–58.

LABRIE, F., BARDEN, N., POIRIER, G. AND DELEAN, A. (1972) Binding of thyrotropin-releasing hormone to plasma membranes of bovine anterior pituitary gland. *Proc. nat. Acad. Sci. (U.S.)*, **69**, 283–287.

LÖFGREN, F. (1959a) New aspects of the hypothalamic control of the adenohypophysis. *Acta morph. neerl. scand.*, **2**, 220–229.

LÖFGREN, F. (1959b) The infundibular recess, a component in the hypothalamoadenohypophyseal system. *Acta morph. neerl. scand.*, **3**, 55–87.

PORTER, J. C., MICAL, R. S., TIPPIT, P. R. AND DRANE, J. W. (1970) Effect of selective surgical interruptions of the anterior pituitary's blood supply on ACTH. *Endocrinology*, **86**, 590–599.

PORTER, J. C., KAMBERI, I. A. AND ONDO, J. G. (1972) Role of biogenic amines and cerebrospinal fluid in the neurovascular transmittal of hypophysiotrophic substances. In *Brain-Endocrine Interaction: Median Eminence: Structure and Function.* Symp., Munich, 1971, K. M. KNIGGE, D. E. SCOTT AND A. WEINDL (Eds.), Karger, Basel, pp. 245–253.

REICHLIN, S., MARTIN, J. B., BOSHANS, R. L., BOLLINGER, J. AND PIERCE, J. W. (1970) Measurement of TSH in plasma and pituitary of the rat by a radioimmunoassay utilizing bovine TSH: Effect of thyroidectomy or thyroxine administration on plasma TSH levels. *Endocrinology*, **87**, 1022–1031.

SCOTT, D. E. AND KNIGGE, K. M. (1970) Ultrastructural changes in the median eminence of the rat following deafferentation of the basal hypothalamus. *Z. Zellforsch.*, **105**, 1–32.

SILVERMAN, A. J. AND KNIGGE, K. M. (1972a) Transport capacity of median eminence, II. Thyroxine transport. *Neuroendocrinology*, **10**, 71–82.

SILVERMAN, A. J. AND KNIGGE, K. M. (1972b) Transport capacity of median eminence, IV. TRF. *Neuroendocrinology*, in press.

SILVERMAN, A. J., KNIGGE, K. M. AND PECK, W. A. (1972) Transport capacity of median eminence, I. Amino acid transport. *Neuroendocrinology*, **9**, 123–132.

SILVERMAN, A. J., KNIGGE, K. M., RIBAS, J. L. AND SHERIDAN, M. N. (1973) Transport capacity of median eminence, III. Amino acid and thyroxine transport of the organ-cultured median eminence. *Neuroendocrinology*, **11**, 107–118.

VALE, W., BURGUS, R. AND GUILLEMIN, R. (1968) On the mechanism of action of TRF: Effects of cycloheximide and actinomycin on the release of TSH stimulated *in vitro* by TRF and its inhibition by thyroxine. *Neuroendocrinology*, **3**, 34–46.

DISCUSSION

STUMPF: We obtained similar localization in our autoradiograms of the median eminence, after the injection of [^{125}I] thyroxine. We observed "streaking" of radioactivity, which we could not explain. It is conceivable that this represents localization of radioactivity in specialized ependyma cells, forming a link between the thyroid, the ventricle, and the primary plexus. Several investigators have observed "thyroxine" in the median eminence, but it was never clear what this meant especially since many substances are known to accumulate in this area.

KNIGGE: It's encouraging to see agreement in this field. With regard to localization of thyroxine or TRF to regions of the hypothalamus other than the median eminence, we do not have substantive information at the present time. I believe Dr. Vaala has some preliminary data on TRF localization in a region along the lower, lateral margin of the arcuate nucleus.

KASTIN: Your finding that in the rat i.v. infusion of TRH (= TRF) does not release any greater amounts of TSH and that the peaks do not differ from when the same dose is injected as a bolus, is of interest. In collaboration with Drs. David Gonzales-Barcena, Schalch, and others we compared the effects of the same dose of TRH infused for 4 h with that injected as a bolus in man. In contrast to your findings in the rat, in man the infusion resulted not only in greater release of TSH, but also a higher maximum which reached a peak later than when TRH was given as a bolus.

KNIGGE: I am aware that this data in the rat is not similar to that described in man and I have no immediate explanation for the discrepancy other than to consider either species differences or details such as infusion rate, time of infusion, *etc.* One possibility may be the rate of inactivation of TRF. Mr. Kubek in our department has been studying the TRF-inactivating enzyme which is present in plasma and there appears to be species differences as well as differences under varying physiological states.

WEINER: First I'd like to say that I am very pleased to see that your data with the TRF agree completely with data that we obtained with LRF following intraventricular injection. One point that I'd like to ask you though is what is the possibility that the substances injected into the third ventricle are transported directly into the portal system. It has been shown that there are long capillary loops which actually come up and make contact with the surface of the third ventricle.

KNIGGE: You are correct about the suggestion of long capillary loops which penetrate the median eminence and reach the ventricular surface. Our studies by Drs. Scott and Weindl suggest that these long ansae may not actually be in contact with the ventricle. They are, furthermore, only seen infrequently, and I would not consider them a major route of transfer of substances between the CSF and portal capillary blood.

SHASKAN: I have two questions. First, you showed that 100 ng (a large dose) of TRF infused intraventricularly resulted in a relatively small release of TSH. Did you use a lower dose of the TRF? My second question relates to the transport of TRF into the median eminence. If I understood correctly, this transport was not temperature-dependent and your studies with metabolic inhibitors suggested that the transport was not dependent on metabolism. Yet at the end of your talk you proposed that specific receptors were involved in this transport process. If so, wouldn't you suspect that an energy-dependent process is involved?

KNIGGE: In answer to your first question, we have not examined thoroughly a wide range of TRF doses administered *via* the intraventricular route. 25 ng of TRF inconsistently gives a detectable response. 100 ng provides a rather consistent and significant response, but one which I believe is not maximal in terms of pituitary response. This dose of TRF is chosen therefore to fit the objectives of our experiment, namely to demonstrate changes in transport by median eminence which may lead to greater or lesser delivery of the TRF to anterior pituitary. In response to your second question, I must emphasize that our *in vitro* studies of the uptake and binding of [^{3}H] TRF by median eminence represent only a demonstration of the presence of some specific TRF-receptor complex. They provide no information on the further steps of the overall transport process. It is entirely likely that further steps of transcellular delivery and release require energy-dependent systems.

MUNSON: Dr. Knigge, in view of the recent trend of thought that the thyroid hormone that acts at the periphery is T_3 rather than T_4 your data on T_4 are especially interesting. Do you have any comparable data on T_3?

KNIGGE: That's an extremely important question, Dr. Munson, but I'm sorry to say we do not, as yet, have any comparable data on T_3 transport.

SACHS: How specific is the uptake of T_4 and TRF into median eminence tissue? Have you done any controls with other neural tissues, for example neural lobe tissue takes up T_4 and T_3 very avidly, what about cerebral cortex or anything else?

KNIGGE: We have used a variety of tissues as "controls" in these *in vitro* studies, including cortex, anterior and posterior pituitary, and pineal. None have an active transport mechanism for thyroxine. TRF binds non-specifically to many tissues, but only anterior pituitary and median eminence thus far appear to have a specific binding mechanism.

SACHS: Ependymal cells have been implicated as being more or less important in neuroendocrine function or in releasing factors release. I wonder if a clear statement or consensus regarding the role of these ependymal cells might be made.

KNIGGE: There is no consensus about this hypothesis of ventricular route of delivery of releasing factors. In my opinion, neurons located perhaps in the periventricular stratum, synthesize TRF. This is axonally delivered to the ventricular wall and released into the CSF; ependyma of median eminence recover the hormone from CSF and deliver it to portal blood. Regulatory mechanisms are present in median eminence which control the rate of delivery.

How Do Neurones Secrete Peptides? Exocytosis and Its Consequences, Including "Synaptic Vesicle" Formation, in the Hypothalamo-Neurohypophyseal System

WILLIAM W. DOUGLAS

Department of Pharmacology, Yale University Medical School, 333 Cedar Street, New Haven, Conn. 06510 (U.S.A.)

The problem of how neurones secrete peptides is, I believe, best addressed by discussing the hypothalamo-neurohypophyseal system secreting the octapeptide hormones oxytocin and vasopressin (ADH). The secretory elements of this system are the archetypical "peptidergic" nerves, and more is known of their function than that of all other such neurones combined.

It has long been suspected that these hypothalamo-neurohypophyseal cells possessing neuronal as well as glandular morphological characteristics generate impulses in response to osmotic or reflex synaptic activation and propagate them to their terminals in the neurohypophysis. This has recently been substantiated by several elegant electrophysiological studies on supraoptic and paraventricular cells positively identified by antidromic stimulation (see Koizumi and Yamashita, 1972).

The questions then are: (*1*) whether impulses provide the adequate stimulus for release of the posterior pituitary hormones; (*2*) if so, how they act; and (*3*) what kind of secretory process is set in motion.

Experiments performed a decade ago when evidence on the electrical properties of the system was embryonic, provided some useful clues. At that time, the elements of what we termed "stimulus-secretion coupling" (Douglas and Rubin, 1961) had become evident in two cell types sharing a common developmental ancestry with the hypothalamo-neurohypophyseal fibres: ordinary nerves and chromaffin cells. The former possessed the electrical characteristics believed present in hypothalamo-neurohypophyseal fibres. The latter had comparable glandular functions and morphology. And in both cells, stimulus-secretion coupling seemed to revolve around depolarization and calcium entry (see Douglas, 1968). It was thus natural to enquire whether this was also true of the neurohypophysis. Affirmative answers were quickly forthcoming when neural lobes *in vitro* were found to release hormone in response to excess potassium, but only when calcium was present. This prompted conjecture that neurohypophyseal secretion "is effected by the arrival of impulses from the supraoptic and paraventricular nuclei which, by depolarizing the endings ... promote calcium influx ..., and that the appearance of free calcium ions somewhere in the endings then causes the release of stored hormone" (Douglas, 1963).

References p. 35–38

Further studies with this simple *in vitro* preparation rapidly accumulated evidence consistent with this scheme. The response to K was found to require no ion other than Ca, to increase with increasing $[Ca]_0$ over a wide range, and to be inhibited by Mg. Moreover, electrical stimulation proved very effective in releasing hormone (Douglas and Poisner, 1964a) and this effect too required Ca and was inhibited by Mg (Mikiten and Douglas, 1965). In addition, ^{45}Ca uptake into neurohypophyses increased with stimulation and Mg reduced this (Douglas and Poisner, 1964b; Ishida, 1967). Impulses in the isolated preparation, of the classical C type characteristic of unmyelinated fibres, fail when Na is removed (Ishida, 1970) or tetrodotoxin (TTX) introduced (Dreifuss *et al.*, 1971b) and clearly depend on the familiar Na entry mechanism. This is an essential link in stimulus-secretion coupling and secretory responses to electrical stimulation are blocked by local anaesthetics (Haller *et al.*, 1965; Mikiten and Douglas, 1965) or TTX (Dreifuss *et al.*, 1971b). However, at the terminal the function of sodium entry seems limited to depolarization. Sodium ions do not contribute directly to release: the response to excess K is not reduced but potentiated in sodium-free media (Douglas and Poisner, 1964a), and secretion to electrical stimulation increases over a wide range as $[Na]_0$ is lowered (Mikiten, 1967; Dreifuss *et al.*, 1971a). And, finally, we have recently found it possible to evoke a massive release of hormones by stimulating electrically in a medium consisting simply of 2–5 mM $CaSO_4$ in isosmotic sucrose (Douglas and Sorimachi, 1971). This response is resistant to TTX but blocked by Mg or Co suggesting the calcium channel most important for secretion corresponds with the late rather than the early component discernable in squid axon (Baker *et al.*, 1971a, 1971b). The main point here, however, is that calcium is sufficient to sustain the secretory response to electrical stimulation. This is reminiscent of the chromaffin cell where secretory responses in the absence of all ions other than calcium were first observed (Douglas and Rubin, 1963) and where intracellular recordings have shown inward calcium current (Douglas *et al.*, 1967). It also resembles the behavior of ordinary nerve endings releasing acetylcholine in "calcium Ringer" (Katz and Miledi, 1969). But this similarity between neurosecretory terminals on the one hand and chromaffin cells and ordinary neurones on the other is but an extension of an already remarkable parallelism in the secretory behavior in these three developmentally related cells emphasized in earlier reviews (Douglas, 1966, 1967, 1968; see also Hubbard, 1970).

There is only one important feature distinguishing the neurosecretory fibre (or ordinary neurone) from the developmentally related chromaffin cell, namely the property of impulse initiation and propagation. But this may be regarded simply as an adaptation serving to telegraph the primitive membrane and ionic events—demonstrably sufficient to induce secretion in the compact chromaffin cell—from the point of reception on the perikaryon to the exceptionally distant "secretory pole" constituted by the axon terminal of the neurosecretory fibre or nerve, the action potential merely imposing on this "secretory pole" the same pattern of depolarization and ionic influx imprinted on the distant cell body by the synaptic transmitter (Fig. 1). Considerations of this sort, coupled with the common developmental origins of these cells and the remarkable ionic and pharmacological parallels between them have been advanced as

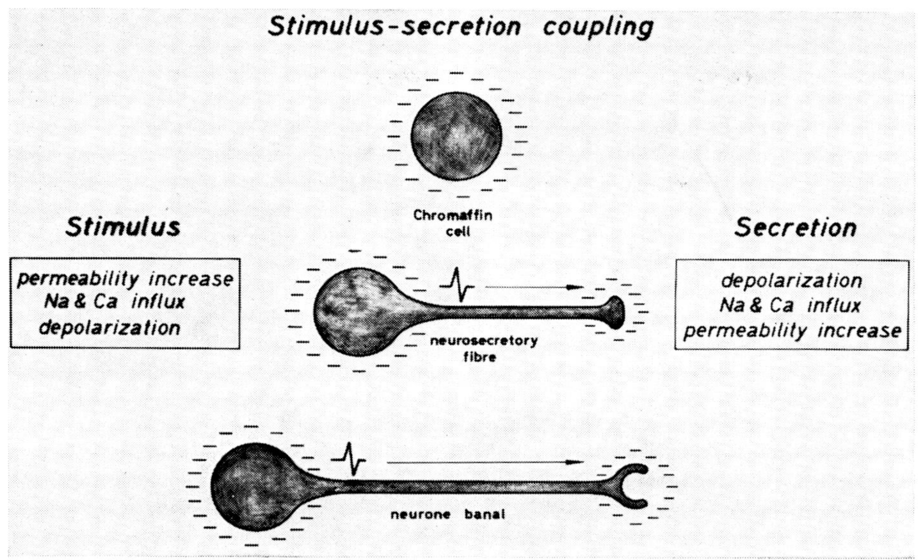

Fig. 1. A schema indicating the unity of the central events in stimulus-secretion coupling in the three developmentally related cells: chromaffin cells, neurosecretory fibres of the hypothalamo-neurohypophyseal tract and ordinary neurones. Impulses in the latter two merely telegraph the basic pattern of depolarization and ion influx impressed directly on the perikarya and chromaffin cell. (After Douglas, 1966)

argument that the calcium-activated secretory process in neurosecretory fibres and neurones must surely be the same as that in the chromaffin cell and involve exocytosis (Douglas and Poisner, 1964a; Douglas, 1966, 1967, 1968). Albeit indirectly based, this line of thought has proved most helpful in defining the intimate nature of neuronal secretion.

MECHANISM OF EXTRUSION OF NEUROHYPOPHYSEAL HORMONES

No secretory cell has been the subject of more diverse speculation concerning its mode of secretion than the hypothalamo-neurohypophyseal fibre. This is largely because of the complexity of the electron-microscopical evidence. In his pioneering study in rats Palay (1957) reported the terminals contained large (about 1500 Å) electron-opaque granules (the elementary neurosecretory granules) which he assumed, correctly, contained posterior pituitary hormones, and also electron-lucent structures of similar size which he supposed were neurosecretory granules emptied of their contents by physiological secretory activity. This opinion that "electron-microscopically empty or only partly filled vesicles are to be considered as granules which have released their contents" (Bargmann, 1968) has won wide acceptance and forms the basis for the oldest and most prevalent view that upon stimulation hormones escape through the membranes of the neurosecretory granules (somehow rendered permeable) to traverse

References p. 35–38

cytoplasm and plasmalemma and reach the extracellular space in the form of a "molecular dispersion" (Palay, 1957; DeRobertis, 1962; Gerschenfeld *et al.*, 1960; Barer and Lederis, 1966; Kurosumi *et al.*, 1964; Ishida, 1967; Bargmann, 1968). Palay's (1957) further discovery that the terminals also contained numerous smaller (about 400 Å) electron-lucent vesicles which he termed "synaptic vesicles" introduced an additional complication. Some authors suggested, by analogy with ordinary nerves, that these vesicles contain a substance such as acetylcholine that is liberated during stimulation to initiate hormone release. Others have maintained they arise by budding or "fragmentation" of neurosecretory granules serving perhaps to ferry hormone to the terminal surface, and consider clusters of vesicles hard against the terminal membrane ("synaptoid figures") as supporting this concept. Or, alternatively, have supposed they result from fragmentation of the larger electron-lucent vesicles (see reviews by Bargmann, 1968; Herlant, 1967; LaBella, 1968). Still other conjectures have arisen from cell fractionation studies yielding hormone (and the binding protein neurophysin) in the supernatant as well as in the large electron-dense granules. This, and other evidence, has prompted the conception that granules are merely reserves and that release occurs from an extragranular cytoplasmic pool, the specific suggestion being made that calcium entering the terminal dissociates an octapeptide–neurophysin complex allowing the former to diffuse out leaving neurophysin behind to be recharged from the granule stores (Thorn, 1965, 1966; Ginsburg *et al.*, 1966; Ginsburg, 1968).

Each scheme is open to criticism. The argument on morphological evidence is indirect and often based on images recent fixation methods indicate as artifactual (Boudier *et al.*, 1970; Douglas *et al.*, 1971a; Santolaya *et al.*, 1972). And "extragranular pools" of hormone may have no existence outside the homogenizer: similar conjectures concerning chromaffin cell secretion have been abandoned as the artifactual nature of the "extragranular pool" has become evident and chromaffin granules shown to void their contents directly to the cell exterior by exocytosis (see reviews by Douglas, 1968; Kirshner and Viveros, 1970).

Exocytosis

The possibility that exocytosis is the physiological mechanism of release of neurohypophyseal hormones has generally been dismissed on the grounds that electron-microscopic evidence for it has been nonexistent. For example, Barer and Lederis (1966) write: "The absence of any appearances suggesting a process akin to reversed pinocytosis or fusion of the elementary granules with the plasma membrane under these conditions (involving stimulation) should also be pointed out" (see also Bargmann, 1968). The contrary opinion that exocytosis (or "reverse micropinocytosis" as it was then called) operates in the neurohypophysis, despite the absence of electron-microscopic evidence (Douglas and Poisner, 1964a; Douglas, 1967, 1968), was generated by argument by analogy with the adrenal medulla and protein-secreting salivary glands each of which had then also been found to require calcium for secretion (Douglas and Rubin, 1961; Douglas and Poisner, 1963). Electron microscopy had by this time, yielded convincing images of exocytosis in exocrine cells and some

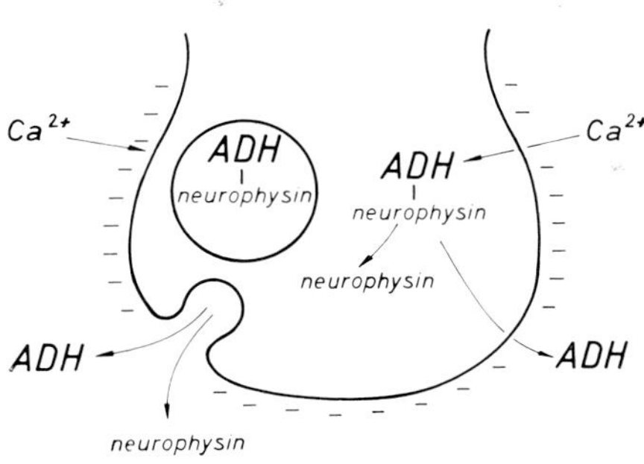

Fig. 2. The "neurophysin test" for distinguishing between different hypotheses of neurohypophyseal secretion (see text). The escape of the protein neurophysin, a molecule unlikely to traverse intact membranes, is held to argue against intracellular "leakage" from granules or dissociation of extragranular neurophysin-hormone complexes, but in favor of exocytosis.

suggestive images in chromaffin cells, and it seemed likely that the common calcium requirement would be accounted for most neatly by a mechanism shared by these diverse cells. Exocytosis appeared to us the only obvious candidate; indeed we suggested that exocytosis wherever it occurred might prove to be calcium-dependent (Douglas and Poisner, 1963). As a general involvement of calcium in exocytotic secretions has become apparent from studies on many cells (see reviews by Douglas, 1968; Rubin, 1970), and as the evidence for exocytosis in the chromaffin cell has become exceptionally strong—this as a result of the introduction of chemical methods (see Douglas, 1966, 1967, 1968; Douglas and Poisner, 1966; Kirshner and Viveros, 1970) and the use of appropriate species for electron microscopy (Diner, 1967)—it seemed increasingly probable that exocytosis must also operate in the neurohypophyseal terminals. As a means of testing this, it was proposed (Douglas, 1967, 1968) that the chemical approaches helpful in defining secretion in the chromaffin cell be extended to the others—specifically that neurophysin should be sought in the effluent from secreting pituitaries since this protein would not be expected to traverse intact membranes and its escape would clearly argue for exocytosis and against all the "intracellular" theories (Fig. 2). When Fawcett *et al.* (1968) detected release of neurophysin (see also Burton *et al.* 1971; Cheng and Freisen, 1970; Legros *et al.*, 1969; Nordmann *et al.*, 1971; Uttenthal *et al.*, 1971; also Norström and Sjöstrand, 1971) we were convinced the absence of electron-microscopic evidence must reflect some technical difficulty. Our conviction was reinforced by the fact that clear images of exocytosis in chromaffin cells had been obtained only in a single species, the hamster. Dr. Nagasawa, Mrs. Schulz and I therefore undertook a fresh electron-microscopic study including neurohypophyses from hamsters. Although scarce, images of exocytosis were clearly present in our material (Fig. 3, A–E) and more abundant in hamsters than rats, and we were able to assemble a series illustrating the classical exocytosis sequence beginning with granules communicating with the extracellular space through a narrow perforation in the melded granule and plasma membranes, passing by way of wider-

References p. 35–38

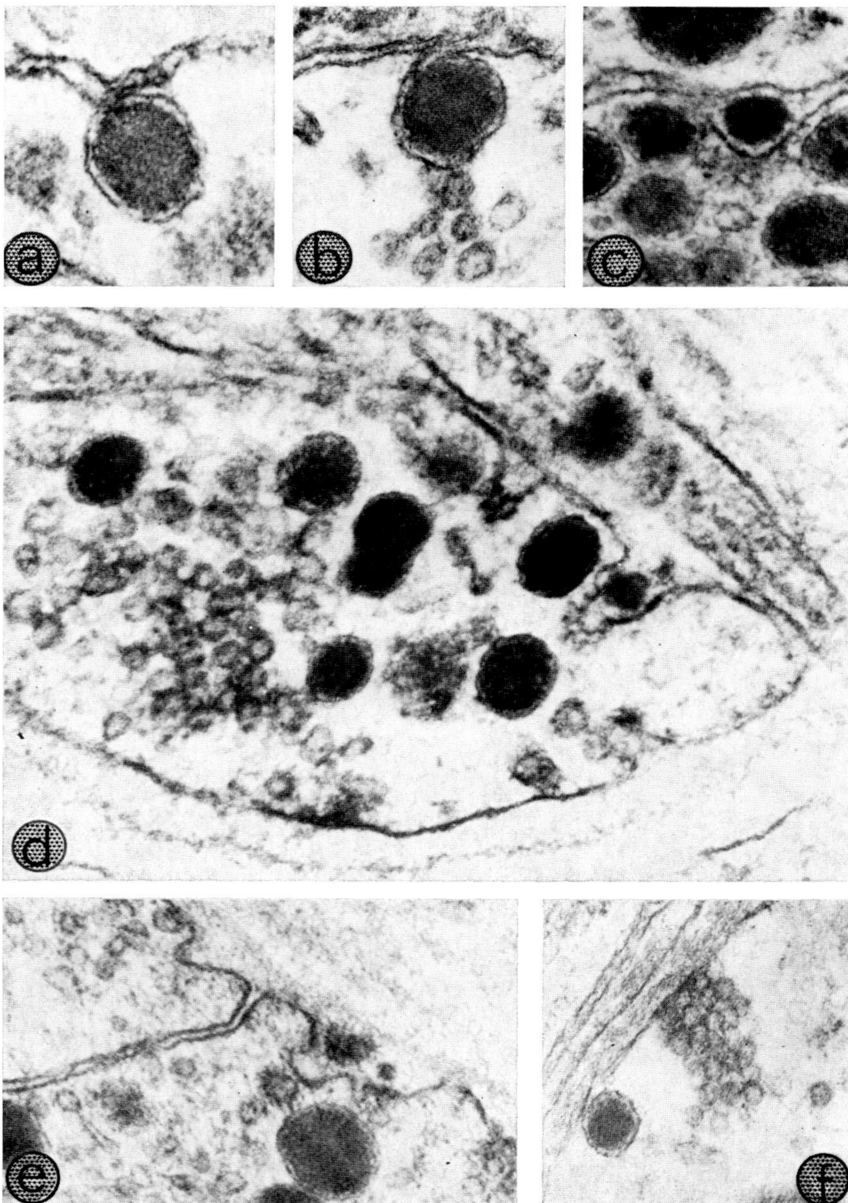

Fig. 3. Electron-microscopic evidence of exocytosis in hypothalamo-neurohypophyseal terminals (a, b, c, d) and formation of microvesicles ("synaptic" vesicles) as a by-product arising by vesiculation (micropinocytosis-like activity) of the exocytotic pit, *i.e.* the depression in the cell surface formed by what was formerly the membrane of a neurosecretory granule (d and e). A "synaptoid figure" believed to arise from such vesiculation is shown in (f). Species: rat (a, b, f), hamster (c, d, e). Magnifications: a, × 100 000; b, c, d, × 80 000; e, × 68 000; f, × 62 000. (From Douglas *et al.*, 1971a)

mouthed figures of the familiar "omega" type to shallow depressions in the terminals containing barely perceptable vestiges of extruded granule contents (Nagasawa *et al.*, 1970; Douglas *et al.*, 1971a). Sparsity of exocytotic images we suggested probably reflects the fleeting nature of the phenomenon and its refractoriness to capture by conventional electronmicroscopic methods: more recently Santolaya *et al.* (1972) have reported greater numbers with freeze etching.

Together then, morphological and chemical evidence indicates that secretion in neurohypophyseal terminals conforms to a rather general pattern, namely calcium-activated exocytosis (Douglas, 1968). Little is known of the chemical events involved in exocytosis in any cell and lengthy discussion is inappropriate in this brief review. Besides calcium, the only common requirement identified is an energy source; and the neurohypophysis is no exception (Douglas *et al.*, 1965). The striking parallels between stimulus-secretion coupling and excitation-contraction coupling to which Rubin and I first drew attention (Douglas and Rubin, 1961) and which my colleagues and I have repeatedly emphasized (see Douglas, 1968) prompted the suggestion that nature has "found calcium entry, or mobilization, a convenient way of initiating secretion or contraction in many cells; and it may further the efforts of us who are engaged in one or other of these fields to see our work within the framework of the more general concept of stimulus-response coupling" (Douglas, 1966). Although efforts to find a "contractile" basis for exocytosis and calcium's involvement have not, as yet, produced any convincing scheme the idea is attractive. A model embracing certain molecular elements of contraction put forward by Poisner and Trifaró (1967)

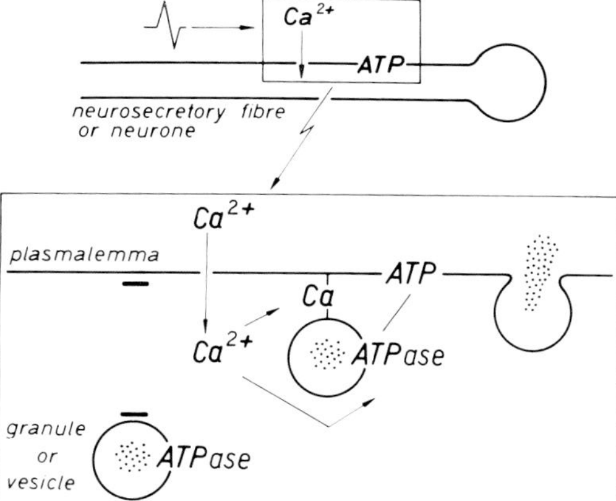

Fig. 4. One speculation on molecular events underlying exocytosis. It is based mainly on evidence that stimulation causes calcium to enter, that ATP is a plasmalemmal constituent (upper part of scheme), that plasmalemma and secretory granule (or synaptic vesicle) both carry net negative surface charges (—) and that the secretory granule membrane contains Mg-dependent ATPase activity (Poisner and Douglas, 1968). It also incorporates more recent evidence that traces of calcium activate the corresponding Mg-dependent ATPase of chromaffin granules (Izumi *et al.*, 1971). The entry of calcium ions is shown: (*1*) annulling net negative surface charges forming cationic bridges and allowing approximation of granule and plasmalemma, and (*2*) activating granule ATPase to split plasmalemmal ATP. These events are somehow supposed to allow melding and rupture of the "granule" membrane and plasmalemma and extrusion of granule contents.

References p. 35–38

has been applied to the posterior pituitary by Poisner and Douglas (1968) and refined in the light of new evidence as illustrated in Fig. 4. Whatever its other merits, this figure will at least serve to illustrate the obvious, that exocytosis involves two factors, movement of the granule to the membrane and interaction between granule membrane and the plasmalemma allowing melding and perforation.

Two other more "macromolecular" contractile hypotheses may also be mentioned. The first holds that microtubules are involved and arose from inhibitory effects of colchicine on the endocrine pancreas (Lacy *et al.*, 1968). However, colchicine depresses neurohypophyseal secretion little (Douglas and Sorimachi, 1972a) and this small effect may be related to axonal transport (Griffin *et al.*, 1972; Jones and Pickering, 1970; Norström *et al.*, 1971) rather than exocytosis. The powerful inhibitory effect of colchicine on chromaffin cell secretion (Poisner and Bernstein, 1971) appears due to some action before the exocytotic step (Douglas and Sorimachi, 1972b; Trifaró *et al.*, 1972). A second hypothesis centering on microfilaments arises from inhibitory effects of cytochalasin on various secretions, including neurohypophyseal (Douglas and Sorimachi, 1972a). But cytochalasin may cause such effects by actions independent of microfilaments.

There has also been much speculation about the possible interaction of calcium with the adenyl cyclase–cyclic AMP system (see Rasmussen, 1971) but nothing concrete has emerged. Dr. Sorimachi and I have found no potent effects of cyclic AMP, dibutyryl cyclic AMP or theophylline on spontaneous or evoked release of neurohypophyseal hormones *in vitro*.

Rather than devote more time to this rather nebulous, albeit exciting area, it seems appropriate to take up the synaptic vesicle problem.

SYNAPTIC VESICLE FORMATION

One satisfying feature of the exocytosis hypothesis is that it offers an explanation for the long-enigmatic "synaptic vesicles". During exocytosis membranes of neurosecretory granules are incorporated into the cell surface and some mechanism must exist to counter this expansion. Our electron-micrographic study indicates that membrane retrieval occurs by a process of vesiculation involving the exocytotic pits which produces "coated" vesicles that rapidly shed their coats to become smooth, classical, "synaptic" vesicles (Figs. 5, 6). The evidence consists of: (*1*) the occurrence, within some exocytotic pits, of caveolae about 400 Å diameter, sometimes clearly displaying the coating indicative of vesiculation, with coated vesicles close-by (Fig. 3, D, E). The appearances are comparable with those noted by Bunt (1969) in crayfish sinus glands, and reminiscent of micropinocytosis (Nagasawa *et al.*, 1970; Douglas *et al.*, 1971a). (*2*) The discovery of exceptionally large numbers of coated vesicles in neurohypophyses fixed during stimulation (Douglas *et al.*, 1971b). (*3*) The presence in such stimulated terminals (Fig. 7) of vesicles with incomplete coatings—the spectrum ranging from near-complete to vestigial—intermingled with alveolate figures characteristic of scraps of shed coating material (Douglas *et al.*, 1971b). (*4*) The demonstra-

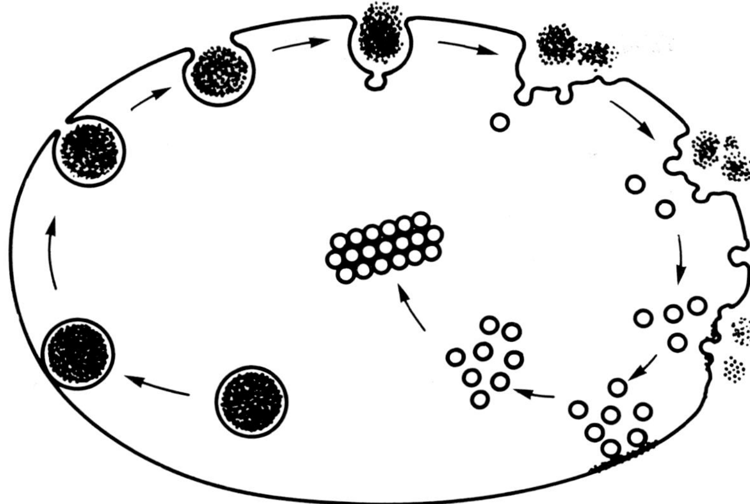

Fig. 5. A schema depicting the proposed exocytosis–vesiculation sequence and suggested origin of microvesicles ("synaptic" vesicles). In the interest of clarity the "coating mechanism" involved in microvesicle formation is here omitted and shown in detail in Fig. 6. The clustered vesicles (centre) are probably digested by lysosomal activity. (From Douglas *et al.*, 1971a)

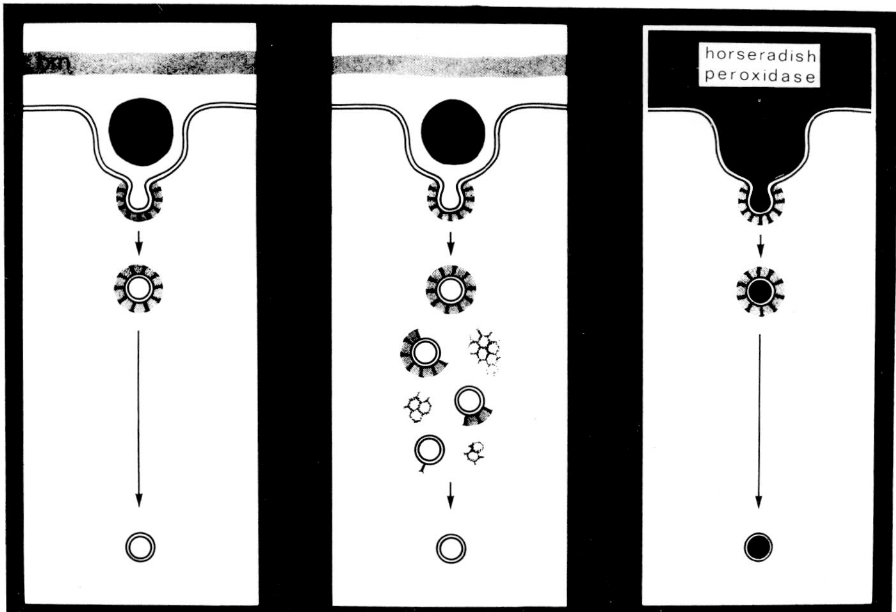

Fig. 6. Schemata summarizing the evidence and suggested origin of smooth microvesicles ("synaptic" vesicles). Left: a coating forms on the exocytotic pit rounds up and pinches off membrane to yield a coated vesicle. This is transformed to a smooth microvesicle by sloughing or shedding of the coat, and the process is repeated until all excess membrane in the terminal is withdrawn (centre). The micropinocytosis-like origin of smooth microvesicles is confirmed (right) by incorporation of horseradish peroxidase.

References p. 35–38

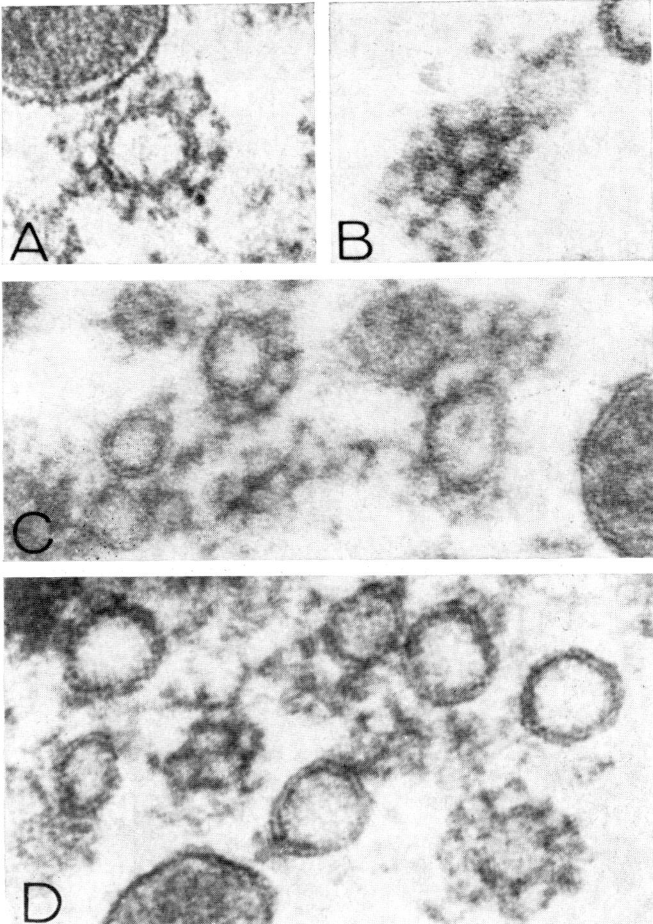

Fig. 7. Electron micrographs of neurohypophyseal terminals indicating smooth microvesicles ("synaptic" vesicles) arise from coated microvesicles. A, a fully coated microvesicle showing the trilaminar core, radiating "bristles" and dense corona. B, a shed coat showing the characteristic alveolar form. C and D, fields showing microvesicles with various amounts of coating ranging from full (D, lower right) through partial, but still substantial (C, the two larger microvesicles), to vestigial, Y-shaped (D, lower centre). Note also alveolate images of shed-coats and some apparently smooth trilaminar microvesicles. Magnification × 200 000. (From Douglas *et al.*, 1971b)

tion (Fig. 8) that horseradish peroxidase, the classical electron-microscopic tracer of pinocytotic activity, finds its way into many smooth "synaptic" as well as coated microvesicles (Nagasawa *et al.*, 1971).

The view that "synaptic" vesicles (perhaps better referred to as smooth microvesicles) arise in the manner we propose (Figs. 5, 6) harmonizes not only with the theoretical requirement for some form of withdrawal of the excess membrane from the cell surface, but with the known characteristics of the synaptic vesicle population: localization to the terminal regions; tendency to increase in number following stimulation; and to appear in clusters (synaptoid figures) under the terminal membrane

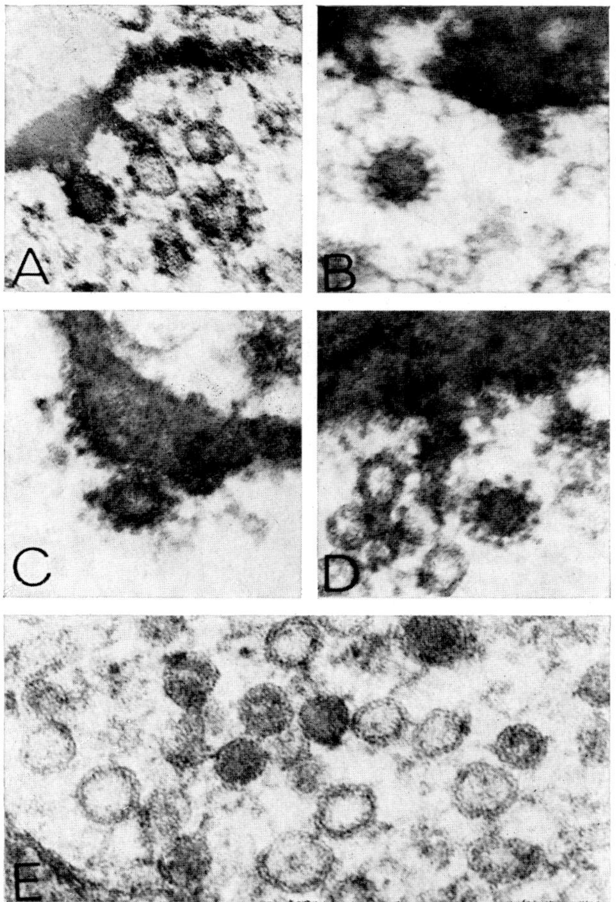

Fig. 8. Demonstration of uptake of horseradish peroxidase (indicated by dense reaction product) into coated (A, B, C, D) and smooth (E) "synaptic" vesicles of neurohypophyseal terminals. Magnification × 128 000. (From Nagasawa *et al.*, 1971)

(Fig. 3, F)—we have calculated that retrieval of the membrane of a single neurosecretory granule would require formation of about 20 microvesicles (Douglas *et al.*, 1971a). From studies on invertebrate material both Weitzman (1969) and Normann (1970) had already suspected that synaptoid figures might arise somehow as a consequence of exocytosis. It may be of functional significance that the volume occupied by the cluster of small vesicles is less than that of a single large vesicle thus allowing entry of fresh neurosecretory granules into the terminal (Douglas *et al.*, 1971a).

It remains to be seen whether all "synaptic" vesicles arise in the way we propose as economy of hypothesis dictates, but clearly many do: we have sometimes found horseradish peroxidase in about 30% despite the fact that vesicles formed before introducing this marker would clearly resist labeling (Nagasawa *et al.*, 1971). However, it could still be argued that unlabeled vesicles are different in origin and function. The old view that "synaptic" vesicles in the neurohypophysis contain a substance such

References p. 35–38

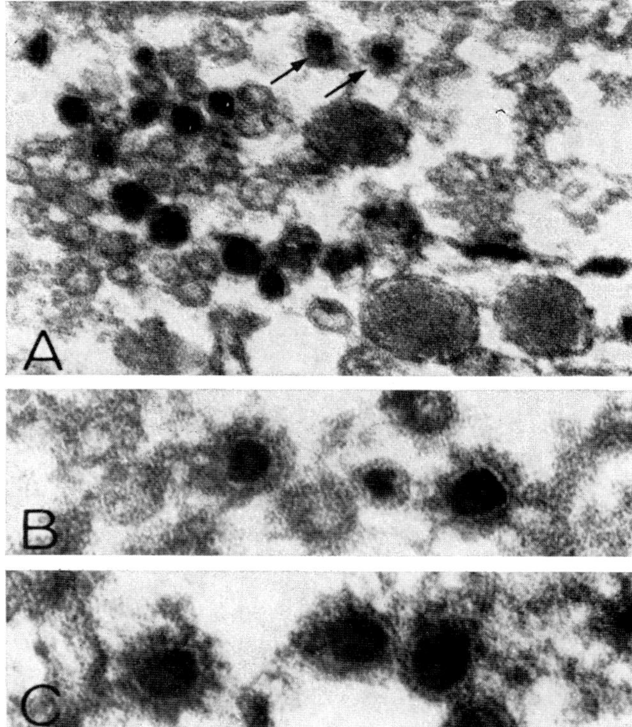

Fig. 9. Demonstration that the Zinc Iodide–Osmic Acid (ZIO) procedure (Kawana *et al.*, 1969) yields electron-dense deposits not only in smooth microvesicles of neurohypophyseal terminals, but also in the "coated" microvesicles (A, arrows: B and C) presumed to arise by membrane vesiculation. ZIO positivity of the former is thus compatible with their origin by membrane vesiculation depicted in Figs. 5, 6. Magnification: A, × 86 500; B and C, × 150 000. Species: rat. (From unpublished work by W. W. Douglas, J. Nagasawa and R. A. Schulz)

as acetylcholine—and are not derived from neurosecretory granules—has recently been revived with the demonstration that they stain preferentially with the zinc iodide–osmic acid (ZIO) procedure as do the classical synaptic vesicles of ordinary nerves (Christ and Bak, 1970; Rufener and Dreifuss, 1970). However, we have discovered that ZIO also stains coated microvesicles (Fig. 9). The basis for the reaction is unknown, but clearly, in the light of this new evidence, ZIO-positivity of "synaptic" vesicles is compatible with our view they arise from the coated forms in turn derived, at least in part, from granule membrane. Although acetylcholine is present in neurohypophyses, Lederis and Livingston (1970) have argued it is not in classical hormone-containing fibres.

VESICULATION COUPLED TO EXOCYTOSIS: A POSSIBLE GENERAL MECHANISM FOR MEMBRANE CONSERVATION

When it seemed likely that the micropinocytosis-like activity in exocytotic pits of neurosecretory terminals functions to retrieve granule membrane, a similar interpretation was placed on corresponding images in chromaffin cells (Douglas and Nagasawa, 1971; Grynszpan-Winograd, 1971). The relative abundance of exocytotic figures and coated caveolae in chromaffin cells has permitted demonstration of incorporation of thorium dioxide (another pinocytotic marker) at such sites (Nagasawa and Douglas, 1972) and provided quantitative evidence of the preferential nature of the phenomenon, coated caveolae in our experiments being about five times more common in exocytotic pits than in surrounding membrane (Douglas and Nagasawa, 1972). Since comparable activity is also discernable at sites of exocytosis in adenohypophyseal and other cells, we have proposed (Douglas and Nagasawa, 1971) that "there exists in a variety of cells a mechanism (perhaps better referred to as "vesiculation" rather than micropinocytosis with its connotation of cell drinking) serving to withdraw from the cell surface the membrane of secretory granules incorporated during exocytosis". And further, that "such specific removal of granule membrane would conserve not only the area of the plasmalemma but also its characteristics associated for example with permeability, excitability, and receptor function".

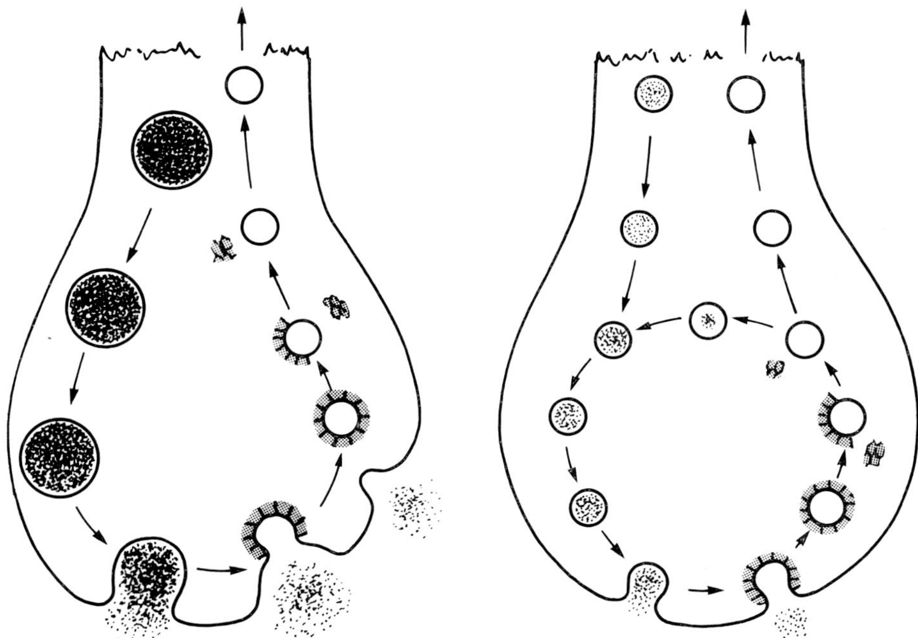

Fig. 10. An illustration of the recycling hypothesis (Douglas *et al.*, 1971a; Douglas and Nagasawa, 1972; Nagasawa *et al.*, 1971) wherein an exocytosis–vesiculation sequence comparable to that detected in neurohypophyseal terminals (left diagram) is postulated in ordinary neurones (right diagram) as a means of recycling membrane of transmitter-containing (true) synaptic vesicles. The essence of the scheme is that retrieval "coupled" to exocytosis would allow recapture of membrane with properties, such as enzymatic activity, appropriate for local synthesis and repackaging of transmitter. "Old" vesicles are seen following the upward directed path of (? lysosomal) degradation as in the neurosecretory terminal. Independently, and on quite different grounds Heuser and Reese (1972) have proposed a comparable scheme for cholinergic neurones.

References p. 35–38

It remains to be determined what induces this "vesiculation coupled to exocytosis": our preliminary experiments have so far revealed no important effect of extracellular ions or transmembrane potential but hint at "induction" of vesiculation by extruded granule contents raising the possibility that this may be the function of granule contents such as ATP or proteins such as chromogranin or neurophysin (Douglas and Nagasawa, 1972).

As to the fate of retrieved granule membrane, we suppose synaptic vesicles in the neurohypophysis are not reused in hormone synthesis and packaging (which occurs in the remote perikaryon) but are degraded by lysosomes or related structures (Douglas *et al.*, 1971a). The abundance of lysosomes in the terminals supports this (Whitaker and LaBella, 1972). In chromaffin cells, too, lysosomal digestion seems likely (Nagasawa and Douglas, 1972). However, we have proposed that a comparable exocytosis–vesiculation sequence might operate in ordinary nerve endings, where there *is* local synthesis and packaging of transmitter, to permit recycling of (true) synaptic vesicles (Fig. 10).

SUMMING UP

Returning now to the main point. The principle events in release of peptide from the neurones of the hypothalamo-neurohypophyseal system can be summarized as follows: impulse generation and propagation through classical sodium-dependent and tetrodotoxin-sensitive spikes → depolarization of the terminal → entry of calcium (the important channel appearing to be that blocked by cobalt and magnesium and not TTX) → induction of exocytosis and extrusion of granule contents directly to the cell exterior → and, finally, retrieval of neurosecretory granule membrane by vesiculation. The challenge that now confronts us is to define the intimate mechanisms involved. It is an exciting challenge for it is now more than ever likely that ordinary neurones also employ the same basic exocytotic mechanism.

SUMMARY

The peptide-secreting nerves of the hypothalamo-neurohypophyseal tract possess the essential electrophysiological attributes of neurones: generation and propagation of impulses by means of the familiar regenerative sodium mechanism sensitive to tetrodotoxin (TTX). The stimulus for release of hormones appears to be depolarization of the neurosecretory terminals with the arrival of these impulses; this, in turn, causing calcium entry and setting in motion the secretory process proper, the release of the posterior pituitary hormones. Such release, to judge from electron-microscopical and chemical evidence, occurs by exocytosis. Following exocytosis the membranes of neurosecretory granules incorporated in the limiting membrane of the neurone appear to be retrieved by a process of vesiculation, superficially resembling micropinocytosis, that produces coated microvesicles which rapidly shed their coats to become smooth. This sequence is held to be the origin of the long-enigmatic "synaptic vesicles" in these terminals. Such "vesiculation coupled to exocytosis" is considered a general mechanism for conservation of the area and chemistry of the cell surface. In neurohypophyseal terminals, granule membrane retrieved in this way is probably destroyed by lysosomes but a comparable mechanism in conventional neurones could permit recycling of synaptic vesicles.

ACKNOWLEDGEMENTS

The work by the author and his colleagues referred to in this paper was supported by grants from the United States Public Health Service.

REFERENCES

BAKER, P. F., HODGKIN, A. L. AND RIDGWAY, E. B. (1971a) Depolarization and calcium entry in squid giant axons. *J. Physiol. (Lond.)*, **218**, 709–755.

BAKER, P. F., MEVES, H. AND RIDGWAY, E. B. (1971b) Phasic entry of calcium in response to depolarization of giant axons of Loligo. *J. Physiol. (Lond.)*, **216**, 70–71P.

BARER, R. AND LEDERIS, K. (1966) Ultrastructure of the rabbit neurohypophysis with special reference to the release of hormones. *Z. Zellforsch.*, **75**, 201–239.

BARGMANN, W. (1968) Neurohypophysis. Structure and function. In *Neurohypophysial Hormones and Similar Polypeptides (Handbook of Experimental Pharmacology, Vol. XIII)*, B. BERDE (Ed.), Springer, Berlin, pp. 1–39.

BOUDIER, J. L., BOUDIER, J. A. AND PICARD, D. (1970) Ultrastructure du lobe postérieur de l'hypophyse du rat et ses modifications au cours de l'excrétion de vasopressine. *Z. Zellforsch.*, **108**, 357–379.

BUNT, A. H. (1969) Formation of coated and "synaptic" vesicles within neurosecretory axon terminals of the crustacean sinus gland. *J. ultrastruct. Res.*, **28**, 411–421.

BURTON, A. M., FORSLING, M. L. AND MARTIN, M. J. (1971) Release of neurophysin oxytocin and arginine vasopressin in the rat. *J. Physiol. (Lond.)*, **217**, 23–24P.

CHENG, K. W. AND FRIESEN, H. G. (1970) Physiological factors regulating secretion of neurophysin. *Metabolism*, **19**, 876–890.

CHRIST, J. F. AND BAK, I. J. (1970) Some structural observations on the small vesicular components in the posterior pituitary nerve fibres of the rabbit. *Z. mikr.-anat. Forsch.*, **81**, 329–344.

DEROBERTIS, E. (1962) Ultrastructure and function in some neurosecretory systems. *Mem. Soc. Endocrinol.*, **12**, 3–20.

DINER, O. (1967) L'expulsion des granules de la médullo-surrénale chez le hamster. *C.R. hebd. Séanc. Acad. Sci., Paris.*, **265**, 616–619.

DOUGLAS, W. W. (1963) A possible mechanism of neurosecretion: release of vasopressin by depolarization and its dependence on calcium. *Nature (Lond.)*, **197**, 81–82.

DOUGLAS, W. W. (1966) Calcium dependent links in stimulus-secretion coupling in the adrenal medulla and neurohypophysis. In *Mechanisms of Release of Biogenic Amines* (Proc. int. Wenner-Gren Symposium, Stockholm, February, 1965), Pergamon, London, pp. 267–290.

DOUGLAS, W. W. (1967) Stimulus-secretion coupling in the adrenal medulla and the neurohypophysis: Cellular mechanisms of release of catecholamines and posterior pituitary hormones. In *Neurosecretion* (4th Int. Symp. Neurosecretion, Strasbourg, July, 1966), F. STUTINSKY (Ed.), Springer, Berlin, pp. 178–190.

DOUGLAS, W. W. (1968) The First Gaddum Memorial Lecture. Stimulus-secretion coupling: the concept and clues from chromaffin and other cells. *Brit. J. Pharmacol.*, **34**, 451–474.

DOUGLAS, W. W. AND NAGASAWA, J. (1971) Membrane vesiculation at sites of exocytosis in the neurohypophysis, adenohypophysis and adrenal medulla: A device for membrane conversation. *J. Physiol. (Lond.)*, **218**, 94–95P.

DOUGLAS, W. W. AND NAGASAWA, J. (1972) Membrane vesiculation following exocytosis. *Proc. Can. Fed. biol. Soc.*, **15**, 757.

DOUGLAS, W. W. AND POISNER, A. M. (1963) The influence of calcium on the secretory response of the submaxillary gland to acetylcholine or to noradrenaline. *J. Physiol. (Lond.)*, **165**, 528–541.

DOUGLAS, W. W. AND POISNER, A. M. (1964a) Stimulus-secretion coupling in a neuro-secretory organ: the role of calcium in the release of vasopressin from the neurohypophysis. *J. Physiol. (Lond.)*, **172**, 1–18.

DOUGLAS, W. W. AND POISNER, A. M. (1964b) Calcium movement in the neurohypophysis of the rat and its relation to the release of vasopressin. *J. Physiol. (Lond.)*, **172**, 19–30.

DOUGLAS, W. W. AND POISNER, A. M. (1966) Evidence that the secreting adrenal medullary chromaffin cell releases catecholamines directly from ATP-rich granules. *J. Physiol. (Lond.)*, **183**, 236–248.

DOUGLAS, W. W. AND RUBIN, R. P. (1961) The role of calcium in the secretory response of the adrenal medulla to acetylcholine. *J. Physiol. (Lond.)*, **159**, 40–57.

DOUGLAS, W. W. AND RUBIN, R. P. (1963) The mechanism of catecholamine release from the adrenal medulla and the role of calcium in stimulus-secretion coupling. *J. Physiol. (Lond.)*, **167**, 288–310.

DOUGLAS, W. W. AND RUBIN, R. P. (1964) The effects of alkaline earths and other divalent cations on adrenal medullary secretion. *J. Physiol. (Lond.)*, **175**, 231–241.

DOUGLAS, W. W. AND SORIMACHI, M. (1971) Electrically evoked release of vasopressin from isolated neurohypophyses in sodium-free media. *Brit. J. Pharmacol.*, **42**, 647P.

DOUGLAS, W. W. AND SORIMACHI, M. (1972a) Effects of cytochalasin B and colchicine on secretion of posterior pituitary and adrenal medullary hormones. *Brit. J. Pharmacol.*, **45**, 143–144P.

DOUGLAS, W. W. AND SORIMACHI, M. (1972b) Colchicine inhibits adrenal medullary secretion evoked by acetylcholine without affecting that evoked by potassium. *Brit. J. Pharmacol.*, **45**, 129–132.

DOUGLAS, W. W., ISHIDA, A. AND POISNER, A. M. (1965) The effect of metabolic inhibitors on the release of vasopressin from the isolated neurohypophysis. *J. Physiol. (Lond.)*, **181**, 753–759.

DOUGLAS, W. W., KANNO, T. AND SAMPSON, S. R. (1967) Influence of the ionic environment on the membrane potential of adrenal chromaffin cells and on the depolarizing effect of acetylcholine. *J. Physiol. (Lond.)*, **191**, 107–121.

DOUGLAS, W. W., NAGASAWA, J. AND SCHULZ, R. A. (1971a) Electron-microscopic studies on the mechanism of secretion of posterior pituitary hormones and significance of microvesicles ("synaptic vesicles"): Evidence of secretion by exocytosis and formation of microvesicles as a by-product of this process. *Mem. Soc. Endocrinol.*, **19**, 353–378.

DOUGLAS, W. W., NAGASAWA, J. AND SCHULZ, R. A. (1971b) Coated microvesicles in neurosecretory terminals of posterior pituitary glands shed their coats to become smooth "synaptic" vesicles. *Nature (Lond.)*, **232**, 340–341.

DREIFUSS, J. J., GRAU, J. D. AND BIANCHI, R. E. (1971a) Antagonism between Ca and Na ions at neurohypophysial nerve terminals. *Experientia*, **27**, 1295–1296.

DREIFUSS, J. J., KALNINS, I., KELLY, J. S. AND RUF, K. B. (1971b) Action potentials and release of neurohypophysial hormones *in vitro*. *J. Physiol. (Lond.)*, **215**, 805–817.

FAWCETT, C. P., POWELL, A. E. AND SACHS, H. (1968) Biosynthesis and release of neurophysin. *Endocrinology*, **83**, 1299–1310.

GERSCHENFELD, H. M., TRAMEZZANI, J. AND DEROBERTIS, E. (1960) Ultrastructure and function in neurohypophysis of the toad. *Endocrinology*, **66**, 741–762.

GINSBURG, M. (1968) Molecular aspects of neurohypophysial hormone release. *Proc. roy. Soc. B.*, **170**, 27–36.

GINSBURG, M., JAYASENA, K. AND THOMAS, P. J. (1966) Preparation and properties of porcine neurophysin and the influence of calcium on the hormone neurophysin complex. *J. Physiol. (Lond.)*, **184**, 387–401.

GRIFFIN, J., KEEN, P. AND LIVINGSTON, A. (1972) Effects of vinblastine and colchicine on oxytocin levels of the posterior pituitary of the rat after saline treatment. *J. Endocrinol.*, **52**, 407–408.

GRYNSZPAN-WINOGRAD, O. (1971) Morphological aspects of exocytosis in the adrenal medulla. *Phil. Trans. roy. Soc. Lond. B*, **261**, 291–292.

HALLER, E. W., SACHS, H., SPERELAKIS, N. AND SHARE, L. (1965) Release of vasopressin from isolated guinea pig posterior pituitaries. *Amer. J. Physiol.*, **209**, 79–83.

HERLANT, M. (1967) Mode de libération des produits de neurosécrétion. In *Neurosecretion*, F. STUTINSKY (Ed.), Springer, Berlin, pp. 20–35.

HEUSER, J. AND REESE, T. S. (1972) Stimulation induced uptake and release of peroxidase from synaptic vesicles in frog neuromuscular junctions. *Anat. Rec.*, **172**, 329–330.

HUBBARD, J. I. (1970) Mechanism of transmitter release. *Progr. Biophys. mol. Biol.*, **21**, 33–124.

ISHIDA, A. (1967) The effect of tetrodotoxin on calcium-dependent link in stimulus-secretion coupling in neurohypophysis. *Jap. J. Physiol.*, **17**, 308–320.

ISHIDA, A. (1970) The oxytocin release and the compound action potential evoked by electrical stimulation on the isolated neurohypophysis of the rat. *Jap. J. Physiol.*, **20**, 84–96.

IZUMI, F., OKA, M. AND KASHIMOTO, T. (1971) Role of calcium for magnesium-activated adenosinetriphosphatase activity and adenosinetriphosphate-magnesium stimulated catecholamine release from adrenal medullary granules. *Jap. J. Pharmacol.*, **21**, 739–746.

JONES, C. W. AND PICKERING, B. T. (1970) Rapid transport of neurohypophyseal hormones in the hypothalamo-neurohypophyseal tract. *J. Physiol.*, **208**, 73P.

KATZ, B. AND MILEDI, R. (1969) Spontaneous and evoked activity of motor nerve endings in calcium Ringer. *J. Physiol.*, **203**, 689–706.

KAWANA, E., AKERT, K. AND SANDRI, C. (1969) Zinc iodide-osmium tetroxide impregnation of nerve terminals in the spinal cord. *Brain Res.*, **16**, 325–331.

KIRSHNER, N. AND VIVEROS, O. H. (1970) Quantal aspects of the secretion of catecholamines and dopamine-β-hydroxylase from the adrenal medulla. In *New Aspects of Storage and Release Mechanisms of Catecholamines*, H. J. SCHÜMANN AND G. KRONBERG (Eds.), Springer, New York, pp. 78–88.

KOIZUMI, K. AND YAMASHITA, H. (1972) Studies of antidromically identified neurosecretory cells of the hypothalamus by intracellular and extracellular recordings. *J. Physiol. (Lond.)*, **221**, 683–706.

KUROSUMI, K., MATSUYAMA, T., KOBAYASHI, Y. AND SATO, S. (1964) On the relationship between the release of neurosecretory substance and lipid granules of pituicytes in the rat neurohypophysis. *Gunma Symp. Endocrinol.*, **1**, 87–118.

LABELLA, F. S. (1968) Storage and secretion of neurohypophyseal hormones. *Canad. J. Physiol. Pharmacol.*, **46**, 335–345.

LACY, P. E., HOWELL, S. L., YOUNG, D. A. AND FINK, C. J. (1968) New hypothesis of insulin secretion. *Nature (Lond.)*, **219**, 1177–1179.

LEDERIS, K. AND LIVINGSTON, A. (1970) Neuronal and subcellular localization of acetylcholine in the posterior pituitary of the rabbit. *J. Physiol. (Lond.)*, **210**, 187–204.

LEGROS, J. J., FRANCHIMONT, P. AND HENDRICK, J. C. (1969) Dosage radioimmunologique de la neurophysine dans le sérum des femmes normales et des femmes enceintes. *C. R. Soc. biol. Paris*, **163**, 2773–2777.

MIKITEN, T. M. (1967) Electrically stimulated release of vasopressin from rat neurohypophyses *in vitro. Ph.D. Thesis*, Yeshiva University, New York.

MIKITEN, T. M. AND DOUGLAS, W. W. (1965) Effect of calcium and other ions on vasopressin release from rat neurohypophyses stimulated electrically *in vitro*. *Nature (Lond.)*, **207**, 302.

NAGASAWA, J. AND DOUGLAS, W. W. (1972) Thorium dioxide uptake into adrenal medullary cells and the problem of recapture of granule membrane following exocytosis. *Brain Res.*, **37**, 141–145.

NAGASAWA, J., DOUGLAS, W. W. AND SCHULZ, R. A. (1970) Ultrastructural evidence of secretion by exocytosis and of "synaptic vesicle" formation in posterior pituitary glands. *Nature (Lond.)*, **227**, 407–409.

NAGASAWA, J., DOUGLAS, W. W. AND SCHULZ, R. A. (1971) Micropinocytotic origin of coated and smooth microvesicles ("synaptic vesicles") in neurosecretory terminals of posterior pituitary glands demonstrated by incorporation of horseradish peroxidase. *Nature (Lond.)*, **232**, 341–342.

NORDMANN, J. J., DREIFUSS, J. J. AND LEGROS, J. J. (1971) A correlation of release of "polypeptide hormones" and of immunoreactive neurophysin from isolated rat neurohypophyses. *Experientia*, **27**, 1344–1345.

NORMANN, T. C. (1970) The mechanism of hormone release from neurosecretory axon endings in the insect *Calliphora erythrocephala*. In *Aspects of Neuroendocrinology* (Vth Int. Symp. Neurosecretion), W. BARGMANN AND B. SCHARRER (Eds.), Springer, New York, pp. 30–42.

NORSTRÖM, A. AND SJÖSTRAND, J. (1971) Effect of haemorrhage on the rapid axonal transport of neurohypophyseal proteins of the rat. *J. Neurochem.*, **18**, 2017–2026.

NORSTRÖM, A., HANSSON, H.-A. AND SJÖSTRAND, J. (1971) Effects of colchicine on axonal transport and ultrastructure of the hypothalamo-neurohypophyseal system of the rat. *Z. Zellforsch.*, **113**, 271–293.

PALAY, S. (1957) The fine structure of the neurohypophysis. In *Ultrastructure and Cellular Chemistry of Neural Tissue*, H. WAELSCH (Ed.), Hoeber, New York, pp. 31–49.

POISNER, A. M. AND BERNSTEIN, J. (1971) A possible role of microtubules in catecholamine release from the adrenal medulla: effect of colchicine, vinca alkaloids and deuterium oxide. *J. Pharmacol. exp. Ther.*, **177**, 102–108.

POISNER, A. M. AND DOUGLAS, W. W. (1968) A possible mechanism of release of posterior pituitary hormones involving adenosine triphosphate and an adenosine triphosphatase in the neurosecretory granules. *Mol. Pharmacol.*, **4**, 531–540.

POISNER, A. M. AND TRIFARÓ, J. M. (1967) The role of ATP and ATPase in the release of catecholamines from the adrenal medulla, I. ATP-evoked release of catecholamines, ATP, and protein from isolated chromaffin granules. *Mol. Pharmacol.*, **3**, 561-565.

RASMUSSEN, H. (1971) Cell communication, calcium ion and cyclic adenosine monophosphate. *Science*, **170**, 404–412.

RUBIN, R. P. (1970) The role of calcium in the release of neurotransmitter substances and hormones. *Pharmacol. Rev.*, **22**, 389–428.

RUFENER, C. AND DREIFUSS, J. J. (1970) Selective ZnIO-OsO_4 impregnation of synaptoid vesicles in the rat neurohypophysis. *Brain Res.*, **22**, 402–405.

SANTOLAYA, R. C., BRIDGES, T. E. AND LEDERIS, K. (1972) Elementary granules, small vesicles and exocytosis in the rat neurohypophysis after acute haemorrhage. *Z. Zellforsch.*, **125**, 277–288.

THORN, N. A. (1965) Role of calcium in the release of vasopressin and oxytocin from posterior pituitary protein. *Acta endocrinol. (Kbh.)*, **50**, 357–364.

THORN, N. A. (1966) *In vitro* studies of the release mechanism for vasopressin in rats. *Acta endocrinol. (Kbh.)*, **53**, 644–654.

THORN, N. A. (1970) Mechanism of release of neurohypophyseal hormones. In *Aspects of Neuroendocrinology* (Vth Int. Symp. Neurosecretion), W. BARGMANN AND B. SCHARRER (Eds.), Springer, New York, pp. 140–152.

TRIFARÓ, J. M., COLLIER, B., LASTOWECKA, A. AND STERN, D. (1972) Inhibition by colchicine and by vinblastine of acetylcholine-induced catecholamine release from the adrenal gland: an anticholinergic action, not an effect on microtubules. *Mol. Pharmacol.*, **8**, 264–267.

WEITZMAN, M. (1969) Ultrastructural study on the release of neurosecretory material from the sinus gland of the land crab *Gecarcinus lateralis*. *Z. Zellforsch.*, **94**, 147–154.

WHITAKER, S. AND LABELLA, F. S. (1972) Ultrastructural localization of acid phosphatase in the posterior pituitary of the dehydrated rat. *Z. Zellforsch.*, **125**, 1–15.

UTTENTHAL, L. O., LIVETT, B. G. AND HOPE, D. B. (1971) Release of neurophysin together with vasopressin by a Ca^{2+}-dependent mechanism. *Phil. Trans. roy. Soc. Lond. B*, **261**, 379–380.

DISCUSSION

LOTT: In stimulating whole-tissue preparations electrically, one cannot assume that only the secretory endings are being altered, indeed the entire preparation may be altered. Therefore, one must take care in describing and explaining the sequence of response or reaction to such stimulation in terms of specific cellular alterations in the preparation. The electrodes in your methods appear to be fairly general; however, this does not subtract from your overall scheme.

DOUGLAS: I agree with your very last statement.

MCCANN: In anterior pituitary cells as in many other secretory cells in the body there is clearly a role for the cyclic AMP system. I am wondering if there is any role for cyclic AMP in the neurohypophyseal secretion mechanism, and, if so, how would you relate it to your secretion coupling hypothesis?

DOUGLAS: Let me say first that I think that cyclic AMP has become one of the most addictive compounds in today's pharmacology and it would be nice to report that there are at least some systems that work perfectly well without it. As soon as this substance appeared on the scene we tried it, the dibutyryl analogue, and theophylline trying to satisfy at least some of the criteria of Sutherland and we obtained no significant results. I think that Howard Sachs probably did similar experiments. Certainly we can generate no enthusiasm for involvement of the adenyl cyclase system in the pituitary.

There are, of course, speculations in great number. I refer you to some by Rasmussen (Science, 170, 404, 1971) on how calcium, membranes and cyclic AMP may be interrelated. But none of us really has the answer. Moreover, I'm not sure that there is any convincing evidence the system is involved in secretion from ordinary nerves; the evidence is not impressive. Finally, I know that Rubin has examined cyclic AMP on the chromaffin cell without results. Maybe we just haven't got the green thumb.

SACHS: First, I would like to corroborate with Bill Douglas about the effects of cyclic AMP or its derivatives on the secretion of vasopressin. We have never been able to show a secretory effect of cyclic AMP, the dibutyryl derivative, or theophylline. In fact, when we measured the levels of cyclic AMP after exposure to 56 mmole of potassium the only thing we ever found was an actual diminution in the cyclic AMP levels in the neural lobe. But I would like to ask Bill a question. Have you any chemical or morphological evidence that microtubules are in any way involved in the secretory phenomenon; have you tried cytocalasin or substances which affect microtubules?

DOUGLAS: That is another entertaining line of speculation. Years ago, following our very first experiments with calcium we coined the phrase stimulus-secretion coupling having in mind the parallels between events in the secretory process and in the contractile process. Since then we have been exploring, along with others, the possibility that there is some sort of contractile element underlying cell secretion as well as muscle contraction. Although the speculation put forward by Lacy *et al.* (Nature 219, 1177, 1968) that microtubules are involved has attracted a lot of attention many of the experimental results held to favor of involvement of microtubules, I must say, are not very impressive. The effect of colchicine on Mast cells, for example, is very small. The most dramatic effect of all is one on the adrenal medulla where colchicine (10^{-3} M) according to Poisner and Bernstein (J. Pharmacol. exp. Ther., 177, 102, 1971) produced a strong inhibition of the response to acetylcholine. We have looked into that as have Trifaró *et al.*, (Mol. Pharmacol., 8, 264, 1972) and it looks as though this effect of colchicine is not on exocytosis. Perhaps colchicine is acting as an anticholinergic agent; certainly its effect is at a stage before the exocytotic event. Colchicine has very little effect on the pituitary and we suspect this could be accounted for by inhibition of migration of granules. I cannot generate much enthusiasm for the idea that microtubules participate in exocytosis. Moreover, morphological evidence shows that the microtubules terminate before reaching the terminal region where secretion is taking place.

Chemistry of Hypothalamic Releasing Factors

ROGER BURGUS, WYLIE VALE, JEAN RIVIER, MICHAEL MONAHAN, NICHOLAS LING, GEOFFREY GRANT, MAX AMOSS AND ROGER GUILLEMIN

The Salk Institute, 10010 North Torrey Pines Road, La Jolla, Calif. 92037 (U.S.A.)

Investigations in recent years have confirmed that substances of hypothalamic origin are involved in the control of secretion of the anterior pituitary hormones. There is now good evidence that hypophysiotrophic hormones or releasing factors from the hypothalamus stimulate the secretion of corticotrophin (ACTH), thyrotrophin (TSH), somatotrophin or growth hormone (GH) and the gonadotrophins, luteinizing hormone (LH) and follicle-stimulating hormone (FSH). There is also some evidence for such factors stimulating the release of prolactin and melanocyte-stimulating hormone (MSH). Other substances called release-inhibiting factors or hormones are involved in tonic inhibition of the secretion of MSH, prolactin and GH. The reports of investigations leading to these conclusions have been reviewed elsewhere (Guillemin, 1971; Vale *et al.*, 1973, Burgus and Guillemin, 1970). It is the purpose of this presentation to review briefly the status of knowledge regarding the chemical structures of the hypothalamic releasing factors in general and to survey some of the recent studies on structure–function relationships of the two hormones, TRF (TSH-releasing factor) and LRF (LH-releasing factor).

STRUCTURES OF THE HYPOTHALAMIC RELEASING FACTORS

Difficulties in the isolation and characterization of the various hypothalamic factors have been twofold: (*1*) the development of specific and reliable bioassays and (*2*) the handling of very small amounts of the hormones usually present in hypothalamic tissue. After several years of arduous work, principally in two laboratories, and collection of several millions of ovine or porcine hypothalamic fragments, the structure of ovine TRF was established in 1969 as the tripeptide pGlu-His-Pro-NH_2 (Burgus *et al.*, 1969, 1970). The porcine hormone was shown to have the same structure (Nair *et al.*, 1970).

In 1971, the luteinizing hormone-releasing factor, LRF, of porcine (Matsuo *et al.* 1971, Baba *et al.*, 1971) and ovine (Burgus *et al.*, 1971, 1972) origin was characterized as the decapeptide pGlu-His-Trp-Ser-Tyr-Gly-Leu-Arg-Pro-Gly-NH_2. TRF and LRF, as well as their synthetic replicates, stimulate the secretion of TSH and LH respectively in a variety of mammalian species, including man (Vale *et al.*, 1973).

References p. 49–50

Other peptides obtained from hypothalamic tissues recently have been characterized. A decapeptide with the primary sequence H-Val-His-Leu-Ser-Ala-Glu-Glu-Lys-Glu-Ala-OH has been isolated from porcine hypothalami and has been proposed as the "growth hormone-releasing hormone, GH-RH" (Schally *et al.*, 1971). The significance of this material as a true releasing factor is open to question primarily because of the vagaries of the bioassay system (Guillemin, 1971). Although it is reported to be active in some bioassay systems, the natural or synthetic product (Veber *et al.*, 1971) is unable to stimulate an increase in levels of radioimmunoassayable growth hormone in plasma. It has been observed that the decapeptide sequence is similar to a fragment of the β-chain of porcine hemoglobin.

Several laboratories have now found that crude or partially purified extracts of hypothalami contain substances which release growth hormone (GRF or SRF) (Frohman *et al.*, 1971; Wilber *et al.*, 1971) and substances which inhibit the release (GIF or SRIF) (Hertelendy *et al.*, 1971) of growth hormone as measured by radioimmunoassay, but nothing regarding the chemical nature of these substances has been published.

It has been reported that the tripeptide H-Pro-Leu-Gly-NH_2 from porcine hypothalamic extracts inhibits the release of MSH (Celis *et al.*, 1971; Nair *et al.*, 1971). This peptide, which corresponds to the C-terminal tripeptide sequence of oxytocin, has been named "MRIH-I". Tocinoic acid, Cys-Tyr-Ileu-Gln-Asn-Cys, the ring structure of oxytocin, has been found in hypothalamic tissue incubated with oxytocin and has been proposed as an inhibitor of MSH release (Hruby *et al.*, 1972). These factors may therefore originate from the action of enzymes in hypothalamic tissue on oxytocin (Celis *et al.*, 1971). A third peptide found in porcine hypothalamus, "MRIH-II", H-Pro-His-Phe-Arg-Gly-NH_2, has also been proposed as an MSH release inhibiting factor (Nair *et al.*, 1972). The situation regarding the specificities of these factors in the various bioassay systems used remains to be clarified.

Recently, it has been shown that the tripeptide TRF, in addition to its role in TSH release, also stimulates the release of prolactin (Tashjian *et al.*, 1971; Bowers *et al.*, 1971; Jacobs *et al.*, 1971). Thus, TRF may be structurally related to the still unidentified prolactin-releasing factor (PRF).

It is now well established (Vale *et al.*, 1973) that the release of the gonadotrophin, FSH, is also stimulated by the LRF decapeptide in several experimental conditions. The question of the possible existence of another specific chemical entity, FSH-releasing factor (FRF), distinct from the LRF is still open.

Although corticotrophin-releasing factor (CRF), which releases ACTH, was the first of the releasing factors to be studied, the chemical nature of hypothalamic CRF is elusive. Not only has it been difficult to establish reliable assay techniques for this substance, but it has also been proposed (Chan *et al.*, 1969) that the factor is chemically unstable. However, substances of posterior pituitary origin which have CRF activity, "α-CRF" and "β-CRF", have been reported to be related but not identical to α-MSH and vasopressin respectively (Burgus and Guillemin, 1970). The relationship of hypothalamic CRF to these substances is uncertain.

The characterization of TRF and LRF as simple polypeptides has led the way to the preparation of synthetic analogues and the study of their structure–function relationship in biological systems.

Structure–activity relationships of TRF

Well over 50 structural analogues of TRF have now been synthesized and tested for biological activity. Many of the results of these studies have been tabulated and discussed elsewhere (Guillemin *et al.*, 1971; Vale *et al.*, 1973). Most of the modifications, which have included the alteration or replacement of every amino acid, have resulted in substantial reduction of the biological activity, measured *in vivo* or *in vitro* (Vale *et al.*, 1973), indicating that every part of the molecule is an essential requirement for biological activity.

Changes at the $pGlu^1$ position of TRF result in a considerable decrease in its ability to induce secretion of TSH. The data suggest the N^α of pGlu is involved as a nucleophile in the action of TRF. Introduction of an N^α methyl function on pGlu gives a compound with reduced biological activity possibly by introducing steric interference at the receptor–substrate complex level, or by interfering with a nucleophilic process involving the N^α of pGlu. Of possible significance to the latter interpretation is that the relative activities of compounds containing replacements of S, O, or C for the N^α of pGlu appear to be a function of the nucleophilicity of the atom in that position. [Pro^1]TRF ought to be more reactive than these three compounds in this series, but the N^α of Pro is protonated at physiological pH, which would reduce its utility as a nucleophile (Monahan *et al.*, 1972b). However, extreme caution must be exercised in interpreting the significance of differences in biological activities of analogues with such low activity ($\leq 1\%$ of TRF).

Substitution of the histidine by more basic amino acids such as arginine, lysine (Gillessen *et al.*, 1971; Rivier *et al.*, 1972), α-γ-diaminobutyric acid (Gillessen *et al.*, 1971), or ornithine (Rivier *et al.*, 1972), yields compounds with little activity. However, there appears to be a requirement for aromaticity at this position as shown by the high activity (10% of TRF) of [Phe^2]TRF (Sievertsson *et al.*, 1972). The marked difference in activity between this compound and [Tyr^2]TRF ($< 0.1\%$ TRF, Rivier *et al.*, 1972) might be explained in terms of steric interactions in the receptor–substrate complex. [Met^2]TRF (Rivier *et al.*, 1972) retains substantial activity (1% TRF), although less than the aromatic substitution, [Phe^2]TRF. CPK models indicate that the side chain of methionine fills almost the same space as the side chain of histidine with the sulfur atom able to occupy nearly the same position as the imidazole π-nitrogen.

Measurements of the pK_a of the imidazole of histidine in several TRF analogues reveal that the pK_a and biological potency appear to correlate (Fig. 1) (Grant *et al.*, 1972). Two points on this plot which fall outside the curve represent compounds which are ionized at physiological pH. Formal charges on the molecule reduce the biological potency considerably. The relationship between pK_a and potency supports the hypothesis that the histidine side chain may be involved in an acid–base capacity either as a general acid in the release mechanism or by stabilizing a particular con-

References p. 49–50

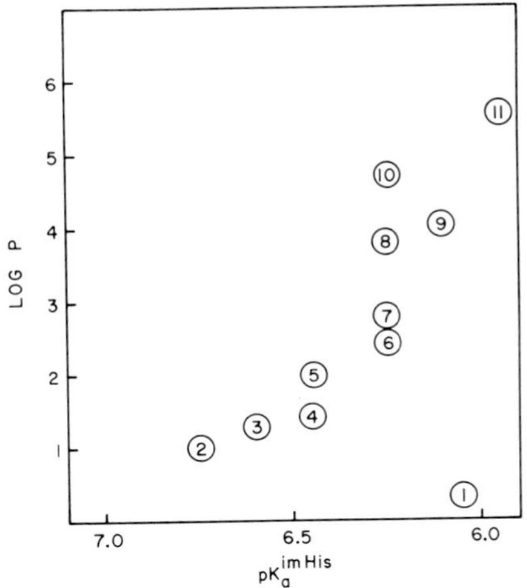

Fig. 1. Logarithm of biological potency (P) *vs.* pK_a of the imidazole of histidine (im His). Numerical designation of points: (1) H-Pro-His-Pro-NH_2; (2) pGlu-His-Pro-OH; (3) pGlu-N^{π}-Me-His-Pro-NH_2; (4) pGlu-His-Pro-N-Et_2; (5) pGlu-His-Pro-N◯; (6) pGlu-His-Pro-N-Me_2; (7) N^{α}-Me-pGlu-His-Pro-NH_2; (8) pGlu-His-Pro-NH-Me; (9) pGlu-His-Pro-OMe; (10) pGlu-His-Pro-NH_2 (TRF); (11) pGlu-N^{τ}-Me-His-Pro-NH_2.

formation of the molecule by internal hydrogen bonding (Grant *et al.*, 1972). Pertinent to the latter point is the observation that [N^{π}-Me-His^2]TRF has a very low biological potency, while [N^{τ}-Me-His^2]TRF is 8 times more active than the parent molecule (Rivier *et al.*, 1972).

Prolineamide substitutions can involve retention of considerable potency. An amide substituent can easily assume a conformation whereby it does not interfere with other groups in the remainder of the molecule (or alternatively, the same could be suggested for interactions in the receptor–substrate complex). Tertiary amides are much less active than the potent secondary amides. The presence of a charged group at the C-terminus as in pGlu-His-Pro-OH, yields a drastic reduction in activity when compared to hydrophobic amide substitutions (Guillemin *et al.*, 1971).

The stereoisomer "L-D-L"-TRF (L-pGlu-D-His-L-Pro-NH_2) exhibited 3% of the biological potency of the native compound, the "L-L-D" and "D-L-L" analogues were much less active, and "D-D-D"-TRF was inactive at the concentrations studied (Wilber and Flouret, 1971). No structural analogues of TRF have been reported to act as inhibitors.

The binding of TRF to whole pituitary cells in culture or plasma cell membrane fractions in competition with [^{3}H]TRF has been studied (Grant *et al.*, 1971; Labrie, 1972; Vale *et al.*, 1973). The binding affinities of the TRF analogues have shown a close correlation with the observed biological activity, suggesting that of the peptides tested the limiting factor in biological activity is the affinity for the receptor.

In summary, we conclude that: the TRF molecule must be hydrophobic; strict stereochemical or bulk properties must be met for each residue; pGlu may act in a nucleophilic capacity; histidine may be involved not only by virtue of its aromatic characteristics but also because of its acid–base properties; and amide substitutions retain high potency except for charged groups or groups of large bulk.

Structure–activity relationships of LRF

Several LRF analogues have been synthesized in our laboratories (Table I). All peptides were obtained as the primary amides. In the first series, referred to as the Gly substitutes of LRF, 8 decapeptides were prepared with the sequence of LRF, each residue normally different from Gly being replaced by Gly. In the case of [Gly^1]LRF, blocking of the N-terminal residue was achieved by preparing the protected decapeptide propionyl-[Gly^1]LRF. In the second series referred to as the des-LRF series, 7 peptides were synthesized, corresponding to the primary sequence of LRF from which one residue, starting at the C-terminus, was subtracted. Other analogues were synthesized with the primary structure of LRF from which specific residues were subtracted (for instance, des-His^2-LRF, thus corresponding to the sequence pGlu-Trp-Ser-Tyr-Gly-Leu-Arg-Pro-Gly-NH_2), or in which substitutions were entered on

TABLE I

LRF ANALOGUES

Compound	*% LRF potency*
pGlu-His-Trp-Ser-Tyr-Gly-Leu-Arg-Pro-Gly-NH_2	100.0
pGlu-His-Trp-Ser-Tyr-Gly-Leu-Arg-Pro-NH_2	10.0
pGlu-His-Trp-Ser-Tyr-Gly-Leu-Arg-NH_2	<0.1
pGlu-His-Trp-Ser-Tyr-Gly-Leu-NH_2	<0.1
pGlu-His-Trp-Ser-Tyr-Gly-NH_2	<0.1
pGlu-His-Trp-Ser-Tyr-NH_2	<0.1
pGlu-His-Trp-Ser-NH_2	<0.1
pGlu-His-Trp-NH_2	<0.1
pGlu-His-NH_2	<0.1
[CH_3CH_2-C(=O)-Gly^1]LRF	0.2
[Gly^2]LRF	*
[Gly^3]LRF	<0.1
[Gly^4]LRF	1.5
[Gly^5]LRF	0.1
[Gly^7]LRF	0.2
[Gly^8]LRF	0.1
[Gly^9]LRF	0.2
des-His^2-LRF	*
[Phe^2]LRF	4.0
[N^{π}-Me-His^2]LRF	2.0
[N^{τ}-Me-His^2]LRF	6.0
[Ala^3]LRF	<0.1
[Phe^3]LRF	2.0
[Ala^6]LRF	1.0

* Antagonist

References p. 49–50

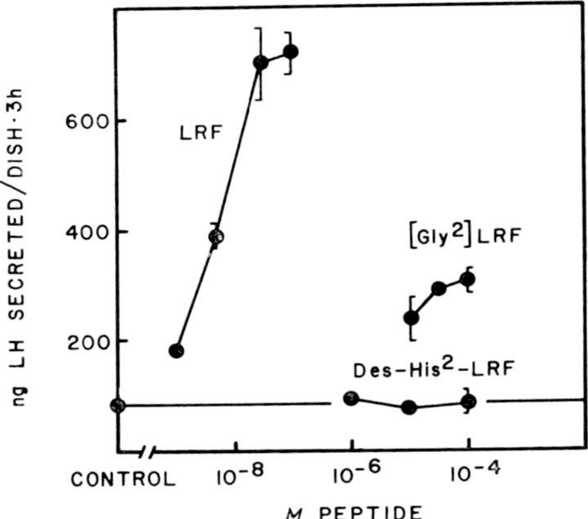

Fig. 2. Dose response curve of LRF and two LRF analogues with alterations in the His[2] position.

specific residues in the otherwise unchanged LRF sequence such as [N^τMe-His^2]-LRF or [N^πMe-His^2]LRF.

In the Gly substitutes of LRF, [Gly$^{2,\ 3,\ 5}$ or ^{8}]LRF (Table I), each have less than 0.1% LRF activity as measured *in vivo* (Amoss and Guillemin, 1968, 1969) or *in vitro* (Vale *et al.*, 1972a). [Gly^4]LRF has a potency of about 1.5% of that of LRF. The des-LRF peptides show less than 0.1% LRF activity with the exception of des^{10}-LRF with a potency of approximately 10% LRF. Neither [N^πMe-His^2]LRF nor [N^τMe-His^2]LRF have increased LRF activity in contradistinction to the increased activity of [N^τMe-His^2]TRF which is 8 times more potent than TRF (Rivier *et al.*, 1972). Des-His^2-LRF had no statistically significant LRF activity at the *in vitro* doses tested (Fig. 2).

When tested in an *in vitro* system by measuring the stimulation of the release of LH by dispersed pituitary cells in tissue cultures (Vale *et al.*, 1972a), [Gly^2]LRF showed a negative interaction with LRF (Fig. 3): At high concentrations, ($3 \cdot 10^{-5}M$–$10^{-4}M$), [Gly^2]LRF did not show additivity in response to low levels ($10^{-9}M$) of LRF; furthermore, it decreased the response to high levels ($10^{-8}M$–$10^{-7}M$) of LRF. The secretion rate of LH as stimulated by LRF was reduced by 50% or more in the presence of 1–4·10^3-fold molar ratios of des-His^2-LRF over LRF (see Fig. 4). Several experiments show that the inhibition of the response to LRF due to either of these analogues mentioned above could be overcome by higher levels of LRF, thereby indicating that each analogue acts as a competitive inhibitor of LRF. In preliminary experiments, *in vivo* des-His^2-LRF has been shown to partially inhibit the response to LRF as measured by radioimmunoassay when injected simultaneously with LRF or perfused prior to injection in castrated rats pretreated with estradiol.

Both [Gly^2]LRF and des-His^2-LRF thus have the ability to antagonize the action of LRF (Monahan *et al.*, 1972a, Vale *et al.*, 1972b). The antagonist activity of [Gly^2]-LRF is less easily demonstrable than that of des-His^2-LRF because of the inherent agonist activity, however slight, of the [Gly^2]LRF analogue. Thus, the antagonism to LRF due to [Gly^2]LRF can be demonstrated only at levels of LRF which stimulate

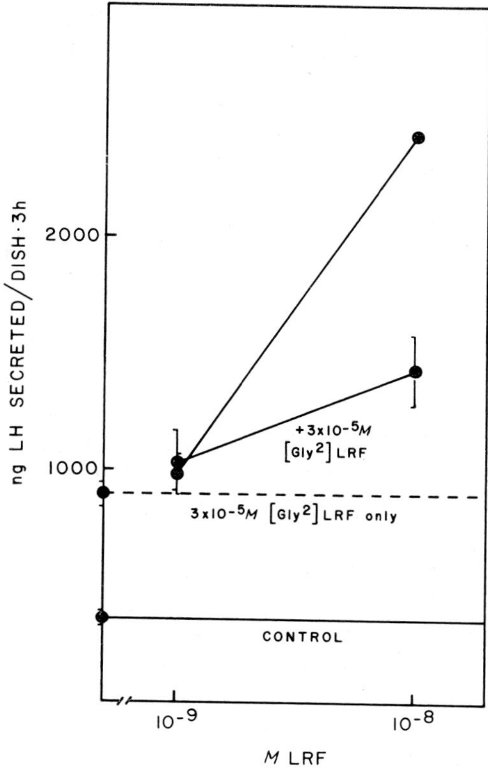

Fig. 3. Antagonism of LRF by [Gly[2]]LRF *in vitro*.

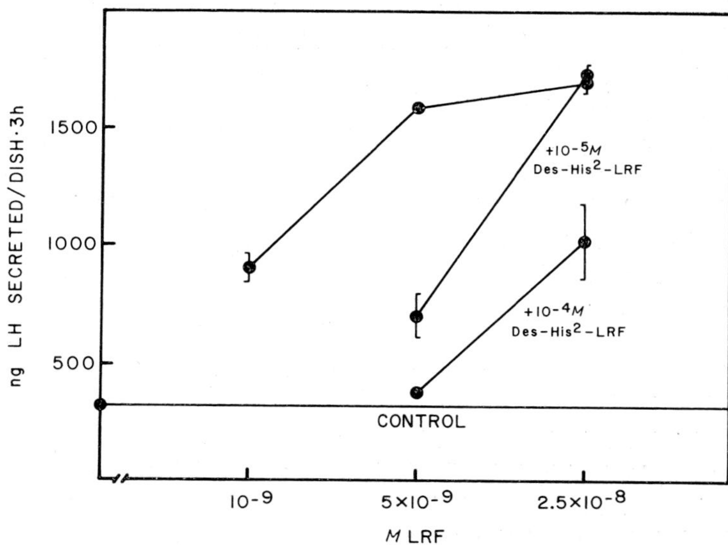

Fig. 4. Antagonism of LRF by des-His[2]-LRF *in vitro*.

References p. 49–50

a greater amount of LH release than that due to the dose of the partial agonist under study. The antagonism of LRF by des-His^2-LRF is more easily visualized because of its low intrinsic activity.

It is obvious that the affinity of the two analogues for the LRF-receptor is considerably less than that of LRF as evidenced by the high (greater or equal to 10^3) molar ratios of antagonist over LRF required for demonstration of the inhibition of LRF. Since des-His^2-LRF has the same or a higher affinity for the LRF receptor than [Gly^2]LRF, it would appear that either the presence of the imidazole ring or an amino acid in the L-configuration in LRF in the second position (pGlu-His^2-...) is important but not obligatory for the binding of LRF to its receptor. Thus, the histidyl residue in LRF is somehow required not only for the recognition of LRF by its receptor but also for full intrinsic activity of the molecule. Although important, the imidazole ring or the presence of an amino acid in the L-configuration, is not obligatory, however, for LRF's intrinsic activity since substitution of glycine for histidine in LRF yields a molecule with almost 50% of the LH releasing activity of LRF.

We cannot ascertain whether the pharmacological properties of the LRF analogues are a result of alteration of functional groups or are secondary to changes in the conformation of the molecule. When confirmational data become available, this point may be clarified.

Interpretation of the results of structure-function studies such as these must be qualified by consideration of the possibility that structural changes that promote biological activity through one part of the mechanism of action of the hormone may negate the overall effect by reducing biological activity in another part of the mechanism; *i.e.*, only the net effect of a given structural change is observed.

The competitive antagonism of LRF by the two analogues [Gly^2]LRF and des-His^2-LRF and the lack of LH releasing activity of des-His^2-LRF at a concentration 10-fold higher than that required to suppress the response to LRF, indicates a dissociation of the binding and secretory processes. This assumption is supported by a preliminary observation showing that des-His^2-LRF competes with [^{3}H-Pro^9]LRF for specific binding to anterior pituitary LRF receptors.

The two LRF analogues described here [Gly^2]LRF and des-His^2-LRF are the first peptides reported to be competitive antagonists of the biological activity of LRF. The physiological significance of these LRF antagonists is now being investigated; more powerful antagonists of LRF than [Gly^2]LRF and des-His^2-LRF will have to be designed and made available before they are considered for potential clinical use.

ACKNOWLEDGEMENTS

We wish to thank H. Anderson, M. Butcher, C. Garcia, W. Hewitt, R. Kaiser, A. Nussey, C. Otto, R. Smith, J. White, P. Wilson and R. Wolbers for their valuable technical assistance. This research is supported by AID (Contract No. AID/csd 2785), the Rockefeller Foundation and the Ford Foundation.

REFERENCES

AMOSS, M. AND GUILLEMIN, R. (1968) Solid-phase radioimmunoassay of ovine, bovine and murine luteinizing hormone. In *Gonadotropins 1968*, E. ROSEMBERG (Ed.), Geron-X, Los Altos, Calif., pp. 313–321.

AMOSS, M. AND GUILLEMIN, R. (1969) Response of plasma LH to hypothalamic LRF in rat and sheep as measured by solid-phase radioimmunoassay (RIA). *Fed. Proc.*, **28**, 381.

BABA, Y., MATSUO, H. AND SCHALLY, A. V. (1971) Structure of the porcine LH- and FSH-releasing hormone, II. Confirmation of the proposed structure by conventional sequential analysis. *Biochem. biophys. res. Commun.*, **44**, 459–463.

BOWERS, C. Y., FRIESEN, H. G., HWANG, P., GUYDA, H. J. AND FOLKERS, K. (1971) Prolactin and thyrotropin release in man by synthetic pyroglutamyl-histidyl-prolinamide. *Biochem. biophys. res. Commun.*, **45**, 1033–1041.

BURGUS, R. AND GUILLEMIN, R. (1970) Hypothalamic releasing factors. *Ann. Rev. Biochem.*, **39**, 499–526.

BURGUS, R., DUNN, T. F., DESIDERIO, D. AND GUILLEMIN, R. (1969) Structure moléculaire du facteur hypothalamique hypophysiotrope TRF d'origine ovine: Évidence par spectrométrie de masse de la séquence PCA-His-Pro-NH_2. *C.R. Acad. Sci. (Paris)*, **269**, 1870–1873.

BURGUS, R., DUNN, T. F., DESIDERIO, D., WARD, D. N., VALE, W. AND GUILLEMIN, R. (1970) Characterization of the hypothalamic hypophysiotropic TSH-releasing factor (TRF) of ovine origin. *Nature*, **226**, 321–325.

BURGUS, R., BUTCHER, M., LING, N., MONAHAN, M., RIVIER, J., FELLOWS, R., AMOSS, M., BLACKWELL, R., VALE, W. AND GUILLEMIN, R. (1971) Structure moléculaire du facteur hypothalamique (LRF) d'origine ovine contrôlant la sécrétion de l'hormone gonadotrope hypophysaire de lutéinisation (LH). *C.R. Acad. Sci. (Paris)*, **273**, 1611–1613.

BURGUS, R., BUTCHER, M., AMOSS, M., LING, N., MONAHAN, M., RIVIER, J., FELLOWS, R., BLACKWELL, R., VALE, W. AND GUILLEMIN, R. (1972). Primary structure of the hypothalamic luteinizing hormone-releasing factor of ovine origin. *Proc. nat. Acad. Sci. (U.S.A.)*, **69**, 278–282.

CELIS, M. E., TALEISNIK, S. AND WALTER, R. (1971) Regulation of formation and proposed structure of the factor inhibiting the release of melanocyte-stimulating hormone. *Proc. nat. Acad. Sci. (U.S.A.)*, **68**, 1428–1433.

CHAN, L. T., SCHAAL, S. M. AND SAFFRAN, M. (1969) Properties of the corticotropin-releasing factor of the rat median eminence. *Endocrinology*, **85**, 644–651.

FROHMAN, L. A., MARAN, J. W. AND DHARIWAL, A. P. S. (1971) Plasma growth hormone responses to intrapituitary injection of growth hormone releasing factor (GRF) in the rat. *Endocrinology*, **88**, 1483–1488.

GILLESSEN, D., PIVA, F., STEINER, H. AND STUDER, R. O. (1971) Über die Bedeutung des Histidins im "Thyrotropin-releasing" Hormon (TRH). *Helv. chim. Acta*, **54**, 1335–1342.

GRANT, G., VALE, W. AND GUILLEMIN, R. (1971) Interaction of thyrotropin releasing factor with membrane receptors of pituitary cells. *Biochem. biophys. res. Commun.*, **46**, 28–34.

GRANT, G., LING, N., RIVIER, J. AND VALE, W. (1972) Orientation restrictions of the peptide hormone, thyrotropin-releasing factor, due to intramolecular hydrogen bonding. *Biochemistry*, **11**, 3070–3073.

GUILLEMIN, R. (1971) Hypothalamic control of secretion of adenohypophysial hormones. In *Advances in Metabolic Disorders (Vol. 5)*, R. LEVINE AND R. LUFT (Eds.), Academic Press, New York, pp. 1–51.

GUILLEMIN, R., BURGUS, R. AND VALE, W. (1971) The hypothalamic hypophysiotropic thyrotropin releasing factor. In *Vitamins and Hormones (Vol. 29)*, P. MUNSON (Ed.), Academic Press, New York, pp. 1–39.

HERTELENDY, F., TODD, H., PEAKE, G. T., MACHLIN, L. J., JOHNSTON, G. J. AND POUNDS, G. (1971) Studies on growth hormone secretion: I. Effects of dibutyryl cyclic AMP, theophylline, epinephrine, ammonium ion and hypothalamic extracts on the release of growth hormone from rat anterior pituitaries *in vitro*. *Endocrinology*, **89**, 1256–1262.

HRUBY, V. J., SMITH, C. W., BOWER, SR. A. AND HADLEY, M. E. (1972) Melanophore stimulating hormone: release inhibition by ring structures of neurohypophysial hormones. *Science*, **176**, 1331–1332.

JACOBS, L. S., SNYDER, P. J., WILBER, J. F., UTIGER, R. D. AND DAUGHADAY, W. H. (1971) Increased serum prolactin after administration of synthetic thyrotropin releasing hormone (TRH) in man. *J. clin. Endocrinol.*, **33**, 996–998.

LABRIE, F., BARDEN, N., POIRIER, G. AND DELEAN, A. (1972) Binding of thyrotropin-releasing hormone to plasma membranes of bovine anterior pituitary gland. *Proc. nat. Acad. Sci. (U.S.A.)*, **69**, 283–287.

MATSUO, H., BABA, Y., NAIR, R. M. G., ARIMURA, A. AND SCHALLY, A. V. (1971) Structure of porcine LH- and FSH-releasing hormone, I. The proposed amino acid sequence. *Biochem. biophys. res. Commun.*, **43**, 1334–1339.

MONAHAN, M. W., RIVIER, J., VALE, W., GUILLEMIN, R. AND BURGUS, R. (1972a) [Gly^2]LRF and des-His^2-LRF. The synthesis, purification and characterization of two LRF analogues antagonistic to LRF. *Biochem. biophys. res. Commun.*, **47**, 551–556.

MONAHAN, M., RIVIER, J., VALE, W., LING, N., GRANT, G., AMOSS, M., GUILLEMIN, R., BURGUS, R., NICOLAIDES, E. AND REBSTOCK, M. (1973) Structure–biological activity relationships of thyrotropin and luteinizing hormone releasing factor analogues. In *Chemistry and Biology of Peptides*, J. MEIENHOFER (Ed.), Ann Arbor Publishers, Ann Arbor, Mich., pp. 601–608.

NAIR, R. M. G., BARRETT, J. F., BOWERS, C. Y. AND SCHALLY, A. V. (1970) Structure of porcine thyrotropin releasing hormone. *Biochemistry*, **9**, 1103–1106.

NAIR, R. M. G., KASTIN, A. J. AND SCHALLY, A. V. (1971) Isolation and structure of hypothalamic MSH-release-inhibiting hormone. *Biochem. biophys. res. Commun.*, **43**, 1376–1381.

NAIR, R. M. G., KASTIN, A. J. AND SCHALLY, A. V. (1972) Isolation and structure of another hypothalamic peptide possessing MSH-release-inhibiting activity. *Biochem. biophys. res. Commun.*, **47**, 1420–1425.

RIVIER, J., VALE, W., MONAHAN, M., LING, N. AND BURGUS, R. (1972) Synthetic thyrotropin-releasing-factor analogues, 3. Effect of replacement or modification of histidine residue on biological activity. *J. med. Chem.*, **15**, 479–482.

SCHALLY, A. V., NAIR, R. M. G., REDDING, T. W. AND ARIMURA, A. (1971) The amino acid sequence of a peptide with growth hormone-releasing activity isolated from porcine hypothalamus. *J. biol. Chem.*, **246**, 6647–6650.

SIEVERTSSON, H., CHANG, J. K. AND FOLKERS, K. (1972) On the role of the histidine moiety in the structure of the thyrotropin-releasing hormone. *J. med. Chem.*, **15**, 219–221.

TASHJIAN, A. H., JR., BAROWSKY, N. J. AND JENSEN, D. K. (1971) Thyrotropin releasing hormone: Direct evidence for stimulation of prolactin production by pituitary cells in culture. *Biochem. biophys. res. Commun.*, **43**, 516–523.

VALE, W., GRANT, G., AMOSS, M., BLACKWELL, R. AND GUILLEMIN, R., (1972a) Culture of enzymatically dispersed anterior pituitary cells: Functional validation of a method. *Endocrinology*, **91**, 562–572.

VALE, W., GRANT, G., RIVIER, J., MONAHAN, M., AMOSS, M., BLACKWELL, R., BURGUS, R. AND GUILLEMIN, R. (1972b) Synthetic polypeptide antagonists of the hypothalamic luteinizing hormone releasing factor. *Science*, **176**, 933–942.

VALE, W., GRANT, G. AND GUILLEMIN, R. (1973) Chemistry of the hypothalamic releasing factors—studies on structure–function relationships in TRF and LRF. In *Frontiers in Neuroendocrinology, 1973*, F. GANONG AND L. MARTINI (Eds.), Oxford University Press, New York, pp. 1–37.

VEBER, D. F., BENNETT, C. D., MILKOWSKI, J. D., GAL, G., DENKEWALTER, R. G. AND HIRSCHMANN, R. (1971) Synthesis of a proposed growth hormone releasing factor. *Biochem. biophys. res. Commun.*, **45**, 235–239.

WILBER, J. F. AND FLOURET, G. (1971) Thyrotropin releasing hormone (TRH) analogues: Stimulation of thyrotropin (TSH) secretion *in vitro*. *Prog. 53rd Meeting of the Endocrine Soc.*, San Francisco, Calif., p. 87 (Abstract).

WILBER, J. F., NAGEL, T. AND WHITE, W. F. (1971) Hypothalamic growth hormone-releasing activity (G.R.A.): Characterization by the *in vitro* rat pituitary and radioimmunoassay. *Endocrinology*, **89**, 1419–1424.

DISCUSSION

HEDGE: I have two related questions, the first being of a very general and perhaps naive nature. You have given us proposed structures for various releasing factors, but I would like to know if all of these peptides have been demonstrated to be present in hypothalamic tissue. Secondly, of a more specific nature, you have shown us that you can slightly modify the structure of TRF and thereby increase its activity. Would you comment on the possibility that some such modified form is also present in the hypothalamus and perhaps released in sufficient quantities so that it might be more important physiologically than what we have thus far been calling TRF?

BURGUS: The answer to your first question is yes. All of the structures that I have presented represent materials from hypothalamic extracts. The TRF and LRF were identified in both bovine and porcine material.

HEDGE: I am aware of the earlier work from which it is clear that TRF and the gonadotrophin-releasing factor can be found in hypothalamic tissue. However, concerning the more recent proposals such as the side chain of oxytocin, tocinoic acid, and growth hormone-releasing factor; are all of these found in the hypothalamus as well or are they perhaps synthetic peptides that just happen to be able to affect pituitary secretion?

BURGUS: The MIF's are found in the hypothalamus. Tocinoic acid has not been as clearly established as the others I mentioned regarding MIF release; it is found to be present after incubation of the hypothalamus with oxytocin. To my knowledge the only ones that have been definitely identified are the Pro-Leu-Gly-NH_2 and the pentapeptide Pro-His-Phe-Arg-Gly-NH_2 by Dr. Schally and Dr. Kastin. We have considered that some of the analogues may be present in the hypothalamus. The methylhistidine analog intrigued us particularly, since there are systems which can methylate histidine in the brain and we have wondered if this isn't perhaps a rat TRF or a TRF in another species. Prolactin-releasing activity seems to be greater for this material also. The difficulty here is the same as it was with TRF itself; the substances are present in very small amounts. We would like to search for them in hypothalamic tissue.

MEYERSON: Do any of your less biologically active analogues compete with the TRF? In other words, does there exist an anti-TRF?

BURGUS: No, we have not yet found an antagonist of TRF.

KNIGGE: May I ask Dr. Burgus two questions? First, regarding the pyroGlu portion of TRF. Is there any evidence that this portion of the molecule may be the site of action of the plasma inactivating enzyme? And secondly, is the "open" tripeptide Glu-His-Pro-amide synthesized in other regions of the brain?

BURGUS: We haven't done any extensive studies on the products of degradation of TRF. The work by Redding and Schally indicates that there is some opening of the ring perhaps during the inactivation process in plasma. In answer to your second question, we haven't searched for these materials in the other parts of the brain. I might comment further though that the open chain compound Glu-His-Pro is completely inactive and that the Gln-His-Pro has been shown by Folkers and his collaborators to have very low activity in TRF bioassays.

KNIGGE: If "open" Glu-His-Pro-NH_2 were synthesized in hypothalamus as well as other regions of the brain, the "uniqueness" of TRF-producing neurons would then only be the possession of an enzyme system which forms the pyro ring.

BURGUS: It's all together possible.

Hormonal Inputs to Releasing Factor Cells, Feedback Sites

WALTER E. STUMPF AND MADHABANANDA SAR

Departments of Anatomy and Pharmacology, Laboratories for Reproductive Biology, University of North Carolina, Chapel Hill, N. C. 27514 (U.S.A.)

We still do not know, *what* releasing factor (RF) cells are and *where* RF cells are located. We also do not know where the feedback sites are, regarding the brain and peripheral glands. A statement that the RF cells and "feedback" sites are located only in the brain—although there is strong belief that this is so—would be presumptuous. Our "knowledge" and concepts are based on indirect evidence. Therefore, in dealing with such a subject, much of what is said will be hypothetical.

Soon after the concept of the hypothalamo-hypophyseal vascular link was created (Harris, 1955), these questions were pursued: what are the hypophysiotrophic substances and where are they produced? While the existence of hypophysiotrophic RFs is now established, their production sites remain obscure. RFs are believed to be manufactured in the "hypophysiotrophic area" (Halász *et al.*, 1962), in *specialized ependymal cells* (Levèque, 1972), or in hormone-neurons in the phylogenetically old *periventricular brain* (Stumpf, 1970a).

Certain peripheral hormones influence the activities of endocrine glands in which they are produced by acting on the pituitary and brain, influencing their own production through the stimulation of the synthesis of peptide messengers. Therefore, a search for the localization of steroid hormones in the brain could provide an answer to the question—where are the substances produced that influence the activities of related endocrine glands? G. Harris made such efforts and reported about it already in his book in 1955. He did not find concentrations of radioactivity in the brain in his radioassays after the injection of [^{14}C]estradiol. This was probably due to the low specific activity of the labeled hormone used. Later, in Harris' laboratory, Glascock and Michael (1962) and Michael (1965) succeeded with [^{3}H]hexestrol to obtain specific localization in neurons of the cat's brain, "involving the lateral septal area, preoptic region and hypothalamus" (Michael, 1965).

Only after the application of the more sensitive dry-mount autoradiographic technique (Stumpf, 1970b, 1971a) it became possible to obtain adequate cellular and subcellular resolution and to map the brain, providing detailed topographic information about the distribution of "estrogen-neurons" (Stumpf, 1968, 1970a), "androgen-neurons" (Stumpf and Sar, 1971), and "glucocorticoid-neurons" (Stumpf, 1971a). G. Harris, aware of the importance of topographic information, organized his last neuroendocrine symposium (which he no longer could attend) around the

References p. 68–70

topic of the hypophysiotrophic structures in the brain (Proceedings Anat. Soc. of Great Britain and Ireland, 1972).

RF-producing cells cannot be identified by the classical stains for "neurosecretion", such as Gomori's trichrome or aldehyde fuchsin. For the identification of the Gomori-negative parvicellular neurosecretory systems, presently no stain is available, no specific histochemical reactions exist, and no clear ultrastructural criteria have been provided. If specific antibodies could be produced, the localization of RFs in their storage and production sites may be accomplished.

EVIDENCE FOR THE "HYPOPHYSIOTROPHIC AREA" AS *THE* RF-PRODUCING SITE

The "hypophysiotrophic area" is the hypothalamic area in which PAS-positive cells are maintained in pituitary grafts (Halász *et al.*, 1962). "In the antero-posterior direction, the area of preserved basophils extends in the level of the optic chiasm from the ventral surface up to the paraventricular nuclei or even slightly above. To the rear the dorsal border gradually comes down in a ventral direction and in the anterior mammillary level the "hypophysiotrophic" effect is limited to a narrow zone around the inframammillary recess of the third ventricle. The medio-lateral extent of the area is 0.5 mm or slightly more, from the midline. Immediately on the basal surface of the hypothalamus the region of preserved basophils is somewhat broader" (Szentágothai *et al.*, 1968). It is noteworthy that the nucleus (n.) paraventricularis, the n. preopticus medialis, the n. interstitialis striae terminalis and apparently also the n. premammillaris ventralis are excluded. Flament-Durand and Desclin (1970) distinguish between areas influencing the gonadotrophs and the thyrotrophs. "Castration cells appeared in all portions of grafts located in the infundibular recess of the third ventricle in contact with the arcuate nuclei, whereas PTU treatment induced the appearance of thyroidectomy cells in all portions of grafts situated in the suprachiasmatic region, the anterior hypothalamic area, the paraventricular nuclei, and the anterior part of the tuberal region" (l.c.). None of these studies provided any evidence regarding the maintenance of corticotrophs in pituitary grafts.

Strong additional indirect evidence has been adduced that the "hypophysiotrophic area" is *the* site of production of RFs. Using the Halász knife to deafferentiate hypothalamic areas, animals with hypothalamic islands, if they survive, continue to have "normal endocrine gland function", except for some modulating nervous influences such as cyclicity (Halász, 1972). No degenerating nerve-fibers could be detected within the median eminence in such hypothalamic islands (Halász, 1972). Furthermore, the fact that RFs can be extracted in the largest amounts from the "median eminence" is considered, perhaps, the strongest supporting evidence that the RFs are produced in the "hypophysiotrophic area".

ARGUMENTS AGAINST THE CONCEPT THAT THE "HYPOPHYSIOTROPHIC AREA" IS *THE* RF-PRODUCING SITE IN THE BRAIN

The fact that basophils are maintained within a narrow strip along the ventral part of the third ventricle may be viewed under the following considerations: How do RFs get to the grafts from RF-producing cells (*e.g.*, pericarya, axons, or nerve endings)? Do they diffuse through membranes, are they transported through the extracellular space or astrocytes, or does the damage of such structures during the experiment permit seepage to the graft? Do the RFs come from the specialized ependyma (Knowles, 1971; Levèque, 1972), with the grafts being placed within the reach of the processes of tanycytes, which extend far into hypothalamic nuclei (Bleier, 1971), *or* do RFs come through the ventricular fluid?

The extraction of highest amounts of RFs from the "median eminence" can be likened to the RF-releasing or -inhibiting substances such as noradrenaline and serotonin. These latter substances are extractable in highest amounts from the "hypothalamus", but the cell bodies, that is, the RF-releasing or -inhibiting neurons are located remotely(!) from the hypothalamus, as has been learned from fluorescence mapping (Fuxe, 1965).

If indeed RF-producing parvocellular neurosecretory cells are located outside of the "hypophysiotrophic area", then deafferentiation should result in endocrine gland dysfunction, and nerve degenerations should become visible at the primary plexus in the median eminence. Experiments of Halász (1972) have failed to show such effects, which is used as support for the concept of the "hypophysiotrophic area" containing *the* RF-producing neurons. However, as conclusive and convincing as the deafferentiation experiments seem, one must bear in mind possible pitfalls. Although the deafferentiation may have resulted in a complete separation of structures, hormonal inputs to the median eminence and pituitary are not excluded. Perhaps, the hypothalamic deafferentiation can be likened to G. Harris' pituitary stalk sections before he put the wax paper between the cut surfaces. As we now know, the results of this deafferentiation were quite different when regeneration of blood vessels and humoral contacts were decreased or eliminated. The non-visibility of degenerating nerve endings in the median eminence does not exclude the possibility of RF-producing neurons existing outside of the "hypophysiotrophic area". Nerve degeneration results need, in general, to be interpreted with caution, especially when links of fine fibers are negated. Also, the possibility remains of a humoral ventriculo-ependymal link between the RF-producing cells and the primary plexus in the median eminence.

HORMONE LOCALIZATION IN THE "HYPOPHYSIOTROPHIC AREA"

Dry-mount autoradiography with radioactively labeled hormones demonstrated populations of neurons which concentrate and retain radioactivity within the "hypophysiotrophic area" of the rat.

[^{3}H]estradiol-concentrating neurons are accumulated within the n. arcuatus, the n. ventromedialis, pars ventrolateralis and the n. periventricularis. In addition, there are dispersed labeled neurons in, for instance, the other parts of the n. ventromedialis, the n. perifornicalis and the area hypothalamica anterior (Stumpf, 1968, 1970a). After the injection of [^{3}H]testosterone, radioactivity was found to be concentrated

References p. 68–70

and retained in nuclei of neurons in the n. arcuatus, the whole n. ventromedialis and the n. periventricularis. Similar to [^{3}H]estradiol, dispersed labeled neurons existed outside of those nuclei which showed accumulations of "androgen-neurons" (Sar and Stumpf, 1971; Stumpf and Sar, 1971). After the injection of [^{3}H]progesterone, as well as [^{3}H]cortisol and [^{3}H]corticosterone, no comparable concentration and retention of radioactivity has been reported so far for the "hypophysiotrophic area". While experiments with both of these hormones are still under way in our laboratory, it is noteworthy that [^{3}H]corticosterone and [^{3}H]cortisol show heavy concentration in nuclei of neurons located in extrahypothalamic sites, for instance, the hippocampus, the dentate gyrus, the piriform cortex and the septum (Stumpf, 1971a and b, 1972; Stumpf and Sar, 1971, 1972), while in the same animals no such concentrations have been observed in neurons of the "hypophysiotrophic area". This is suggestive that the "feedback" sites for glucocorticoids are largely extrahypothalamic (Stumpf, 1971a and b). Regarding the failure to specifically localize [^{3}H]progesterone or metabolites of it, the rapid metabolism of this hormone must be considered. From the known hormone effects, progestin-binding sites can be expected to exist inside as well as outside the "hypophysiotrophic area" (Pasteels and Ectors, 1971). In order to be able to demonstrate them biochemically or autoradiographically, special experimental manipulations may be required.

[^{125}I]thyroxin, injected into intact or thyroidectomized rats failed to localize in specific neurons in our autoradiograms. There was no accumulation of radioactivity within the "thyrotrophic area". However, radioactivity existed within the neuropil of the median eminence and at the bottom of the third ventricle (Stumpf and Sar, unpublished observations). This localization had already been reported earlier by Jensen and Clark (1951) and later by Sturm and Wernitz (1956). This lack of concentration of radioactivity within the "thyrotrophic area" does not exclude feedback actions of thyroid hormones at this or other sites in the brain. The mechanism of thyroid hormone action may not include lasting and detectable binding as is the case in certain steroid target tissues, or there may be a rapid intracellular turnover. The statement needs to be reiterated that, in principle, lack of detectable binding of a hormone does not exclude action, just as binding or deposition of a substance does not by itself imply action. Regarding the brain, additional functional evidence is needed, as can be derived from hormone implantation, lesion or electrical stimulation. For this reason, some implantation data from the literature have been compiled in Table I for estrogens, in Table II for androgens and in Table III for glucocorticoids. Regarding these hormones, there is, in general, fair agreement between the areas as defined by dry-autoradiographic hormone localization and the effective feedback sites as defined by hormone implantation, although the topographic information provided through autoradiography is much more detailed and precise. Major discrepancies, however, seem to exist between the effects of hypothalamic glucocorticoid implants (Table III) and the so far available autoradiographic data.

TABLE I

EFFECTS OF ESTROGEN IMPLANTS IN THE FEMALE RAT BRAIN ON REPRODUCTIVE FUNCTION

Hormone	*Site of implants*	*Effect*	*References*
Estradiol	Arcuate nucleus, mammillary bodies	Atrophy of the genital tract and gonads	Lisk, 1960
	Preoptic regions, anterior hypothalamus, medial hypothalamus	No significant effect on genital tract and gonads	
Estradiol	Basal tuberal hypothalamus	Prevented post castration elevation in plasma and hypophysial LH and evoked adenohypophysial enlargement	Ramirez, Abrams and McCann, 1963
	Suprachiasmatic region, posterior hypothalamus, globi palladi	No effect	
Estradiol	Preoptic area, lateral hypothalamus, basolateral amygdala, fornix-hippocampus, caudate-putamen, subarachnoidal space	No effect on COH	Littlejohn and DeGroot, 1963
	Mammillary complex (peduncle)	Inhibited COH	
	Anterior or anteromedial amygdala	Greater than normal COH	
Estradiol	Median eminence or pituitary	Increased release and synthesis of prolactin by the adenohypophysis	Ramirez and McCann, 1964
Estradiol benzoate[a] (acute)	Anterior hypothalamic preoptic region	Advanced vaginal opening: ovaries, uteri, and cycles normal	Smith and Davidson, 1968
	Median eminence	No apparent effect	
Estradiol benzoate (chronic)	Median eminence	Inhibited uterine and ovarian development	
Estradiol	Median eminence	Precocious opening of the vagina, ovulation, reduction in pituitary LH, increase of plasma LH levels, increase in uterine weight	Motta, Fraschini, Giuliani and Martini, 1968

References p. 68–70

TABLE I

EFFECTS OF ESTROGEN IMPLANTS IN THE FEMALE RAT BRAIN ON REPRODUCTIVE FUNCTION *(continued)*

Hormone	*Site of implants*	*Effect*	*References*
	Habenular region	Retardation of puberty, reduction of the weight of ovaries and uteri, increased pituitary LH stores, plasma LH undetectable	
Estradiol benzoate	Amygdala	No effect on the vaginal opening	Davidson, 1969
Estradiol	Cortical amygdaloid nucleus or hypothalamic preoptic area	Tendency to stimulate LH secretion	Lawton and Sawyer, 1970
	Arcuate-ventromedial nuclear region	Depressed LH secretion	
Estradiol benzoate (unilateral)	Preoptic anterior hypothalamic area	Elevated plasma LH at 6 h	Kalra and McCann, 1972
Estradiol benzoate (bilateral)	Median eminence, arcuate region, amygdala	Increased plasma level of LH and FSH at 30 h	
Estradiol benzoate	Dorsal and ventral hippocampus	Significant decrease of only plasma FSH at 30 h	

[a]Intact 26-day immature rats were used.
COH, compensatory ovarian hypertrophy.
FSH, follicle-stimulating hormone.
LH, luteinizing hormone.

TABLE II

EFFECTS OF ANDROGEN IMPLANTS IN THE RAT BRAIN ON REPRODUCTIVE FUNCTION

Hormone	*Site of implants*	*Effect*	*References*
Testosterone	Basal tuberal median eminence region, arcuate nucleus	Atropy of the ventral prostate and seminal vesicles	Lisk, 1962
	Lateral hypothalamus, anterior pituitary	No effect	
	Arcuate region[e]	Some atrophies of the ovaries	
Testosterone propionate[a]	Hypothalamus	Androgen sterilization	Wagner, Erwin and Critchlow, 1966

TABLE II

EFFECTS OF ANDROGEN IMPLANTS IN THE RAT BRAIN ON REPRODUCTIVE FUNCTION *(continued)*

Hormone	*Site of implants*	*Effect*	*Reference*
Testosterone propionate[b]	Median eminence	Atrophy of the testis, seminal vesicle and prostate	Smith and Davidson, 1967a
Testosterone propionate[c]	Median eminence	Retardation of puberal development of the testis and accessory sex glands	Smith and Davidson, 1967b
Testosterone propionate	Arcuate nucleus	Decreased testicular biosynthesis of testosterone, atrophy of the seminal vesicles and urethral bulbs	Matsuyama, 1970
	Preoptic area	Slight increase in the weight of the accessory sex organs	
Testosterone propionate[d]	Ventromedial-arcuate nucleus area	More effective in androgen sterilization	Nadler, 1971
	Basal-preoptic suprachiasmatic region	Less effective in androgen sterilization	

[a]Female rats, 4 days old; [b]Hypophysectomized rat with renal pituitary graft; [c]Prepuberal; [d]Female rats, 5 days old; [e]Female rats, mature. Except for [a], [d] and [e], all experiments listed in this table were done with male rats.

TABLE III

EFFECTS OF ADRENOCORTICOID IMPLANTS IN THE BRAIN ON ADRENAL FUNCTION[a]

Species	*Hormone*	*Site of implants*	*Effect*	*Reference*
Rat, Cat	Cortisone	Basomedial hypothalamus	Inhibits adrenal secretion (at rest) and prevents the increase caused by operative stress	Endröczi, Lissak and Tekeres, 1961
Rabbit	Corticosterone	Basal hypothalamus, anterior portion of median eminence	Inhibits stress response to rise in plasma corticoids	Smelik and Sawyer, 1962
		Anteromedial hypothalamus	Less inhibition	
		Post. hypothalamus, mesencephalon	No effect	
		Adenohypophysis	No effect on blood corticoid level	

References p. 68–70

TABLE III

EFFECT OF ADRENOCORTICOID IMPLANTS IN THE BRAIN ON ADRENAL FUNCTION[a] *(continued)*

Species	*Hormone*	*Site of implants*	*Effect*	*Reference*
Rat	Cortisol, hydrocortisone acetate	Median eminence, anteromedial hypothalamus	Abolish CAH and the AAAD in the remaining gland following unilateral adrenalectomy	Davidson and Feldman, 1963
		Midbrain, anterior forebrain	Slight or no inhibition of CAH	
		Posterior diencephalon, cerebellum	Normal CAH	
		Pituitary	No effect	
Rat	Cortisol acetate	Median eminence	Adrenal atrophy, inhibition of AAAD	Chowers, Feldman and Davidson, 1963
		Pituitary	No effect	
Rat	Corticosterone	Anterobasal hypothalamus	Decreased stress-induced ACTH secretion, plasma corticosterone level. Small decrease in adrenal weight	Smelik, 1965
Rat	Dexamethasone, cortisol	Median eminence	Reduced plasma and adrenal corticosterone levels. Decreased adrenal weight. (Cortisol did not reduce adrenal weight)	Corbin, Mangili, Motta and Martini, 1965
	Dexamethasone	Pituitary	No effect	
		Cerebral cortex	No effect	
		Midbrain, lateral reticular formation	Lower plasma and adrenal corticosterone levels. Reduced adrenal weight	
Rat	Cortisol, corticosterone	Median eminence	Block of stress response to increased adrenal corticoids	Davidson, Jones and Levine, 1965

TABLE III

EFFECTS OF ADRENOCORTICOID IMPLANTS IN THE BRAIN ON ADRENAL FUNCTION[a] *(continued)*

Species	*Hormone*	*Site of implants*	*Effect*	*Reference*
Rat	Cortisol	Median eminence	Decreased adrenal weight. Depression of adrenal corticosterone	Slusher, 1966
		Midbrain reticular formation, ventral hippocampus	Decreased level of adrenal corticosterones. No change in adrenal weight	
Rat	Cortisol	Median eminence	Substantial suppression of the stress-induced ACTH release	Bohus, 1968
		Mesencephalic reticular formation	Moderate suppression of the stress-induced ACTH release	
Rat	Cortisol, corticosterone	Median eminence	Decrease in rise of plasma corticosterone following ether stress	Grimm and Kendall, 1968
Rat	Cortisol acetate	Median eminence	Depressed adrenal function, adrenal atrophy	Kendall and Allen, 1968
Rabbit	Corticosterone	Hippocampus: CA2 and CA3 and part of fascia dentata	Adrenocortical biosynthetic activity increased as measured by [1-^{14}C] acetate incorporation into corticosterone	Kawakami, Seto and Yoshida, 1968
		CA1	No influence	
		Amygdala: nucleus centralis, nucleus basolateralis, nucleus medialis	Decreased corticosterone synthesis	
		nucleus corticalis	No change	
Rat	Dexamethasone	Hypothalamus	Marked suppression of diurnal peak in non-stress plasma corticosterone levels	Zimmerman and Critchlow, 1969
		Ventral diencephalon, rostral midbrain	Suppressed non-stressed corticosteroid level	

References p. 68–70

TABLE III

EFFECTS OF ADRENOCORTICOID IMPLANTS IN THE BRAIN ON ADRENAL FUNCTION[a] *(continued)*

Species	*Hormone*	*Site of implants*	*Effect*	*Reference*
		Amygdala	No suppression	
		Pituitary	No suppression	
Rat	Dexamethasone, cortisol, corticosterone, 11-dehydrocorticosterone, 11-deoxycorticosterone	Anterior median eminence region	Suppression of ACTH release in response to stress	Bohus and Strashimirov, 1970
	11-Deoxycortisol, tetrahydrocortisol, pregnenolene, progesterone, testosterone	Anteromedian eminence region	No effect	
	Dexamethasone, cortisol, 11-deoxycorticosterone	Infundibular region	Suppressed ACTH release	
	Dexamethasone, 11-deoxycorticosterone	Anterior pituitary (bilateral implants)	Suppressed ACTH release	

[a]Animals other than rat are included in this table, because only few studies on extrahypothalamic implants have been reported.
AAAD, adrenal ascorbic acid depletion. ACTH, corticotrophin. CAH, compensatory adrenal hypertrophy.

ESTROGEN-NEURONS, ANDROGEN-NEURONS AND GLUCOCORTICOID-NEURONS IN THE PERIVENTRICULAR BRAIN

The autoradiographic data mentioned here, were obtained in our laboratory. The results published from other laboratories in part confirm our data, but also disagree to a varying extent. The discrepancies in the hormone localization reported by others have been discussed (Stumpf, 1969, 1971a, 1972).

Our present knowledge regarding the topographic distribution of steroid hormone concentrating neurons in the rat brain is schematically represented in Figs. 1–3. The information available to date is incomplete and more detailed qualitative, as well as quantitative data are required.

Most detailed information exists for *estradiol* (Stumpf, 1968, 1970a; Stumpf and Sar, 1971). Estradiol-concentrating neurons (estrogen-neurons) are found within, as well as outside the "hypophysiotrophic area". Accumulations of estrogen-neurons are found, for instance, not only in the n. arcuatus and the ventrolateral n. ventro-

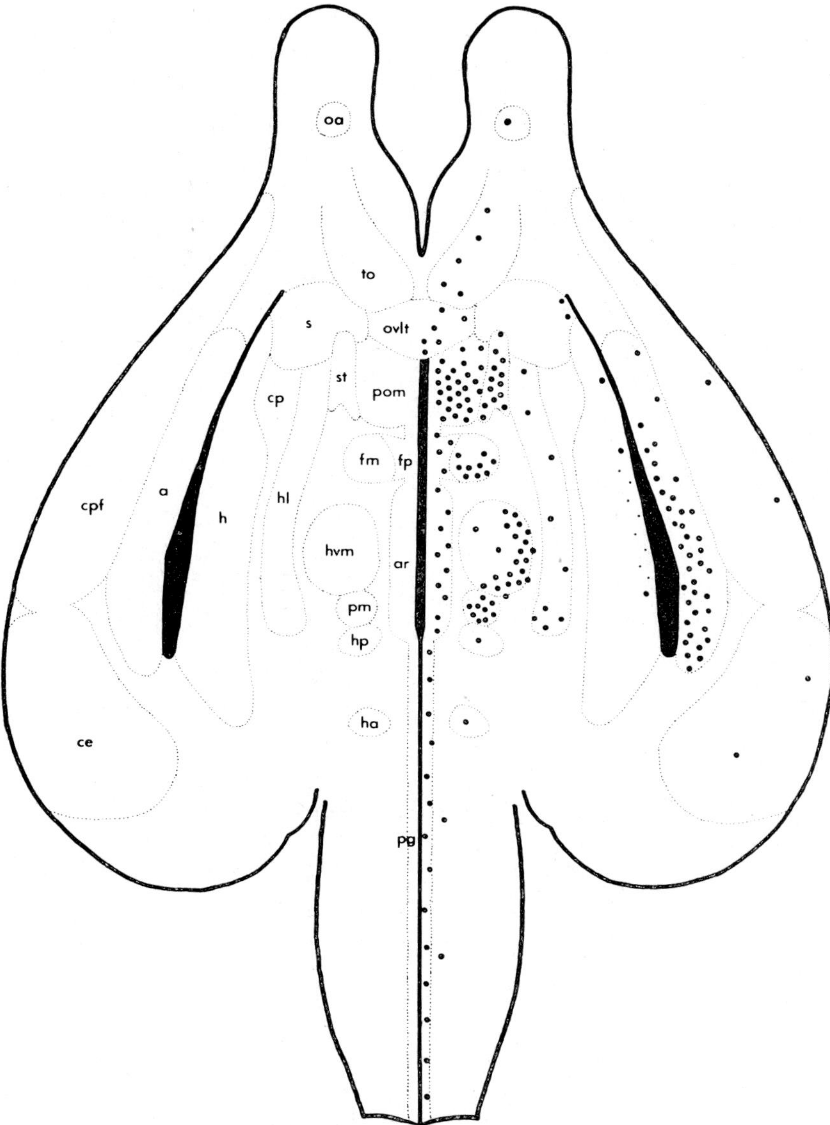

Fig. 1. Topographic distribution of estrogen-neurons in rat brain, obtained after dry-autoradiography, projected on hypothetical horizontal plane. Schematic.
Right-half: the spacing of dots indicates the frequency of occurrence of estradiol-concentrating neurons; the size of dots indicates the intensity of radioactive labeling.
Left half with designation of structures: a, n. amygdaloideus; ar, n. arcuatus; ce, cortex entorhinalis; cp, n. caudatus putamen; cpf, cortex piriformis; fm, n. paraventricularis, pars magnocellularis; fp, n. paraventricularis, pars parvocellularis; h, hippocampus; ha, n. lateralis habenulae; hl, n. lateralis hypothalami; hp, n. posterior hypothalami; hvm, n. ventromedialis hypothalami; oa, n. olfactorius anterior; ovlt, organon vasculosum lamina terminalis; pg, periventricular gray; pm, n. premammillaris; pom, n. preopticus medialis; s, septum; st, n. stria terminalis; to, tuberculum olfactorium.

References p. 68–70

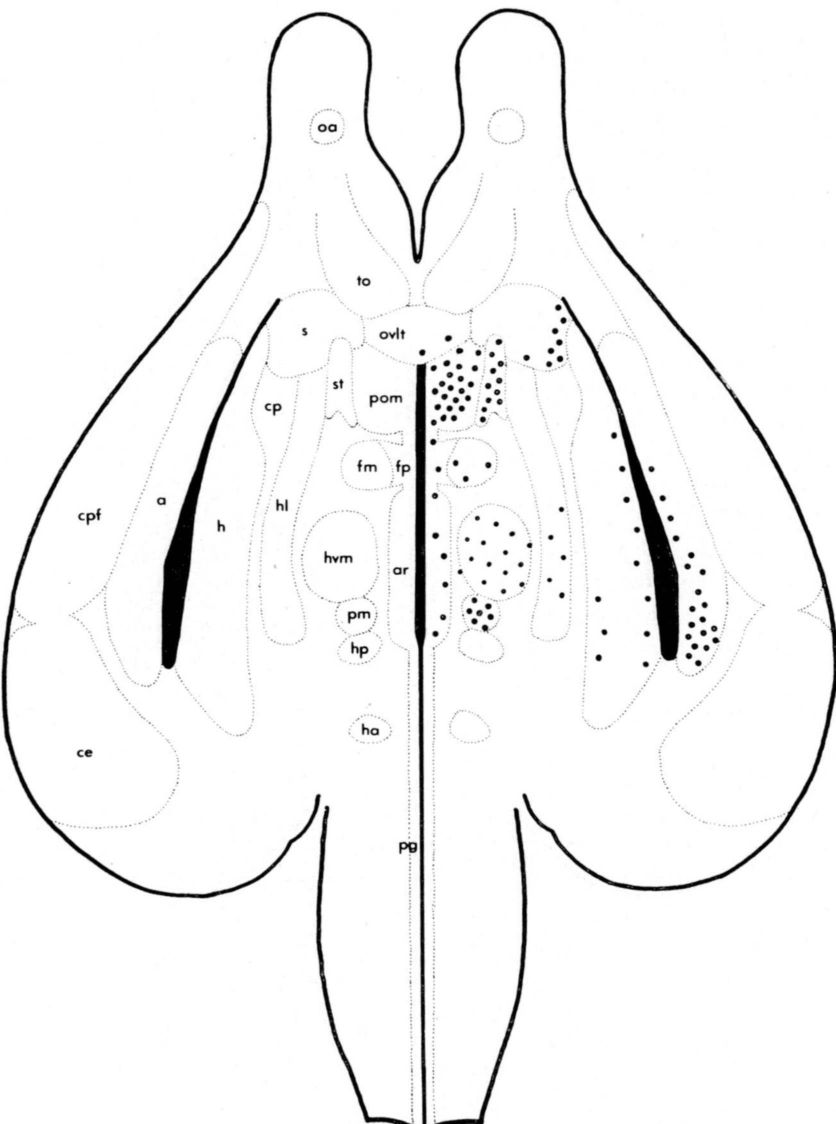

Fig. 2. Topographic distribution of androgen-neurons in rat brain (incomplete), obtained after dry-autoradiography with [^{3}H]testosterone, projected on hypothetical horizontal plane. Schematic. Right half: the spacing of dots indicates the frequency of occurrence of neurons which concentrate radioactivity after the injection of [^{3}H]testosterone; the size of dots indicates the intensity of radioactive labeling.
Left half: designation of structures (see Fig. 1).

medialis, but also in the immediate vicinity of the "hypophysiotrophic area" in the n. paraventricularis, the n. preopticus medialis, the bednucleus of the stria terminalis, the n. premammillaris ventralis and the posterior lateral hypothalamus. These structures, as well as the many other areas in the brain where estrogen-neurons are

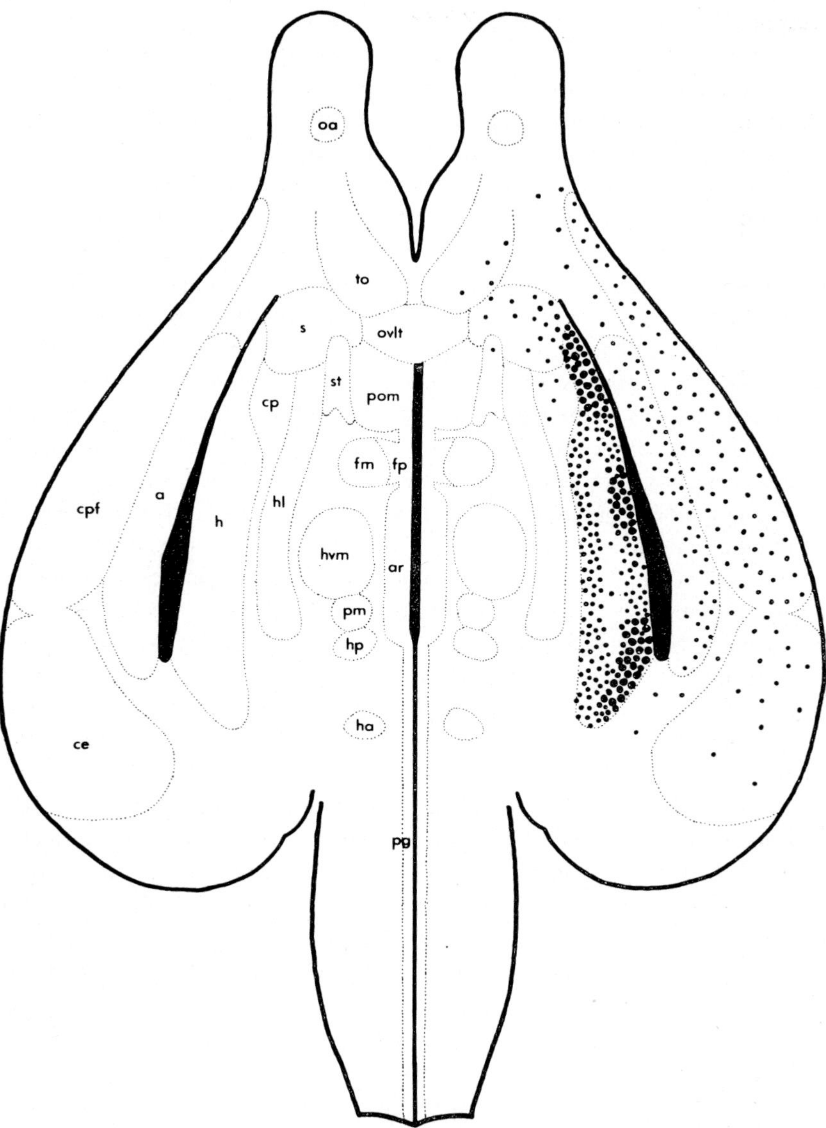

Fig. 3. Topographic distribution of glucocorticoid-neurons in rat brain (incomplete), obtained after dry-autoradiography with [^{3}H]corticosterone and [^{3}H]cortisol, projected on hypothetical horizontal plane. Schematic.

Right half: the spacing of dots indicates the frequency of occurrence of neurons which concentrate glucocorticosteroids. The size of dots indicates the intensity of radioactive labeling, which is highest in portions of the hippocampus, *i.e.* area CA1 > CA3 > CA2 > CA4. Heavy labeling, comparable to area CA1, exists also in neurons of the precommissural hippocampus anterior and the supra-commissural hippocampus, the indusium griseum. Neurons of the gyrus dentatus and area CA4 of the hippocampus show less heavy concentration of radioactivity (M-type of neurons).

Left half: designation of structures (see Fig. 1).

found, are candidates for "feedback" or other effects of estradiol. This is supported by the implantation data compiled in Table I, but also by the results of lesion and electrical stimulation experiments reviewed elsewhere (Sawyer, 1969).

Successful mapping of *androgen*-concentrating neurons (androgen-neurons) has been accomplished only recently (Sar and Stumpf, 1971, 1973). Fig. 2 represents schematically the sites where androgen-neurons are found. The areas of androgen-neuron accumulation overlap in part with those of estrogen-neuron accumulation as can be recognized by a comparison of Figs. 1 and 2. Table II provides a functional correlate to the autoradiographic data in the regions of the hypothalamus.

Reports on the existence and topographic distribution of *glucocorticoid*-concentrating neurons (glucocorticoid-neurons) in the rat brain, using [^{3}H]cortisol and [^{3}H]corticosterone, have first been published from our laboratory in 1971, describing glucocorticoid-neurons in the hippocampus, the dentate gyrus, the indusium griseum and in parts of the septum and amygdala (Stumpf, 1971a, 1971b; Stumpf and Sar, 1971). More recently, Gerlach and McEwen (1972) reported localization of [^{3}H]-corticosterone in the hippocampal complex and neocortex. However, these authors did not mention specific concentrations of this hormone in other areas of the brain. Continued studies in our laboratory indicate that glucocorticoid-neurons have a rather wide distribution in the brain (Stumpf and Sar, 1972; see Fig. 3). The topographic distribution of glucocorticoid-neurons is different from the sex steroids, estrogen and androgen. In contrast to the latter, glucocorticoid-neurons are mainly found, perhaps exclusively, at extrahypothalamic sites, such as the archicortex and paleocortex, including the related adjacent cortical areas, further, in the dorsal septum, the olfactory tubercle and in parts of the amygdala.

Concentration and retention of glucocorticoids in cells of the basal tuberal region is, if it exists, very low. Ongoing experiments need to provide a more definite answer to the question of whether or not glucocorticoid-neurons exist in the "hypophysiotrophic area". The functional significance of extrahypothalamic glucocorticoid-neurons for "feedback" regulation can be recognized in some of the results of the hormone implantation studies compiled in Table III. The effective intrahypothalamic hormone implants seem to be in disagreement with our presently available autoradiographic information. Further studies need to be done. The effects of tuberal implants, however, need to be viewed under the possibility of diffusion to the pituitary, which has been shown to contain glucocorticoid-concentrating cells (Stumpf, 1971a and b).

The intensity of radioactive labeling of glucocorticoid-neurons varies within different areas of the hippocampus, with the heavily labeled "H-type" glucocorticoid-neurons existing in area CA1 and the moderately labeled "M-type" neurons in, for instance, area CA4 and the dentate gyrus.

Regarding the intensity of radioactivity concentration in groups of neurons, the labeled neurons may be classified into three different types. After the injection of radioactively labeled estradiol, testosterone or corticosterone, areas of neurons with relatively high (H), medium (M) or low (L) subcellular silver grain concentration have been observed and reported for [^{3}H] estradiol (Stumpf, 1970a) with, for instance, very weak labeling, L-type estrogen-neurons, in parts of the hippocampus and the n. supraopticus, when compared to the heavily labeled H-type estrogen-neurons in the n. preopticus medialis.

In the case of androgen distribution, most heavily labeled H-type androgen-neurons have been observed, for instance, in the n. preopticus medialis, the bednucleus of the stria terminalis and the n. medialis of the amygdala, while the n. ventromedialis of the hypothalamus seemed to contain M-type androgen-neurons (Sar and Stumpf, 1973).

Since the differences in neuronal hormone binding between specific areas of the brain are striking, it can be expected that they are of functional relevance regarding hormone effects on the different structures of the brain, depending on hormone blood levels. For instance, "overlap feedback" and "cross feedback", or even positive and negative feedback effects of the same hormone may be linked to the observed quantitative *characteristics of topographic hormone binding in the brain*. The deficiencies, as well as the heuristic value of the above H, M, L designations are obvious. More quantitative studies, considering different hormonal states, are required. Selective topographic changes in hormone binding affinities can be expected (Stumpf, Sar and Prasad, unpublished).

SUMMARY AND CONCLUSIONS

In this brief review of hormone localization and hormone feedback effects in the brain, with special reference to the "hypophysiotrophic area", it appears that there is little agreement between the sites of pituitary graft preservation and hormone localization. Therefore, no support can be given for the contention that the "hypophysiotrophic area" is *the* site where RFs are produced, provided hormone target sites in the brain can be further established to be feedback sites and that such feedback sites produce RFs. Some of the cited hormone implantation data, as well as results from lesion experiments, electrical recording and stimulation, as well as metabolic studies—not listed in this paper—suggest that this may be so. From the implantation data compiled in the tables it appears that hormone effects in the "median eminence" may be related to a "negative feedback", while in other parts of the brain, sites for "positive feedback" as well as "negative feedback" seem to exist. The nuclear concentration of the mentioned steroids has been interpreted as suggesting a *stimulatory feedback* (Stumpf, 1970) which could result in a variety of effects, related to, for instance, the production of releasing or inhibiting factors, the stimulation of protein synthesis to affect membrane potentials, electrical thresholds and conductivity, or even the production of the more classical neurotransmitters—all of which could be instrumental in hormone-induced alterations of emotion, sex behavior, memory and various vegetative functions.

References p. 68–70

ACKNOWLEDGEMENTS

This work has been supported by PHS grant NS 09914, AEC grant AT-(40-1)-4057, and a grant from the Rockefeller Foundation to the Laboratories for Reproductive Biology, Chapel Hill, North Carolina. We acknowledge the technical assistance of Gerda Michalsky and Anu Turnbull and the help rendered by Don Keefer in preparing the drawings and for reading the manuscript.

REFERENCES

BLEIER, R. (1971) The relations of ependyma to neurons and capillaries in the hypothalamus. A Golgi–Cox study. *J. comp. Neurol.*, **142**, 439–463.

BOHUS, B. (1968) Pituitary ACTH release and avoidance behavior of rats with cortisol implants in mesencephalic reticular formation and median eminence. *Neuroendocrinology*, **3**, 355–365.

BOHUS, B. AND STRASHIMIROV, D. (1970) Localization and specifity of corticosteroid "Feedback receptors" at the hypothalamo-hypophyseal level. Comparative effects of various steroids implanted in the median eminence or the pituitary of the rat. *Neuroendocrinology*, **6**, 197–209.

CHOWERS, I., FELDMAN, S. AND DAVIDSON, J. M. (1963) Effects of intrahypothalamic crystalline steroid on acute ACTH secretion. *Amer. J. Physiol.*, **205**, 671–673.

CORBIN, A., MANGILI, C. AND MARTINI, L. (1965) Effects of hypothalamic and mesencephalic steroid implantations on ACTH feedback mechanism. *Endocrinology*, **76**, 811–818.

DAVIDSON, J. M. (1969) Feedback control of gonadotropin secretion. In *Frontiers in Neuroendocrinology*. W. F. GANONG AND L. MARTINI (Eds.), Oxford University Press, New York, pp. 343–388.

DAVIDSON, J. M. AND FELDMAN, S. (1963) Cerebral involvement in the inhibition of ACTH secretion by hydrocortisone. *Endocrinology*, **72**, 936–964.

DAVIDSON, J. M., JONES, L. E. AND LEVINE, S. (1965) Effects of hypothalamic implantation of steroids on plasma corticosterone. *Fed. Proc.*, **24**, 191. (Abstract)

ENDRÖCZI, E., LISSAK, K. AND TEKERES, M. (1961) Hormonal feedback regulation of pituitary adrenocortical activity. *Acta physiol. acad. sci. hung.*, **18**, 291–299.

FLAMENT-DURAND, T. AND DESCLIN, L. (1970) The hypophysiotropic area. In *The Hypothalamus*, L. MARTINI, M. MOTTA AND F. FRASCHINI (Eds.), Academic Press, New York, pp. 245–257.

FUXE, K. (1965) Evidence for the existence of monoamine neurons in the central nervous system, IV. The distribution of monoamine nerve terminals in the central nervous system. *Acta. physiol. scand.*, **64**, Suppl. 247, 37–85.

GLASCOCK, R. F. AND MICHAEL, R. P. (1962) The localization of oestrogen in a neurological system in the brain of the female cat. *J. Physiol.*, **163**, 38–39.

GERLACH, J. L. AND MCEWEN, B. S. (1972) Rat brain binds adrenal steroid hormone: radioautography of hippocampus with corticosterone. *Science*, **175**, 1133–1136.

GRIMM, Y. AND KENDALL, J. W. (1968) A study of feedback suppression of ACTH secretion utilizing glucocorticoid implants in the hypothalamus. The comparative effects of cortisol, corticosterone and their 21-acetates. *Neuroendocrinology*, **3**, 55–63.

HALÁSZ, B. (1972) Proceedings of the Anatomical Society of Great Britain and Ireland. *Symp. Neuroendocrinol.*, in press.

HALÁSZ, B., PUPP, L. AND UHLARIK, S. (1962) Hypophysiotrophic area in the hypothalamus. *J. Endocrinol.*, **25**, 147–154.

HARRIS, G. W. (1955) *Neural Control of the Pituitary Gland*. Edward Arnold, London.

JENSEN, J. M. AND CLARK, D. E. (1951) Localization of radioactive L-thyroxine in the neurohypophysis. *J. lab. clin. Med.*, **38**, 663–670.

KALRA, P. S. AND MCCANN, S. M. (1972) Effect of CNS implants of ovarian steroids on gonadotropin release. IVth Int. Congr. Endocrinol. *Excerpta Medica ICS*, **256**, 118. (Abstract)

KAWAKAMI, M., SETO, K. AND YOSHIDA, K. (1968) Influence of corticosterone implantation in limbic structure upon biosynthesis of adrenocortical steroid. *Neuroendocrinology*, **3**, 340–354.

KENDALL, J. W. AND ALLEN, C. W. (1968) Studies on the glucocorticoid feedback. *Endocrinology*, **82**, 397–405.

KNOWLES, F. G. W. (1971) Secretory cells in the ependyma. *Mem. Soc. Endocrinol.*, **19**, 875–881.

LAWTON, I. E. AND SAWYER, C. H. (1970) Role of amygdala in regulating LH secretion in the adult female rat. *Amer. J. Physiol.*, **218**, 622–626.

LEVÈQUE, T. F. (1972) The medial prechiasmatic area in the rat and LH secretion. In *Brain–Endocrine Interaction*, K. KNIGGE, D. SCOTT AND A. WEINDL (Eds.) Karger, Basel, pp. 298–305.

LISK, R. D. (1960) Estrogen-sensitive centers in the hypothalamus of the rat. *J. exp. Zool.*, **145**, 197–208.

LISK, R. D. (1962) Testosterone-sensitive centers in the hypothalamus of the rat. *Acta endocrinol.*, **41**, 195–204.

LITTLEJOHN, B. M. AND DEGROOT, J. (1963) Estrogen sensitive areas in the rat brain. *Fed. Proc.*, **22**, 571. (Abstract)

MATSUYAMA, S. (1970) Effects of brain implantation of androgen, estrogen and an androgen antagonist on the reproductive organs of male rat. *Nippon Seirigaku Zasshi*, **32**, 152–164.

MICHAEL, R. P. (1965) The selective accumulation of estrogens in the neural and genital tissues of the cat. *Proc. 1st Int. Congr. hormonal Steroids, Milan*, **2**, 469–481.

MOTTA, M., FRASCHINI, F., GIULIANI, G. AND MARTINI, L. (1968) The central nervous system, estrogen and puberty. *Endocrinology*, **83**, 1101–1107.

NADLER, R. D. (1971) Sexual differentiation following intrahypothalamic implantation of steroids. In *Influence of Hormones on the Nervous System* (Proc. int. Soc. Psychoneuroendocrinology, Brooklyn), Karger, Basel, pp. 306–321.

PASTEELS, J. L. AND ECTORS, F. (1971) Identical localization of oestrogen and progestogen-sensitive hypothalamic areas. In *Basic Actions of Sex Steroids on Target Organs*, P. O. HUBINONT, R. LEROY AND P. GALAND (Eds.), Karger, Basel, pp. 200–207.

RAMIREZ, V. D. AND MCCANN, S. M. (1964) Induction of prolactin secretion by implants of estrogen into the hypothalamo-hypophysial regions of female rats. *Endocrinology*, **75**, 206–214.

RAMIREZ, V. D., ABRAMS, R. M. AND MCCANN, S. M. (1963) Effects of estrogen implants in the hypothalamo-hypophysial region on the secretion of LH in the rat. *Fed. Proc.*, **22**, 506 (Abstract).

SAR, M. AND STUMPF, W. E. (1971) Androgen localization in the brain and pituitary. *Fed. Proc.*, **30**, 363. (Abstract)

SAR, M. AND STUMPF, W. E. (1973) Autoradiographic localization of radioactivity in the rat brain after the injection of 1,2-^{3}H-testosterone. *Endocrinology*, **92**, 251–256.

SAWYER, C. H. (1969) Regulatory mechanisms of secretion of gonadotrophic hormones. In *The Hypothalamus*, W. HAYMAKER, E. ANDERSON AND W. T. H. NANTA (Eds.), Thomas, Springfield, Ill., pp. 389–430.

SLUSHER, M. A. (1966) Effects of cortisol implants in the brain stem and ventral hippocampus on diurnal corticosteroid level. *Exp. Brain Res.*, **1**, 184–194.

SMELIK, P. G. (1965) The regulation of ACTH secretion. *Acta physiol. pharmacol. neer.*, **13**, 370–371.

SMELIK, P. G. AND SAWYER, C. H. (1962) Effects of implantation of cortisol into the brain stem or pituitary gland on the adrenal response to stress in rabbit. *Acta Endocrinol.*, **41**, 561–570.

SMITH, E. R. AND DAVIDSON, M. (1967a) Testicular maintenance and its inhibition in pituitary-transplanted rats. *Endocrinology*, **80**, 725–734.

SMITH, E. R. AND DAVIDSON, M. (1967b) Differential response to hypothalamic testosterone in relation to male puberty. *Amer. J. Physiol.*, **212**, 1385–1390.

SMITH, E. R. AND DAVIDSON, J. M. (1968) Role of estrogen in the cerebral control of puberty in female rats. *Endocrinology*, **82**, 100–108.

STUMPF, W. E. (1968) Estradiol concentrating neurons: topography in the hypothalamus by dry-mount autoradiography. *Science*, **162**, 1001–1003.

STUMPF, W. E. (1969) Too much noise in the autoradiogram? *Science*, **163**, 958–959.

STUMPF, W. E. (1970a) Estrogen-neurons and estrogen-neuron systems in the periventricular brain. *Amer. J. Anat.*, **129**, 207–218.

STUMPF, W. E. (1970b) Localization of hormones by autoradiography and other histochemical techniques, a critical review. *J. Histochem. Cytochem.*, **18**, 21–29.

STUMPF, W. E. (1971a) Autoradiographic techniques and the localization of estrogen, androgen and glucocorticoid in pituitary and brain. *Amer. Zool.*, **11**, 725–739.

STUMPF, W. E. (1971b) Estrogen, androgen and adrenal hormone attracting neurons in the periventricular brain. *Fed. Proc.*, **30**, 309. (Abstract)

STUMPF, W. E. (1972) Hypophyseotrophic neurons in the periventricular brain: topography of estradiol concentrating neurons. In *Steroid Hormones and Brain Function*, C. H. SAWYER AND R. A. GORSKI (Eds.), Univ. of California Press, Los Angeles, pp. 215–227.

STUMPF, W. E. AND SAR, M. (1971) Localization of steroid hormones in the brain. In *Proceedings of the Third International Congress on Hormonal Steroids, Hamburg*. Excerpta Medica, Amsterdam, pp. 503–507.

STUMPF, W. E. AND SAR, M. (1972) Topography of extrahypothalamic glucocorticosteroid "feedback" sites in the rat brain. IVth Int. Congr. Endocrinol., *Excerpta Medica ICS*, **256**, 120–121. (Abstract)

STURM, A. AND WERNITZ, W. (1956) Hormonjod im Gehirn. *Acta neuroveget.*, **13**, 50–62.

SZENTÁGOTHAI, J., FLERKO, B., MESS, B. AND HALÁSZ, B. (1968) *Hypothalamic Control of the Anterior Pituitary*, 3rd ed., Akademiai Kiado, Budapest.

WAGNER, W., ERWIN, W. AND CRITCHLOW, V. (1966) Androgen sterilization produced by intracerebral implants of testosterone in neonatal female rats. *Endocrinology*, **79**, 1135–1142.

ZIMMERMAN, E. AND CRITCHLOW, V. (1969) Effects of intracerebral dexamethasone on pituitary-adrenal levels in female rats. *Amer. J. Physiol.*, **217**, 392–396.

DISCUSSION

MCCANN: I have been very interested in Dr. Stumpf's work and would like to relate to it some work that has been going on in our laboratory. We have exerted a great deal of effort over the last few years in attempting to localize the releasing factors by a simple technique of cutting frozen sections through the hypothalamus and then assaying extracts made from these sections. The work was done by Drs. Watanabe, Creighton, and Schneider, and more recently by Drs. Krulich and Quijada. The important point about this work is that many of the localizations correspond to the regions which Dr. Stumpf has just told us take up estrogen. LRF, for example, is found in a region starting in the medial pre-optic area and extending down to the median eminence arcuate region. Dr. Stumpf found uptake of estrogen in the preoptic area and also down in the arcuate nucleus. TRF can be found in the region extending from the bednucleus of the stria terminalis caudally to the dorsomedial nucleus and ventrally to the median eminence. There are probably interrelationships between estrogen and TSH release and this might be related to the uptake of estrogen in these areas. GRF is found in the ventromedial nucleus. This agrees with the localization for the GH-controlling area based upon both stimulation and lesion experiments. Again, this region takes up estrogen and estrogen alters GH release. Thus we know that the RFs are localized in discrete regions of the hypothalamus and that several of these regions take up estrogen. However, we cannot determine where the RFs are produced using this technique. The fact that they are found in regions somewhat removed from ependymal cells makes it likely that the ependymal cells are not the sole producers of RFs.

REITER: Are there any anatomical relationships between the sites that localize radioactive hormones and the tanycytes lining the third ventricle? For example, do tanycytes concentrated in this area have processes extending from the ventricular wall to the bednucleus of the stria terminalis or to any other nuclear group that you mentioned?

STUMPF: I cannot answer this question satisfactorily, perhaps Dr. Knigge will add something later. As far as I know the lining of the lateral ventricle does not have these types of tanycytes. The tanycytes from the bottom of the third ventricle extend into the ventromedial nucleus as well as into the arcuate nucleus region. This is where we find strong localization of sex steroids. I would like to emphasize that the histology of the ependyma is different in different areas of the third ventricle. The interrelationship between the morphology of the specialized ependyma and hormone-neurons needs to be studied further.

KNIGGE: I would like to support Dr. Stumpf's comments that the ependyma in this region of the third ventricle are not all of the same type. The ones he cited from Dr. Bleier's work, for example, are located primarily on the roof of the ventricular recess and along the vertical portion of the ventricular wall at the level of the arcuate nucleus. The processes of these ependyma sweep laterally into and through the arcuate nucleus. We have reported that many of these ependymal processes terminate in rather unusual saccular or bulbous endings; the function of such cells remains obscure. These ependyma are clearly very different from the ones in median eminence which we consider to be concerned in thyroxine and TRF transport.

In response to your suggestion, Dr. Stumpf, that ependyma may be involved in the synthesis of releasing factors, I would report our feeling against this possibility. Drs. Silverman, Joseph and I reported in Dallas earlier this year that median eminence does not biosynthesize TRF. Our biosynthesis studies suggest that an anterior, dorsal and medial region of the hypothalamus may be the area responsible for production of this releasing factor. These results would be in agreement with the data just mentioned by Dr. McCann.

MESS: You have quoted the work of Dr. Martini and myself involving hypothalamic lesions. I would like to point out that our results are in close agreement with those mentioned by Dr. McCann. I continued our experiments in Pecs in regard to TRF localization. We clearly demonstrated that different lesions inside the hypophysiotrophic area decreased TRF concentration of the hypothalamus, whereas lesions outside the hypophysiotrophic area, but inside the hypothalamus (for example in the dorsomedial nucleus, or in the lateral hypothalamic area) did not decrease TRF concentration of the hypothalamus. This experiment shows that TRF-producing cells are localized inside the hypophysiotrophic area.

LOTT: In relation to trying to locate the sites of the releasing factor cells in the hypothalamic areas alone, I am reminded of the story of the drunk who lost a button and was looking for it under a lighted lamp. When asked why was he looking for it under the lamp he replied that that is where all the light is. I was wondering if there should be more experiments done in search of possible extra-hypothalamic or indeed extra CNS sites of releasing factor cells?

STUMPF: We have tried to climb up the pole in order to adjust the lamp shade, so that the light can also cover other areas, perhaps, where the button is. There is increasing evidence that extrahypothalamic sites are involved in endocrine regulation. The rhinencephalon is involved and also areas of the brain stem, probably even special structures of the spinal cord. I tried to encompass these structures in the concept of the periventricular brain (Amer. J. Anat., 1970). This periventricular brain relates to the ventricular system, that is, a population of hormone-neurones which are located in more central parts of the brain, at least a large portion of it, and which is probably phylogenetically older than the "canal neurones". One of the points of my presentation was to focus attention on the extrahypothalamic sites. The fact that one does not find large amounts of releasing factors outside the hypothalamus is no argument against the concept that cell bodies of RF-producing cells are located there, considering the serotonin and noradrenaline analogy, where the cell bodies are remote from the hypothalamus, the site of maximal concentration of these substances.

MCCANN: I have just one comment on what Dr. Stumpf said. I think there is obvious input from other areas into the hypothalamus but to my knowledge there has been no good localization of any releasing factor outside the preoptic and hypothalamic regions, so until proven otherwise I would rather think of these other areas as areas which project to the hypothalamus and modulate its activity but do not contain RF-secreting elements.

Input to Releasing Factor Cells*

ONEIDA M. CRAMER** AND JOHN C. PORTER

Department of Physiology, The University of Texas Southwestern Medical School, Dallas, Tex. 75235 (U.S.A.)

INTRODUCTION

The hypothalamus, median eminence, and pituitary contain the various cellular elements necessary for transforming neural inputs into hormonal outputs. The outputs of the hypothalamus are the hypothalamic hypophysiotrophic hormones which are involved in the regulation of the release of trophic hormones from the anterior pituitary (McCann and Porter, 1969). Although much is known about the release of anterior pituitary hormones, little is known about the mechanisms regulating the secretion of the hypothalamic hypophysiotrophic hormones (also called releasing factors or releasing hormones).

However, Jewell and Verney (1957) have demonstrated the presence of osmoreceptors, a type of strain receptor, in the hypothalamus. These osmoreceptors are characterized by a capacity to respond to changes in osmotic pressure and in doing so control the secretory activity of the hypothalamic cells involved in the release of the neurohypophysial hormone, vasopressin. These facts have led us to consider the possibility that strain receptors may also have a role in the control of the secretion of other hypothalamic hormones. Subsequently, we will present preliminary evidence to support the hypothesis that distortion of brain tissue in the vicinity of the third ventricle may affect the secretion of certain hypophysiotrophic hormones.

Although neurotransmitters, *e.g.*, certain biogenic amines, are believed to act as modulators linking neural stimuli and the cells which produce hypophysiotrophic substances (Glowinski, 1970; Page and Carlsson, 1970), the precise role of such transmitters is equivocal. For example, Fuxe and Hökfelt (1969) propose that dopamine (3,4-dihydroxyphenylethylamine) is an inhibitor of the secretion of luteinizing hormone-releasing factor (LRF). Yet, some other investigators suggest

* This investigation has been supported by research grant No. AM01237 from the National Institutes of Health, Bethesda, Md. and by a research grant from The Population Council, New York, N.Y. (U.S.A.).

** NIH Postdoctoral Research Fellow, Neurological Diseases and Stroke, Bethesda, Maryland, Fellowship No. 1F02 NS50809-01 NSRB.

Future address: Department of Physiology, The University of Maryland School of Medicine, Baltimore, Md. 21201 (U.S.A.).

References p. 82–84

that dopamine stimulates LRF secretion (Kordon and Glowinski, 1969, 1970; Kamberi *et al.* 1970; Schneider and McCann, 1970a). Serotonin (5-hydroxytryptamine) is thought by some to inhibit gonadotrophin release (Fraschini *et al.*, 1971; Kordon, 1971; Kordon *et al.*, 1968; Kamberi *et al.*, 1970; Labhsetwar, 1971); however, Brown (1967) believes that serotonin stimulates gonadotrophin release in some conditions. The functions of adrenaline and noradrenaline as transmitters acting on releasing factor cells have also been disputed (Rubinstein and Sawyer, 1970; Kamberi *et al.*, 1970; Donoso and Stefano, 1967; Kurachi and Hirota, 1969).

The confusion and discrepancies which revolve around neurotransmitters as modulators of releasing factor cells may be due in part to the use of different experimental conditions and different animal models. For example, it is known that modifications of an animal's hormonal state alter the hypothalamic composition of endogenous catecholamines and indoles (Lichensteiger *et al.*, 1969; Kato, 1960; Donoso and Stefano, 1967; Donoso *et al.*, 1967, 1969; Fuxe *et al.*, 1969, 1971; Kurachi *et al.*, 1968). Furthermore, it is recognized that the efficacy of an exogenous transmitter may be influenced by certain barriers which separate initially the transmitter from its site of action. Some evidence indicates that monoamines placed in a ventricle may not penetrate more than 300 μ into the periventricular tissue (Fuxe and Ungerstedt, 1968). Thus, it seems probable that the distance between the site of injection and the site of action of a neurotransmitter may limit its effectiveness. The distance variable assumes added significance when one considers that adrenergic and serotonergic neurons have been demonstrated only in discrete regions of the brain (Fuxe, 1965; Björklund *et al.*, 1970). Furthermore, ventricularly administered catecholamines and indoles are for the most part incorporated into their respective neurons (Fuxe and Ungerstedt, 1968; Constantinidis *et al.*, 1971; Glowinski, 1970). Since the capacity of adrenergic and serotonergic neurons to incorporate exogenous neurotransmitters may be modified by various hormones, it would not be surprising if the response of neural elements to neurotransmitters were also modified by hormones.

MATERIALS AND METHODS

Male rats weighing 350 to 500 g were divided into three groups. One group received no experimental manipulation prior to use; another group received subcutaneously 200 μg estradiol-17β in sesame oil daily for 3 days before the experiment; and a third group was castrated 15 to 25 days before use. The experiments were conducted under pentobarbital anesthesia. Each animal received oxygen through an endotracheal tube connected to a rodent respirator and was infused intravenously with 0.1% heparin–Ringer lactate solution (200 μl/min).

The ventral hypothalamus was exposed by a parapharyngeal approach as described by Porter and Smith (1967). All test solutions were administered by injection into the third ventricle using a microcannula. In some animals, the cannula was inserted in the third ventricle by forcing the tip through the dura mater, arachnoid, and ventromedial hypothalamus. Such rats sustained no loss of cerebrospinal fluid (CSF), and pressure in the subarachnoid space appeared to be minimally affected, or not at all. In other animals, the dura and arachnoid over the ventral hypothalamus were incised and reflected to expose the median eminence. In these rats, CSF was lost; and the pressure in the subarachnoid space over the median eminence fell to atmospheric pressure. These two subgroups are identified as rats with intact or rats with incised dura mater and arachnoid. In all cases, the cannula entered the third ventricle at the anterior extremity of the median eminence. The test solutions which were injected into the third ventricle through the cannula were prepared immediately before use and contained a small quantity of lissamine green which served as a dye marker. The location of the tip of the cannula in the ventricle was confirmed by observing the distribution of the dye beneath the median eminence. In rats with intact meninges, the dye usually disappeared from the third ventricle within 10 min or less; but the disappearance of dye in animals with incised meninges was more variable and frequently slower, requiring as much as 30 min in some rats.

After the cannula was placed in the ventricle but before the test solution was injected, a sample of blood was withdrawn from a femoral artery. This sample was called the 0-min collection or resting sample. After injecting the test solution, additional samples of arterial blood were collected during the succeeding 120 min of the experiment. After centrifugation of the blood sample, the erythrocytes were suspended in 0.15 *M* NaCl and returned to the donor. The plasma was used in the determination by radioimmunoassay of luteinizing hormone (LH), follicle-stimulating hormone (FSH), and prolactin according to the procedures of Niswender *et al.* (1968), Parlow *et al.* (1969), and Niswender *et al.* (1969). NIAMD (Natl. Inst. of Arthritis and Metabolic Diseases) reference preparations were used as standards.

RESULTS AND DISCUSSION

Are strain receptors involved in the release of anterior pituitary hormones?

The demonstration of osmoreceptors in the hypothalamus which regulate the release of the antidiuretic hormone from the neurohypophysis (Jewell and Verney, 1957) led us to consider the hypothesis that strain receptors may be involved in the release of trophic hormones from the anterior pituitary. We examined this hypothesis in estrogen-treated, in untreated, and in castrated rats since the sensitivity of such strain receptors, if they exist, may be modified by gonadal hormones.

First, it should be noted that the resting levels in plasma of LH, FSH, and prolactin were affected differently by different hormonal states (Figs. 1, 2). The plasma level of prolactin in estrogen-treated animals was twofold greater than that found in untreated rats. However, the LH levels did not differ in the two groups. Although Debeljuk *et al.* (1972) did not observe suppression of plasma FSH levels with 20 μg of estradiol benzoate, the large amount of estrogen used in this study did reduce FSH levels in plasma. Castration, on the other hand, greatly increased the resting LH and FSH

References p. 82–84

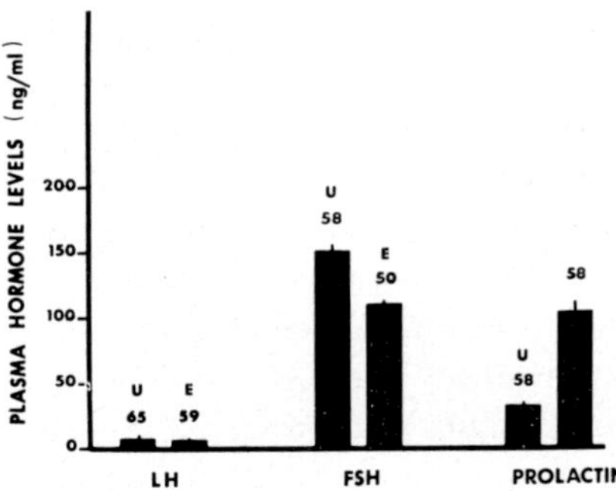

Fig. 1. Hormone levels in untreated rats (U) and estrogen-treated rats (E). The mean values and magnitudes of the standard errors of the means are represented by the vertical bars and lines, respectively. The number of animals is presented above each bar.

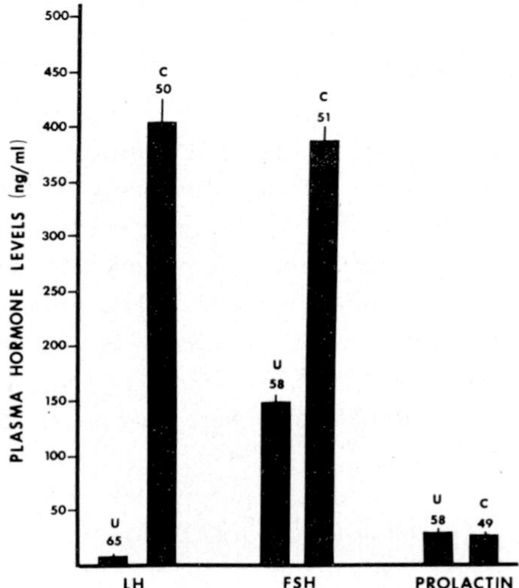

Fig. 2. Hormone levels in untreated rats (U) and in castrated rats (C). The mean values and the magnitudes of the standard errors of the means are represented by the vertical bars and lines, respectively. The number of animals is presented above each bar.

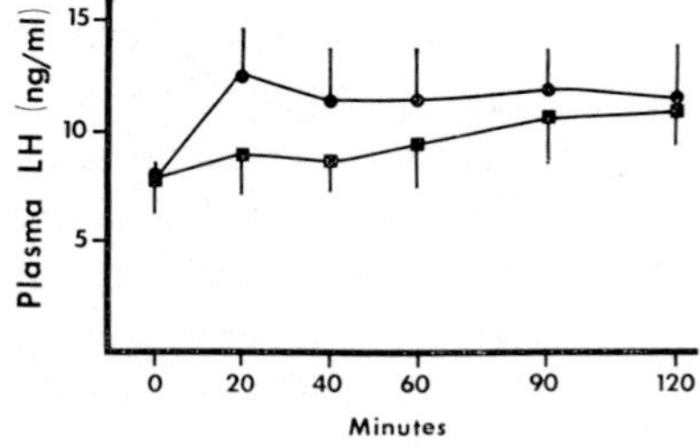

Fig. 3. Effect on LH release of 2 μl of 0.15 M NaCl injected into the third ventricle of untreated rats. Closed circles represent mean levels in animals with intact meninges; $N = 9$. Closed squares represent mean levels in rats in which the dura mater and arachnoid were incised; $N = 7$. Vertical lines represent the magnitudes of the standard errors of the means.

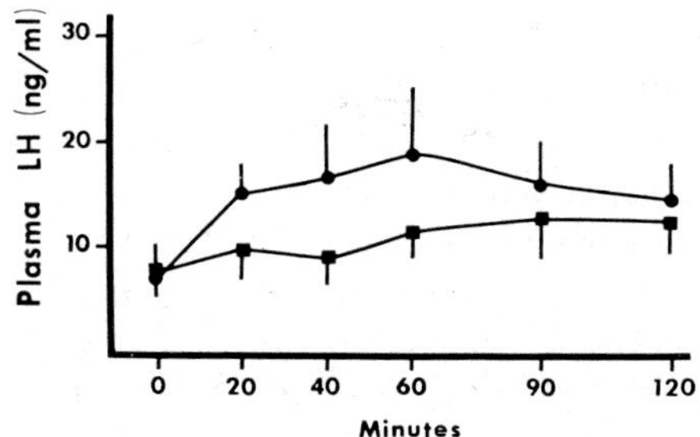

Fig. 4. Effect on LH release of 2 μl of 0.15 M NaCl injected into the third ventricle of estrogen-treated rats. Closed circles represent mean levels in rats with intact meninges; $N = 13$. Closed squares represent mean levels in rats in which the dura mater and arachnoid were incised; $N = 12$. Vertical lines represent the magnitudes of the standard errors.

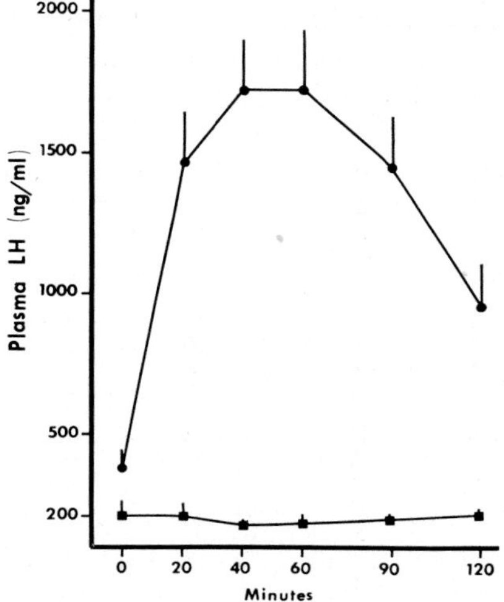

Fif. 5. Effect on LH release of 2 μl of 0.15 M NaCl injected into the third ventricle in castrated rats. Closed circles represent mean levels in rats with intact meninges; $N = 10$. Closed squares represent mean levels in rats in which the dura mater and arachnoid were incised; $N = 4$.

levels but did not affect that of prolactin. Gay and Midgley (1971) and Blackwell and Amoss (1971) have also observed that castration increases plasma LH and FSH levels.

The injection of 2 μl of 0.15 M NaCl into the third ventricle of untreated rats with an intact dura and arachnoid caused within 20 min a small but transient release of LH as indicated by an increase in the plasma level of this hormone (Fig. 3). However, the injection of 2 μl of 0.15 M NaCl into untreated animals with incised meninges had no effect on the release of LH (Fig. 3).

The injection of 2 μl of 0.15 M NaCl into estrogen-treated rats with intact dura and arachnoid also increased the release of LH (Fig. 4). 20, 40, and 60 min after the injection, the plasma LH was increased 2.3-, 2.5-, and 2.9-fold over the resting LH concentration. The injection of isotonic saline into the third ventricle of estrogen-treated rats with incised meninges appeared to have no effect on LH release.

References p. 82–84

The injection of 2 μl of 0.15 *M* NaCl into the third ventricle of castrated rats also had no effect on the release of LH providing the dura and arachnoid had been incised. However, the injection of 2 μl of isotonic saline into the ventricle of castrated animals with intact meninges caused a marked increase in the release of LH (Fig. 5). Within 20 min, the plasma LH rose from a resting level of 370 $\pm$ 59 ng/ml (mean and S.E.M.) to 1460 $\pm$ 185 ng/ml. At 40 and 60 min, the LH concentrations were 1736 $\pm$ 173 and 1732 $\pm$ 210 ng/ml, respectively. Thereafter, the level began to fall (Fig. 5).

The injection of 2 μl of 0.15 *M* NaCl into the third ventricle had no effect on the release of FSH regardless of the hormonal state of the animal or whether the meninges were intact or incised. These results are summarized in Fig. 6, but the results from the animals with intact and with incised meninges have been combined.

The presence of intact or of incised meninges had no effect on the release of prolactin following the injection of 2 μl of 0.15 *M* NaCl. However, the hormonal state of the rats did affect the response of the animal to the injection *per se*. As shown in Fig. 7, the plasma prolactin levels in estrogen-treated rats remained constant throughout the period of observation, varying little from the resting level of approximately 100 ng/ml.

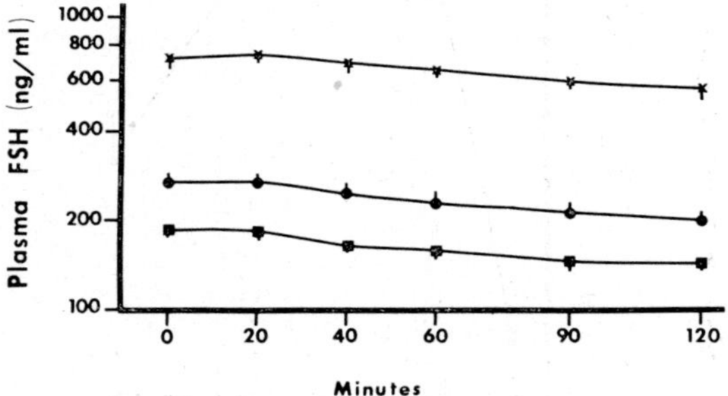

Fig. 6. Effect on FSH release of 2 μl of 0.15 *M* NaCl injected into the third ventricle of untreated rats (closed circles), of estrogen-treated rats (closed squares), and of castrated rats (crosses). The vertical lines represent the magnitudes of the standard errors.

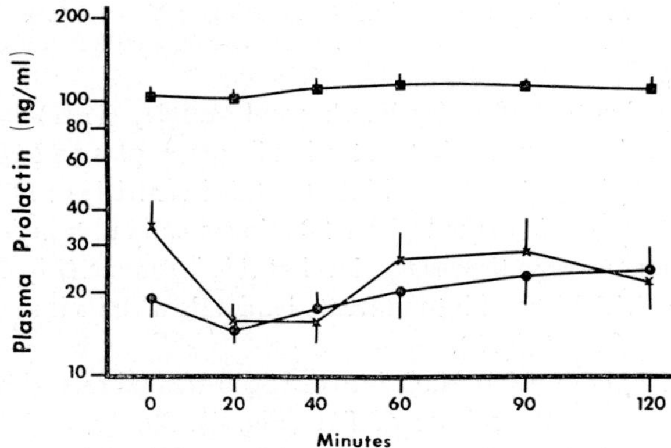

Fig. 7. Effect on prolactin release of 2 μl of 0.15 *M* NaCl injected into the third ventricle of untreated rats (closed circles), of estrogen-treated rats (closed squares), and of castrated rats (crosses). The vertical lines represent the magnitudes of the standard error.

The injection of 2 μl of isotonic saline into untreated animals caused a slight but insignificant fall in plasma prolactin (Fig. 7). However, 2 μl of 0.15 *M* NaCl injected into castrated rats caused a significant ($P < 0.02$) fall in prolactin within 20 min (Fig. 7).

It is interesting to speculate about the meaning of these observations. The brain is covered by the relatively nondistensible dura mater, is filled with an incompressible fluid, *viz.*, CSF in the ventricles, and is surrounded almost entirely by the same fluid, *viz.*, CSF in the subarachnoid space. This arrangement imparts a certain rigidity to the entire brain including the ventricles. Consequently, an expansion of the volume of the third ventricle, albeit small, probably increases markedly the ventricular pressure. This pressure can be dissipated partially by distortion of all the periventricular tissue. Such distortion could stimulate strain receptors in the periventricular region. If such receptors were involved in the release of some anterior pituitary hormones, an expanded third ventricle could thereby be expected to release hormones from the anterior pituitary. Our results are in agreement with this view. When the dura and arachnoid were intact, LH release was stimulated by expansion of the third ventricle (Figs. 3, 4, 5).

We believe that failure of ventricular expansion to cause LH release when the dura and arachnoid were incised also supports the view that strain receptors are involved in the release of LH, but, in this instance, such strain receptors were not stimulated. They were not stimulated for these reasons: When the dura mater and arachnoid covering the ventral hypothalamus are removed, the floor of the third ventricle becomes more distensible, particularly in the region of the thin median eminence. When a small volume of a solution is injected into the third ventricle, the median eminence, made distensible by the absence of the dura and arachnoid, bulges outward, and pressure changes in the third ventricle are damped. Consequently, there is little distortion of the periventricular tissue excluding the median eminence. Indeed, when the dura and arachnoid were incised, no effect was observed on the release of LH after expansion of the third ventricular volume (Figs. 3, 4, 5). These results also suggest that strain receptors are located not in the median eminence *per se* but in another region around the third ventricle, perhaps near the supraoptic region.

FSH release is unaffected by the injection of 2 μl of 0.15 *M* NaCl into the third ventricle regardless of the state of the meninges, suggesting that FSH release may be controlled by a mechanism that is different from that for LH.

Injection of 2 μl of 0.15 *M* NaCl had no effect on the release of prolactin except in the castrated rats in which prolactin release was inhibited. Strain receptors may not be involved in the release of prolactin, however, since the presence or absence of the dural and arachnoid coverings of the ventral hypothalamus did not seem to be an important variable.

Are neurotransmitters involved in the release of anterior pituitary hormones?

The levels of catecholamines in the hypothalamus seem to change with alterations of the endocrine state of the animal. Donoso *et al.* (1967) observed an increase in nor-

References p. 82–84

adrenaline and a decrease in dopamine concentrations in the anterior hypothalamus following castration. After steroid treatment, the levels returned to those seen in intact animals (Donoso and Stefano, 1967). Fuxe *et al.* (1969) observed that dopamine turnover in the median eminence remained unchanged after orchidectomy but increased if the castrated rats were given estrogen or testosterone (Fuxe *et al.*, 1971). Yet, the role of catecholamines and indoles in anterior pituitary regulation is unclear; and conflicting results are frequently reported (Brown, 1967; Fuxe and Hökfelt, 1969; Kordon, 1969; Kordon and Glowinski, 1969, 1970; Schneider and McCann, 1970a, 1970b; Kamberi *et al.*, 1970, 1971a, 1971b, 1971c; Labhsetwar, 1971; Rubinstein and Sawyer, 1970). Many of these studies were performed in animals in different hormonal states. Consequently, the hypothalamic monoamine and indole composition in the brain may not have been comparable. Therefore, after observing that the injection of 2 μl of 0.15 *M* NaCl into the third ventricle induced various responses depending not only upon the hormonal state of the animal but also on the presence or absence of an intact dura and arachnoid over the hypothalamus, we expanded this investigation to include a study of the efficacy of neurotransmitters in the stimulation of release of the gonadotrophins and prolactin in rats in different hormonal states.

Effect of catecholamines and indoles on prolactin release

Adrenaline bitartrate (100 μg in 2 μl of 0.15 *M* NaCl) injected into the third ventricle inhibited the release of prolactin in estrogen-treated, in castrated, and in untreated male rats. Noradrenaline bitartrate (100 μg in 2 μl of 0.15 *M* NaCl) also inhibited prolactin release in all three groups. The inhibitory effect of each catecholamine on prolactin release was especially pronounced in castrated rats. In general, these data agree with previous results from our laboratory using intact rats; but no convincing evidence linking dopamine and prolactin release was demonstrated in this study (Kamberi *et al.*, 1971b).

Serotonin and melatonin have been implicated in the regulation of prolactin release (Kamberi *et al.*, 1971c). In the present investigation, *N*-acetylserotonin (50 μg in 4 μl of 0.15 *M* NaCl) as well as serotonin creatinine sulfate (50 μg in 2 μl of 0.15 *M* NaCl) stimulated prolactin release in intact male rats and in estrogen-treated rats. However, in castrated rats, neither serotonin nor *N*-acetylserotonin stimulated prolactin release appreciably. The potency of these indoles on prolactin release would seem to be dependent upon the hormonal state of the animal.

Effect of catecholamines and indoles on LH release

Adrenaline bitartrate stimulates the release of LH slightly in untreated rats, but noradrenaline bitartrate was ineffective. In estrogen-treated rats, adrenaline stimulated the release of LH but the response was quite variable. Again, noradrenaline was ineffective. When a comparison is made with the results seen in the saline-treated controls, adrenaline as well as noradrenaline appears to have an inhibitory effect on the release of LH in castrated animals.

Intraventricularly administered dopamine produced no change in plasma LH in either intact or estrogen-treated animals. But, dopamine appeared to act as a potent inhibitory agent in the castrated male rats, inhibiting the release of LH normally seen following ventricular injections of 0.15 *M* NaCl. These results conflict with those reported by Kamberi *et al.* (1970). Although we have no explanation for the discrepancy, it is of interest that Rubinstein and Sawyer (1970) were able to induce ovulation in anesthetized, proestrous rats with adrenaline, but not with dopamine or noradrenaline.

The effects of indoles on LH release were surprising. Serotonin markedly stimulated the release of LH in untreated rats, was less effective in estrogen-treated animals, and was ineffective in castrated rats. *N*-acetylserotonin inhibited the release of LH in all groups, and its inhibitory effects were especially pronounced in castrated and in estrogen-treated animals. It is of interest that *N*-acetylserotonin appeared to be a more potent inhibitor of LH release than was serotonin. Since *N*-acetyltransferase, the enzyme that converts serotonin to *N*-acetylserotonin, is widely distributed in the brain (Ellison *et al.*, 1972), the inhibitory effects observed after injections of serotonin (Fraschini *et al.*, 1971; Labhsetwar, 1971) or after procedures which increase the serotonin content of the brain (Kordon, 1969; Kordon *et al.*, 1968) may be due to increased levels in the brain of *N*-acetylserotonin and not of serotonin.

Effect of catecholamines and indoles on FSH release

Plasma FSH concentrations were not influenced by catecholamines or indoles injected into the third ventricle. These findings conflict with those reported by Kamberi *et al.* (1971a, 1971c).

SUMMARY

The results of this investigation show:

(*1*) Estrogen treatment suppresses FSH levels, elevates prolactin levels, and has little or no effect on LH levels.

(*2*) Castration elevates plasma LH and FSH levels, but has little effect on prolactin levels.

(*3*) Injection of 2 μl of 0.15 *M* NaCl into the third ventricle stimulates LH release in untreated rats, in estrogen-treated rats, and in castrated rats, providing the dura and arachnoid are intact, but has no effect when these meninges are incised.

(*4*) Injection of 2 μl of 0.15 *M* NaCl into the third ventricle has no effect on FSH release regardless of whether the animals are untreated, estrogen-treated, or castrated or whether the dura and arachnoid are intact or incised.

(*5*) Injection of 2 μl of 0.15 *M* NaCl into the third ventricle has no effect on prolactin release in estrogen-treated rats, a slight but insignificant inhibitory effect in castrated rats, but a significant inhibitory effect on prolactin release in untreated rats.

References p. 82–84

(*6*) Adrenaline or noradrenaline inhibits prolactin release in untreated, in castrated, and in estrogen-treated rats.

(*7*) Serotonin and *N*-acetylserotonin stimulate prolactin release in untreated and in estrogen-treated rats, but not in castrated rats.

(*8*) Dopamine has no influence on prolactin release.

(*9*) Adrenaline stimulates LH release in estrogen-treated rats and in untreated rats, but inhibits LH release in castrated rats.

(*10*) Noradrenaline does not alter LH release in untreated or in estrogen-treated rats, but inhibits LH release in castrated rats.

(*11*) Serotonin stimulates LH release in untreated rats and in estrogen-treated rats.

(*12*) *N*-acetylserotonin inhibits LH release in castrated, in estrogen-treated, or in untreated rats.

(*13*) FSH release is not affected by catecholamines or indoles.

ACKNOWLEDGMENTS

The authors are indebted to Dr. G. D. Niswender for antiserum to LH and to the National Institute of Arthritis and Metabolic Diseases Rat Pituitary Hormone Program for reagents used in the radioimmunoassay of rat FSH and prolactin.

REFERENCES

Björklund, A., Falck, B., Hromek, F., Owman, C. and West, K. A. (1970) Identification and terminal distribution of the tuberohypophyseal monoamine fibre systems in the rat by means of stereotaxic and microspectrofluorimetric techniques. *Brain Res.*, **17**, 1–23.

Blackwell, R. E. and Amoss, M. S., Jr. (1971) A sex difference in the rate of rise of plasma LH in rats following gonadectomy. *Proc. Soc. exp. Biol. Med.*, **136**, 11–14.

Brown, P. S. (1967) The effect of 5-hydroxytryptamine and two of its antagonists on ovulation in the mouse. *J. Endocrinol.*, **37**, 327–333.

Constantinidis, J., Gaillard, J. M., Geissbuhler, F. and Tissot, R. (1971) Passage into the rat brain of dopa and dopamine injected into the lateral ventricle. *Brit. J. Pharmacol.*, **43**, 32–38.

Debeljuk, L., Arimura, A. and Schally, A. V. (1972) Effect of testosterone and estradiol on the LH and FSH release induced by LH-releasing hormone (LH–RH) in intact male rats. *Fed. Proc.*, **31**, 212 (Abstract).

Donoso, A. O. and Stefano, F. J. E. (1967) Sex hormones and concentration of noradrenalin and dopamine in the anterior hypothalamus of castrated rats. *Experientia*, **23**, 665–666.

Donoso, A. O., Stefano, F. J. E., Biscardi, A. M. and Cukier, J. (1967) Effects of castration on hypothalamic catecholamines. *Amer. J. Physiol.*, **212**, 737–739.

Donoso, A. O., De Gutierrez Moyano, M. B. and Santolaya, R. C. (1969) Metabolism of noradrenaline in the hypothalamus of castrated rats. *Neuroendocrinology*, **4**, 12–19.

Ellison, N., Weller, J. L. and Klein, D. C. (1972) Development of a circadian rhythm in the activity of pineal serotonin N-acetyltransferase. *J. Neurochem.*, **19**, 1335–1342.

Fraschini, F., Collu, R. and Martini, L. (1971) Effects of pineal indoles on the hypothalamic-pituitary-gonadal axis. In *Proceedings of the Third International Congress on Hormonal Steroids*, V. H. T. James and L. Martini (Eds.), Excerpta Medica, Amsterdam, pp. 830–838.

Fuxe, K. (1965) Distribution of monoamine nerve terminals in the central nervous system. *Acta physiol. scand.*, **64**, Suppl. 247, 37–85.

Fuxe, K. and Ungerstedt, U. (1968) Histochemical studies on the distribution of catecholamines and 5-hydroxytryptamine after intraventricular injections. *Histochemie*, **13**, 16–28.

FUXE, K. AND HÖKFELT, T. (1969) Participation of central monoamine neurons in the regulation of anterior pituitary function with special regard to the neuro-endocrine role of tubero-infundibular dopamine neurons. In *Aspects of Neuroendocrinology*, W. BARGMANN AND B. SCHARRER (Eds.), Springer, Berlin, pp. 192–205.

FUXE, K., HÖKFELT, T. AND NILSSON, O. (1969) Castration, sex hormones, and tuberoinfundibular dopamine neurons. *Neuroendocrinology*, **5**, 107–120.

FUXE, K., HÖKFELT, T. AND JONSSON, G. (1971) The effect of gonadal steroids on the tuberoinfundibular dopamine neurons. In *Proceedings of the Third International Congress on Hormonal Steroids*, V. H. T. JAMES AND L. MARTINI (Eds.), Excerpta Medica, Amsterdam, pp. 806–813.

GAY, V. L. AND MIDGLEY, A. R., JR. (1971) Response of the adult rat to orchidectomy and ovariectomy as determined by radioimmunoassay. *Endocrinology*, **84**, 1359–1364.

GLOWINSKI, J. (1970) Storage and release of monoamines in the central nervous system. In *Handbook of Neurochemistry, Vol. 4 (Control Mechanisms in the Nervous System)*, A. LAJTHA (Ed.), Plenum, New York, pp. 91–114.

JEWELL, P. A. AND VERNEY, E. B. (1957) An experimental attempt to determine the site of the neurohypophysial osmoreceptors in the dog. *Physiol. Trans. royal Soc. London (Series B)*, **240**, 197–324.

KAMBERI, I. A., MICAL, R. S. AND PORTER, J. C. (1970) Effect of anterior pituitary perfusion and intraventricular injection of catecholamines and indoleamines on LH release. *Endocrinology*, **87**, 1–12.

KAMBERI, I. A., MICAL, R. S. AND PORTER, J. C. (1971a) Effect of anterior pituitary perfusion and intraventricular injection of catecholamines on FSH release. *Endocrinology*, **88**, 1003–1011.

KAMBERI, I. A., MICAL, R. S. AND PORTER, J. C. (1971b) Effect of anterior pituitary perfusion and intraventricular injection of catecholamines on prolactin release. *Endocrinology*, **88**, 1012–1020.

KAMBERI, I. A., MICAL, R. S. AND PORTER, J. C. (1971c) Effects of melatonin and serotonin on the release of FSH and prolactin. *Endocrinology*, **88**, 1288–1293.

KATO, R. (1960) Serotonin content of rat brain in relation to sex and age. *J. Neurochem.*, **5**, 202.

KORDON, C. (1969) Effects of selective experimental changes in regional hypothalamic monoamine levels on superovulation in the immature rat. *Neuroendocrinology*, **4**, 129–138.

KORDON, C. (1971) Involvement of catecholamines and indoleamines in the control of pituitary gonadotropin release. *J. neuro-visc. Relations*, Suppl. **10**, 41–50.

KORDON, C. AND GLOWINSKI, J. (1969) Selective inhibition of superovulation by blockage of dopamine synthesis during the "critical period" in the immature rat. *Endocrinology*, **85**, 924–931.

KORDON, C. AND GLOWINSKI, J. (1970) Role of brain catecholamines in the control of anterior pituitary functions. In *Neurochemical Aspects of Hypothalamic Function*, L. MARTINI AND J. MEITES (Eds.), Academic Press, New York, pp. 85–100.

KORDON, C., JAVOY, F., VASSENT, G. AND GLOWINSKI, J. (1968) Blockade of superovulation in the immature rat by increased brain serotonin. *Europ. J. Pharmacol.*, **4**, 169–174.

KURACHI, K. AND HIROTA, K. (1969) Catecholamine metabolism in rat's brain related with sexual cycle. *Endocrinol. japon.*, Suppl. **1**, 69–73.

KURACHI, K., IWATA, R. AND HIROTA, K. (1968) Experimental studies on the metabolism of catecholamine in rat brain and sexual function. *Integr. Mech. Neuroendocr. Syst.*, **1**, 151–163.

LABHSETWAR, A. P. (1971) Effects of serotonin on spontaneous ovulation: A theory for the dual hypothalamic control of ovulation. *Acta endocrinol.*, **68**, 334–344.

LICHENSTEIGER, W., KORPELA, K., LANGEMANN, H. AND KELLER, P. J. (1969) The influence of ovariectomy, estrogen, and progesterone on the catecholamine content of hypothalamic nerve cells in the rat. *Brain Res.*, **16**, 199–214.

MCCANN, S. M. AND PORTER, J. C. (1969) Hypothalamic pituitary stimulating and inhibiting hormones. *Physiol. Rev.*, **49**, 240–284.

NISWENDER, G. D., MIDGLEY, A. R., JR., MONROE, S. E. AND REICHERT, L. E., JR. (1968) Radioimmunoassay for rat luteinizing hormone with antiovine LH serum and ovine LH-^{131}I. *Proc. Soc. exp. Biol. Med.*, **128**, 807–811.

NISWENDER, G. D., CHEN, C. L., MIDGLEY, A. R., JR., MEITES, J. AND ELLIS, S. (1969) Radioimmunoassay for rat prolactin. *Proc. Soc. exp. Biol. Med.*, **130**, 793–797.

PAGE, I. H. AND CARLSSON, A. (1970) Serotonin. In *Handbook of Neurochemistry, Vol. 4 (Control Mechanisms in the Nervous System)*, A. LAJTHA (Ed.), Plenum, New York, pp. 251–262.

PARLOW, A. F., DAANE, T. A. AND SCHALLY, A. V. (1969) Quantitative, differential measurement of rat serum FSH, LH, and hypothalamic FSH–RH and LH–RH with specific radioimmunoassays. *Prog. 51st Meeting of the Endocrine Society, New York*, p. 83 (Abstract).

PORTER, J. C. AND SMITH, K. R. (1967) Collection of hypophysial stalk blood in rats. *Endocrinology*, **81**, 1182–1185.

RUBINSTEIN, L. AND SAWYER, C. H. (1970) Role of catecholamines in stimulating the release of pituitary ovulating hormone(s) in rats. *Endocrinology*, **86**, 988–995.

SCHNEIDER, H. P. G. AND MCCANN, S. M. (1970a) Luteinizing hormone-release factor discharged by dopamine in rats. *J. Endocrinol.*, **46**, 401–402.

SCHNEIDER, H. P. G. AND MCCANN, S. M. (1970b) Mono- and indoleamines and control of LH secretion. *Endocrinology*, **86**, 1127–1133.

DISCUSSION

KASTIN: Do you think, Dr. Cramer, that your observation of catecholamine injection causing a differential release of LH and FSH constitutes evidence against the concept that LH–RH releases both LH and FSH? Does it raise the possibility that these amines, perhaps in conjunction with the sex steroids, may interact with LH–RH at the pituitary level? An additional comment I would like to make provides evidence in support of your concept in rats that prolactin and gonadotrophin release are differentially controlled. In collaboration with Drs. Friesen, Jacobs, Schalch, Arimura, Schally and Daughaday we recently showed in man that LH–RH, while elevating LH and FSH levels, does not affect the release of prolactin.

CRAMER: This study does not rule out the possibility that the biogenic amines could have interacted with the steroids and LH–RH at the pituitary level to alter the release of LH and FSH. FSH release, however, was consistently unaffected by any treatment whereas LH release responded to a variety of treatments regardless of the steroid condition of the animal. Therefore, I am more inclined to think that FSH and LH release are controlled by different hypothalamic mechanisms and that those modulators of FSH release were not excited by the injections of biogenic amines.

DICKEY: In some experiments which we did last year, we gave L-DOPA in an attempt to cause release of FSH or LH in humans. These experiments are bedeviled by the fact that there is considerable hour to hour variation in FSH and LH as shown by Yen *et al.* However, we did see an apparent increase in FSH in women, particularly those in mid-cycle and much less increase in FSH in women who were anovulatory. When given to normal men, we saw no increase in FSH. When given to normal men pre-treated with estrogen we did see an increase in FSH. There was no comparable increase of LH in any of these subjects. This would seem to corroborate the differential you've seen in FSH and LH release.

SHASKAN: I would like to emphasize caution in interpreting results obtained by placing catecholamines or serotonin into ventricles, especially with regard to the concentrations of these amines. If, in the study where you used 50 μg or 100 μg of serotonin or noradrenaline, these amines were evenly distributed within the median eminence, they far exceed the endogenous concentration of these amines. My work with Snyder, (J. Pharm. exp. Therap., 175, 404, 1970), would suggest that a great proportion of the serotonin you used would enter catecholamine-containing neurons, and would compete with the endogenous inactivating mechanisms for catecholamines. I feel that when you inject serotonin at these high concentrations there is an inhibition of catecholamine uptake thus allowing more catecholamine to reach the receptor site, possibly the LRF-producing cells. The evidence that serotonin is not an inhibitory input on LH release could otherwise be interpreted that, in fact, it is the noradrenaline or dopamine neurons that are facilitatory.

CRAMER: Our results following third-ventricle injection of serotonin were quite surprising and the facilitatory effects of serotonin may be attributed to the mechanism you have just described. However, adrenaline was the only catecholamine which was able to induce LH release when injected into the third ventricle. If dopamine or noradrenaline were the stimulating agents, I feel that injections of these two catecholamines into the third ventricle should have stimulated a release of LH.

SAWYER: I was delighted to see adrenaline and noradrenaline come back into prominence in this field. We used these many years ago, as many of you may know, in stimulating ovulation in the rabbit. In our hands dopamine was ineffective, and more recently we have been preceding intraventricular injections of noradrenaline with injections of dopamine. We find that the earlier injection of dopamine inhibits the action of the subsequent infusion of noradrenaline into the ventricle relative to stimulating LH release in the rabbit. These results are also consistent with Weiner's results in electrical recording from the rat median eminence on the infusion of these agents in our laboratory, but I wonder where this leaves the earlier work from Dr. Porter's laboratory in which it seemed that dopamine was the important agent rather than noradrenaline or adrenaline.

PORTER: My position, Dr. Sawyer, is confused at present. We are now observing results with dopamine which conflict with earlier findings. We cannot account for the discrepancy. It may be simply that the findings in one of the studies are wrong. It is also possible that different effector cells are involved. One set may be stimulated whereas the other may be inhibited. This was found to be the case for serotonin. Beyond this, I have no satisfactory explanation; and I am at the moment quite perplexed by our inability to repeat the earlier findings.

MESS: Dr. Cramer, do you think it is possible that *N*-acetylserotonin might act as a melatonin precursor? Have you tried, for example, to perform the same experiment in pinealectomized animals, where the main source of hydroxyindole-*O*-methyltransferase, *i.e.*, the transformation site of *N*-acetylserotonin into melatonin, is removed? I wonder whether in this case *N*-acetylserotonin would still exert its LH-inhibitory effect.

CRAMER: We have not tried injecting indoles into pinealectomized animals. However, we have put melatonin into the third ventricle of intact, estrogen-treated and castrated male rats and have received responses from these animals which were not appreciably different from the responses to injections of the diluent.

REITER: Just in comment to the question that Dr. Mess raised, it is possible that the *N*-acetylserotonin could have been converted to melatonin which then had the anti-gonadotrophic effect. Unfortunately, pinealectomy may not solve our problem considering that hydroxyindole-*O*-methyltransferase, the enzyme that converts *N*-acetylserotonin to melatonin has also been found in the retina and in the Harderian gland of the mammal. Thus, melatonin can presumably be formed in these organs as well.

Glucocorticoid Binding Sites in Rat Brain: Subcellular and Anatomical Localizations

BRUCE S. McEWEN

Rockefeller University, New York, N.Y. (U.S.A.)

INTRODUCTION

Steroid hormones act directly on the brain to regulate pituitary hormone secretion and influence behavior (for review, see McEwen *et al.*, 1972b). Thus, from the point of view of neuroendocrinology and physiological psychology, the brain is a target organ for steroid hormones, but the chemistry of the hormone–brain interaction has only recently come under intensive investigation. We have studied the chemistry of glucocorticoid action in brain by following the interaction of the hormone itself with this organ. This approach has provided information as to the subcellular and neuroanatomical location within the rat brain of glucocorticoid binding sites—presumptive "receptors"—located in the cell nuclei and soluble portion of the tissue. The results serve to direct attention to a particular cellular mechanism of hormone action and to certain brain regions for further neurochemical and physiological studies.

EXPERIMENTAL PROCEDURE

Male Sprague-Dawley rats (Charles River Breeding Labs., Wilmington, Mass.) of 250 to 450 g body weight were used in these experiments. Adrenalectomies were performed in our laboratory, and adrenalectomized animals were maintained on 0.8% saline. All animals were maintained on Purina Lab Chow *ad libitum*.

[1,2-^{3}H]Corticosterone (New England Nuclear Corp., Boston, Mass., 20 Ci/mmole) was injected intraperitoneally in 50% ethanol–saline at a dose of 100 μCi (0.7 μg). Purity checks of the steroid were carried out by thin-layer chromatography, as described previously (McEwen *et al.*, 1969, 1970a). Unless indicated otherwise, injected animals were sacrificed one h after injection either by decapitation or by perfusion with 6% Dextran in 0.85% saline (Abbott Labs., Chicago, Ill.) under Diabutal anesthesia.

Dissection of the brain into anatomically defined regions was performed as described elsewhere (McEwen and Pfaff, 1970). All tissue samples were chilled on ice during dissection and the subsequent treatment. Preparation and counting of cytosol and purified cell nuclei from animals injected with [^{3}H]corticosterone were carried out as

References p. 95–96

described elsewhere (McEwen *et al.*, 1972a). Salt extraction of bound radioactivity from isolated nuclei and chromatography on Sephadex G200 are also described in another publication (McEwen and Plapinger, 1970).

Cytosol for *in vitro* binding studies was prepared by homogenizing perfused whole brain tissue in buffer G (5% glycerol, 5 m*M* Tris [trishydroxymethylaminomethane], 1 m*M* EDTA [ethylene diaminetetraacetate, disodium salt], 1 m*M* 2-mercapto-ethanol, adjusted to pH 7.4 with hydrochloric acid) and centrifuging at 105000 × *g* for 60 min. Serum was diluted with the same buffer for comparison of binding with cytosol. Cytosol binding *in vitro* was measured with Dextran-coated charcoal (see Baxter and Tomkins, 1971).

Cytosol for *in vitro* cytosol–nuclear transfer experiments was prepared by homogenizing perfused whole brain, kidney, or liver tissue in buffer H (0.25 *M* sucrose, 30 m*M* HEPES [*N*-2-hydroxyethylpiperazine *N'*-2-ethanesulfonic acid], 1.5 m*M* EDTA, and 1 m*M* dithiothreitol, adjusted to pH 7.4 with hydrochloride acid) and centrifuging at 105 000 × *g* for 60 min. Cell nuclei for these experiments were prepared from perfused brain (minus cerebellum) by a procedure described elsewhere (McEwen and Zigmond, 1972). In this procedure, in contrast to *in vivo* labelling experiments, Triton-X-100 was omitted from the homogenizing medium and 1 m*M* $MgCl_2$ was present in all isolation solutions in place of 3 m*M* $MgCl_2$. Cytosols in buffer H were incubated for 2 h at 0–4° with $1 \cdot 10^{-8}$ *M* [^{3}H]corticosterone. An equal volume of nuclei, resuspended in buffer H, was added to the cytosol and incubation was continued for 30 min at 25°. Nuclei were sedimented at 1500 × *g* for 10 min and washed twice with 0.25 *M* sucrose, 3 m*M* $MgCl_2$ and then collected on 0.45 μ Millipore filters with additional washing. The washed filters with the nuclear pellet were transferred to scintillation vials and counted in a toluene-based scintillator (160 μl Liquifluor, New England Nuclear, in 8 pints of toluene AR) in a Packard Model 3375 scintillation counter at 38% efficiency. Filters were recovered from the vials and washed in ethanol, and the DNA was hydrolyzed in 3% perchloric acid (85° for 30 min) and determined colorimetrically by the diphenylamine procedure of Burton (1956).

Brain tissue slices were prepared with a McIlwain tissue chopper (Mickle Labs., Great Britain, distributed by Brinkman Instruments) at a thickness of 300 μ and incubated with [^{3}H]corticosterone in a Krebs-Ringer bicarbonate buffer equilibrated with 95% O_2 5% CO_2 for 30 min. Slices were recovered by centrifugation at 12 000 × *g* for 10 min and nuclei were isolated from the slices and counted by the standard procedure used in *in vivo* uptake studies (McEwen *et al.*, 1970a; Zigmond and McEwen, 1970).

RESULTS

A. Hippocampal concentration of corticosterone

When 0.7 μg of [^{3}H]corticosterone is administered to adrenalectomized male rats 1 h before sacrifice, considerable radioactivity is found to have entered all parts of the

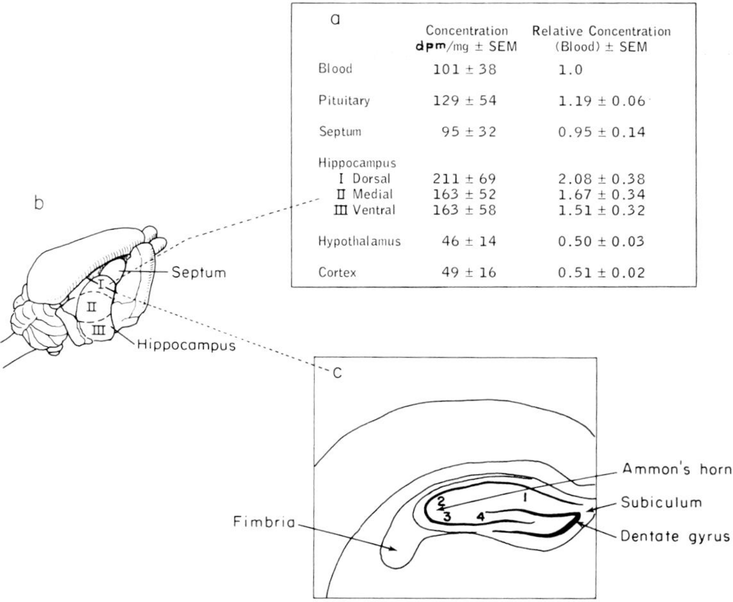

a

	Concentration dpm/mg ± SEM	Relative Concentration (Blood) ± SEM
Blood	101 ± 38	1.0
Pituitary	129 ± 54	1.19 ± 0.06
Septum	95 ± 32	0.95 ± 0.14
Hippocampus		
I Dorsal	211 ± 69	2.08 ± 0.38
II Medial	163 ± 52	1.67 ± 0.34
III Ventral	163 ± 58	1.51 ± 0.32
Hypothalamus	46 ± 14	0.50 ± 0.03
Cortex	49 ± 16	0.51 ± 0.02

Fig. 1. Hippocampal structure in relation to uptake of [^{3}H]corticosterone. (a) [^{3}H]Corticosterone distribution in hippocampus compared with other brain regions (see McEwen *et al.*, 1969). (b) Position of hippocampus in the rat brain. (c) Cross section of dorsal hippocampus showing cell layers and designating Ammon's horn subdivisions CA1–CA4 as 1–4. (From McEwen *et al.*, 1972b.)

brain (McEwen *et al.*, 1969). Studies of this uptake have revealed that a considerable part of it has a stereospecificity and limited capacity for corticosterone (McEwen *et al.*, 1969). The largest amount of this limited-capacity binding occurs in the hippocampus (McEwen *et al.*, 1969). Fig. 1 summarizes some of this work, illustrating the location of the hippocampus in the rat brain (Fig. 1b) and showing that the concentration of radioactivity in the hippocampus 1 h after injection of [^{3}H]corticosterone is several times higher than that in hypothalamus or cerebral cortex (Fig. 1a). In addition, the concentration of radioactivity is uniform along the length of the hippocampus (Fig. 1a). However, the hippocampus has a characteristic cellular organization in cross section (Fig. 1c) which is the same *along* the length of this structure, so that any differences in hormone uptake are likely to go undetected in lengthwise measurements. Thus we embarked on autoradiographic studies the better to localize corticosterone binding in the hippocampus. This technique has shown this uptake to be due to binding by pyramidal neurons, particularly those of CA1 and CA2 (designated 1 and 2 in Fig. 1c) and by many granule cells of the dentate gyrus (Gerlach and McEwen, 1972).

Several other species have been investigated for hippocampal binding of glucocorticoids. The rat, mouse, and hamster all concentrate [^{3}H]corticosterone in cell nuclei of hippocampus and amygdala (Kelley and McEwen, unpublished). Of particular interest is the observation by Rhees *et al.* (1972) that the hippocampus and

References p. 95–96

septum of the Pekin duck concentrate [^{3}H]corticosterone. It remains to be seen if such observations can be extended to other species, particularly primates.

B. Nuclear and soluble binding proteins for corticosterone

Further biochemical studies of the corticosterone uptake revealed that the limited-capacity, stereospecific part of it is due to protein-binding sites located in the cell nuclei (McEwen *et al.*, 1970a) and soluble (cytosol) fraction of the tissue (Grosser *et al.*, 1971; McEwen *et al.*, 1972a). Corticosterone binding protected the hormone from metabolism and at least 90% of the bound radioactivity was recovered as unmetabolized corticosterone (McEwen *et al.*, 1972a). Autoradiography supported the nuclear localization of much of the bound corticosterone (Gerlach and McEwen, 1972). Fig. 2 shows an example of this localization in a pyramidal neuron of hippocampus. Note particularly the absence of radioactivity in the region of the nucleolus (arrow in Fig. 2). Cell nuclear binding was shown to be due at least in part to binding proteins extractable by 0.4 *M* NaCl (McEwen and Plapinger, 1970). The fractionation of these 0.4 *M* salt extracts on Sephadex G200 columns is illustrated in Fig. 3. Bound radioactivity coincides with a peak of protein eluting after the void volume. By treating the bound material with various lytic enzymes, it was shown that the binding macromolecule is most likely a protein (McEwen and Plapinger, 1970).

Cytosol binding of corticosterone is also due to a protein which can be distinguished

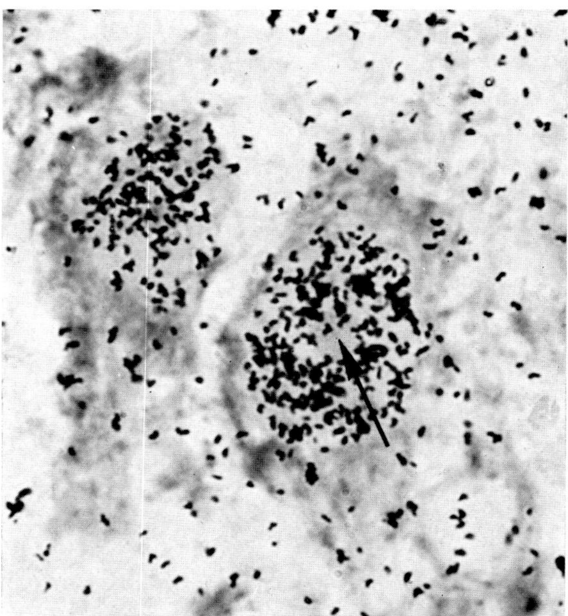

Fig. 2. Autoradiograph of [^{3}H]corticosterone localization in a pyrimidal neuron of hippocampus. Grains are located primarily over the cell nucleus and absent from the nucleolus (arrow). Autoradiography by Mr. John Gerlach.

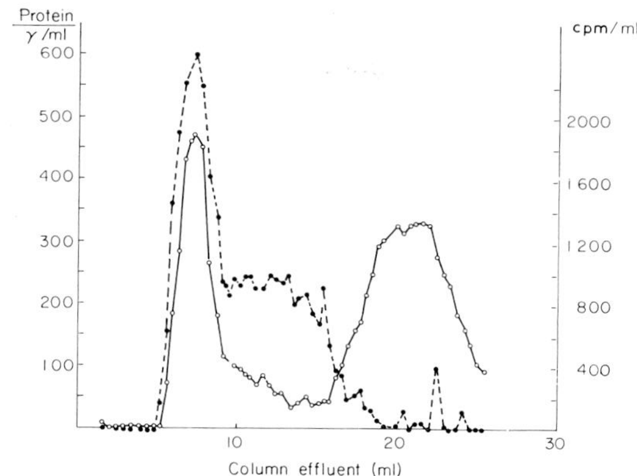

Fig. 3. Sephadex G200 chromatography of 0.4 *M* NaCl extract of rat brain cell nuclei labelled by *in vivo* injection of [^{3}H]corticosterone. Conditions as described in McEwen and Plapinger (1970). Open circles: radioactivity; closed circles: protein.

TABLE I

BRAIN CYTOSOL AND NUCLEAR BINDING OF [^{3}H]CORTICOSTERONE

Bound radioactivity in cytosol and isolated cell nuclei is presented as dpm/mg protein ± SEM. Perfusion indicates removal of cerebral blood by perfusion as described in EXPERIMENTAL PROCEDURE. Data from McEwen *et al.* (1972a).

Structure	*Perfusion*	*Cytosol*	*Nuclei*
Hippocampus	−	3730 ± 390	18900 ± 4000
	+	5300 ± 1200	28600 ± 7700
Hypothalamus	−	1250 ± 230	1700 ± 300
	+	600 ± 140	2200 ± 300
Amygdala	−	1860 ± 140	5300 ± 1400
	+	1200 ± 300	6400 ± 1400

TABLE II

EXCHANGE OF BOUND [^{3}H]CORTICOSTERONE WITH UNLABELLED STEROIDS

Cytosol or serum from adrenalectomized male rats was incubated with $1 \cdot 10^{-8}$ *M* [^{3}H]corticosterone for 2 h in an ice bath. Exchange was carried out by adding $1.25 \cdot 10^{-5}$ *M* unlabelled corticosterone or dexamethasone and allowing the incubation to proceed in the cold for 2 more hours. Binding was measured by charcoal adsorption (Baxter and Tomkins, 1971).

Steroid	*Exchange in 2 h at 4 ° (% of control)*	
	Serum	*Cytosol*
Control	100	100
Corticosterone ($1.25 \cdot 10^{-5}$ *M*)	2	39
Dexamethasone ($1.25 \cdot 10^{-5}$ *M*)	106	49

References p. 95–96

from another binding protein, the serum factor, transcortin, on the basis of a number of physical properties (McEwen *et al.*, 1972a). First, the brain protein is present after perfusion of the brain at sacrifice with a Dextran–saline solution (Table I). Second, it is precipitated by protamine sulfate under conditions in which very little of the serum-binding protein is precipitated, even when serum and cytosol extracts are mixed (McEwen *et al.*, 1972a). Third, it migrates differently from the serum-binding proteins in glycerol density gradients and can be separated completely from serum-binding protein on polyacrylamide gels containing glycerol (McEwen *et al.*, 1972a). Finally, brain cytosol protein exchanges bound [^{3}H]corticosterone for unlabelled dexamethasone as well as corticosterone whereas the serum protein exchanges bound [^{3}H]corticosterone with unlabelled corticosterone and not with unlabelled dexamethasone (Table II).

C. *In vitro studies of cell nuclear [^{3}H]corticosterone binding*

We attempted to simplify the study of cell nuclear binding of [^{3}H]corticosterone by developing *in vitro* systems for measuring this binding. In view of recent success in other hormone target tissues in demonstrating sequential transfer of radioactive hormone from cytosol to nuclei in both intact (Jensen *et al.*, 1968; Shyamala and Gorski, 1969) and cell-free systems (O'Malley *et al.*, 1972), we attempted to demonstrate uptake of radioactive [^{3}H]corticosterone from brain cytosol by isolated nuclei. In order to recognize the appearance of specific binding, we compared nuclear uptake in cytosols incubated in [^{3}H]corticosterone along with nuclear uptake in cytosols incubated in [^{3}H]corticosterone plus a 1000-fold excess of unlabelled corticosterone (referred to as competition). We concluded that specific nuclear uptake had occurred when the radioactivity of the sample exceeded that of the "competition" sample. Results of these experiments are summarized in Table III. Nuclei incubated in buffer

TABLE III

NUCLEAR BINDING OF [^{3}H]CORTICOSTERONE *in vitro*

Cytosol or the indicated serum albumin, serum, or buffer solution was incubated for 2 h at 0–4 ° with $1 \cdot 10^{-8}$ *M* [^{3}H]corticosterone. Aliquots of isolated nuclei were then added and the incubation was continued for 30 min at 25 °. Nuclei were then reisolated, washed, and counted as described in EXPERIMENTAL PROCEDURE. Each experiment consisted of duplicate determinations of each condition. Results are expressed as dpm bound per μg of DNA.

Medium	*Number of expts.*	*Bound radioactivity*		
		Control	*Competed*	*Δ*
Buffer	6	33 ± 4	31 ± 6	2 ± 3
Serum	2	24	18	6
		20	23	−3
Serum albumin	1	29	26	3
Brain cytosol	7	71 ± 11	16 ± 1	55 ± 10
Liver cytosol	4	85 ± 19	23 ± 2	59 ± 27
Kidney cytosol	3	35 ± 9	16 ± 4	19 ± 6

TABLE IV

$[^3H]$CORTICOSTERONE UPTAKE BY 300 μ BRAIN TISSUE SLICES

Incubation of tissue slices was for 30 min at 25° in the presence of 0.5–1.0 · 10^{-8} *M* $[^3H]$corticosterone (see EXPERIMENTAL PROCEDURE). Radioactive concentrations are presented as dpm/μg protein in the nuclear fraction (N) or whole homogenate (WH).

		$[^3H]$Corticosterone concentration · 10^{-8}	*Unlabelled corticosterone · 10^{-7}*	*Concentration of radioactivity*		
				N	*WH*	*N/WH*
Hippocampus	25°	0.5	—	14.9	39.2	0.38
		1.0	—	24.3	53.7	0.45
		0.5	2.5	1.3	32.8	0.04
Hypothalamus	25°	0.5	—	5.5	37.6	0.14
		1.0	—	8.7	57.8	0.15
		0.5	2.5	0.4	31.8	0.01
Hippocampus	0°	1.0	—	2.8	25.0	0.11
	25°	1.0	—	24.3	53.7	0.45
	37°	1.0	—	5.7	52.0	0.11

TABLE V

REGIONAL CELL NUCLEAR BINDING OF $[^3H]$CORTICOSTERONE

Radioactive concentration is expressed as dpm/mg protein in the nuclear pellet. N/WH is the ratio of nuclear concentration to concentration in the whole homogenate. Data are taken from McEwen *et al.* (1970b).

Brain region	*Nuclear concentration dpm/mg protein*	*N/WH*
Hippocampus	19800 ± 4350	6.8 ± 1.1
Hypothalamus	1750 ± 360	1.7 ± 0.2
Amygdala	5550 ± 1200	3.9 ± 0.4
Cerebral cortex	2350 ± 860	2.5 ± 0.4
Midbrain + brain stem	1410 ± 410	1.4 ± 0.3
Cerebellum	980 ± 260	1.0 ± 0.1

alone, diluted serum, or serum albumin solution showed no specific corticosterone uptake. Nuclei incubated in brain cytosol did show specific uptake. Liver cytosol was as good as brain cytosol in promoting *brain nuclear* binding, while kidney cytosol was only slightly less effective. This apparent lack of tissue specificity between cytosols raises questions as to how similar are corticosteroid binding molecules in various tissues. If they are indeed identical, wherein lies the specificity of the hormone effect on each tissue?

Another *in vitro* technique which we are developing involves the incubation of slices 300 μ thick of fresh brain tissue prepared with a McIlwain tissue chopper, in a

References p. 95–96

Krebs-Ringer bicarbonate buffer containing $0.5–1 \cdot 10^{-8}$ *M* [^{3}H]corticosterone. After incubation at room temperature, the slices are collected by centrifugation, and cell nuclei are isolated for determination of bound radioactive steroid. Concentrations of radioactive corticosterone in isolated nuclei and unfractionated tissue are summarized in Table IV. Optimal incubation temperature was found to be around 25°. Incubation at 0° reduced nuclear as well as whole tissue uptake, but nuclear uptake was reduced to a greater degree as indicated by a reduction in the concentration ratio nuclear fraction/whole homogenate (N/WH). The *in vitro* uptake of [^{3}H]corticosterone by brain slices is higher in slices of hippocampus than hypothalamus, in agreement with *in vivo* uptake results (see below). Unlabelled corticosterone saturates the nuclear binding sites in hippocampus and hypothalamus without affecting tissue uptake, as indicated by a fall in the concentration ratio N/WH (Table IV).

D. Distribution of corticosterone binding sites in rat brain

Biochemical studies of nuclear and cytosol binding of [^{3}H]corticosterone revealed that hormone-binding sites were not confined to the hippocampus (McEwen *et al.*, 1970b, 1972a). This is illustrated in Table I for nuclear and cytosol binding and in Table II for nuclear binding alone. Following the hippocampus are the amygdala, cerebral cortex, hypothalamus, midbrain and brainstem, and cerebellum. Autoradiography has provided additional support for these observations by showing labelled neurons—generally less numerous and less intensely labelled than in hippocampus—in amygdala, septum, cerebral cortex, among other structures. In many instances, the silver grains over a neuron are clearly localized over the cell nucleus (Gerlach and McEwen, 1972). Nuclear [^{3}H]corticosterone accumulation in all of these structures is subject to competition by unlabelled corticosterone.

DISCUSSION

The regional neuroanatomical distribution of corticosterone-binding sites can be compared with the regional distribution of estradiol-binding sites in rat brain (for review, see McEwen *et al.*, 1972b). Like corticosterone, estradiol binds to brain cell nuclei but, in contrast, these cell nuclear estradiol-binding sites are located in hypothalamus, preoptic area, and amygdala (Zigmond and McEwen, 1970). The sites of estradiol binding are also sites where implanted estrogen exerts feedback effects on gonadotrophin secretion and facilitates the lordosis reflex (see McEwen *et al.*, 1972b). Thus, estradiol binding to brain cell nuclei may be the first step in neuroendocrine and behavioral effects of this hormone.

Can the same be said of corticosterone binding sites? The first problem is to delineate the nature of glucocorticoid effects on neuroendocrine regulation and behavior. Glucocorticoid feedback on corticotrophin (ACTH) secretion occurs when hormone implants are made in hypothalamus, septum, hippocampus, and amygdala (for review, see McEwen *et al.*, 1972b). Glucocorticoids implanted in many of these same brain areas also facilitate extinction of conditioned avoidance responding (Bohus, 1970). Other neural events in which glucocorticoids participate include the interplay between paradoxical sleep and ACTH secretion (Slusher, 1966; Hellmann *et al.*, 1970; Johnson and Sawyer, 1971) and the detection and recognition of sensory stimuli (Henkin, 1970). Underlying some or all of these neural effects of glucocorticoids may be changes in neuronal electrical activity which have been attributed to circulating glucocorticoids (Pfaff *et al.*, 1971).

Cell nuclear binding of corticosterone in brain points to a mechanism of action of this hormone mediated by the genome. Direct experiments are needed to demonstrate genomic regulation in brain by corticosterone. However, in other glucocorticoid target tissues such as thymus and liver, and in target tissues for estradiol, progesterone, dihydrotestosterone, and aldosterone such genomic effects have been documented together with the existence of hormone-specific cytosol and cell nuclear "receptor" proteins (for review, see McEwen *et al.*, 1972b). Subsequent studies of the glucocorticoid-mediated neural effects referred to in the previous paragraph might well be directed not only toward understanding the role of particular brain regions but also the possible involvement of the genome.

SUMMARY

Studies of the uptake and binding of [^{3}H]corticosterone in rat brain are reviewed and brought up to date with data from recent experiments. Protein binding sites for this hormone are shown to occur in cell nuclei of neurons and in the soluble portion of the tissue. The soluble binding protein differs from that in blood and appears able to transfer [^{3}H]corticosterone to isolated cell nuclei *in vitro*. Nuclear uptake is also demonstrated in brain tissue slices and is shown to be strongly temperature-dependent. Binding of [^{3}H]corticosterone is highest in the hippocampus and amygdala and lower but not insignificant in hypothalamus, cerebral cortex, cerebellum, and midbrain and brain stem. The possible functional correlates of this binding are briefly considered.

ACKNOWLEDGEMENTS

This research was supported by grants NS 07080 and MH 13189 from the United States Public Health Service. The author would like to acknowledge the efforts of Mr. John Gerlach in preparation and photography of the autoradiographs and the excellent technical assistance of Mrs. Carew Magnus, Miss Linda Plapinger, and Mrs. Gislaine Wallach.

REFERENCES

BAXTER, J. D. AND TOMKINS, G. M. (1971) Specific cytoplasmic glucocorticoid hormone receptors in hepatoma tissue culture cells. *Proc. nat. Acad. Sci. (U.S.)*, **68**, 932–937.

BOHUS, B. (1970) Central nervous structures and the effect of ACTH and corticosteroids on avoidance behavior: A study with intracerebral implantation of corticosteroids in the rat. *Progr. Brain Res.*, **32**, 171–183.

BURTON, K. A. (1956) A study of the conditions and mechanism of the diphenylamine reaction for the colorimetric estimation of DNA. *Biochem. J.*, **62**, 315–323.

GERLACH, J. L. AND MCEWEN, B. S. (1972) Rat brain binds adrenal steroid hormone: Radioautography of hippocampus with corticosterone. *Science*, **175**, 1133–1136.

GROSSER, B. I., STEVENS, W., BRUENGER, F. W. AND REED, D. J. (1971) Corticosterone binding by rat brain cytosol. *J. Neurochem.*, **18**, 1725–1732.

HELLMAN, L., NAKADA, F., CURTIZ, J., WEITZMAN, E. D., KREAM, J., ROFFWARG, H., ELLMAN, S., FUKUSHIMA, D. K. AND GALLAGHER, T. F. (1970) Cortisol is secreted episodically by normal men. *J. clin. endocrin. Metab.*, **30**, 411–422.

HENKIN, R. I. (1970) The effects of corticosteroids and ACTH on sensory systems. *Progr. Brain Res.*, **32**, 270–293.

JENSEN, E. V., SUZUKI, T., KAWASHIMA, T., STUMPF, W. E., JUNGBLUT, P. W. AND DESOMBRE, E. R. (1968) A two-step mechanism for the interaction of estradiol with rat uterus. *Proc. nat. Acad. Sci. (U.S.)*, **59**, 632–638.

JOHNSON, J. H. AND SAWYER, C. H. (1971) Adrenal steroids and the maintenance of a circadian distribution of paradoxical sleep in rats. *Endocrinology*, **89**, 507–512.

MCEWEN, B. S. AND PFAFF, D. W. (1970) Factors influencing sex hormone uptake by rat brain regions: I. Effects of neonatal treatment, hypophysectomy, and competing steroid on estradiol uptake. *Brain Res.*, **21**, 1-16.

MCEWEN, B. S. AND PLAPINGER, L. (1970) Association of corticosterone-1,2-H^3 with macromolecules extracted from brain cell nuclei. *Nature (Lond.)*, **226**, 263–264.

MCEWEN, B. S. AND ZIGMOND, R. E. (1972) Isolation of brain cell nuclei. In *Methods of Neurochemistry*, N. MARKS AND R. RODNIGHT (Eds.), Plenum, New York, pp. 140–161.

MCEWEN, B. S., WEISS, J. M. AND SCHWARTZ, L. S. (1969) Uptake of corticosterone by rat brain and its concentration by certain limbic structures. *Brain Res.*, **16**, 227–241.

MCEWEN, B. S., WEISS, J. M. AND SCHWARTZ, L. S. (1970a) Retention of corticosterone by nuclei from brain regions of adrenalectomized rats. *Brain Res.*, **17**, 471–482.

MCEWEN, B. S., ZIGMOND, R. E., AZMITIA, E. C., JR. AND WEISS, J. M. (1970b) Steroid hormone interaction with specific brain regions. In *Biochemistry of Brain and Behavior*, R. E. BOWMAN AND S. P. DATTA (Eds.), Plenum, New York, pp. 123–167.

MCEWEN, B. S., MAGNUS, C. AND WALLACH, G. (1972a) Soluble corticosterone-binding macromolecules extracted from rat brain. *Endocrinology*, **90**, 217–226.

MCEWEN, B. S., ZIGMOND, R. E. AND GERLACH, J. L. (1972b) Sites of steroid binding and action in the brain. In *Structure and Function of the Nervous System*, Vol. 5, G. H. BOURNE (Ed.), Academic Press, New York, pp. 205–291.

O'MALLEY, B. W., SPELSBURG, T. C., SCHRADER, W. T., CHYTIL, F. AND STEGGLES, A. W. (1972) Mechanisms of interaction of a hormone-receptor complex with the genome of a eukaryotic target cell. *Nature (Lond.)*, **235**, 141–144.

PFAFF, D. W., SILVA, M. T. A. AND WEISS, J. M. (1971) Telemetered recording of hormone effects on hippocampal neurons. *Science*, **172**, 394–395.

RHEES, R. W., ABEL, J. H., JR. AND HAACK, D. W. (1972) Uptake of tritiated steroids in the brain of the duck *(Anas platyrhynchos)*. An autoradiographic study. *Gen. comp. Endocr.*, **18**, 292–300.

SHYMALA, G. AND GORSKI, J. (1969) Estrogen receptors in the rat uterus: Studies on the interaction of cytosol and nuclear binding sites. *J. Biol. Chem.*, **244**, 1097–1103.

SLUSHER, M. A. (1966) Effects of cortisol implants in the brainstem and ventral hippocampus on diurnal corticosterone levels. *Exp. Brain Res.*, **1**, 184–194.

ZIGMOND, R. E. AND MCEWEN, B. S. (1970) Selective retention of oestradiol by cell nuclei in specific brain regions of the ovariectomized rat. *J. Neurochem.*, **17**, 889–899.

DISCUSSION

JACOBY: Is there a relationship between the dose of corticosterone that you gave and the concentration at different sites within the brain, and how does this concentration compare with normal physiologic levels of corticosterone?

McEwen: I could give you two answers to that. In the first place, if we inject corticosterone into adrenalectomized animals we find that we can saturate the binding sites in the hippocampus with a dose of approximately 200 micrograms given i.p. If we are dealing with an *in vitro* system, which I didn't have time to describe, the concentration at which the binding sites are saturated is approximately $2 \cdot 10^{-8}$ *M*. The apparent affinity constant for corticosterone is in the range reported for proteins in other tissues which bind estradiol and other steroid hormones, and is such that the binding sites would be saturated by the levels of endogenous corticosterone reached during stress.

Jacoby: Have you attempted to see if there is a difference with time of day with respect to uptake of corticosterone?

McEwen: We have not. I would assume that there would be such a variation. It is technically difficult to do this kind of experiment because when we inject labelled hormone into the animal we stimulate the secretion of endogenous corticosterone and this competes for binding sites.

Kitay: How can you distinguish an increased apparent binding capacity after castration or after adrenalectomy as being due to a reduction in cold hormone competition from the possibility that these treatments lead to new or more binding sites *per se*?

McEwen: There are several ways, using mainly *in vitro* methods. We have evidence which suggests that there is an increase in the binding capacity beginning about 1 day after adrenalectomy. This increase appears to be independent of the desaturation of the binding sites from the endogenous hormone. Thus the brain-binding protein may respond to absence of adrenal hormone by increasing in amount in much the same way as transcortin.

Kitay: There seems to be at least an hour's latency time in the response of hippocampal neurones to the injection of 1 mg of corticosterone. In our hands hypothalamic neurones respond in considerably shorter time to the administration of corticosterone, the latency being 7 to 10 min. on the average and I wondered if you had any comments about the functional significance of the long latency in your studies?

McEwen: I really cannot comment on this, except to say that the longer latency and duration of the effect may indicate mediation by intracellular binding of the hormone.

Steroid Feedback Mechanisms in Pituitary-Adrenal Function

P. G. SMELIK AND E. PAPAIKONOMOU

Department of Pharmacology, Free University Medical Faculty, Amsterdam (The Netherlands)

In this paper an attempt is made to describe the pituitary-adrenal system as a biological control system, and to include in the description the features on which a fair agreement exists in the literature. Controversial opinions have often been expressed on the role of the feedback loop in this system. It is hoped that the new results and their discussion may contribute towards setting the controversy.

A SCHEMATIC VIEW OF THE SYSTEM

We may start from a simplified scheme of the pituitary-adrenal system, in which only the most essential elements are indicated (Fig. 1). In this scheme the central nervous system is represented by "neural inputs", and peripheral mechanisms modulating

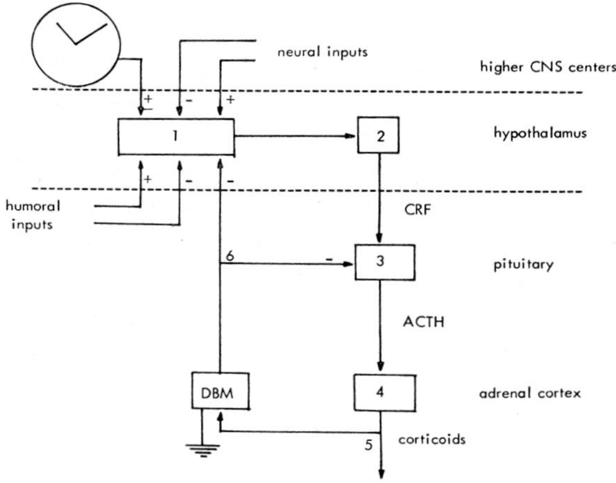

Fig. 1. A simplified block-diagram of the pituitary-adrenal control system. CRF, corticotrophin-releasing factor; ACTH, corticotrophin; DBM, distribution-binding metabolism; CNS, central nervous system.

References p. 108–109

corticoid blood levels are summarized by one distribution-binding-metabolism (DBM) element. These aspects will not be considered in this paper.

No full discussion is needed of the feedforward part of the system. A stimulus will reach the cells that produce corticotrophin-releasing factor (CRF) in the hypothalamus, which can be considered as a transducer, releasing a neurohumoral signal to the anterior pituitary. This organ, which may also have an amplifier function (see below), produces the hormone corticotrophin (ACTH), which activates the adrenal cortex. Digital signals (neuronal firing) are converted to an analog signal (continuous production of corticoid) by these transducers. In this system the blood level of glucocorticoids is thought to be the controlled variable.

The feedback part of the system is the main subject of this paper, and will be discussed in more detail.

It is a common feature of control systems that the controlled variable is fed back to the controller, so that the system is forced to adjust its level of activity to the actual demands. If this level is to be kept constant, we can speak of a homeostatic device or regulator; if the system has to follow changing conditions, it should be called a servomechanism.

The question of set-point

There is much confusion in the literature on set-point. Older theories, like that of Sayers (1950), considered the pituitary-adrenal axis as a closed-loop system with a fixed set-point, and its function was thought to be the preservation of a constant glucocorticoid level, which would be disturbed by the increase in peripheral corticoid utilization during stress. After a period in which the system seemed rather to be considered as an open-loop system, the idea of a variable set-point was introduced by Yates *et al.* (1961). In this concept the system was thought of as a servomechanism, which follows the changing need for glucocorticoids.

It seems to us that this idea better fits the experimental data. Blood levels of corticoids are far from constant, but show considerable variations. Not only is there a rather fixed pattern of circadian rhythms, which seems to be correlated with the sleep–wake cycle, but also a great number of emotional and other stimuli frequently appears to activate the system. Since the pituitary-adrenal system is a typical adaptation system, it should not be surprising that its activity is permanently adjusted to the changing demands of the environment. Of course, the continuously changing activity of the system may serve to preserve the constancy (homeostasis) of the internal environment by counteracting any force endangering the equilibrium. But this does not make the pituitary-adrenal system itself a homeostatic device. If the system follows changing conditions, it should be called a servo-system. And if that is so, there is no need for a variable set-point. Hence, in our scheme a set-point or reference value is omitted. Instead, a comparator is introduced, being the simplest device which in our opinion can explain satisfactorily what happens in the controlling structure. This comparator processes all excitatory and inhibitory inputs, and its output is the net outcome of this summation, which is directly translated in the amount of CRF released. The incoming stimuli can be either neural or humoral, and one of these stimuli is the level of circulating corticoids. It is supposed here that the comparator has corticoid receptors, although it cannot be excluded that the humoral feedback signal is first partly or completely translated into neural signals, *e.g. via* higher brain structures.

In this view there is only a quantitative difference between "basal" and "stress" conditions. We think it is now justified to avoid the use of the word stress in this context. There is a complete continuous scale from zero to peak activity of the system, induced by a great number of minor emotional disturbances, variable blood levels of powerful endogenous factors such as histamine and adrenaline, and metabolic changes induced by food, exercise and so on. Other factors, such as anticipation of harm (fear), cold, bacterial invasions, tissue damage and drugs, complete this picture of permanently changing stimulatory inputs to the system.

Feedback has low capacity

Another consequence of this approach is that the corticoid feedback is only one of the inputs to the comparator, so that one may expect it to be easily overridden by other inputs. This is in accordance with the experimental data. The capacity of the feedback signal is rather restricted, and supraphysiological blood levels are needed to prevent the response of the system to noxious stimuli. Since most of the older work has been done with very high doses of corticoids, this has been recognized only when careful studies were done on the relation between the actual corticoid blood levels and the intensity of the activating stimulus. There is now general agreement that inhibition of the system depends on the balance between the strength of the stimulus and the amount of circulating free corticoids, and that even maximal (endogenous) corticoid levels can counterbalance only very moderate stimuli.

The presence of this stabilizing feedback will operate especially at lower levels of activity of the system and keep the system near a certain activity level until a new stimulus alters this level. This can be demonstrated in a simple way (Papaikonomou, 1972). A correlation exists between the amount of CRF released and the level of

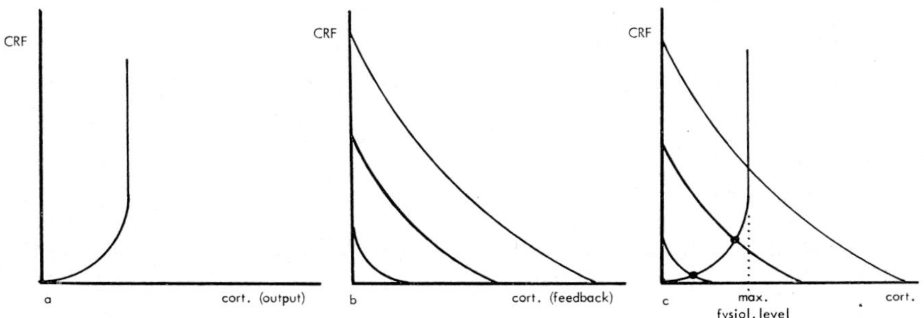

Fig. 2. Theoretical steady-state characteristics of the pituitary-adrenal system (feedback only on the hypothalamus). (a) steady-state relationship between CRF and corticoid production (cort.); (b) hypothalamic feedback characteristics in the steady-state; (c) combination of a and b, resulting in stable activity levels.

References p. 108–109

circulating corticoids, until maximal corticoid production has been reached (Fig. 2a). At the same time, an inverse relationship exists between these variables, because any corticoid level is a minus signal for the comparator (Fig. 2b). Since both characteristics hold simultaneously, they should be combined, and this results in a theoretical point at which the system finds its stability (Fig. 2c). However, higher rates of release of CRF can only be matched by supraphysiological corticoid levels, so that the physiological capacity of the system appears to be limited.

At a certain level of CRF production the maximal capacity of adrenocortical production is reached, so that saturation occurs. This does not mean that at that moment saturation of the feedback receptor is reached; a further increase in corticoid levels by administration of corticoids may be able to prevent the effect of stronger stimuli, but this is beyond the physiological range. In our opinion, stimuli of any intensity can be blocked if the amount of administered corticoids is high enough. Consequently, the system will not operate at high levels as an open-loop system, as has been argued by Yates *et al.* (1969), but it will be less sensitive, because reduction in CRF production will only result in lower adrenocortical activity, when that part of the curve has been reached where a dose–effect relationship exists.

Feedback at the pituitary level

There is, however, another aspect of the feedback loop. It has been shown by several groups that the effect of CRF preparations can be blocked by corticoids, particularly by dexamethasone (De Wied, 1964, Russell *et al.*, 1969). This demonstrates the existence of a feedback site at the pituitary level, apart from feedback receptors within the central nervous system.

The problem is whether both sites are of physiological importance and if so, which

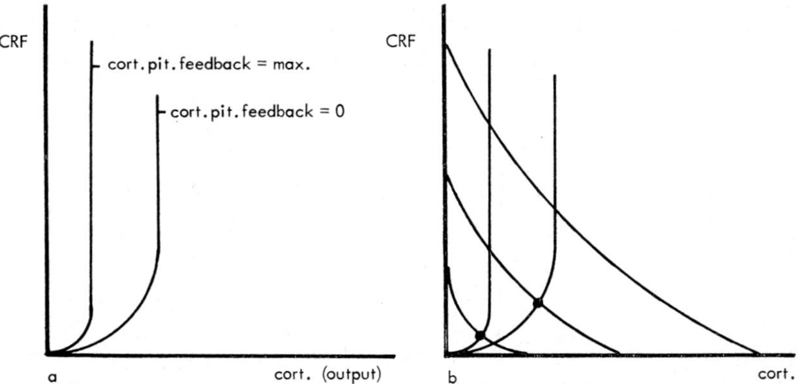

Fig. 3. Theoretical steady-state characteristics of the pituitary-adrenal system (feedback on both hypothalamus and pituitary). (a) steady-state relation between CRF and corticoid (cort.) production, at different levels of pituitary sensitivity (induced by cort. feedback); (b) combination of (a) with Fig. 2b, resulting in stable activity levels; system's sensitivity is reduced compared to that in the case of Fig. 2c.

one plays the predominant role. We are not aware of any study that presents evidence for a pituitary feedback site for endogenous corticoids within the physiological range. Most work has been done with the synthetic steroid preparation dexamethasone phosphate, which is water-soluble but has a low lipid solubility. It may be, therefore, that dexamethasone is more easily taken up by anterior pituitary tissue than by brain tissue, but that the reverse is true for cortisol and corticosterone.

Anyway, it appears that corticoids may alter the sensitivity of the ACTH-producing cells for the CRF. This has been included in our graphs (Fig. 3a). The pituitary can be considered as a kind of amplifier, whose sensitivity can be modified by the level of circulating corticoid.

Maximal physiological levels of circulating corticoids will reduce pituitary sensitivity to some extent, and this results in a limitation of adrenocortical stimulation. As a consequence, saturation is reached earlier, and the system becomes even more insensitive (Fig. 3b). It can easily be seen from these curves that pharmacological amounts of corticoids may be capable of reducing pituitary sensitivity ultimately to zero, causing a complete blockade of the system at the pituitary level. It remains to be demonstrated experimentally that maximal plasma corticosterone levels reduce pituitary sensitivity for CRF, but the work with synthetic steroids suggests the possibility.

The temporal aspect

So far, we have only considered the relationship between degree of inhibition and concentration of corticoids in the blood, without paying attention to the temporal aspect. The time variable also appears to be important. If the response of the system to noxious stimulation is to be blocked, a pharmacological dose of corticosterone has to be administered 1 to 2 h before the stress (Smelik, 1963). Even when dexamethasone is given intravenously, it takes 45 to 90 min before elevated corticoid levels are depressed. The time lag appears to be dependent on the intensity of the stimulation (De Kloet, unpublished results).

There is no explanation for this delay at present. It cannot be attributed to slow penetration of the receptor cells or conversion to an active metabolite, since it applies to both corticosterone and dexamethasone. It may be, however, that the feedback action is on CRF and/or ACTH synthesis rather than on the release mechanism (Hedge and Smelik, 1969).

Feedback and circadian rhythm

Theoretically it is possible that circadian variations in corticoid levels can be caused by intrinsic oscillations of the system, in which the delayed level-sensitive feedback would play a major role. The available evidence suggests, however, that the circadian rhythm is induced by periodic neural inputs from higher centers. This would be in accordance with recent data, indicating that the hypothalamic CRF content shows a circadian rhythm in adrenalectomized and hypophysectomized rats (Takebe *et al.*,

References p. 108–109

1971). These findings do not exclude the possibility that these inputs are rather sensitive to corticoid feedback, because of their slow character and the low activity levels at which they operate.

Rate-sensitive feedback?

Recently it has been claimed that, apart from the delayed level-sensitive type of feedback, a fast rate-sensitive feedback may also exist (Dallman and Yates, 1969; Dallman *et al.*, 1971; Jones and Neame, 1971, 1972).

The evidence stems mainly from observations that during the increase in plasma concentration of infused corticosterone, the system does not respond to stimuli like laparotomy or histamine. As soon as the steady-state level has been reached the system is responsive again, until the level-sensitive feedback inhibition appears 1–2 h later. After cessation of the infusion of corticosterone a decrease in corticosterone levels occurs, whose slope is less steep than that of the rise at the beginning of the

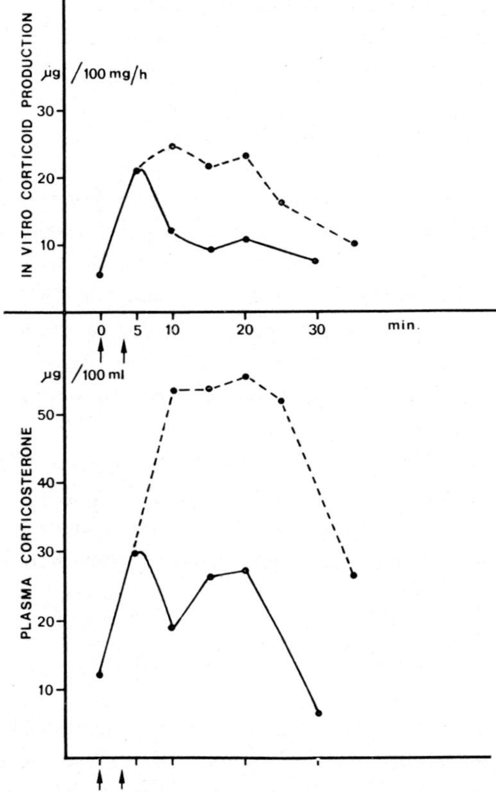

Fig. 4. Time course of plasma free corticosterone levels and *in vitro* corticoid production by incubated adrenals after intravenous injection of ACTH (0.8 mU), under pentobarbital anesthesia. The second injection of ACTH was given 3 min later, during the steep rise in adrenal activity. ●——●, ACTH i.v. at 0 min; ●- - -●, ACTH i.v. at 0 min + ACTH i.v. at 3 min.

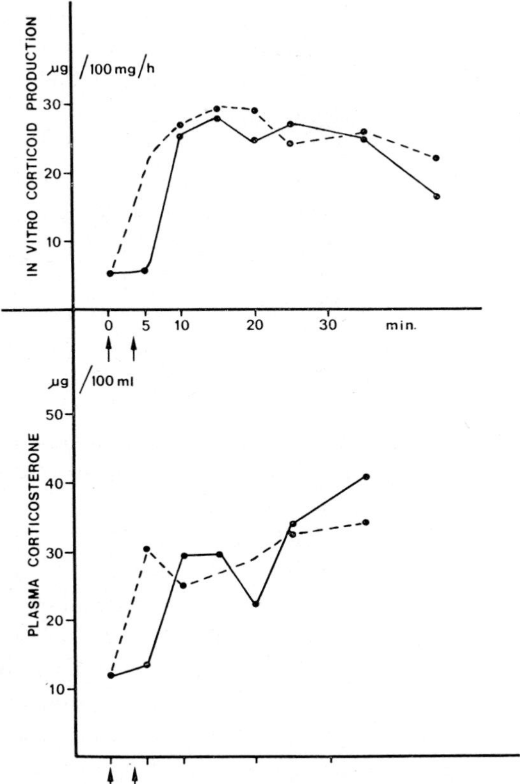

Fig. 5. Time course of plasma free corticosterone levels and *in vitro* corticoid production after surgery (laparotomy = lap.) under pentobarbital anesthesia. ACTH or saline was given i.v. 3 min before laparotomy. ●——●, saline i.v. at 0 min + lap. at 3 min; ●- - -●, ACTH i.v. at 0 min + lap. at 3 min.

infusion. During the falling slope an essentially normal stress response was noted. It was therefore assumed that the rate-sensitive feedback is unidirectional (Dallman and Yates, 1969). The fast feedback phenomenon has not been found with dexamethasone according to Yates (unpublished).

Rate sensitivity means that the slope of the rise or fall in blood concentration will determine whether or not inhibition occurs. If the slope is not steep enough, no inhibition will be found. From the available evidence it appears that the rate of rise should exceed 1.3 μg corticosterone/100 ml/min (Jones and Neame, 1972), which it often does when a stressful stimulus is applied. This suggests that this type of feedback may play a physiological role. After the response of the system to a stimulus, the system would then be unresponsive to another stimulus for a short time. This refractory period would be present from the time the blood levels begin to rise until the peak has been reached, which is about 20 min later. We have studied this question as follows. Instead of by a corticosterone infusion, corticosterone levels were elevated by intravenous injection of ACTH, in such a dose that the rate of rise was sufficient but that

References p. 108–109

the peak was well below saturation. Since it would be possible that an actively producing adrenal is less sensitive to ACTH, a second injection of ACTH was given during the rise in corticosterone blood levels. A further increase in adrenal corticoid production and blood levels was found, indicating that no inhibition occurred at the adrenal level (Fig. 4).

In a second series of experiments a noxious stimulus was applied during the rise in corticosterone levels. However, here, too, the adrenal response was not blocked (Fig. 5).

It is not yet possible to give an explanation for the discrepancy between results obtained from corticosterone infusions and our results from stimulated adrenocortical production.

Oscillations of the system

A different approach to the problem can be made in cannulated animals, in which the corticosterone blood levels are followed by taking frequent small blood samples. However, such preparations have the disadvantage that the system operates on a "stress" level owing to the surgical procedures.

When a T-shaped cannula was brought into one carotid artery, thus ensuring undisturbed circulation, the blood corticosterone levels became stable within 20 min (Fig. 6), but immediately after removal of one adrenal the blood level of corticosterone started to oscillate with a period of about 12 min (Fig. 7). In another experiment a delay in the output of one adrenal was brought about by cannulating the adrenal vein and connecting this cannula with the femoral vein *via* a long piece of tubing. In this way the contribution of one adrenal was switched off during 24 min, namely 2 cycles of oscillation. This induced oscillations as well, and the arrival of the adrenal vein blood in the circulation appeared to reactivate this oscillating behavior (Fig. 8).

In acutely hypophysectomized animals infused with ACTH, the removal of one adrenal did not induce oscillations (Fig. 9), indicating that they are not caused by peripheral mechanisms. It may be, therefore, that the observed oscillations are caused

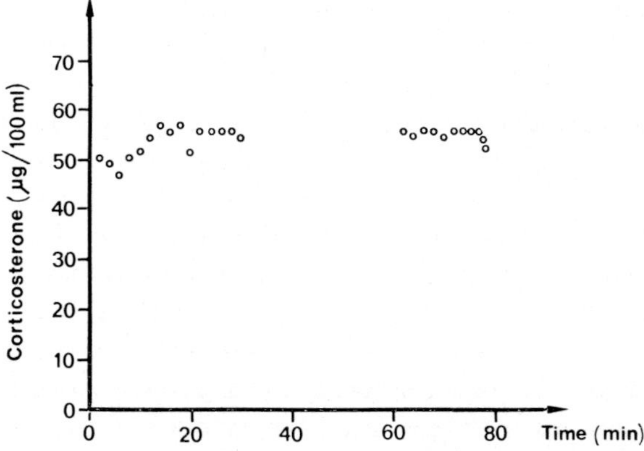

Fig. 6. Plasma corticosterone levels in a rat with a T-shaped cannula in one carotid artery under pentobarbital anesthesia.

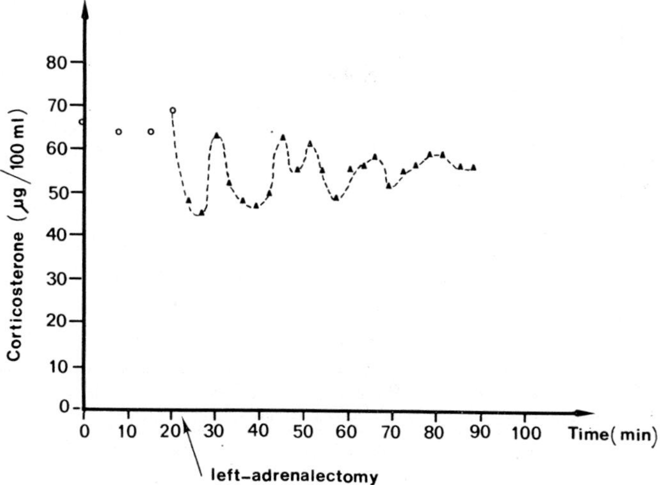

Fig. 7. Plasma corticosterone levels in a cannulated rat under pentobarbital anesthesia, in which one adrenal gland is removed.

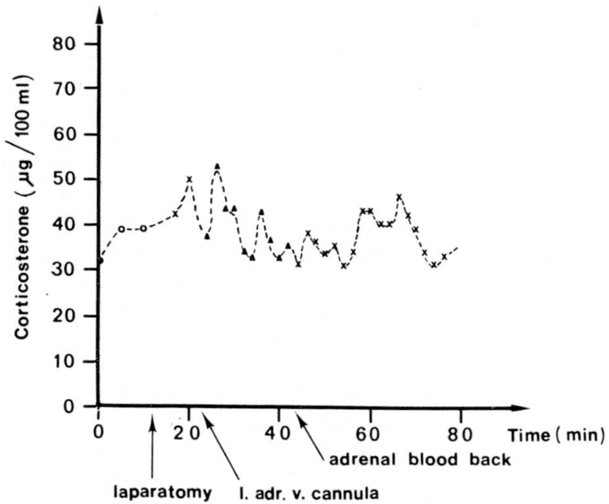

Fig. 8. Plasma corticosterone levels in a cannulated rat under pentobarbital anesthesia, in which the return to the systemic circulation of the output of one adrenal gland was delayed for 24 min.

by short pulses of CRF release, which are induced by the rapid falls in corticosterone levels. This would mean that a fast differential or derivative feedback control mechanism does exist, but sensitive only for negative rates of change.

The few data which exist at the moment on fast feedback phenomena cannot permit us to draw any definite conclusions. They only indicate that rate sensitivity may exist, without demonstrating its significance for the normal functioning of the pituitary-adrenal system.

References p. 108–109

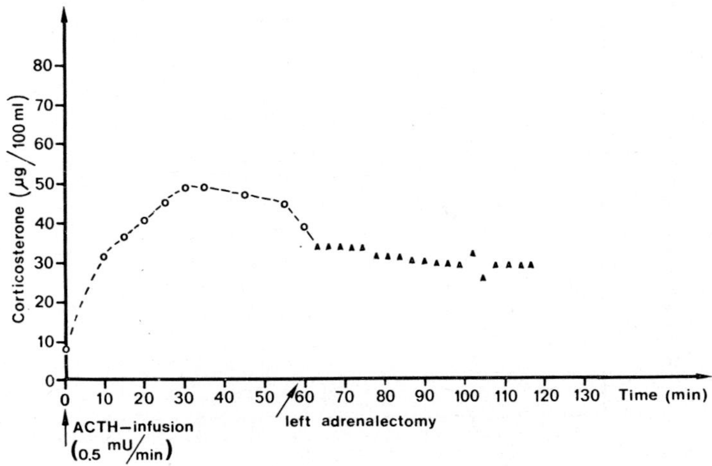

Fig. 9. Plasma corticosterone levels in a cannulated hypophysectomized rat infused with ACTH, under pentobarbital anesthesia, in which one adrenal gland is removed.

SUMMARY

Several aspects of the role of corticoid feedback in the control of the pituitary-adrenal system are discussed. The following tentative conclusions have been reached.

(*1*) The system does not operate with a fixed or variable set-point, but should be considered as a servomechanism, which follows the variable needs for glucocorticoids.

(*2*) The amount of CRF released depends on a summation by a hypothalamic comparator of neural and humoral stimuli, which can be positive or negative.

(*3*) There is no qualitative difference between the basal state and stress conditions.

(*4*) The capacity of the feedback signal is rather small, so that it has only a stabilizing function.

(*5*) High corticoid blood levels not only act as a negative humoral signal to the comparator, but also depress pituitary sensitivity.

(*6*) The long delay of level-sensitive feedback cannot be explained satisfactorily at present.

(*7*) Although a fast, rate-sensitive feedback has been found, it remains to be seen whether any physiological role can be attributed to this phenomenon.

REFERENCES

DALLMAN, M. F. AND YATES, F. E. (1969) Dynamic asymmetrics in the corticosteroid feedback path and distribution-metabolism-binding elements of the adrenocortical system. *Ann. N.Y. Acad. Sci.*, **156**, 696–721.

DALLMAN, M. F., JONES, M. T., VERNIKOS-DANELLIS, J. AND GANONG, W. F. (1971) Feedback control of ACTH secretion: early effects of adrenalectomy on plasma ACTH in the rat. *Fed. Proc.*, **30**, 311.

DE WIED, D. (1964) The site of the blocking action of dexamethasone on stress-induced pituitary ACTH release. *J. Endocrinol.*, **29**, 29–37.

HEDGE, G. A. AND SMELIK, P. G. (1969) The action of dexamethasone and vasopressin on hypothalamic CRF production and release. *Neuroendocrinology*, **4**, 242–253.

JONES, M. T. AND NEAME, R. L. B. (1971) Evidence in favour of a fast feedback control of ACTH secretion by corticosterone. *J. Physiol.*, **216**, 74–75 P.

JONES, M. T. AND NEAME, R. L. B. (1972) Some characteristics of the fast feedback control of corticotrophin secretion. *J. Physiol.*, **220**, 12–13 P.

PAPAIKONOMOU, E. (1972) A cybernetic approach to the hypothalamo-pituitary-adrenal system. *Progr. Brain Res.*, **38**, 293–302.

RUSSELL, S. M., DHARIWAL, A. P. S., MCCANN, S. M. AND YATES, F. E. (1969) Inhibition by dexamethasone of the *in vivo* pituitary response to corticotropin-releasing factor (CRF). *Endocrinology*, **85**, 512–521.

SAYERS, G. (1950) The adrenal cortex and homeostasis. *Physiol. Rev.*, **30**, 241–320.

SMELIK, P. G. (1963) Relation between blood level of corticoids and their inhibiting effect on the hypophyseal stress response. *Proc. Soc. exp. Biol. Med.*, **113**, 616–619.

TAKEBE, K., SAKAKURA, M., HORIUCHI, Y. AND MASHIMO, K. (1971) Persistence of diurnal periodicity of CRF activity in adrenalectomized and hypophysectomized rats. *Endocr. jap.*, **18**, 451–455.

YATES, F. E., LEEMAN, S. E., GLENISTER, D. W. AND DALLMAN, M. F. (1961) Interaction between plasma corticosterone concentration and adrenocorticotropin-releasing stimuli in the rat: evidence for the reset of an endocrine feedback control. *Endocrinology*, **69**, 67–80.

YATES, F. E., BRENNAN, R. D. AND URQUHART, J. (1969) Adrenal glucocorticoid control system. *Fed. Proc.*, **28**, 71–83.

DISCUSSION

HODGES: Several years ago Joan Vernikos-Danellis and I emphasized that ACTH secretion can be inhibited only by very high non-physiological doses of corticosteroids and that high circulating ACTH levels occur in adrenalectomized animals only after a considerable time delay. One objection to our data was that our assay technique for plasma ACTH was too insensitive to detect small but significant changes in the concentration of corticotrophin in the blood. My colleague Julia Buckingham has now shown, using the exquisitively sensitive assay method of Chayen *et al.*, that after adrenalectomy ACTH remains remarkably constant and does not begin to rise until after five days. In spite of the work which Dr. Smelik has presented, I still believe that while corticosteroids may control the basal level of ACTH secretion and corticotrophin synthesis, a feedback mechanism controlling stress induced ACTH secretion is of little physiological significance.

Effects of Adrenal Steroids on Brain Function and Behavior

L. KORÁNYI

Institute of Physiology, University Medical School, Pécs (Hungary)

I am interested in the effects of corticotrophin (ACTH) and adrenal steroids on elementary neural processes, brain function and behavior (Lissák *et al.*, 1957; Lissák and Endröczi, 1965; Korányi and Endröczi, 1967, 1970; Korányi *et al.*, 1965, 1966, 1967, 1969). Therefore, I have continued and extended the experimental work in which the hormonal influences on multiple unit activity have been studied (Korányi *et al.*, 1971a, 1971b). The behavior of multiple unit activity (MUA) was studied during the process of habituation, and the action was analyzed of pituitary-adrenocortical hormones on this mechanism in diverse subcortical structures, namely, that of the mesencephalic reticular formation, the preoptic area, the medial forebrain bundle, the nucleus fornicis and the non-specific thalamic nuclei.

One of the most suggestive findings seemed to be the gradual decrease of the average MUA level in the above brain structures in the course of the process of habituation to a novel environmental situation. By contrast, the dynamics of the sleep–wakefulness cycle in individual brain structures did not show changes; that is, whereas the MUA was high during attentive behavior and low during slow-wave sleep, it increased in paradoxical sleep to markedly higher levels than those observed during quiet wakefulness, both before and after habituation.

Administration of adrenocortical steroid resulted in a decrease of MUA levels both in non-habituated and habituated cats. However, the decreasing effect proved to be significantly pronounced in non-habituated animals. I conclude from these experiments that the process of habituation to a novel environment is based on neural mechanisms which are only secondarily modified or influenced by the hormones.

The present paper is devoted to studying the behavior of MUA in the course of habituation to the environment and of habituation to sensory stimuli. The effect of adrenocortical steroids is also analyzed in some subcortical structures known to be involved both in the complex regulation of the function of the pituitary-adrenal axis and the integration of behavioral events. Studies of forebrain-limbic structures, as well as the brain stem, are reported with special regard to the different rates in tendency of MUA changes.

We have chosen the technique of MUA recording because of its several advantages. Though activity of the central nervous system (CNS) can also be assessed by the analysis of behavioral manifestations using behavioral methods, the changes of MUA

References p. 121–123

levels reflect the state of CNS excitation or depression more specifically. Behavioral shifts are characteristically associated with MUA changes. Correlation has been found between MUA and the sleep–wakefulness cycles (Evarts *et al.*, 1962; Goodman and Mann, 1967; Huttenlocker, 1961; Manohar *et al.*, 1972; *etc.*), rage reaction, aggressive behavior, orienting reaction, diverse phases of attentive behavior and habituation (Guzmán-Flores and Garcia-Castells, 1970; Hirano *et al.*, 1970; Korányi *et al.*, 1971a, 1971b; Winters and Wallach, 1970).

Even though the simultaneous activity of activatory and inhibitory neurons may overlap, the MUA technique offers the advantage that it indicates the firing rate of both types of neuron or the suppression of their activity. Moreover, depending on the adjustment of the amplitude discriminator, the electronic window detector, not only the activity, but also the similarity of response patterns to hormonal changes from a small neuronal pool can be recorded.

GENERAL METHOD

The experiments were carried out on adult male cats, and on male rats of R-Amsterdam strain.

In each animal 8 electrodes were aimed at the following structures: the mesencephalic reticular formation (MRF), the area hypothalami posterior (PH), the basal nuclear group of the amygdala (AMY), the area septalis (SEPT), the dorsal hippocampus (HIPP) and three electrodes in the area hypothalami anterior (AH).

The basic methods for implanting of fixed probes for simultaneous electroencephalogram (EEG) and MUA recording, chronic derivation of MUA, and the amplification systems have been previously described (Guzmán-Flores and Alcaraz, 1970). Briefly, the neuronal spikes of a chosen height were selected at the start of each experiment and the identical electronic window detector was used throughout a session for the same animal. The output of the spike discriminator was fed to a

	PROGRAMS				
	I.	II.	III.	IV.	V.
CHANNEL 1	MRF	MRF	MRF	AMY	AMY
2	PH	AH_1	AH_1	PH	PH
3	SEPT	SEPT	AH_2	AH_2	SEPT
4	AH_3	HIPP	HIPP	HIPP	AH_3

Table I. MUA recording programs for the analysis of eight different subcortical structures with the four-channel MUA analyser.
MRF, mesencephalic reticular formation; AMY, amygdala; PH, area hypothalami posterior; SEPT, area septalis; HIPP, dorsal hippocampus; AH_1, AH_2, AH_3, the three electrodes in the area hypothalami anterior.

staircase generator and multivibrator system which drove the pen of the EEG apparatus and reset to zero every 16 pulses. This produced a saw-toothed line on the EEG channel. The raw MUA of two structures was monitored on a dual beam oscilloscope.

The analyzer device, built of operational amplifier circuits, analyzed MUA from four subcortical structures simultaneously. Our modification made it possible to record activity from eight structures alternately. For the experiments the following five programs were used (Table I). The programs, lasting for 10 min each, allowed us to study the MUA of eight neuronal pools in several combinations in the same animal.

Experiment I: Rats

Rats were housed in individual cages. Each spent 22 h in a living-cage and 2 h in the experimental situation which consisted of a plexiglass box (30 cm × 15 cm × 15 cm).

The experiments were performed on consecutive days on the strictest schedule to minimize behavioral variability due to the circadian rhythm. During the sessions both cages were put into an electrically shielded, sound-attenuated, dimly illuminated chamber with a glass front which allowed the observation of the behavior of the animals. Recording was done for 2 h in the living cage and for 2 h in the experimental situation during a session.

The MUA base levels showed a stable low rate in all structures, while the recording was made in the living-cage, but showed an increased activity in the novel situation both during wakefulness and sleep cycles. In the novel situation, at the early period of habituation, only short periods or episodes of slow-wave sleep could be recorded because the animals showed the typical behavioral manifestations that are characteristic of the rat in an open-field test. It took two, sometimes three, sessions before one or more complete sleep–wakefulness cycles could be recorded in the experimental situation. The high MUA base levels showed a gradual decrease in the course of habituation. The experimental schedule was continued for 20 days in each animal. During that time the MUA tended to approach the level of activity initially recorded in the living-cage.

Figs. 1a and 1b demonstrate the consecutive changes of MUA levels in the MRF and AH in the course of 12 sessions in both the novel situation and the living-cage. The MRF showed a gradual decrease of activity, but a sharp decrease was characteristic of the MUA recorded from the AH. The activity of the PH showed a similarity to the MRF. On the other hand, the AMY was similar to the AH. The MUA rate of the hippocampus and septal area took an intermediate position.

Earlier, we found (Korányi *et al.*, 1971a) that injection of corticosteroids to non-habituated cats resulted in a more significant decrease of MUA in all structures than in environmentally habituated animals. This observation suggested the possibility that adrenal steroids, beyond their specific action on some subcortical structures, produced a generalized non-specific effect as well. To study the changes of MUA after administration of corticosterone (1 mg per animal) in rats that were completely

References p. 121–123

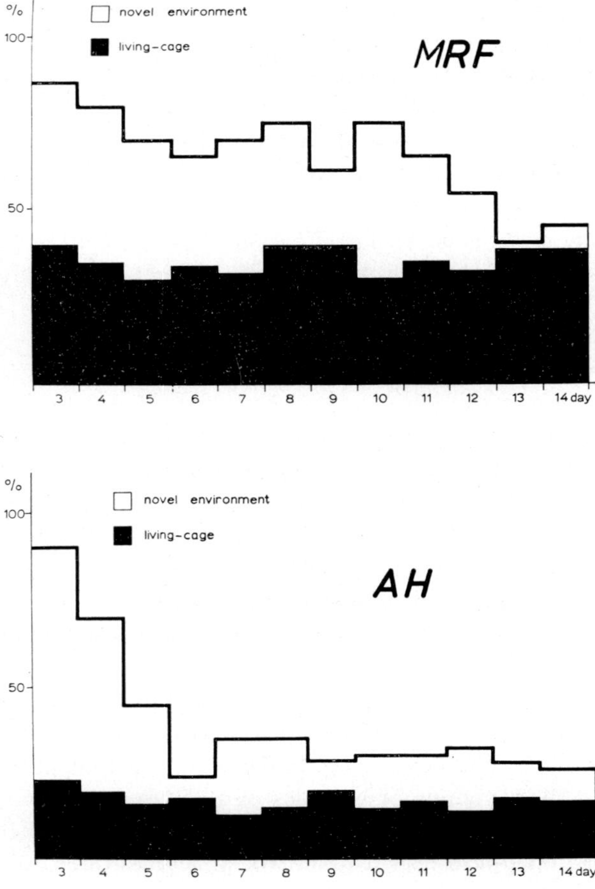

Fig. 1a and 1b. Changes of average MUA during slow-wave sleep in the mesencephalic reticular formation (MRF) and area hypothalami anterior (AH) in the course of consecutive habituation sessions. MUA is calculated as per cent value of the average activity recorded during quiet wakefulness of the rat on the 3rd day in the novel environment (white). Black columns represent the average activity during slow-wave sleep in the living-cage.

habituated to the environment, recordings were made from animals remaining in the living-cage, after a reasonable time of habituation to the experimental procedure (*e.g.* handling, injection of physiological saline solution and attachment to cable).

The MUA base levels showed a marked decrease in the AH and AMY, whereas the activity of other structures did not change significantly (Fig. 2). Any increase or decrease of activity was noted throughout the experiments, if the change was greater than 20% of the starting base level. Some changes were observed in the PH, SEPT and HIPP, but not until 24 or 48 h after the treatment. Possibly these changes were not due to the direct influence of the corticosterone, but were the results of some secondary mechanism.

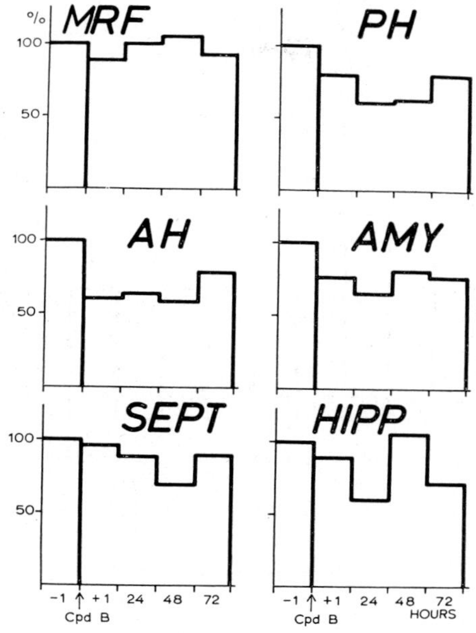

Fig. 2. The effect of corticosterone (Cpd.B) on MUA of rat. For abbreviations see Table I.

Experiment II: Cats

Cats were habituated to the environment and to the experimental procedure as mentioned above. I studied the changes of MUA during this process, and focused my

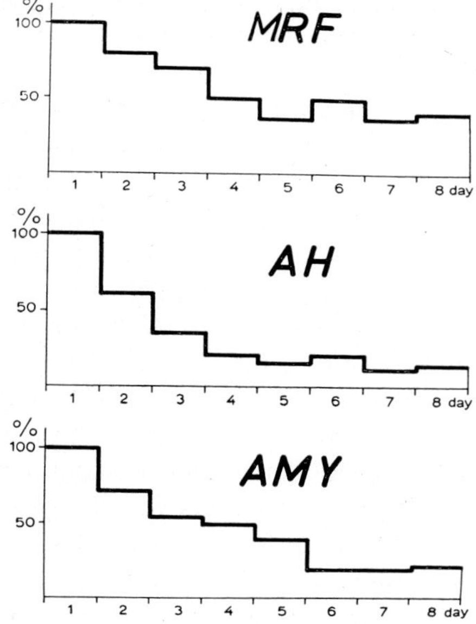

Fig. 3. Changes of average MUA during slow-wave sleep in the course of habituation of the cat.

References p. 121–123

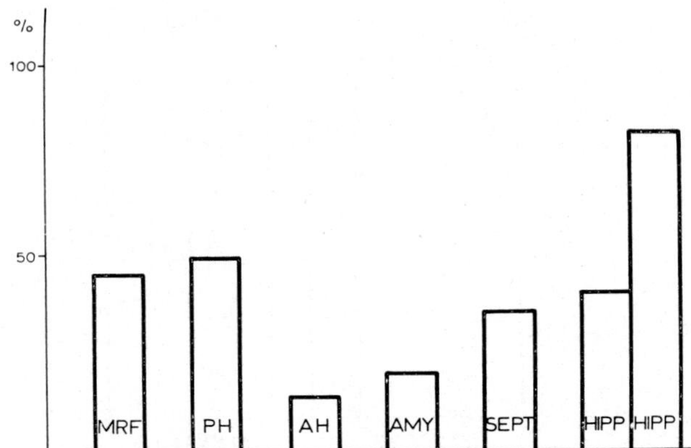

Fig. 4. MUA base levels in different structures at the advanced stage of habituation of the cat. MUA levels are calculated as per cent values of the average activity recorded during the animal's slow-wave sleep in the first session. For abbreviations see Table I.

attention on the different rates of decrease that occurred among the diverse subcortical structures.

Fig. 3 illustrates changes in the MUA base level in three subcortical structures in the course of consecutive habituation sessions to the environment. As compared with the MRF, a sharp and significant decrease of MUA was characteristic of the behavior of neuronal pools in the AH and AMY. In a comparison of the activity rates of different structures at the final stage of habituation to MUA base levels which had been registered at the start of the experiment, the low levels in the AH and AMY groups of cells were conspicuous. Hippocampal cells did not show typical changes. The changes in MUA were calculated as percentage values of the average activity recorded during the animal's slow-wave sleep in the course of the first session (Fig. 4).

The presentation of acoustic stimuli to cats was started after the animals had already been environmentally habituated, and 240 stimuli were given during a session. As we reported earlier (Korányi *et al.*, 1972) the MUA analysis showed that it took 4 to 5 sessions for habituation to an acoustic signal of high intensity (85 to 88 db) to be established. This slow habituation of the cats proved to be a suitable model for testing the changes of responsiveness of diverse subcortical structures after administration of hydrocortisone (10 mg per kg body weight).

Some individual records showed EEG and MUA changes during the second session of the acoustic signal habituation of a cat. On the first record (Fig. 5a) the EEG arousal was accompanied by a marked increase of MUA in all structures. In a later period, the firing rate was also increased during spindle sleep, as illustrated on the second record (Fig. 5b). The decreasing tendency of responsiveness of the population of neurons in the advanced stage of habituation was also observed (Fig. 5c).

Figs. 6a and 6b show the changes of MUA in the MRF and the AH during quiet wakefulness and slow-wave sleep. Black columns represent the average activity recorded during intertrial intervals (ITI) and the white ones the average MUA during the presentation of five acoustic stimuli (200 Hz lasting for 4.8 sec). These figures also

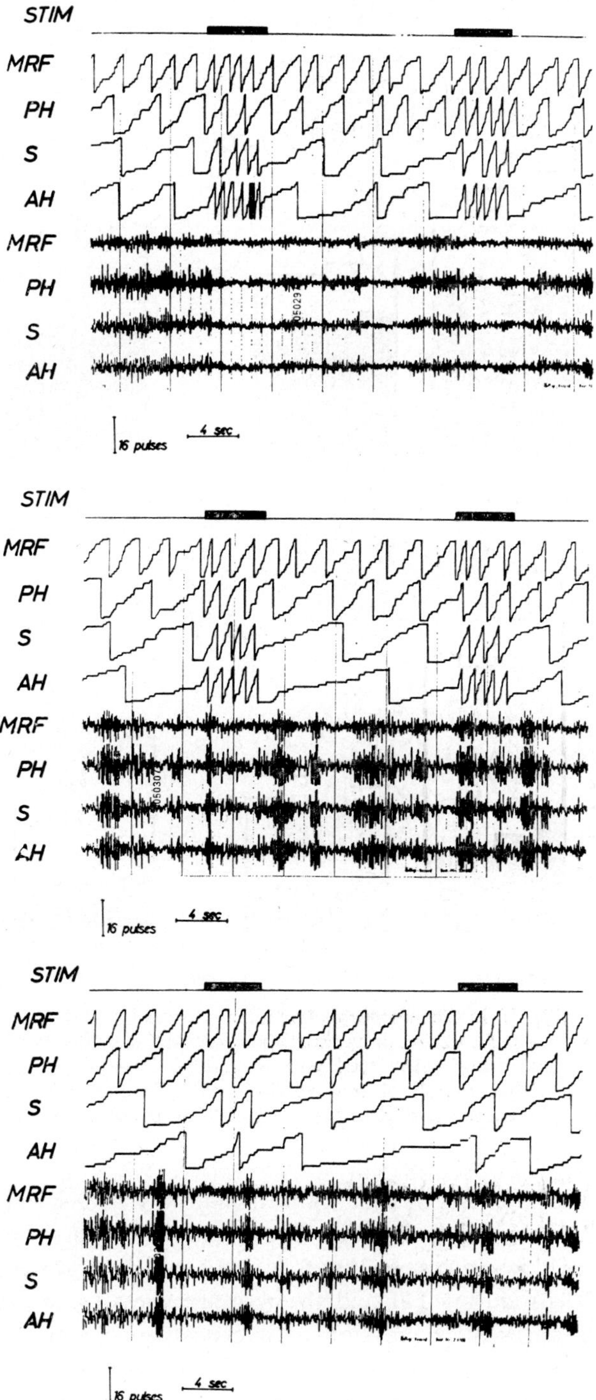

Fig. 5a, 5b, 5c. MUA (upper four channels) and EEG (four channels below) changes in response to acoustic stimulation (STIM: 200 Hz acoustic signal of 88 db intensity), in the course of a session. MRF, mesencephalic reticular formation; PH, area hypothalami posterior; S, area septalis; AH, area hypothalami anterior. For details see text.

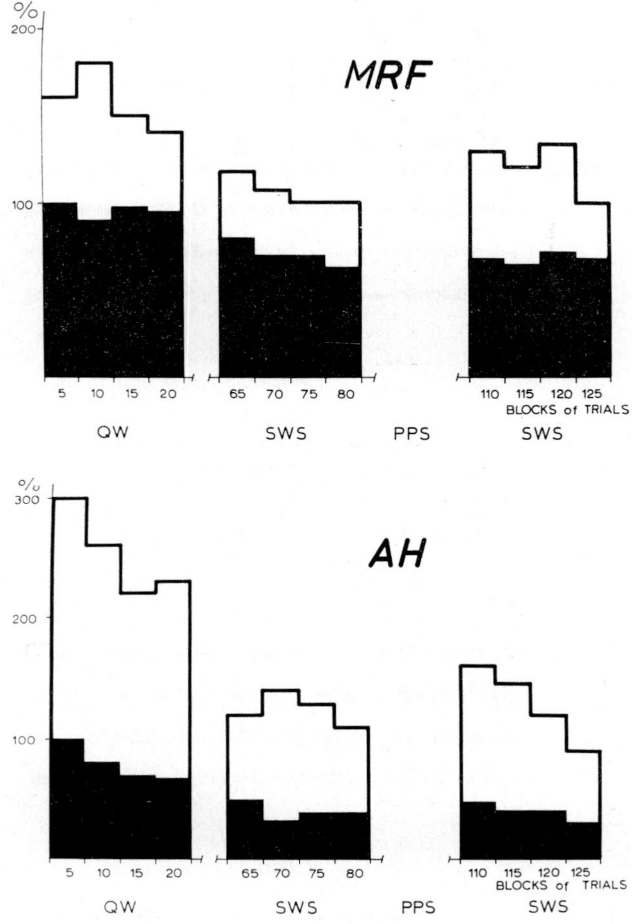

Fig. 6a, 6b. Changes of MUA in the mesencephalic reticular formation (MRF) and area hypothalami anterior (AH) in the course of a session of habituation to acoustic stimulus. Black columns represent the average activity recorded during intertrial intervals and the white ones the MUA during stimulation. QW, quiet wakefulness; SWS, slow wave sleep; PPS: paradoxical sleep. MUA levels are calculated as per cent values of the average activity recorded during QW at the start of the experiment.

demonstrate that AH groups of cells show significantly higher responsiveness than that of the MRF. Moreover, a slight increase of activity was usually observed during the first minutes of slow-wave sleep that followed a paradoxical sleep cycle.

The average MUA during ITI and the responsiveness to the acoustic stimulus showed typical changes after injection of hydrocortisone (Fig. 7). Generally the changes of firing of neurons in different regions during ITI were similar to those observed in the rats after administration of corticosterone. The spontaneous firing rates significantly decreased, first of all in the AH and AMY neuronal pools, as far as the ITI levels were concerned. On the other hand, the responsiveness of all structures was markedly altered. Accordingly, the steroid treatment markedly suppressed

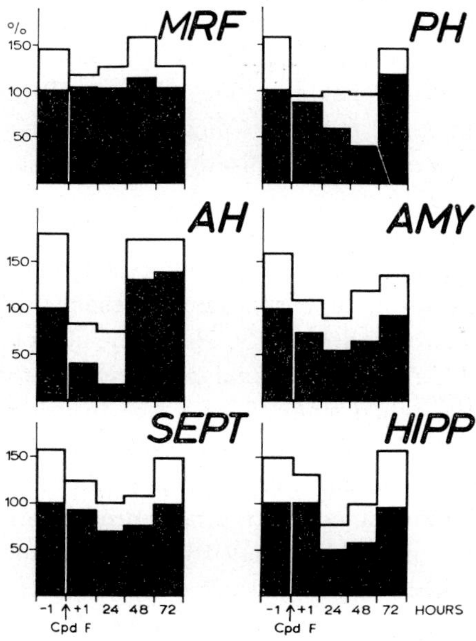

Fig. 7. The average MUA during ITI (black) and the responsivity to acoustic stimulation (white), before and after hydrocortisone (Cpd.F) injection. For abbreviations see Table I.

the reactivity of MRF and PH, but the AH and AMY neurons continued to respond to the stimulus, though at a lower base level.

DISCUSSION

The interpretation of the results presented here is difficult and should be done with caution. Nevertheless, I should like to point out two important phenomena. First, as compared with the findings in forebrain and limbic structures, as well as the brain stem, a striking decrease of MUA is observed in the AH during the processes of habituation (both environmental and signal habituation), which at the same time reflects the high responsiveness of the neuronal population in this region. This can probably be correlated with the mild stress response resulting from the novel situation. Second, as far as the effect of corticosteroids is concerned, the sensitivity of the hypothalamic area to steroids is conspicuous, and it is manifested in a further decrease of activity. However, the maintenance of responsiveness to a certain sensory modality was observed, whereas the base levels were set to a lower level of activity. Possibly the neural mechanism of the maintenance of responsiveness in the AH is distinct from the neuroendocrine events.

Steiner (1970) found steroid-sensitive neurons in the brain stem and anterior hypothalamus and pointed out that no conspicuous difference of steroid-sensitive neuron density has been observed. Feldman and Dafny (1970) reported changes in the responsiveness of the hypothalamus anterior and posterior after injection of steroid.

References p. 121–123

McEwen *et al.* (1968) pointed to the observation that some forebrain-limbic structures are able to accumulate corticosteroids, which might have functional significance in regulation of the pituitary-adrenal axis. De Wied (1969) called attention to the possibility that certain thalamic structures might also be involved in this regulatory mechanism. That is, with a certain simplification, one may say that almost the entire brain but the cerebral cortex (Korányi *et al.*, 1969; Steiner, 1970) has neuron sensitive to adrenocortical steroids scattered over it.

These findings would explain our earlier observation that, at an early stage of habituation, the administration of corticosteroid resulted in a marked change of activity in almost all subcortical structures. However, our present observations also suggest that there is a "differential functional sensitivity" of the groups of cells that is possibly a function of the actual state of the CNS. In other words, it seems to be characteristic that, in animals completely habituated to the environment, administration of adrenocortical steroid markedly suppresses the responsiveness of MRF and PH neurons, whereas the spontaneous firing rates are left practically unaltered.

Feldman (1964), Dafny and Feldman (1970) and Sarne and Feldman (1971) have demonstrated that a considerable convergence of somatosensory, acoustic and visual projections exists on the same hypothalamic neurons. This leads to the conclusion that through this mechanism the various exteroceptive modalities, as well as sensory and psychic influences, play an important role in the modification of the autonomic regulatory function of the hypothalamus, and in the control of the pituitary and target organ axes.

Several attempts have been made to clarify the pathways responsible for the transmission of various exteroceptive stimuli to the hypothalamus. Wolf and DiClara (1971) have demonstrated the existence of the reticulo-hypothalamic pathway which is distinct from the dorsal longitudinal fasciculus and from the medial forebrain bundle. The authors have concluded that this pathway, which is a component of the ascending reticular system, enters the hypothalamic area and may also participate in the transmission of sensory information which modulates hypothalamic visceral and behavioral functions.

Some considerations raise the possibility of the existence of the so-called multisensory cells which would be responsible for the interaction, integration and association of stimulus patterns which converge from different sources on the same cell. These cells are present in all brain regions and respond to more than one type of sensory stimulus (Yoshii and Ogura, 1960; O'Brien and Fox, 1969). As far as the neurons of the area hypothalami anterior and/or the hypophysiotrophic area are concerned, at the moment it would be unwise to draw final conclusions with respect to their multisensory or multilateral functional characteristics. Yet this is the structure that could be considered as a final common pathway for the integration and organization of both neuroendocrine and behavioral events. Moreover, these events are modified by the limbic system which is involved in these processes. The limbic influences have decisive importance in the determination of both neuroendocrine and behavioral resultants.

Theoretical considerations and experimental findings have led several authors (Gerstein and Mandelbrot, 1964; Guzmán-Flores and Garcia-Castells, 1970; Iso,

1965; Oomura *et al.*, 1969) to suggest that the analysis of the patterns of interval distribution and the patterns of cell discharges are initially important in the assessment of functional characteristics of CNS neuronal behavior.

Consideration of the findings presented here permits the formulation of the future perspectives of the main problem as follows: the hypothalamic neurons show high responsiveness to several sensory modalities, which through complex mechanisms in return, manifest in diverse, though specific humoral activation (pituitary-adrenal axis, pituitary-thyroid axis or pituitary-gonadal system), and in specific behavioral reactions as well (fight, flight, sexual behavior, *etc.*). It can be assumed that the specific humoral and behavioral responses are not dependent on the cell firing rate of the hypothalamus itself, but on the patterns of cell discharges, which are the function of inputs coming from the ascending reticular system and are modulated by the neural codes of the limbic system.

SUMMARY

Experiments were carried out on chronically implanted freely moving rats and cats. MUA of the brain stem and forebrain-limbic structures was studied during habituation to a novel environment as well as to habituation to sensory stimuli. A gradual marked decrease was found in the MUA levels in the brain stem and hippocampus while a sharp decrease was characteristic of the activity recorded from the anterior hypothalamus and amygdala during habituation to the environment. In response to stimulation the anterior hypothalamic groups of cells showed significantly higher responsiveness than that of the brain stem. In environmentally completely habituated animals, corticosteroid administration resulted in a significant decrease of MUA level first of all in the anterior hypothalamic and amygdalar neuronal pools, whereas the spontaneous firing rates in the brain stem were practically unaltered. On the other hand, the responsiveness to sensory stimulation was markedly suppressed in the brain stem, but anterior hypothalamic and amygdalar neurons continued to respond, though at a lower fuse level.

Results indicate that the high responsiveness of the neuronal population in the anterior hypothalamic area are probably correlated with a mild stress response resulting from the novel situation, and suggest that the neural mechanisms of the maintenance of responsiveness in this area are distinct from neuroendocrine events. Moreover, results suggest that there is a differential functional sensitivity of the groups of neurons which is a function of the actual state of the CNS.

REFERENCES

Dafny, N. and Feldman, S. (1970) Unit response and convergence of sensory stimuli in the hypothalamus. *Brain Res.*, **17**, 243–257.

De Wied, D. (1969) Effects of peptide hormones on behavior. In *Frontiers in Neuroendocrinology*, W. F. Ganong and L. Martini (Eds.), Oxford University Press, London, pp. 97–140.

EVARTS, E. V., BENTAL, E., BIHARI, B. AND HUTTENLOCKER, P. R. (1962) Spontaneous discharge of single neurons during sleep and waking. *Science*, **153**, 726–728.

FELDMAN, S. (1964) Visual projections to the hypothalamus and preoptic area. *Ann. N.Y. Acad. Sci.*, **117**, 53–68.

FELDMAN, S. AND DAFNY, N. (1970) Effects of adrenocortical hormones on the electrical activity of the brain. In *Pituitary, Adrenal and the Brain* (Progress in Brain Research, vol. 32), D. DE WIED AND J. A. W. M. WEIJNEN (Eds.), Elsevier, Amsterdam, pp. 90–101.

GERSTEIN, G. L. AND MANDELBROT, B. (1964) Random walk models for the spike activity of a single neuron. *Biophys. J.*, **4**, 41–68.

GOODMAN, S. J. AND MANN, P. E. G. (1967) Reticular and thalamic multiple unit activity during wakefulness, sleep and anesthesia. *Exp. Neurol.*, **19**, 11–24.

GUZMÁN-FLORES, C. AND ALCARAZ, M. (1970) A technique for recording and integrating unit activity. *Bol. Inst. Estud. méd. biol. Méx.*, **25**, 8.

GUZMÁN-FLORES, C. AND GARCIA-CASTELLS E. (1970) Análisis de la actividad eléctrica de los nucleos amigdalinos y la conducta emocional. *Bol. Inst. Estud. méd. biol. Méx.*, **26**, 331.

HIRANO, T., BEST, P. AND OLDS, J. (1970) Units during habituation, discrimination learning and extinction. *Electroenceph. clin. Neurophysiol.*, **28**, 127–135.

HUTTENLOCKER, P. R. (1961) Evoked and spontaneous activity in single units of the medial brain stem during natural sleep and waking. *J, Neurophysiol.*, **24**, 451–468.

ISO, Y. (1965) Threshold elements and random process, I. The first passage problem for Erling's system. *Rep. Kyushu Inst. Tech.*, **15**, 13–22.

KORÁNYI, L., ENDRÖCZI, E. (1967) The effect of ACTH on nervous processes. *Neuroendocrinology*, **2**, 65–75.

KORÁNYI, L., ENDRÖCZI, E. (1970) Influence of pituitary-adrenocortical hormones on thalamo-cortical and brain stem-limbic circuits. In *Pituitary, Adrenal and the Brain* (Progress in Brain Research, vol. 32), D. DE WIED AND J. A. W. M. WEIJNEN (Eds.), Elsevier, Amsterdam, pp. 120–130.

KORÁNYI, L., ENDRÖCZI, E. AND TÁRNOK, F. (1965/66) Sexual behavior in the course of avoidance conditioning in male rabbits. *Neuroendocrinology*, **1**, 144–157.

KORÁNYI, L., ENDRÖCZI, E., LISSÁK, K. AND SZEPES, É. (1967) The effect of ACTH on behavioral processes motivated by fear in mice. *Physiol. Behav.*, **2**, 439–445.

KORÁNYI, L., ENDRÖCZI, E., TAMÁSY, V. (1969) Influence of pituitary-adrenocortical hormones on the central nervous system. Electrophysiological and behavioral studies on rats and chicks. *Acta physiol. Acad. Sci. hung.*, **36**, 73–82.

KORÁNYI, L., BEYER, C., GUZMÁN-FLORES, C. (1971a) Multiple unit activity during habituation, sleep-wakefulness cycle and the effect of ACTH and corticosteroid treatment. *Physiol. Behav.*, **7**, 321–329.

KORÁNYI, L., BEYER, C. AND GUZMÁN-FLORES, C. (1971b) Effect of ACTH and hydrocortisone on multiple unit activity in the forebrain and thalamus in response to reticular stimulation. *Physiol. Behav.*, **7**, 331–335.

KORÁNYI, L., TAMÁSY, V. AND LISSÁK, K. (1972) Multiple units in the brainstem and limbic structures during habituation to acoustic stimulus. *Acta physiol. Acad. Sci. hung.*, in press.

LISSÁK, K. AND ENDRÖCZI, E. (1965) *The Neuroendocrine Control of Adaptation.* Pergamon, Oxford, pp. 139–159.

LISSÁK, K., ENDRÖCZI, E. UND MEDGYESI, P. (1957) Somatische Verhalten und Nebennierenrinden-tätigkeit. *Arch. ges. Physiol.*, **117**, 265–273.

MANOHAR, S., NODA, H. AND ADEY, R. W. (1972) Behavior of mesencephalic reticular neurons in sleep and wakefulness. *Exp. Neurol.*, **34**, 140–157.

MCEWEN, B. S., WEISS, J. M. AND SCHWARTZ, L. S. (1968) Selective retention of corticosterone by limbic structures in rat brain. *Nature (Lond.)*, **220**, 911–912.

O'BRIEN, J. AND FOX, S. (1969) Single cell activity in cat motor cortex, I. Modification during classical conditioning procedures. *J. Neurophysiol.*, **32**, 267–284.

OOMURA, Y., OOYAMA, H., NAKA, F., YAMAMOTO, T., ONO, T. AND KOBAYASHI, N. (1969) Some stochastical patterns of single unit discharges in the cat hypothalamus under chronic condition. *Ann. N.Y. Acad. Sci.*, **157**, 666–689.

SARNE, Y. AND FELDMAN, S. (1971) Sensory evoked potentials in the hypothalamus of the rat. Electro-enceph. clin. *Neurophysiol.*, **30**, 45–51.

STEINER, F. A. (1970) Effects of ACTH and corticosteroids on single neurons in the hypothalamus.

In *Pituitary, Adrenal and the Brain* (Progress in Brain Research, vol. 32), D. DE WIED AND J. A. W. M. WEIJNEN (Eds.), Elsevier, Amsterdam, pp. 102–107.

WINTERS, W. D. AND WALLACH, M. B. (1970) Drug induced states of CNS excitation: a theory of hallucinosis. In *Psychomimetic Drugs*, D. H. EFRON (Ed.), Raven, New York, pp. 193–228.

WOLF, G. AND DICLARA, L. V. (1971) A third ascending hypothalamo-petal pathway. *Exp. Neurol.*, **33**, 69–77.

YOSHII, N. AND OGURA, N. (1960) Studies on the unit discharge of brain stem reticular formation in the cat. *Med. J. Osaka Univ.*, **11**, 1–17.

DISCUSSION

CARROLL: Did you find any evidence for a diurnal variation in response of these multiple units to the stress stimuli? Stimuli like vasopressin have differential effects at different times of day.

KORÁNYI: In order to have standard circumstances, we tested our animals only in the morning. I don't know how the responsiveness changes as compared to the afternoon.

SAWYER: My colleagues, Terkel and Johnson, have noted a marked circadian rhythm in multiple-unit activity in the rat's preoptic region and septum, a much higher activity occurring in the dark period. This rhythm was reduced and eventually lost after adrenalectomy.

HAGINO: By what pathway does acoustic stimulus increase multiunit activity in anterior hypothalamus and amygdala?

KORÁNYI: I assume that the medial forebrain bundle, reticulo-hypothalamic pathway, and possibly also the dorsal longitudinal fasiculus are involved.

HAGINO: Is the hippocampal-septal complex sensitive to corticosterone? Your results show multiunit activity changes 24 h after injection. We are recording changes in unit spontaneous activity in the septal area 15 min after injection of 15 μg dexamethasone.

KORÁNYI: We have not tried dexamethasone.

TAYLOR: Dr. Korányi, what dose of steroid did you use in the rat? I ask this because in our experiments with Dafny and Phillips (Fed. Proc. 30, 203 and 311, 1971) we not only observed differential central effects of cortisol on spontaneous single unit activity, but also observed dose-related effects. Low doses of cortisol (1.0–4.0 mg/kg) produced primarily facilitation of unit activity in anterior hypothalamus, midbrain reticular formation, and dorsal hippocampus and inhibition of unit discharge and ventromedial hypothalamus. Higher doses of the cortisol (8.0 and 16.0 mg/kg) produced a majority of inhibitory effects at each of these sites.

KORÁNYI: We used 4.0 mg/kg.

Changes in Multiunit Electrical Activity (MUA) in Rat Brain During the Estrous Cycle and After Administration of Sex Steroids

MASAZUMI KAWAKAMI, EI TERASAWA, FUKUKO KIMURA, TAKASHI HIGUCHI AND NOBUHIDE KONDA

Second Department of Physiology, Yokohama City University School of Medicine, Yokohama (Japan)

It has long been known that the secretion of pituitary gonadotrophins is controlled in some way by the steroid hormones produced by the gonads. As early as 1932, Hohlweg and Junkmann postulated the existence in the hypothalamus of a "sex center" that controls the release of pituitary gonadotrophin and that is affected by the feedback action of sex steroids. Everett and Sawyer (1950) showed that the activity of neural elements controlling ovulation undergoes 24-h periodicity and that neural activity during a "critical period" is essential for release of the ovulatory surge of gonadotrophic hormone. Since this finding, numerous investigations have elucidated the role of the brain in triggering ovulation. The medial basal hypothalamus serves as a final common pathway for neural control of basal secretion of gonadotrophin (Flerko, 1953; Bogdanove *et al.*, 1955; Critchlow, 1958) while the preoptic anterior hypothalamus controls cyclic release of gonadotrophin (Flerko and Bardos, 1960; Everett, 1964; Gorski, 1968; Barraclough, 1968; Halász, 1969). Both brain regions are known to be sensitive to ovarian steroids (Dörner and Döcke, 1967; Davidson, 1969; Kawakami *et al.*, 1968, 1970).

Recent work from several laboratories suggests that limbic structures also participate importantly in reproductive physiology, especially at the onset of puberty and ovulation (Terasawa and Timiras, 1968; Velasco and Taleisnik, 1969a and b; Kawakami *et al.*, 1970, 1971, 1972b). However, the role of the limbic structures in the control of cyclic pituitary secretion is not clear. It therefore seemed important to study further the relationships between limbic structures and the medial preoptic anterior hypothalamus during normal reproductive cycles. This report describes observed changes in multiunit activity (MUA) in several brain regions during the estrous cycle and/or after administration of sex hormone to the rat. An attempt is made in the DISCUSSION to correlate these changes with cyclic gonadotrophin secretion and ovulation in this species.

MATERIALS AND METHODS

Adult female Wistar rats were housed in an air-conditioned room with fluorescent

References p. 132–134

light from 5:00 *a.m.* to 7:00 *p.m.*, and maintained with ordinary laboratory chow and water *ad libitum*. Vaginal smears were taken daily around 10:00 *a.m.* and only rats showing 2 consecutive 4-day cycles were used. In one study rats were ovariectomized about 2 weeks before the experiment.

Recording of MUA was done through chronically implanted electrodes, which were made of No. 00 stainless steel insect pins with stainless steel attachments and insulated with epoxylite except for an exposed tip of 20–40 μ in diameter. The electrodes were inserted into several regions in the brain according to the atlas by Albe-Fessard *et al.* (1966), fixed by dental cement to the skull and soldered to an ITT Cannon plug for leading to the preamplifier. Recording was performed under unanesthetized and unrestrained conditions, after animals regained their estrous cycles. Integrated levels of MUA were recorded on paper throughout the experimental period, and the basal levels of activity during cortical electroencephalogram (EEG) sleep were compared for every 10 min. Further details of recording procedures are described elsewhere (Kawakami *et al.* 1970). Sites of recording were confirmed by the histological study.

Estrogen (200 μg of estradiol-17β) or progesterone (2 mg of progesterone propionate) was injected subcutaneously at 10:00 *a.m.* and at 2:00–3:00 *p.m.*, respectively, on the day of diestrus I.

Ovulation was determined by identification of ova in the oviducts.

RESULTS

(A) Changes of MUA in the arcuate nucleus (ARC) (Fig. 1)

During the estrous cycle basal levels of MUA in the ARC were lowest in the afternoon of diestrus I, and the low level lasted until late afternoon of diestrus II. A gradual elevation of basal MUA started at about 4:00 *p.m.* on the day of diestrus II and reached the first maximum at about 8:00 *p.m.* on the same day. The high level decreased slightly in the early morning of proestrus, and it rose again reaching the maximum between 8:00 and 12:00 *p.m.* on the day of proestrus. Although the level decreased slightly in the early morning of estrus, a relatively high level lasted throughout the day of estrus to the day of diestrus I.

Injection of estrogen at 10:00 *a.m.* on the day of diestrus I induced elevation of MUA in the ARC with a latency of 30 min, reaching a peak by about 4 h. The high level lasted about 16 h, and then decreased gradually to the preinjection level. The response to estrogen in the ARC on the day before diestrus II was similar to the spontaneous change of MUA in the late afternoon to the evening of diestrus II. A 1-day advance in the vaginal smear and slight dilation of ampullae were observed in these estrogen-primed rats, but no ova were found in the oviduct. Progesterone injection at 3:00 *p.m.* on the day of diestrus I lowered the basal level of MUA in the ARC with a latency of 1 h. The low level lasted more than 8 h. Furthermore, progesterone inhibited the spontaneous elevation in the late afternoon of diestrus II and delayed ovulation by one day. In contrast with the change of MUA in the medial part

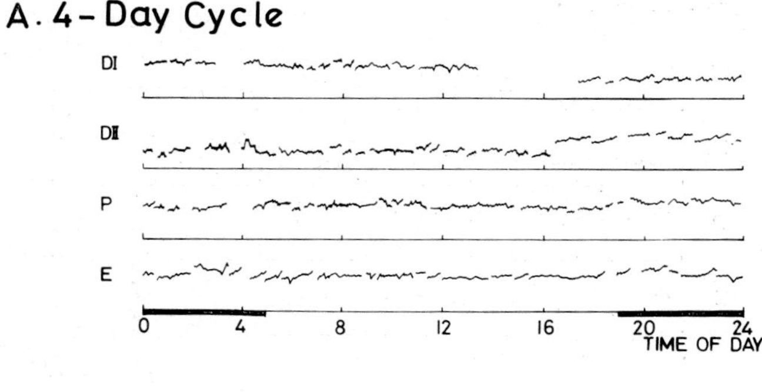

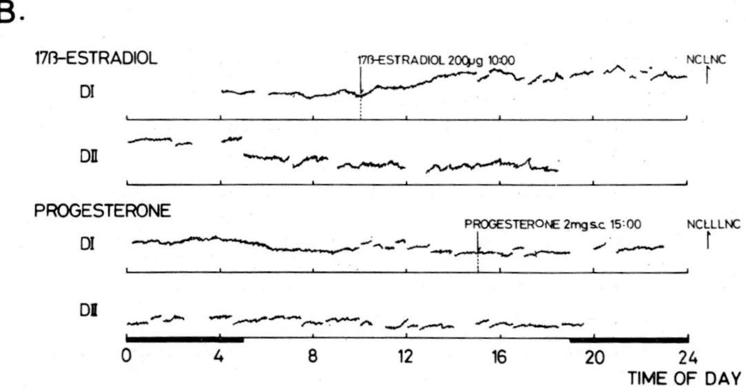

Fig. 1. Changes of integrated multiunit activity in the arcuate nucleus during estrous cycle (A) and effect of estradiol-17β (200 μg) or progesterone (2 mg) injection (s.c.) at 10:00 *a.m.* or at 15:00 *p.m.* on the day of diestrus I, respectively (B).

of the ARC, MUA in the lateral ARC was decreased after injection of estradiol-17β. This decrease started 8 h after the injection and lasted for 12–14 h.

(B) Changes of MUA in the periventricular preoptic area (PVA) (Fig. 2)

The lowest level of the basal MUA in this brain region, particularly the medial prechiasmatic area, was observed from the evening of the day of estrus through the day of diestrus I. The level started to increase gradually in the late afternoon of diestrus I reaching a high level by late afternoon on the day of diestrus II. The level continued to increase and reached a maximum during the critical period on the day of proestrus. At 4:00 *p.m.* on the day of proestrus, the level suddenly dropped and remained low until the morning of estrus. The level increased somewhat during the day of estrus but fell again to low levels by evening.

In the rats bearing neural transection at the level of the anterior commissure (AC) made with an L-shaped knife (the knife blade was 2 mm wide), the MUA in this region did not exibit such a characteristic change as mentioned above. And the vaginal smear of the transected rats showed irregular cyclicity for about 30 days after transection.

References p. 132–134

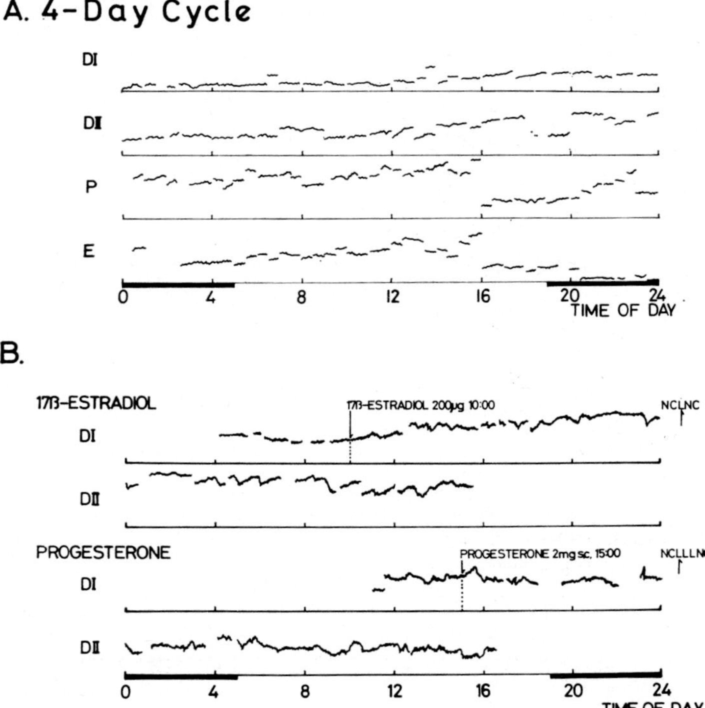

Fig. 2. Changes of integrated multiunit activity in the periventricular preoptic area during estrous cycle (A) and effect of estradiol-17β (200 μg) or progesterone (2 mg) injection at 10:00 *a.m.* or at 15:00 *p.m.* on the day of diestrus I, respectively (B).

Administration of estrogen at 10:00 *a.m.* on the day of diestrus I induced a marked elevation of MUA in the PVA with a latency of about 6 h. This increased level lasted more than 14 h and appeared to extend into the late afternoon of diestrus II. Progesterone injection on the day of diestrus I did not induce any marked changes of MUA in this region.

(C) Changes of MUA in the medial preoptic region (MPO)

The basal level of MUA in the MPO was relatively higher in the morning (8:00 *a.m.* to 1:00 *p.m.*) than in the afternoon throughout the estrous cycle. Changes of MUA in the MPO during the estrous cycle were somewhat similar to those observed in the PVA, so that the highest level was observed on the day of proestrus.

Injection of estrogen at 10:00 *a.m.* on diestrus I induced an elevation of MUA with a latency of 5–10 h. An elevated level of MUA lasted for 9–13 h and returned to the preinjection level in the morning of diestrus II. Progesterone injection at 2:00 *p.m.* on the day of diestrus I did not induce changes in this region during the 18–24-h period of observation following injection.

(D) Changes of MUA in the septal complex

The septal nuclei proper. A marked increase in MUA in the lateral part of the septum was observed after injection of estradiol-17β, and a slight increase was observed in the medial part. In both regions the basal level of MUA rose with a latency of about 30 to 60 min, and the high level lasted for about 16 h. It then decreased to a level below the preinjection level. Progesterone injection did not induce any marked changes in the MUA of this area. Therefore, the response of the septal nuclei to estradiol-17β was biphasic, as was that observed in the ARC, although the septal nuclei did not show any sensitivity to progesterone.

The basal level of MUA in the region adjacent to the lateral septum increased slightly 8 h after estradiol-17β, and this increase continued for about 12 h; subsequently it decreased to the preinjection level. Progesterone injection depressed MUA in this region, and the low level lasted at least 28 h.

Posterior part of nucleus accumbens (ACC). Injection of estradiol-17β decreased the MUA in the ACC with a latency of about 1 h. The decrease lasted for about 12 h and was subsequently followed by increased MUA for several hours. The high level of MUA returned to the preinjection level at 24 h, on the morning of diestrus II. Thus, a biphasic response to the estradiol-17β was observed in this region, although the first elevation was not as marked as those observed in the septal nuclei proper.

Bed nucleus of anterior commissure (BAC). An increase of MUA was observed in the BAC 6 h after injection of estradiol-17β. The elevated MUA lasted for 12 h and subsequently returned to the preinjection level. A rise of MUA was also observed with progesterone injection with a latency of about 2.5 h. The high level continued for 14 to 16 h and then returned to the preinjection level. The response to progesterone in this area was more marked than that to estradiol.

(E) Changes of MUA in the amygdala (AMYG)

Injection of estradiol-17β induced a rise of MUA in both medial and central nuclei of the AMYG with a latency of about 18–20 h. The elevated level lasted for 8–20 h and peaked at 20–40 h after estrogen. Injection of progesterone induced a decrease in MUA with a latency of about 13 h. The low level of MUA lasted for 4–8 h and gradually returned to the preinjection level by about 20 h.

(F) Changes of MUA in the hippocampus (HPC)

In the dorsal HPC of both cycling and ovariectomized rats, the basal level of MUA was relatively higher during the day-time (5:00 *a.m.*–5:00 *p.m.*) than that during the night. This diurnal fluctuation was especially apparent on both days of diestrus. After injection of estradiol-17β on the day of diestrus I, no change in the activity was observed. However, in the ovariectomized rats, the activity in this region started to

References p. 132–134

decrease 44 h after the administration, and this decreased level lasted for more than 60 h.

(G) Effect of estradiol-17β on MUA in the neural transected rats

Estrogen injection at 10:00 *a.m.* on the day of diestrus I in the rats bearing the neural transection at the level of the AC with an L-shaped knife (the knife blade was 1 mm wide) markedly increased the MUA in the ARC with a latency of about 1 h. A gradual increase persisted, reaching its peak at about 40 h, and the high level lasted for about 80 h.

DISCUSSION

The results of these studies show a similar pattern of changes in MUA in several basal forebrain regions which correlates with the estrous cycle in the rat. This pattern, observed in medial ARC, PVA and MPO of 4-day cycling animals, was characterized by low levels of MUA from the evening of diestrus I through the afternoon of diestrus II. MUA in these areas appeared to increase during the evening of diestrus II, and elevated levels were achieved and maintained on the following day. Thereafter, levels fell somewhat but remained elevated until the afternoon or evening of the day of estrus. The close temporal correlation between vaginal cornification and the presence of tubal ova suggests that these changes in MUA are associated with neural events underlying cyclic secretion of pituitary gonadotrophins. This possibility is consistent with a large body of experimental evidence indicating that the medial preoptic anterior hypothalamus participates in hormonal regulation of cyclic gonadotrophin section in the rat (Everett, 1964; Gorski, 1968, Halász, 1969).

The basis for the cyclic pattern of MUA in the ARC, MPO and PVA is not known. However, this pattern does not represent a generalized shift in neural activity since it is not observed in cortical EEG or extrahypothalamic subcortical electrical activity. This characteristic pattern of MUA appears to be localized in regions known to be particularly sensitive to the feedback action of gonadal steroids. The possibility that sex steroids are in some way responsible for the observed changes in MUA is consistent with reported changes in circulating levels of estrogen during the estrous cycle in the rat (Kobayashi, *et al.*, 1969a, b and c). The possibility is further supported by the observed effects of administration of estrogen on MUA in the present studies. Although the latencies of its effect differed somewhat, estrogen injection on the morning of diestrus I induced an increase of MUA in the ARC, MPO and PVA which corresponded to the spontaneous rise in MUA that occurred normally one day later on the evening of diestrus II. Thus it appeared as though estrogen injection on the day of diestrus I induced a 1-day advance of the brain activity, although the occurrence of ovulation was not observed. However, injection of estrogen resulted in a biphasic effect of MUA changes in the ARC, septum and AMYG, increasing at first and decreasing subsequently. Most changes occurred within 30 h after injection. Since estrogen induced a prolonged increase of MUA in the ARC, MPO and AMYG of ovariectomized rats (Kawakami *et al.*, 1970), the possibility must be considered that estrogen injection on the day of diestrus I in the present studies facilitated the release of gonadotrophin which may stimulate the ovary further to increase the ovarian steroids in the circulation. Both gonadotrophin [luteinizing hormone (LH), follicle-stimulating hormone (FSH) and prolactin] and ovarian steroids (estrogen and progesterone) are known to change brain activity (Kawakami and Sawyer, 1959; Kawakami and Terasawa, 1967; Kawakami and Saito, 1967; Ramirez *et al.*, 1967; Terasawa and Timiras, 1968; Terasawa *et al.*, 1969; Terasawa and Sawyer, 1970; Kawakami *et al.*, 1970).

Köves and Halász (1970) found that 9 out of 13 rats with interruption of the bilateral, anterior and superior connections of the preoptic anterior hypothalamic region continued to ovulate and that some rats showed nearly normal vaginal cycles whereas others showed predominantly diestrous smears. Therefore, the possibility remains that regions outside of the preoptic anterior hypothalamus, such as the septal complex, AMYG and HPC, may be involved in triggering release of gonadotrophin in the normal cycling rat, although the medial preoptic anterior hypothalamus seems to be sufficient for inducing ovulation even in the neural disconnected condition.

In view of this possibility, it is interesting that the MUA responses of the septal complex, particularly the area surrounded by the anterior part of the optic chiasm and the anterior commissure, were as great as that observed in the ARC, and more than in the MPO. Electrical stimulation of this region induced ovulation (Everett, *et al.*, 1964; Terasawa and Sawyer, 1969; Kawakami *et al.*, 1970); and deafferentation of this region on the day of diestrus I prevented the expected events of proestrus and estrus. In addition, the effects of estrogen on the MUA in the ARC in the neural transected rats were much prolonged as compared with intact rats. These findings suggest that the septal complex participates in the cyclic release of gonadotrophin and may function as an important site of the feedback action of estrogen.

The importance of limbic structures in the regulation of gonadotrophin secretion in the rat is suggested by several lines of evidence. Previous work from our laboratory indicates that the HPC is a neural structure responsible for release of FSH in normal cycling rats and prepuberal rats (Kawakami *et al.*, 1971, 1972a and b; Kawakami and Terasawa, 1972), in which FSH may induce the secretion of estrogen, at least, at the initiation of cyclicity or onset of puberty. Under appropriate conditions, surgical interruption of both fornix and stria terminalis prevented vaginal cornification, uterine distension and ovulation, and blocked ovulation induced by injection of 200 μg estradiol-17β. However, damage to adjacent neural structures, including the lateral septum, in these animals was extensive. Stimulation of the AMYG increased serum LH and FSH on the day of proestrus, but did not induce any change in pituitary contents. Both the MPO and medial AMYG decreased serum prolactin by stimulation throughout the cycle. Stimulation of the dorsal hippocampus (d-HPC) increased both pituitary and serum levels of FSH on the day of estrus, but decreased serum FSH on the day of diestrus II. The stimulation also decreased serum prolactin on the days of proestrus and estrus. Pituitary and serum contents of LH did not change on stimulation of the d-HPC. However, if it was applied simultaneously with the MPO stimulation, the d-HPC stimulation inhibited the increase of pituitary LH, serum LH and FSH, which normally follows MPO stimulation. Moreover, such d-HPC stimulation inhibited the decrease of pituitary prolactin, which ordinarily follows MPO stimulation. Thus, the influence of d-HPC on gonadotrophin secretion is variable and its inhibitory influence appears to be exerted on neural elements responsible for the increase or decrease of gonadotrophin secretion. Thus, limbic structures, especially the HPC, appear to act as modulators of the medial preoptic anterior hypothalamus with respect to the release of gonadotrophin from the pituitary.

SUMMARY

A characteristic pattern of MUA in the ARC, PVA and MPO appears to correlate with the estrous cycle in the rat. MUA in these regions also shows characteristic changes in response to administration of estrogen. Injection of estrogen on the day of diestrus I advances the evening rise of MUA in these regions by one day. The increase of MUA after estrogen administration appears to correspond to the facilitatory effect of estrogen on gonadotrophin secretion. The septal complex appears to act primarily as a site of the feedback action of estrogen whereas MPO, ARC and PVA constitute the central integrative mechanism responsible for the cyclic release of gonadotrophin.

ACKNOWLEDGMENTS

The authors wish to thank Dr. K. Wakabayashi for his kind advice and Dr. Yanase, Mr. Mochizuki and Miss Konno for secretarial assistance.

REFERENCES

ALBE-FESSARD, D., STUTINSKY, F. AND LIBOUBAN, S. (1966) *Atlas Stéréotaxique du Diencéphale du Rat Blanc*. Éd. CNRS, Paris.

BARRACLOUGH, C. A. (1968) Alterations in reproductive function following prenatal exposure to hormones. In *Advances in Reproductive Physiology*, A. MCLAREN (Ed.), Logos, London, pp. 81–112.

BOGDANOVE, E. M., SPIRTOS, B. N. AND HALMI, N. S. (1955) Further observations on pituitary structure and function in rat bearing hypothalamic lesions. *Endocrinology*, **57**, 302–315.

CRITCHLOW, B. V. (1958) Ovulation induced by hypothalamic stimulation in the anesthetized rat. *Amer. J. Physiol.*, **195**, 171–174.

DAVIDSON, J. M. (1969) Feedback control of gonadotropin secretion. In *Frontiers in Neuroendocrinology*, 1969, W. F. GANONG AND L. MARTINI (Eds.), Oxford University Press, New York, pp. 343–388.

DÖRNER, G. AND DÖCKE, F. (1967) The influence of intrahypothalamic and intrahypophyseal implantation of estrogen or progestogen on gonadotrophin release. *Endocrinol. exp.*, **1**, 65–71.

EVERETT, J. W. (1964) Central neural control of reproductive functions of the adenohypophysis. *Physiol. Rev.*, **44**, 373–431.

EVERETT, J. W. AND SAWYER, C. H. (1950) A 24-hour periodicity in the "LH-release apparatus" of female rats, disclosed by barbiturate sedation. *Endocrinology*, **47**, 198–218.

EVERETT, J. W., RADFORD, H. M. AND HOLSINGER, J. (1964) Electrolytic irritative lesions in the hypothalamus and other forebrain areas: Effects on luteinizing hormone release and the ovarian cycle. In *Steroid, Biochemistry, Pharmacology and Therapeutics*, L. MARTINI (Ed.), Academic Press, New York, pp. 251–258.

FLERKO, B. (1953) Einfluss experimenteller Hypothalamusläsionen auf die Funktion des Sekretionsapparates im weiblichen Genitaltrakt. *Acta morph. hung.*, **3**, 65–86.

FLERKO, B. AND BARDOS, V. (1960) Pituitary hypertrophy after anterior hypothalamic lesions. Acta endocrinol. (Kbh.), **35**, 375–380.

GORSKI, R. A. (1968) The neural control of ovulation. In *Biology of Gestation, Vol. I, The Maternal Organism*, N. S. Assali (Ed.), Academic Press, New York, pp. 1–66.

HALÁSZ, B. (1969) The endocrine effects of isolation of the hypothalamus from the rest of the brain. In *Frontiers in Neuroendocrinology*, 1969, W. F. GANONG AND L. MARTINI (Eds.), Oxford University Press, New York, pp. 307–342.

HOHLWEG, W. AND JUNKMANN, K. (1932) Die hormonal-nervöse Regulierung der Funktion des Hypophysenvorderlappens. *Klin. Wschr.*, **11**, 321–323.

KAWAKAMI, M. AND SAITO, H. (1967) Unit activity in the hypothalamus of the cat: Effect of genital stimuli, luteinizing hormone and oxytocin. *Jap. J. Physiol.*, **17**, 466–486.

KAWAKAMI, M. AND SAWYER, C. H. (1959) Neuroendocrine correlates of changes in brain activity thresholds by sex steroids and pituitary hormones. *Endocrinology*, **65**, 652–668.

KAWAKAMI, M. AND TERASAWA, E. (1967) Differential control of sex hormone and oxytocin upon evoked potentials in the hypothalamus and midbrain reticular formation. *Jap. J. Physiol.*, **17**, 65–93.

KAWAKAMI, M. AND TERASAWA, E. (1972) Electrical stimulation of the brain on gonadotropin secretion in the female prepubertal rat. *Endocr. jap.*, **19**, 335–347.

KAWAKAMI, M., SETO, K. AND YOSHIDA, K. (1968) Influences of the limbic structure on biosynthesis of ovarian steroids in rabbits. *Jap. J. Physiol.*, **18**, 356–372.

KAWAKAMI, M., TERASAWA, E. AND IBUKI, T. (1970) Changes in multiple unit activity of the brain during the estrous cycle. *Neuroendocrinology*, **6**, 30–48.

KAWAKAMI, M., TERASAWA, E., SETO, K. AND WAKABAYASHI, K. (1971) Effect of electrical stimulation of the medial preoptic area on hypothalamic multiple unit activity in relation to LH release. *Endocr. jap.*, **18**, 13–21.

KAWAKAMI, M., KIMURA, F. AND WAKABAYASHI, K. (1972a) Electrical stimulation of the hippocampus under the chronic preparation and changes of LH, FSH and prolactin levels in serum and pituitary. *Endocr. jap.*, **19**, 85–96.

KAWAKAMI, M., SETO, K., TERASAWA, E. AND KIMURA, F. (1972b) Role of the limbic-hypothalamic system in relation to ovulation and ovarian steroid-genesis in the rats. *Med. J. Osaka Univ.*, **23**, 57–75.

KOBAYASHI, F., HARA, K. AND MIYAKE, T. (1969a) Effects of steroids on the release of luteinizing hormone in the rat. *Endocr. jap.*, **16**, 251–260.

KOBAYASHI, F., HARA, K. AND MIYAKE, T. (1969b) Causal relationship between luteinizing hormone release and estrogen secretion in the rats. *Endocr. jap.*, **16**, 261–267.

KOBAYASHI, F., HARA, K. AND MIYAKE, T. (1969c) Further studies on the causal relationship between the secretion of estrogen and the release of luteinzing hormone in the rat. *Endocr. jap.*, **16**, 501–506.

KÖVES, K. AND HALÁSZ, B. (1970) Location of the neural structures triggering ovulation in the rat. *Neuroendocrinology*, **6**, 180–193.

RAMIREZ, V. D., KOMISARUK, B. R., WHITMOYER, D. I. AND SAWYER, C. H. (1967) Effects of hormones and vaginal stimulation on the EEG and hypothalamic units in rats. *Amer. J. Physiol.*, **212**, 1376–1384.

TERASAWA, E. AND SAWYER, C. H. (1969) Changes in electrical activity in the rat hypothalamus related to electrochemical stimulation of adenohypophyseal function. *Endocrinology*, **85**, 143–149.

TERASAWA, E. AND SAWYER, C. H. (1970) Diurnal variation in the effects of progesterone on multiple unit activity in the rat hypothalamus. *Exp. Neurol.*, **27**, 359–374.

TERASAWA, E. AND TIMIRAS, C. S. (1968) Electrophysiological study of the limbic system in the rat at onset of puberty. *Amer. J. Physiol.*, **215**, 1462–1467.

TERASAWA, E., WHITMOYER, D. L. AND SAWYER, C. H. (1969) Effects of luteinizing hormone on multiple unit activity in the rat hypothalamus. *Amer. J. Physiol.*, **217**, 1119–1126.

VELASCO, M. E. AND TALEISNIK, S. (1969a) Release of gonadotropins induced by amygdaloid stimulation in the rat. *Endocrinology*, **84**, 132–139.

VELASCO, M. E. AND TALEISNIK, S. (1969b) Effect of hippocampal stimulation on the release of gonadotropin. *Endocrinology*, **85**, 1154–1159.

DISCUSSION

SAWYER: Your demonstration that hippocampal stimulation can induce FSH release but not LH release is a further argument for a separate releasing factor for each hormone.

KAWAKAMI: Yes, I might say that there seems to exist separate mechanisms releasing LH and FSH in the limbic-hypothalamo-pituitary system. We recently found that an extract of hypothalamus from an animal given electrical stimulation of the dorsal hippocampus on the day of estrus tended to increase FSH secretion while it had no effect on LH secretion. This might also support that assumption.

KALRA: We found that implants of estradiol in estrogen-pretreated spayed female rats caused dissociation of LH and FSH release when put into the hippocampus. We got a release of LH whereas FSH was inhibited. But with implants in the amygdala we got release of both FSH and LH.

KAWAKAMI: Thank you for your comment.

Mechanisms of Action of Sex Steroids on Behavior; Inhibition of Estrogen-Activated Behavior by Ethamoxy-Triphetol (Mer-25), Colchicine and Cycloheximide

BENGT J. MEYERSON

Department of Pharmacology, Biomedicum, Box 573, 75123 Uppsala (Sweden)

Estrogen produces in the female rat an increase of locomotor activity (see Reed, 1947), a specific urge to seek sexual contact (sexual motivation) (see Meyerson and Lindström, 1970) and the characteristic performance related to the copulatory act (see Young, 1961). It is generally accepted that the hormone exerts its effect directly on the brain. In several species, including the rat, implants of minute amounts of estrogen into the hypothalamus activate estrous behavior without producing detectable stimulation of peripheral estrogen target tissue (Harris *et al.*, 1958; Lisk, 1962; Sawyer, 1963; Harris and Michael, 1964; Palka and Sawyer, 1966). Radiochemical studies show that estrogen is taken up and concentrated in certain cerebral neuronal systems (Glascock and Hoeksta, 1959; Michael, 1965; Eisenfeld and Axelrod, 1967; Kato and Willee, 1967; Stumpf, 1968; Pfaff, 1968; Zigmond and McEwen, 1970). This uptake and the functional effects of estradiol (induction of estrous behavior) can be inhibited by estrogen antagonists (Eisenfeld and Axelrod, 1967; Arai and Gorski, 1968; Meyerson and Lindström, 1968; Meyerson, 1971). A study on the capacity of optical isomers of estrogen to produce estrous behavior in the female rat suggests that the system by which estrogens produce such behavior is highly stereospecific (Meyerson, 1971). A comparison of the efficiency of different estrogens in activating estrous behavior and a vaginal response suggests that the "receptor site" in the brain has recognition characteristics for estrogen similar to the estrogen-binding sites in the vagina (Meyerson, 1971).

Accumulating evidence suggests that there exist estrogen "receptor sites" in the brain. However, only little is known about the biochemical mechanisms whereby estrogen produces its effect in the central nervous system. The already established female copulatory behavior is sensitive to changes in monoaminergic and cholinergic activity. Increased monoaminergic activity decreases the hormone-activated copulatory behavior in the female rat (Meyerson, 1964, 1968; Meyerson and Lewander, 1970), mouse, hamster and rabbit (Meyerson, 1970, 1972a). Moreover, muscarinic drugs such as pilocarpine and oxotremorine inhibit the copulatory response in the female rat (Lindström and Meyerson, 1967) and hamster (Lindström, 1972). Although monoaminergic and cholinergic mechanisms seem to be involved in sexual behavior, and changes in monoamine levels have been reported to fluctuate during the estrous cycle

References p. 145–146

and to be influenced by estrogen treatment (Stefano and Donoso, 1967; Donoso *et al.*, 1969; Lichtensteiger, 1969; Fuxe and Hökfelt, 1969; Tonge and Greengrass, 1971), there still are no explicit data on a causal relationship between the estrogen mechanism of action on sexual behavior and changed monoaminergic and cholinergic activities.

The time it takes from the moment a submaximal dose of estradiol benzoate has been given until *e.g.* wheel running activity, lordotic behavior or sexual motivation has reached its maximal level is rather long—a matter of 48 h or more. Implications of protein synthesis in the action of sex steroids on behavior have been proposed (Thiessen and Yahr, 1970; Quandagno *et al.*, 1971; Wallen *et al.*, 1972; Meyerson, 1972b), the hypothesis being partly based upon results that show how estrogen acts on peripheral target tissue (see De Angelo and Gorski, 1970).

The present investigation is concerned with the effects on estrogen-activated behavior by the estrogen antagonist ethamoxytriphetol (Mer-25) (Lerner *et al.*, 1958), by colchicine which is known to impair microtubular functions (Borisy and Taylor, 1967) and by the protein synthesis inhibitor cycloheximide (Sisler and Siegel, 1967). Emphasis was put on the effects of these compounds before the estrogen response was fully developed. Estradiol benzoate (EB), progesterone and ethamoxytriphetol (Mer-25) were dissolved in olive oil and injected in a volume of 0.2–0.3 ml. Cycloheximide (cyclohex) and colchicine were dissolved in saline and injected in a volume of 0.2–0.3 ml. All injections were given subcutaneously (s.c.)

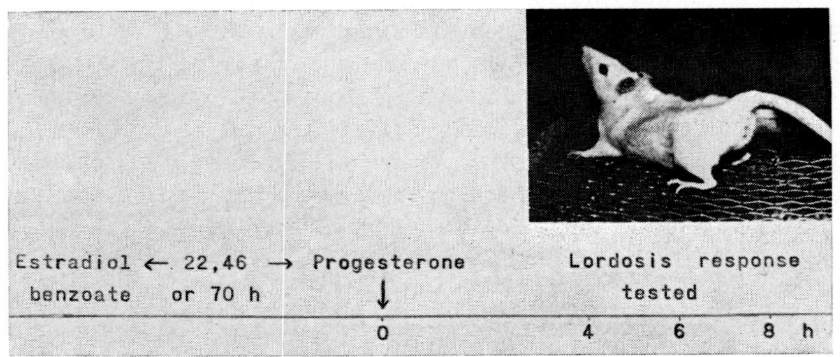

TABLE I

LORDOSIS RESPONSE ACTIVATED BY ESTRADIOL BENZOATE (EB) AND PROGESTERONE GIVEN 22, 46 OR 70 h APART

Treatment				*Results*	
EB μg/kg	*Progesterone mg/rat*			*Lordosis response*	
at 0 h	*at 22 h*	*46 h*	*70 h*	%	*N*
10	0.4			63	71
10		0.4		81	72
10			0.4	67	36

THE ESTROGEN-PROGESTERONE ACTIVATED COPULATORY BEHAVIOR (LORDOSIS RESPONSE)

Ovariectomized Sprague-Dawley rats (250–300 g) were exposed to a reversed day–night regime with light off from 9 *a.m.* to 9 *p.m.* EB was injected at 10 *a.m.* followed by progesterone (0.4 mg/animal) given either 22, 46, or 70 h after the injection of estrogen. The females were transferred to an observation cage, which held a sexually active male, and tested for lordosis response on mounting by the male. Each female was subjected to 6 mounts per test and tests were performed 4, 6 and 8 h after the progesterone injection. The estimate of the percentage lordosis response was based on the number of subjects showing a clearcut lordosis reflex after at least 2 out of the 6 mounts, in two tests or the last test performed. Table I shows the time relationship between the administration of the EB and the appearance of the lordosis response. The maximal response was obtained in the 46-h experiment. Previous studies have shown that the peak of the response also occurs at this time when other estrogens than EB are used to activate the behavior (Meyerson, 1971).

THE EFFECT OF THE ESTROGEN ANTAGONIST Mer-25

We know from earlier studies that the anti-estrogen Mer-25 inhibits the EB + progesterone activated lordosis response provided the compound is given in connection with the estrogen injection (Meyerson and Lindström, 1968). When given 24 h after the EB treatment the anti-estrogen was ineffective (Table II). In previous experiments the optimal time between the EB and progesterone injections was used (48 h). In the present study we were concerned with the extent of inhibition achieved by Mer-25 when the behavior was elicited by progesterone earlier than at the time when a full response could be expected. Progesterone was given 22, and for comparison at 46, h after the EB treatment, and Mer-25 at 150 or 75 mg/kg was injected 2 h before

TABLE II

THE EFFECT OF THE ANTI-ESTROGEN ETHAMOXYTRIPHETOL (Mer-25) ON ESTRADIOL BENZOATE (EB) + PROGESTERONE-ACTIVATED LORDOSIS RESPONSE IN OVARIECTOMIZED RATS

EB 5 μg/kg s.c. was given at 0 h.

Mer-25 mg/kg	*Treatment*		*Lordosis response*		
	h before (−) or after (+) EB inj.	*Progesterone 0.4 mg/rat*	*Controls %*	*Exptls % of controls*	*N*
150	− 2	at 22 h	50	18[a]	22
150	− 2	at 46 h	63	13[a]	24
75	− 2	at 22 h	50	34[a]	22–24
75	− 2	at 46 h	63	53[a]	24
150	+24	at 46 h	73[b]	87[b]	23

[a]Indicates statistical significance $p < 0.01$ (χ^2-test).
[b]Data taken from Meyerson and Lindström (1968).

References p. 145–146

the EB injection. Table II shows that Mer-25 inhibited the response in the 22- as well as 46-h experiment; the degree of inhibition was about the same in the two experiments.

THE EFFECT OF COLCHICINE

By a strong binding to the microtubule protein (Borisy and Taylor, 1967), colchicine interferes with a number of cell functions dependent on microtubules including movements of intraaxonal amine storage granules in sympathetic nerves in the rat (Dahlström, 1968), acetylcholine esterase in the sciatic nerve of the rat (Kreutzberg, 1969) and protein in the rabbit optic nerve (Karlsson and Sjöstrand, 1969). Lundberg

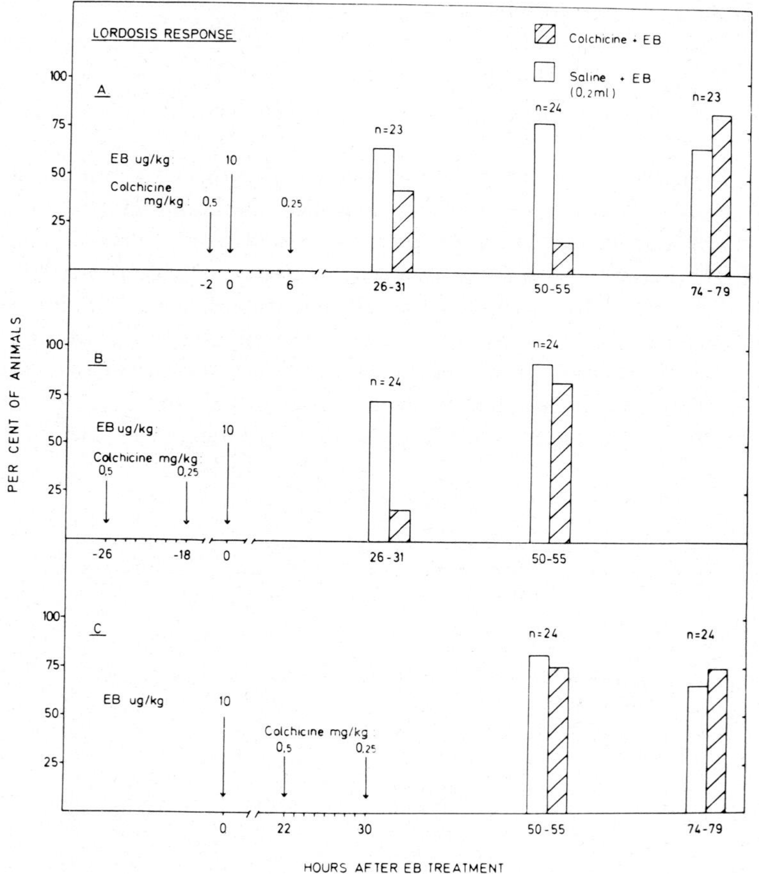

Fig. 1. The effect of colchicine on estradiol benzoate (EB) + progesterone-activated lordosis response in ovariectomized rats. Progesterone, 0.4 mg/animal was given at 22, 46 or 70 h after the EB treatment. See also Table I.

(1970) showed that colchicine at 1.0 mg/kg s.c. was effective in delaying degeneration release of sympathetic transmitter in conscious rats.

In the present experiments, colchicine was dissolved in saline and injected subcutaneously, at 0.5 mg/kg and 0.25 mg/kg, the two doses being given 8 h apart. This regime brought about a maximal effect on the overt behavior after about 48 h. The locomotor activity was decreased to the exent that in some subjects no spontaneous activity was seen but they moved readily during the tests for lordotic behavior. Most animals had diarrhea. At about 24 h the effects were hardly detectable and after 72 h the animals had almost recovered. In experiment A (Fig. 1A) colchicine was given 2 h before (0.5 mg/kg) and 6 h after (0.25 mg/kg) the EB treatment. Progesterone was injected either 22, 46 or 70 h after the EB (10 μg/kg) injection. A slight but insignificant ($p > 0.05$) decrease of the lordosis response was seen in tests performed at 26–31 h after the estrogen treatment. The inhibitory effect of colchicine, however, was obvious in the 50–55 h tests.

Two analogous experiments were performed with colchicine given at the same time of day but one day before (Fig. 1B) or one day after (Fig. 1C) the EB treatment. When given one day before the EB treatment the inhibitory effect was now obvious in the 26–31-h test but no effect was seen in the 50–55-h tests. In experiment C no inhibitory effect was obtained at the 50–51-h nor at the 74–79-h tests. Thus, colchicine inhibited the EB + progesterone-activated copulatory behavior. The effect appeared 2 days after the colchicine treatment regardless of whether colchicine was given one day before or in connection with the EB treatment. When given one day after the EB treatment, colchicine was not effective in inhibiting the lordosis response.

THE EFFECT OF THE PROTEIN SYNTHESIS INHIBITOR CYCLOHEXIMIDE

Glutarimide derivatives such as cycloheximide interfere with protein synthesis by a direct action on the protein synthesis system at the ribosomal level. It is generally thought that cycloheximide stops ongoing protein synthesis, but does not significantly affect DNA or RNA synthesis (Sisler and Siegel, 1967). Quantitative results have been obtained on the inhibitory effect of cycloheximide *in vivo*. Cycloheximide at 0.5 mg/kg i.p. significantly reduced the leucine incorporation in the rat brain 7 h after treatment (Yeah and Shils, 1969). In the present experiments cycloheximide, 1.0 mg/kg, was dissolved in saline and given s.c. This treatment produced alterations in the overt behavior of the rats. They became irritable, slightly aggressive, and females which were not sexually receptive vigorously kicked at the male with the hindlegs on his mounting attempts. A few of the cycloheximide-treated females had ruffled fur, and most subjects had obvious diarrhea. The symptoms were most evident 24 h after the treatment, clearly less pronounced at 48 h, and the subjects had almost recovered 72 h after the treatment.

(A) Copulatory behavior

Cycloheximide given 2 h before the EB treatment (Fig. 2A and B) significantly

References p. 145–146

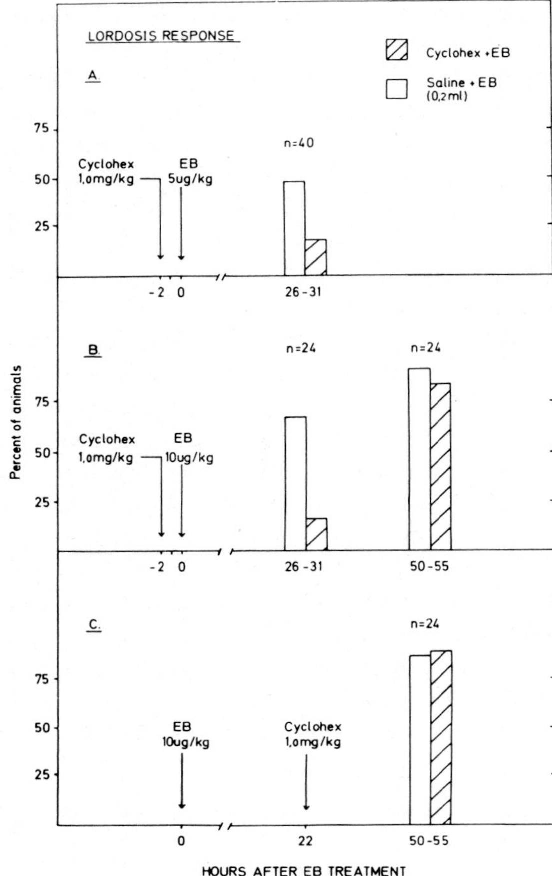

Fig. 2. The effect of cycloheximide (cyclohex.) on EB + progesterone-activated lordosis response in ovariectomized rats. Progesterone, 0.4 mg/animal was given at 22 or 46 h after the EB treatment. See also Table I.

decreased the number of females that displayed lordosis response in the 26–31-h tests. When progesterone was given 46 h after EB (Fig. 2B), in an otherwise analogous experiment, no difference was obtained between cycloheximide- and only hormone-treated animals. The effect on the overt behavior was more pronounced in the 26–31-h tests than at the 50–55-h tests. However, the effect on the lordosis response when cycloheximide was given 22 h after EB, *i.e.* 28–33 h before the behavior tests, was not significant (Fig. 2C). It appears that the inhibitory effect of cycloheximide on the lordosis response is not coupled with the effect on the overt behavior but rather related to the time of the estrogen treatment.

(B) Wheel running activity

Estrogen produces an increase in wheel running activity. This effect is not dependent

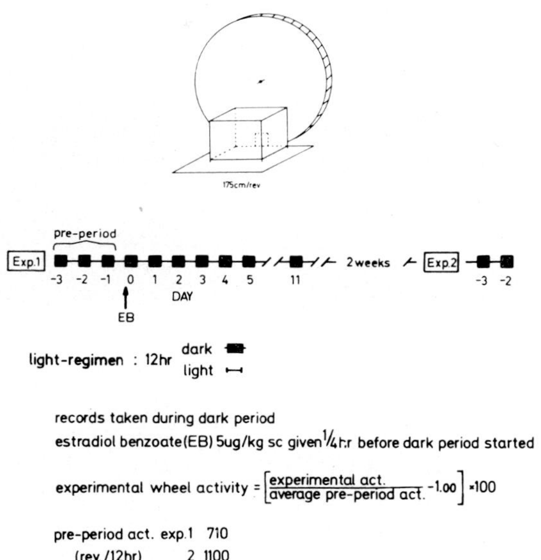

Fig. 3. Wheel running activity—experimental design. EB, 5 μg/kg s.c. was given at day 0 in Exp. 1 and 2. Cycloheximide, 1 mg/kg s.c. was given 2 h before the EB treatment in Exp. 2.

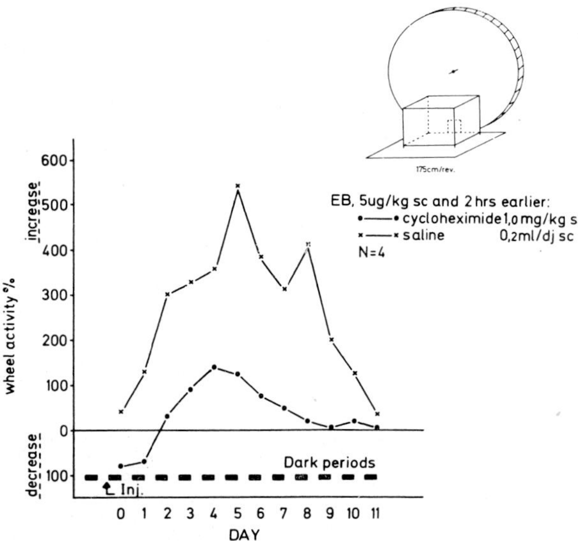

Fig. 4. Wheel running activity. The effect of cycloheximide on estradiol benzoate (EB)-activated wheel running activity in ovariectomized rats. Treatment at day 0. See also Fig. 3.

on a subsequent administration of progesterone. Four ovariectomized Sprague-Dawley females were used that had been housed in running wheels for at least 2 months before the experiment. The running wheel was adjoined by a 25 cm × 25 cm × 25 cm chamber in which the animal had free access to food and water. Each revolution

References p. 145–146

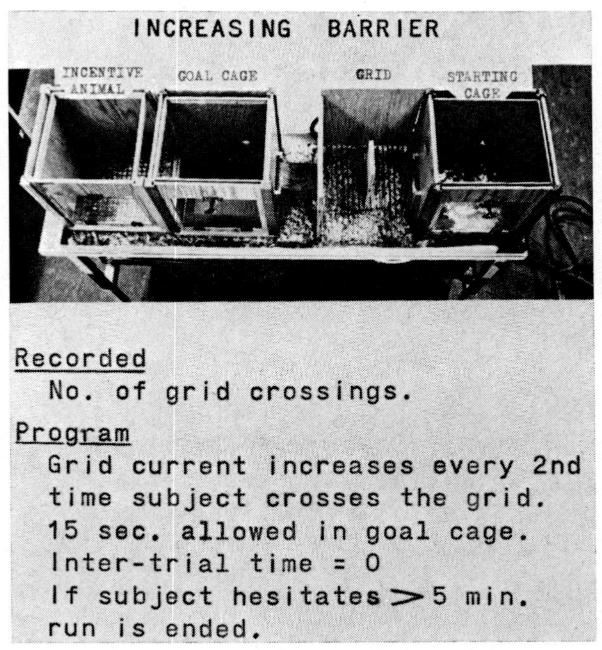

Fig. 5. Increasing-barrier technique to measure the urge of the female to seek contact with a sexually active male.

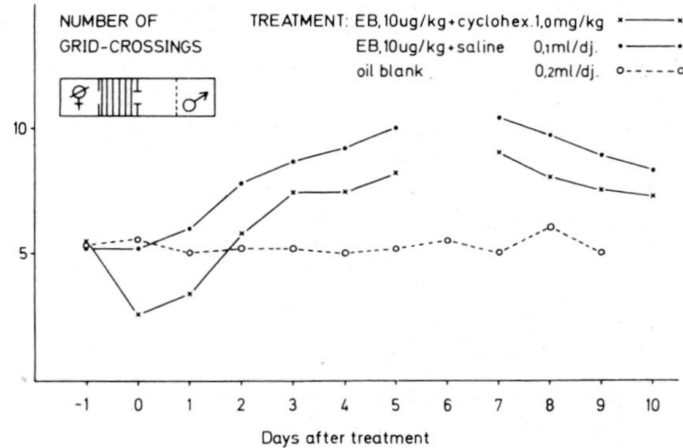

Fig. 6. Increasing-barrier technique. The effect of cycloheximide on EB-activated sexual motivation in ovariectomized rats. Cycloheximide was given 2 h before the EB treatment at day 0. N = 24.

(175 cm) triggered a print out recorder (Sodeco) which printed the number of revolutions performed during 6 h. The injection schedule and experimental procedure are evident from Fig. 3. EB: 5 μg/kg produced an increase in the wheel running activity which reached a peak value around day 4–6 after treatment (Fig. 4). Cychloheximide, 1.0 mg/kg, given 2 h before the EB treatment, clearly reduced the activity on the day of treatment (day 0) and the day after the treatment had been given. On day 2 the

activity increased and reached a peak value around days 4 and 5. The maximal response was clearly less than when the animals had estrogen only.

(C) Sexual motivation

By the use of three different techniques to measure sexual motivation it was recently demonstrated that EB induced a clearcut urge in the ovariectomized female rat to seek sexual contact with a vigorous male (Meyerson and Lindström, 1970). In the present investigation we used the increasing barrier technique which means that the subject had to pass from a starting cage *via* an electric grid to a second cage to establish contact with the male. The intensity of the current was increased stepwise every second time the animal passed. The amount of barrier shock (number of crossings) the subject was willing to take was recorded (Fig. 5). The technique is described in detail elsewhere (Meyerson and Lindström, 1973). 24 ovariectomized Sprague-Dawley rats were used. They were kept under the same laboratory conditions as were the animals used in the study of the lordosis response. EB, 10 μg/kg s.c. was given at day 0, and cycloheximide was given 2 h before the EB injection (Fig. 6). The effect of cycloheximide resembled the effect seen in the wheel running experiment. Cycloheximide-treated females crossed the grid less than oil-treated controls on days 0 and 1. The response then increased but never reached the level of the hormone-only treated females.

DISCUSSION

The three compounds used in this investigation—Mer-25, colchicine and cycloheximide—all inhibited the EB + progesterone activated lordosis response in the ovariectomized rat. The inhibitory effect was seen when the compounds were given before or in connection with the EB treatment. The same dose regimen was ineffective in decreasing the copulatory behavior when given about 24 h after the EB treatment. Colchicine and cycloheximide influenced the overt behavior to an extent which could be expected to interfere with the sexual behavior. However, the experiments in which the agents were given after the EB treatment (Figs. 1 and 2C) demonstrate that the subjects were also fully capable of displaying lordotic behavior at the time the overt behavior was most influenced by the colchicine (at about 48 h after treatment) or cycloheximide (at about 24 h after injection) treatment. The observation that the compounds did not inhibit the lordosis response if the estrogen was allowed to act for about 24 h suggests that the agents used interfered with the production of the lordotic behavior rather than that they affected the already established response.

A further interpretation of the results obtained is likely to go beyond what the available data allow. Dose– and time–effect relationships have to be further investigated before comparisons between the effects of the compounds can be made and before the effects on the different estrogen-activated patterns can be compared. However, even in the present state of this investigation it might be justifiable to comment on the dissimilarity between the effect of Mer-25 and the two other agents

References p. 145–146

used and also the differences between the effect of cycloheximide on the lordosis response and the other two estradiol-activated behavior patterns (wheel running activity and grid crossings to reach the male). Mer-25 inhibited the lordotic behavior elicited by progesterone 22 and 46 h respectively after the EB injection to almost the same extent (Table II). This is to be expected by a competitive estrogen antagonist. This feature was not seen in the cycloheximide or the colchicine experiments. In spite of a reduced response when progesterone was given at 22 h a full response was obtained when the progesterone treatment was delayed to 44 h. Cycloheximide interferes with estradiol uptake and retention in peripheral estrogen target tissue *in vitro* and *in vivo* (McGuire and Lisk, 1968; Maurer, 1970). If cycloheximide and/or colchicine interfere with the binding of estradiol in the brain at the dose levels used in the present experiments, this interaction seems to be different from that obtained from an estrogen antagonist such as Mer-25.

The initial decrease of the wheel running activity and grid crossings (the increasing barrier technique) after cycloheximide should most likely be ascribed to a non-specific effect, *i.e.* the gross behavior was affected to the extent that the estradiol-activated response was impaired. However, the total response over several days was also reduced. In this sense the results contrast with the effect obtained from cycloheximide on the lordosis response which was delayed but finally appeared. It is likely that cycloheximide interferes with the estradiol-activated behavior by more than one mechanism of action.

The predominant action of the compounds used in this investigation is receptor blockade (Mer-25), inhibition of protein synthesis (cycloheximide) and impaired microtubular function (colchicine). A comparison of the effects of these and similar compounds on hormone-activated behavior might be useful tools in the investigation of the mechanism of action of sex steroids on the behavior. However, this usefulness will be affected by whether different schedules of treatment are used, different hormone-activated behavior patterns studied and the specificity of the drug effects obtained are further controlled by compounds with analogous actions.

SUMMARY

The modification of estrogen-activated behavior by an estrogen antagonist (Mer-25), protein synthesis inhibitor (cycloheximide) and agent known to impair microtubular functions (colchicine) was studied. All three compounds inhibited EB + progesterone-activated copulatory behavior in the ovariectomized rat. The compounds did not inhibit the behavior if the estrogen was allowed to act for 24 h, which suggests that the agents used interfered with the production of the copulatory behavior rather than that they affected the already established response.

ACKNOWLEDGEMENTS

The author wishes to thank Ing. Asta Palis, Miss Ann-Kristin Söderlund and Miss

Marita Berg for efficient technical assistance. EB and progesterone were gifts from Organon (through Erco, Stockholm) and Mer-25 was kindly supplied by Wm.S. Merrel Comp., Cincinnati, Ohio. The work was supported by NIH grant RO1-HD04108-03 and Swedish Medical Research Council grant 14x-64-08.

REFERENCES

ARAI, Y. AND GORSKI, R. A. (1968) Effect of anti-estrogen on steroid induced sexual receptivity in ovariectomized rats. *Physiol. Behav.*, **3**, 351–353.

BORISY, G. G. AND TAYLOR, E. W. (1967) The mechanism of action of colchicine. *J. cell. Biol.*, **34**, 525–533.

DAHLSTRÖM, A. (1968) Effect of colchicine on transport of amine storage in sympathetic nerves of rat. *Europ. J. Pharmacol.*, **5**, 111–113.

DE ANGELO, A. B. AND GORSKI, J. (1970) Role of RNA synthesis in the estrogen induction of a specific uterine protein. *Proc. nat. Acad. Sci. (U.S.A.)*, **66**, 693–700.

DONOSO, A. O., DE GUTIERREZ MOYANG, M. B. AND SANTOLAYA, R. L. (1969) Metabolism of noradrenaline in the hypothalamus of castrated rats. *Neuroendocrinology*, **4**, 12–19.

EISENFELD, A. J. AND AXELROD, J. (1967) Evidence for estradiol binding sites in the hypothalamus-effect of drugs. *Biochem. Pharmacol.*, **16**, 1781–1785.

FUXE, K. AND HÖKFELT, T. (1969) Catecholamines in the hypothalamus and the pituitary gland. In *Frontiers in Neuroendocrinology*, W. F. GANONG AND L. MARTINI (Eds.), Oxford Univ. Press, New York, p. 47.

GLASCOCK, R. F. AND HOEKSTRA, W. G. (1959) A selective accumulation of tritium labeled hexoestrol by the reproductive organs of immature female goats and sheep. *Biochem. J.*, **72**, 673–682.

HARRIS, G. W. AND MICHAEL, R. P. (1964) The activation of sexual behavior by hypothalamic implants of oestrogen. *J. Physiol. (Lond.)*, **171**, 275–301.

HARRIS, G. W., MICHAEL, R. P. AND SCOTT, P. P. (1958) Neurological site of action of stilboestrol in eliciting sexual behaviour. In *Neurological Basis of Behaviour*, G. E. W. WHOLSTENHOLME AND C. M. O'CONNOR (Eds.), Churchill, London, p. 236.

KARLSSON, J. O. AND SJÖSTRAND, J. (1969) The effect of colchicine on the axonal transport of protein in the optic nerve and tract of the rabbit. *Brain Res.*, **13**, 617–619.

KATO, J. AND VILLEE, C. A. (1967) Preferential uptake of estradiol by the anterior hypothalamus of the rat. *Endocrinology*, **80**, 567–575.

KREUTZBERG, G. (1969) Neuronal dynamics and axonal flow, IV. Blockade of intra-axonal enzyme transport by colchicine. *Proc. nat. Acad. Sci. (U.S.A.)*, **62**, 722–725.

LERNER, L. J., HOLTHAUS, F. J. AND THOMPSON, C. R. (1958) A non-steroidal estrogen antagonist 1-(*p*-2-diethylaminoethoxyphenyl)-1-phenyl-2-*p*-methoxyphenyl ethanol. *Endocrinology*, **63**, 295–318.

LICHTENSTEIGER, W. (1969) Cyclic variations of catecholamine content in hypothalamic nerve cells during the estrous cycle of the rat, with a concommitant study of the substantia nigra. *J. Pharmacol. exp. Ther.*, **105**, 204–215.

LINDSTRÖM, L. (1972) The effect of pilocarpine and oxotremorine on hormone activated copulatory behaviour in the ovariectomized hamster. *Naunyn-Schmiedeberg's Arch. Pharmacol.*, **275**, 233–241.

LINDSTRÖM, L. AND MEYERSON, B. J. (1967) The effect of pilocarpine, oxotremorine and arecoline in combination with methylatropine or atropine on hormone-activated oestrous behaviour in ovariectomized rats. *Psychopharmacologia (Berl.)*, **11**, 405–413.

LISK, R. D. (1962) Diencephalic placement of estradiol and sexual receptivity in the female rat. *Amer. J. Physiol.*, **203**, 493–496.

LUNDBERG, D. (1970) Colchicine-induced delay of degeneration release of sympathetic transmitter in the conscious rat. *Acta. physiol. scand.*, **80**, 430–432.

MAURER, H. R. (1970) Prolonged *in vitro* retention of oestradiol by cycloheximide in rat uterus. *Endocrinology*, **56**, 257–266.

MCGUIRE, J. L. AND LISK, R. D. (1968) Estrogen receptors in the intact rat. *Proc. nat. Acad. Sci. (U.S.A.)*, **61**, 497–503.

MEYERSON, B. J. (1964) Central nervous monoamines and hormone induced estrus behaviour in the spayed rat. *Acta physiol. scand.*, **63**, suppl. 241.

MEYERSON, B. J. (1968) Amphetamine and 5-hydroxytryptamine inhibition of copulatory behavior in the female rat. *Ann. med. exp. fenn.*, **46**, 394–398.

MEYERSON, B. J. (1970) Monoamines and hormone activated oestrous behaviour in the ovariectomized hamster. *Psychopharmacologia (Berl.)*, **18**, 50–57.

MEYERSON, B. J. (1971) Optical isomers of estrogen and estrogen inhibitors as tools in the investigation of estrogen action on the brain. In *Steroid Hormones and Brain Function* (UCLA Forum, Med. Sci. No. 15, Calif.), R. A. GORSKI AND C. H. SAWYER (Eds.), Univ. of California Press, Los Angeles.

MEYERSON, B. J. (1972a) Monoamines and female sexual behaviour. In *C.I.N.P. Symp. on Drugs for Treatment of Sexual Disorders, Psychopharmacologia (Berl.)*, **265**, Suppl. 132.

MEYERSON, B. J. (1972b) Change of estrogen activated behaviour by cycloheximide in the female rat. *Acta pharmacol. toxicol.*, **31**, Suppl. 1.

MEYERSON, B. J. AND LEWANDER, T. (1970) Serotonin synthesis inhibitors and estrous behavior in female rats. *Life Sci.*, **9**, 661–671.

MEYERSON, B. J. AND LINDSTRÖM, L. (1968) Effect of an estrogen antagonist ethamoxy-triphetol (MER-25) on oestrous behaviour in rats. *Acta endocrinol. (Kbh.)*, **59**, 41–48.

MEYERSON, B. J. AND LINDSTRÖM, L. (1970) Sexual motivation in the estrogen treated ovariectomized rat. In *Hormonal Steroids.* Excerpta Med. Int. Congr. Ser. No. 219, pp. 731–737.

MEYERSON, B. J. AND LINDSTRÖM, L. (1973) Sexual behaviour in the female rat. A methodological study applied to the investigation of the effect of estradiol benzoate. *Acta physiol. scand.*, Suppl. No. 389.

MICHAEL, R. P. (1965) Oestrogens in the central nervous system. *Brit. med. Bull.*, **21**, 87–90.

PALKA, Y. S. AND SAWYER, C. H. (1966) The effects of hypothalamic implants of ovarian steroids on oestrous behaviour in rabbits. *J. Physiol.*, **185**, 251–269.

PFAFF, D. W. (1968) Uptake of ^{3}H estradiol by the female rat brain. An autoradiographic study. *Endocrinology*, **82**, 1141–1155.

QUANDAGNO, D. M., SHRYNE, J. AND GORSKI, R. A. (1971) The inhibition of steroid-induced sexual behavior by intrahypothalamic actinomycin-D. *Hormones Behav.*, **2**, 1–10.

REED, J. D. (1947) Spontaneous activity of animals: A review of the literature since 1929. *Physiol. Bull.*, **44**, 393–412.

SAWYER, C. H. (1963) Induction of estrus in the ovariectomized cat by local hypothalamic treatment with estrogen. *Anat. Rec.*, **145**, 280.

SISLER, H. D. AND SIEGEL, M. R. (1967) Cycloheximide and other glutarimide antibiotics. In *Antibiotics, Vol. 1*, D. GOTTLIEB (Ed.), Springer, Berlin, p. 283.

STEFANO, F. J. E. AND DONOSO, A. O. (1967) Norepinephrine levels in the rat hypothalamus during the estrous cycle. *Endocrinology*, **81**, 1405–1406.

STUMPF, W. E. (1968) Estradiol-concentrating neurons: topography in the hypothalamus by dry-mount autoradiography. *Science*, **162**, 1001–1003.

THIESSEN, D. D. AND YAHR, P. (1970) Central control of territorial marking in the mongolian gerbil. *Physiol. Behav.*, **5**, 275–278.

TONGE, S. R. AND GREENGRASS, P. M. (1971) The acute effects of oestrogen and progesterone on the monoamine levels of the brain in ovariectomized rats. *Psychopharmacologia (Berl.)*, **21**, 374–381.

WALLEN, K., GOLDFOOT, D. A., JOSLYN, W. D. AND PARIS, C. A. (1972) Modification of behavioral estrus in the guinea pig following intracranial cycloheximide. *Physiol. Behav.*, **8**, 221–223.

YEH, S. D. J. AND SHILS, M. E. (1969) Quantitative aspects of cycloheximide inhibition of amino acid incorporation. *Biochem. Pharmacol.*, **18**, 1919–1926.

YOUNG, W. C. (1961) The hormones and mating behavior. In *Sex and Internal Secretions, Vol. II*, W. C. YOUNG (Ed.), Williams and Wilkins, Baltimore, pp. 1173–1239.

ZIGMOND, R. E. AND MCEWEN, B. S. (1970) Selective retention of estradiol by cell nuclei in specific brain regions of the ovariectomized rat. *J. Neurochem.*, **17**, 889–899.

DISCUSSION

DE WIED: What was the influence of estradiol or cyclohexamide on shock sensitivity of your rats?

MEYERSON: I doubt that the low dose of estradiol necessary to activate this behavior influences the shock sensitivity. The estrogen treatment increased the grid crossings only if the incentive animal was a male, significantly less if run against a female one. Estrogen-treated rats did not cross more than untreated controls when the goalbox was empty. The cycloheximide effect on shock sensitivity should be considered, but very similar effects were obtained with the wheel-running method.

McEwen: Did you measure the extent of inhibition of protein synthesis in the brain at, for example, 1 or 2 h after the dose you gave?

Meyerson: No, we are not set up in my laboratory for estimation of protein synthesis. According to Yen and Shils (Biochem. Pharmacol., 18, 1919, 1969) cyclohexamide will decrease the incorporation of leucine in brain tissue by 30% after a dose half the size of that which we used in these experiments.

Bohus: Does "reinforcement" by a full copulation behavior reduce the sexual motivation of estradiol-treated female?

Meyerson: We have only preliminary results on this but it seems not so. Neither copulation before trial nor direct contact with the male in the goal-box seems to change the urge to seek contact.

Perinatal Effects of Sex Steroids on Brain Development and Function

ROGER A. GORSKI

Department of Anatomy and Brain Research Institute, UCLA School of Medicine, Los Angeles, Calif. 90024 (U.S.A.)

Distinct sex differences in brain function are reflected in the regulation of reproduction in the adult rat (Gorski, 1971a). In the male testosterone and spermatazoa are produced at a relatively constant rate and specific masculine behavioral patterns will be displayed with a sexually receptive partner essentially at any time. In contrast, the female rat exhibits cyclic reproductive activity. Cyclic changes in ovarian steroid secretion, which produce the vaginal cycle, are in turn the result of cyclic fluctuations in the hypothalamic secretion of gonadotrophin (GTH) releasing factors. Sexual behavior of the female rat, in addition to being cyclic in its appearance, is quite distinct from that of the male. The subject of the present chapter can be summarized by the question: "What brings about these functional differences in brain activity?".

Although the mature gonad may play an important role in maintaining some sex differences (for example, the pattern of GTH secretion of the ovariectomized rat does not exhibit the cyclicity of the intact female (Gay and Rees Midgley, 1969; Taleisnik *et al.*, 1971)), the subject of this chapter are those sex differences in brain function which can be demonstrated even under similar hormonal conditions. One might argue that such differences are the direct result of neuronal genetic expression. However, this is not true; rather these differences are due to the perinatal hormone environment. Specifically, the development of the masculine pattern of neuroendocrine function is due to the *permanent* action of androgen during a critical phase in neuronal development.

The permanent action of gonadal hormones during the perinatal period is unique and led to the proposal that gonadal steroids, can have two types of action depending on the state of development of the central nervous system, either "organizational" or "activational" (Phoenix *et al.*, 1959). However, Beach (1971) has critically reviewed the use of the term "organizational" to describe the permanent action of gonadal hormones, particularly with respect to behavioral parameters. We will refer to this action of gonadal hormones in terms of the physiological process in which they act, namely, the development of sexual differences in brain function, or the sexual differentiation of the brain.

Although sexual differentiation applies to both the control of pituitary GTH activity and of sexual behavior, we shall first consider the former system. Because ovulation

References p. 160–162

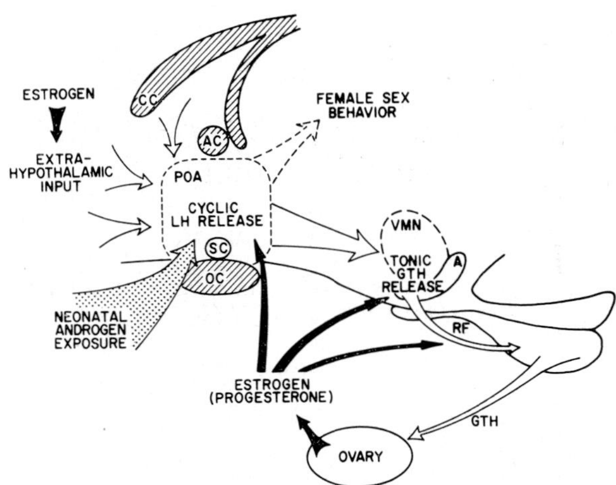

Fig. 1. Schematic concept of the localization of the neural control of GTH release projected on a parasagittal diagram of the rat brain. Black arrows indicate possible sites of feedback of ovarian hormones. Stippled arrow indicates the possible site of the permanent perinatal action of androgen. Abbreviations: A, arcuate nucleus; AC, anterior commissure; CC, corpus callosum; GTH, gonadotrophin; OC, optic chiasm; POA, preoptic area; RF, releasing factors; SC, suprachiasmatic nucleus; and VMN, ventromedial nucleus. Reprinted from Gorski (1970).

establishes the cyclic pattern of reproductive neuroendocrine regulation in the female (Schwartz, 1969), the main sex difference is the ability of the brain of the female to initiate the cyclic release of luteinizing hormone (LH) necessary for ovulation. Therefore, how the brain regulates ovulation is central to a discussion of sexual differentiation of the brain. Fig. 1 illustrates schematically the generally accepted concept that ovulation is regulated by a cyclic release mechanism for LH for which the preoptic area (POA) appears to be a key region (Gorski, 1968b, 1970; Everett, 1972).

Although recent studies suggest that the POA may be able to initiate spontaneous ovulation autonomously (Köves and Halász, 1970; Kaasjager *et al.*, 1971), the POA is certainly not the only area of the brain involved in the ovulatory process (see Donovan, 1971; Gorski, 1971b; Taleisnik and Carrer, 1972). The amygdala, hippocampus, and the midbrain have all been shown to have the potential to modify the ovulatory release of LH. Although the POA takes up and retains labelled estrogen, other regions of the brain also have this capacity (Pfaff, 1971; Stumpf, 1971). The POA represents an integrative system which is essential for ovulation, but which is subject to a modulating influence from numerous areas of the brain. The POA also contains neural elements essential for the display of sexual behavior (see Lisk, 1967). Fig. 1 suggests that the POA is an important site of the perinatal action of androgen responsible for sexual differentiation.

This view forms the basis for our current concept of the sexual differentiation of the neural control of GTH secretion (Fig. 2). Since the supporting experimental evidence has been reviewed recently (Gorski, 1971a), this concept will be only summarized briefly. A major difference between the brain of the female and male is the ability of the POA system, when ovarian tissue is present, to support a cyclic pattern

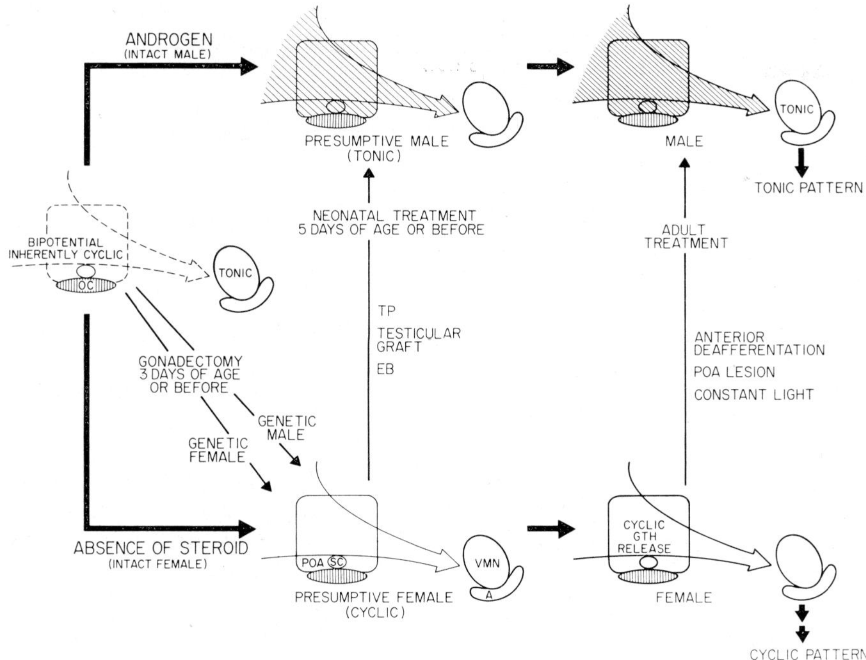

Fig. 2. A concept of the sexual differentiation of the neural control of GTH secretion in the rat. Abbreviations: EB, estradiol benzoate; TP, testosterone propionate; others as in Fig. 1. Reprinted from Gorski (1971b).

of GTH release in the female but not in the male. However, the genetic male does have the *capacity* to develop the typical female pattern as shown by the fact that after castration of the male rat within the first few days of postnatal life, he, just like the female, will release GTH cyclically and support ovulation in ovarian grafts. The stimulus for sexual differentiation of the brain is the presence of gonadal steroids during a period of neuronal sensitivity, as seen by the fact that a single injection of testosterone propionate (TP), or estradiol benzoate (EB), permanently blocks ovulation in the genetic female, and also in the male that has been castrated perinatally.

Thus, the concept of sexual differentiation of the regulation of the pituitary states that the POA system is either undifferentiated at birth in the rat, or is inherently female. In the absence of gonadal steroids the POA system matures and if ovarian tissue is provided, ovulation is possible irrespective of genetic sex. On the other hand, if the brain develops in the presence of testicular androgen in the male, or if exogenous steroids are administered, the animal when adult and provided with ovarian tissue cannot ovulate.

Although the process of androgen-induced "masculinization" of the brain is physiological only for the male, the fact that exogenous androgen can duplicate this process in the female (androgenization) is an important observation. The neonatal rat testis does produce testosterone (Resko *et al.*, 1968), but the temporal aspects of

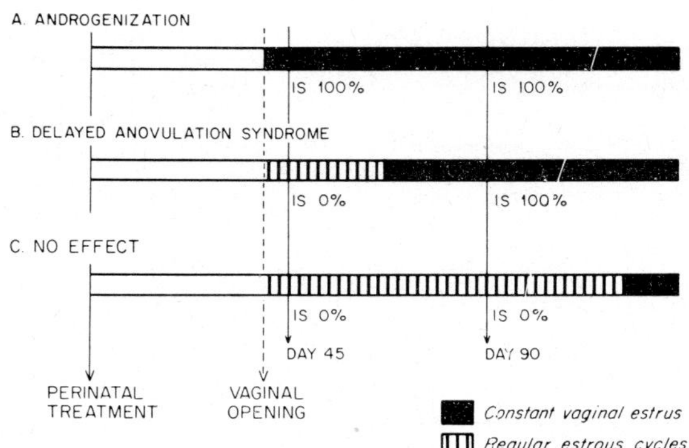

Fig. 3. A representation of the three possible effects on ovarian function of the perinatal injection of androgen to the intact female rat.

its activity are virtually unknown. In the female the experimenter can control the identity of an exogenous hormone, its dose, and the time of its injection.

There are three possible effects on ovarian function of the perinatal injection of androgen to the intact female rat (Fig. 3). The first effect is that of androgenizationl In this case the female is unable to ovulate and enters a state of persistent vagina. estrus at the time of vaginal opening. In contrast, some animals, although injected perinatally with TP, exhibit normal ovulatory vaginal cycles for a period of time after puberty, but after this delay develop anovulatory persistent vaginal estrus. We have called this response to androgen the delayed anovulation syndrome (DAS; Gorski, 1968a).

Finally, there may be no apparent effect of TP injection. Although such a female may eventually develop the anovulatory condition, this is a common occurrence in old normal rats. In our laboratory most rats, if injected with an adequate dose of TP perinatally, will become anovulatory by about 90 days of age. These different effects can be produced at will by varying the dose of TP or the age at injection. For example, rats treated with 30, 10, or 5 μg TP on day 5 of life will be androgenized, show the DAS, or continue normal ovarian function, respectively (Gorski, 1966). On the other hand, although many rats treated with 10 μg TP on day 5 develop the DAS, this same dose administered on day 2 leads to immediate postpubertal anovulatory persistent vaginal estrus (Gorski, 1968a). This observation that the effect of perinatal TP injection may vary is important for the interpretation of experiments in which we have attempted to analyse the possible mechanism of androgenization by identifying drugs which could protect against TP.

Since progesterone, reserpine, and chlorpromazine had been shown to inhibit androgenization, we initially attempted to confirm these reports by injecting one of these agents simultaneously with TP (Arai and Gorski, 1968a). As shown in Table I these agents did reduce the incidence of sterility (IS) at 60 days of age, although the effect of chlorpromazine did not reach statistical significance ($p = 0.06$). However, when the rats reached 120 days of age, sufficient numbers had shown the DAS so that there no longer was a significant effect of these potential inhibitors. Although we had

TABLE I

PROTECTION AGAINST ANDROGENIZATION

Injection(s) on day 5 of age	*Incidence of sterility*			
	at 60 days of age		*at 120 days of age*	
	Number anovulatory/ number injected	%	*Number anovulatory/ number injected*	%
30 μg TP + oil vehicle	10/11	91	10/11	91
30 μg TP + reserpine vehicle	7/8	88	8/8	100
30 μg TP + 2500 μg progesterone	2/10[a]	20[b]	7/10[a]	70[d]
30 μg TP + 10 μg reserpine	6/16	37[c]	11/16	69[d]
30 μg TP + 500 μg chlorpromazine	5/12	42[d]	9/12	75[d]
2500 μg progesterone	1/5	20	1/5	20
10 μg reserpine	0/5	0	0/5	0
500 μg chlorpromazine	0/6	0	0/6	0

[a]Incidence of sterility at 45 and 90 days of age.
[b]$p < 0.01$ *vs.* TP control.
[c]$p < 0.05$ *vs.* TP control.
[d]Not significant *vs.* TP control, Fisher Exact Probability Test.

TABLE II

PROTECTION BY THE BARBITURATES PENTOBARBITAL (PB) AND PHENOBARBITAL (PhB) AGAINST ANDROGENIZATION BY TESTOSTERONE PROPIONATE (TP)

Injection(s) on day 5 of age	*Incidence of sterility*			
	at 45 days of age		*at 90 days of age*	
	Number anovulatory/ number injected	%	*Number anovulatory/ number injected*	%
30 μg TP + saline	13/16	81	15/16	94
30 μg TP + PB[a]	0/15[e]	0	4/15[e]	27
30 μg TP + PB[a] + Metrazol[b]	18/25	72	7/10	70
30 μg TP + PhB[c]	2/17[e]	12	4/17[e]	23
30 μg TP + Metrazol[d]	5/6	83	4/6	83
PB[a]	0/12	0	0/12	0
PhB[c]	0/9	0	0/9	0

[a]Two injections (0.3 mg/rat) given 4–5 h apart.
[b]Two injections (2 mg/rat) given with PB.
[c]Single injection (0.5 mg/rat).
[d]Single injection (0.5 mg/rat).
[e]$p < 0.001$ *vs.* respective TP control group, Fisher Exact Probability Test.

hoped to demonstrate complete inhibition of androgenization, the appearance of the DAS following the injection of a highly effective dose of TP does indicate that the action of androgen had been partially inhibited or attenuated.

More complete inhibition of androgenization was obtained when the injection of TP was combined with either pentobarbital (PB) or phenobarbital (PhB). These barbiturates significantly protected against TP as determined by the IS at both 45 and

References p. 160–162

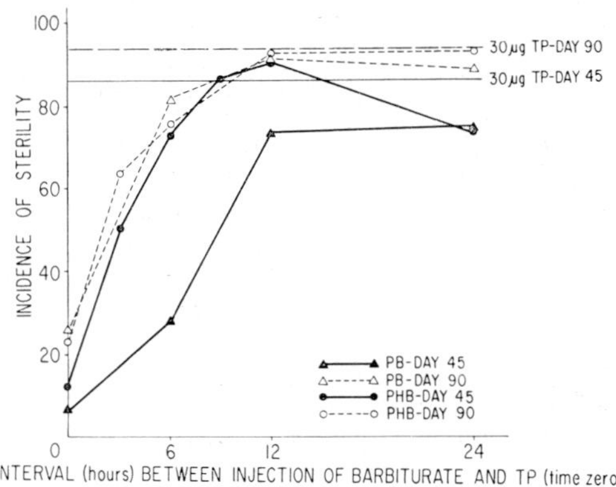

Fig. 4. Incidence of sterility at 45 and 90 days of age following the injection of 30 μg TP alone (horizontal lines), simultaneously with, or at various times prior to PB or PhB administration to the 5-day-old female rat. Reprinted from Arai and Gorski (1968b).

90 days of age (Table II; Gorski, 1971a). The inhibitory action of PB could be counteracted by the simultaneous injection of 2 mg pentylenetetrazol (Metrazol). Note that not every perturbation of brain function during the period of TP exposure will inhibit androgenization. When 0.5 mg Metrazol was injected simultaneously with TP, androgenization was not inhibited even though these animals were markedly stimulated and hyperexcitable (Table II; Sutherland and Gorski, 1972).

Since barbiturates effectively inhibited the action of TP, these drugs were used to elucidate the temporal pattern of androgenization. In this experiment the barbiturates were injected at varying intervals after the administration of an effective dose of TP. Although 30 μg TP induced anovulatory sterility in more than 80% of the animals by 45 days of age the simultaneous injection of either PB or PhB significantly inhibited androgenization (Fig. 4). When the injection of PB was delayed by 6 h, significant inhibition was still observed, but after 12 h PB was no longer effective in interfering with TP (Arai and Gorski, 1968b). Thus, a PB-sensitive component of androgen action is completed between 6–12 h after TP injection. The development of the DAS by day 90 (Fig. 4) favors the shorter interval.

Although these results suggest that the brain need be exposed to TP for a brief period of only 6 h, note that when PhB was used as the potential inhibitor, even a 3-h delay was sufficient to render this drug ineffective. The fact that these drugs have different temporal patterns of effectiveness, suggests that they may act on different (but unidentified) components of the androgenization process.

Because the perinatal action of TP is permanent, it is likely that it involves an alteration in fundamental neuronal biochemical processes. To investigate the possible nature of these biochemical processes, we studied the ability of the subcutaneous (s.c.) injection of actinomycin-D or puromycin to inhibit the action of s.c. TP. Although we did observe attenuation of androgenization, the temporal pattern of this inhibition was complex and we could provide no evidence that these toxic antibiotics were interacting specifically with an androgen-sensitive process in the brain (Kobayashi

TABLE III

INFLUENCE OF THE INTRAHYPOTHALAMIC IMPLANTATION OF VARIOUS AGENTS IN COCOA BUTTER AT 5 DAYS OF AGE ON SUBSEQUENT OVARIAN FUNCTION IN THE ADULT FEMALE RAT

Subcutaneous injection	*Intrahypothalamic implant*		*Incidence of sterility*			
			At 45 days of age		*At 90 days of age*	
	Substance	*Total dose (μg)*	*Number anovulatory/ number injected*	%	*Number anovulatory/ number injected*	%
30 μg TP	–	–	29/37	78	34/37	92
–	Cocoa Butter	–	0/6	0	1/6	17
–	Actinomycin-D	0.2	1/6	17	1/6	17
–	Chloramphenicol	16.0	0/5	0	0/5	0
–	Cycloheximide	14.0	0/2	0	0/2	0
–	Puromycin	1.4	0/2	0	0/2	0
–	Rifampicin	15.0	0/6	0	0/6	0
–	Sarkomycin	12.0	0/7	0	0/7	0
–	Streptomycin Sulfate	18.0	0/6	0	0/6	0
–	Atropine	11.0	0/2	0	0/2	0
–	Procaine	15.0	0/2	0	0/2	0

and Gorski, 1970). To circumvent these problems we acutely implanted various antibiotics directly into the POA of 5-day-old rats under cold anesthesia, and immediately after recovery injected TP s.c. (Gorski and Shryne, 1972).

At this point it is necessary to consider the theoretical role of genetic mechanisms in sexual differentiation of the brain. Although it is clearly established that the rat, male or female, is born with the *potential* to develop the cyclic pattern of GTH secretion, nothing is known about the normal maturation of this system even in the female. It is possible that genetically regulated processes are required to *establish* the adult female pattern. Androgen might act by inhibiting these processes. If true, one would predict that specific antibiotics when placed in the developing brain might also inhibit these same processes and mimic the action of TP. However, sarkomycin, a DNA

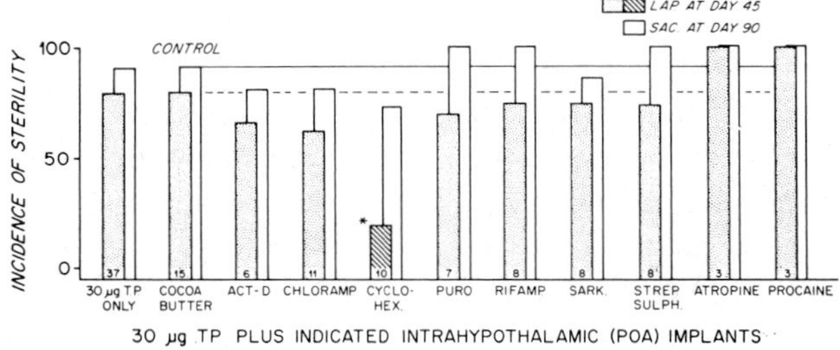

Fig. 5. Influence of the implantation into the POA in the 5-day-old rat of cocoa butter pellets containing various agents upon the effectiveness of a simultaneous subcutaneous injection of TP as measured by the IS at 45 and 90 days of age. The IS resulting from the control procedure is represented by horizontal lines. Figures at the base of each bar indicate the number of rats per group. Asterisk indicates that cycloheximide (combined results from two dosages) significantly ($p < 0.01$) attenuated TP action (Fischer Exact Probability Test). Reprinted from Gorski and Shryne (1972).

References p. 160–162

synthesis inhibitor; actinomycin-D, rifampicin, RNA synthesis inhibitors; or the protein synthesis inhibitors, chloramphenicol, cycloheximide, puromycin or streptomycin sulfate, did not cause anovulatory sterility in animals treated s.c. only with oil (Table III). Thus, these antibiotics and at the doses employed, do not mimic the action of TP when implanted in the POA.

On the other hand, TP might activate genetic mechanisms which ultimately *inhibit* the development of the female cyclic pattern or perhaps *induce* mechanisms specifically responsible for the tonic pattern of GTH secretion. In this case one would predict that an appropriate antibiotic would inhibit androgenization. When these same antibiotics were implanted into the POA of 5-day-old rats also injected s.c. with TP, only cycloheximide was found to attenuate androgen action (note that by day 90 even these animals had developed the DAS; Fig. 5). In a limited number of rats intrahypothalamic implants of atropine or procaine were not able to inhibit androgenization (Gorski and Shryne, 1972). These results suggest that androgenization may require protein synthesis. Several experiments support this possibility. Shimada and Gorbman (1970) reported that the forebrain of the androgenized female rat possesses a unique species of RNA. Clayton *et al.* (1970) demonstrated a unique amino acid uptake response of the POA (and also the amygdala) following the neonatal injection of androgen. Finally, Salaman (1970) has observed that androgenization alters the rate of RNA labelling in the anterior hypothalamus.

Unfortunately, the fact that androgen may act through protein synthesis does not clarify the precise mechanism of androgenization. Androgen may alter the brain morphologically particularly with respect to neuronal connectivity. This concept has received support from the recent demonstration of a morphological sex difference within the POA (Raisman and Field, 1971). It is also possible that androgenization alters transmitter function. Ladosky and Gaziri (1970) have suggested that serotonin metabolism may play an important role in androgenization. They believe that critical steps in sexual differentiation occur after the tenth day of life. Although this appears to contradict the results with barbiturate injection which suggest a rapid effect of androgen, it must be emphasized that functional neuronal development is complex. It may be that androgenization which is initiated by TP exposure very early in postnatal life, takes many weeks to complete. At each stage one might be able to inhibit androgenization with a different and specific agent.

Finally, it is possible that androgenization involves the development of the neuronal steroid receptor system. It has been reported that the adult androgenized female takes up and retains less labelled estrogen (see Lisk, 1971; Gorski, 1971a). Vértes and King (1971) and Lobl (1972) reported that neuronal nuclear uptake of estrogen is altered by androgenization. Since the outcome of sexual differentiation of the brain requires gonadal hormones for expression (*i.e.*, ovarian tissue must be present to detect the presence or absence of cyclic GTH release, and the androgenization of sexual behavior is also dependent on the presence of gonadal steroids), it is probable that androgenization involves an alteration in the synthesis, maintenance, or function of steroid receptor mechanisms in the brain.

Although this chapter has focused on GTH secretion, sexual differentiation of the regulation of sexual behavior appears to be a more widespread phenomenon and has been reported for the rat (see Whalen, 1968; Dorner, 1970; Gorski, 1971a), guinea pig (Phoenix *et al.*, 1959), hamster (Ciaccio and Lisk, 1971; Paup *et al.*, 1972), monkey (at least with reference to mounting behavior; Goy and Phoenix, 1971), and perhaps man (Money, 1971). Although the male and female rat normally exhibit distinct behavioral patterns, the concept of the differentiation of behavioral mechanisms

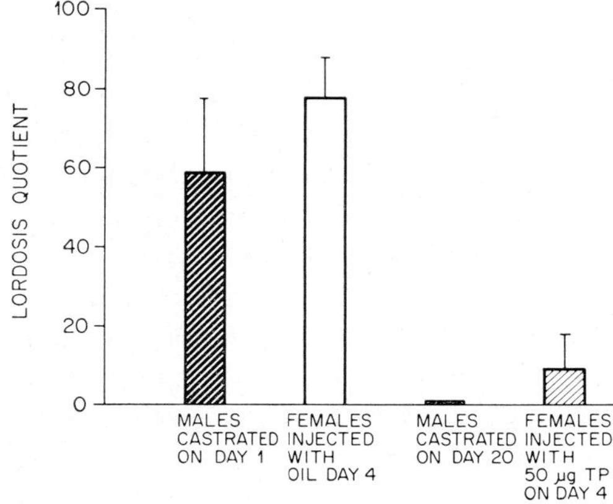

Fig. 6. The perinatal influence of endogenous or exogenous androgen on the sex difference in the display of lordosis behavior by estrogen-progesterone primed gonadectomized adult rats. Males castrated on day 20 and androgenized females exhibited a significantly ($p < 0.001$) reduced LQ. Data from Quadagno *et al.* (1972).

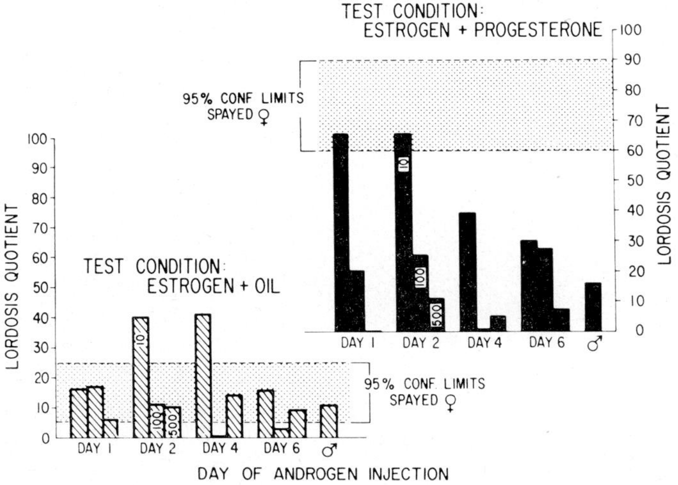

Fig. 7. Influence of 10, 100, or 500 μg TP administered to female rats of various ages on their adult display of the lordosis response subsequent to ovariectomy and priming with estrogen and progesterone (solid bars) or with estrogen alone (shaded bars). The mean response of the male orchidectomized as an adult, as well as the 95% confidence limits for the response of normal ovariectomized females similarly primed with ovarian hormones, are also indicated. Based on data from Clemens *et al.* (1969, 1970) and reprinted from Gorski (1971c).

implies that one cannot necessarily identify the genetic sex of an animal by its sexual behavior under experimental conditions. Consideration of the lordosis response, a major component of female sexual behavior, will illustrate this point. Although there is a clear sex difference in the display of lordosis behavior following priming with EB and progesterone, this difference is not genetic but is established by the perinatal hormone environment. In Fig. 6 female sexual behavior is expressed in terms of the lordosis quotient (LQ) which is the percent of the mounts by a stud male accompanied by lordosis of the test animal. The ovariectomized female, when primed with EB and progesterone, displays a high LQ, while the male castrated as an adult (or as early as day 10; Grady, *et al.*, 1965) and primed with similar doses of EB and progesterone, will only rarely exhibit lordosis. Androgenization of the female rat inhibits lordosis behavior of the adult, while early postnatal castration of the male produces a genetic male capable of attaining female levels of lordosis behavior (Quadagno *et al.*, 1972).

The suppression of lordosis behavior by the perinatal injection of TP in the female is both dose- and age-dependent (Fig. 7). Treating the neonatal female with increasing doses of TP within the first 6 days of life causes a more marked suppression of lordosis behavior (Clemens *et al.*, 1969, 1970). Because the suppression of lordosis behavior was determined following priming with both EB and progesterone, it is difficult to specify the cause of this behavioral deficit. However, when lordosis behavior is studied following priming only with EB the androgenized females as well as the normal male attain an LQ not less than that of the normal female (Fig. 7). Although the LQ of the normal female primed only with EB is quite low, the similar behavior of the androgenized female led to the conclusion that androgenization may lower the progesterone sensitivity of the brain. In fact, it is possible that the androgenized female can be more responsive to EB behaviorally than the normal female (Clemens *et al.*, 1969).

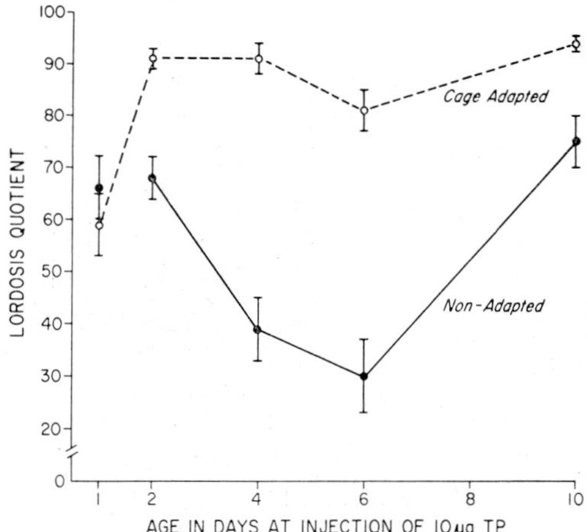

Fig. 8. Facilitation of the LQ of adult females injected with 10 μg TP at different ages induced by a 2-h "adaptation" to the mating arena. The closed circles indicate the mean LQ of these same animals when not allowed the pretest adaptation period. All behavioral tests were performed on ovariectomized rats following estrogen-progesterone priming. Based on data from Clemens *et al.* (1969) and reprinted from Gorski (1971a).

The apparent decrease in progesterone sensitivity following androgenization is particularly interesting since progesterone may act in the mesencephalic reticular formation to facilitate lordosis behavior (Ross *et al.*, 1971). It is possible that the site of the perinatal action of TP in the rat may not be restricted to the POA as indicated in Fig. 2, but may influence the development of other brain regions as diverse as the reticular formation.

Beach (1971) has argued that the concept of the perinatal "organizational" action of androgen is potentially misleading. The data illustrated in Fig. 8 support this view. Treatment of the 4- or 6-day-old female rat with 10 μg TP markedly suppresses the LQ when these animals are tested following ovariectomy and replacement with ovarian hormones. The concept of the "organizational" action of TP would suggest that the neural substrate for lordosis behavior did not develop properly in these animals. That this is not true, however, is demonstrated by the observation that when the testing conditions are altered (*i.e.*, the females are allowed a period to adjust to the testing arena (adaptation)), these same animals exhibit normal female levels of lordosis behavior (Clemens *et al.*, 1969). As Beach has suggested, it is likely that perinatal androgen exposure alters the *responsiveness* of the rat to environmental and hormonal influences, rather than anatomically organizing or disorganizing neuronal circuits.

Table IV summarizes the concept of sexual differentiation in the rat. Although the development of the testis or ovary is directly dependent on genetics, further masculine differentiation of the sexual ducts, the genitalia, and the brain appears to depend on

TABLE IV

SEXUAL DIFFERENTIATION IN THE RAT

Dependent on genetics	*Dependent on a testicular factor*		*Dependent on testicular androgen*		
	Prenatal differentiation		*Postnatal differentiation*		
Testis	Development of wolffian derivatives	Development of male genitalia	Suppression of hypothalamo-hypophyseal cyclicity (in presence of an ovary)	Suppression of capacity to respond to *ovarian hormones and mounting stimuli* with lordosis	Alteration in unknown parameters of brain function
	Apparently independent of perinatal gonadal factors				
Ovary	Development of mullerian derivatives	Development of female genitalia	Development of hypo-thalamo-hypophyseal cyclicity (in presence of an ovary)	Development of full capacity to respond to *ovarian hormones and mounting stimuli* with lordosis	Alteration in unknown parameters of brain function

References p. 160–162

the activity of the testes. The fact that the cyclic release of GTH and the display of lordosis behavior require ovarian hormones in the adult, is consistent with the view that androgenization involves a permanent change in the brain's ability to respond to these hormones. In the case of lordosis, and possibly GTH release, androgenization may alter the response of the brain to environmental factors as well. Our studies with drugs and antibiotics suggest that it will be possible with further study to characterize the process of androgenization temporally and in terms of possible alterations in neurochemical development. However, the elucidation of the precise mechanism(s) of androgenization requires much additional study. It is also important to note that the full extent of the effect of androgen on the developing brain is unknown. The perinatal hormone environment may influence adult social behavior (Goy and Phoenix, 1971; Quadagno *et al.*, 1972), open field and emergence behavior (Pfaff and Zigmond, 1971), agressive behavior (Vale *et al.*, 1972), and the regulation of body weight (see Wade, 1972). Certainly in the case of the latter process (and probably in all) the dose of androgen is again an important variable (Tarttelin and Gorski, unpublished observations). The physiological or pharmacological significance of these possible effects of gonadal hormones on the developing brain awaits further study.

SUMMARY

The concept that the perinatal steroid environment determines sexual differences in neuroendocrine function is reviewed both with respect to the control of pituitary activity and of female sexual behavior. Various drugs were used to elucidate the possible mechanism(s) of exogenous androgen in "masculinizing" the brain. These studies suggest that exposure of the brain to androgen for a relatively brief perinatal period induces complex changes in neural development which may involve protein synthesis among other possible biochemical changes. However, the precise nature and the full extent of the action of androgen on the developing brain are unknown and require further study.

ACKNOWLEDGEMENT

The original research of the author has been supported by USPHS Grant HD-01182 and by the Ford Foundation. The excellent technical assistance of J. Shryne and E. Freiberg is gratefully acknowledged.

REFERENCES

Arai, Y. and Gorski, R. A. (1968a) Protection against the neural organizing effect of exogenous androgen in the neonatal rat. *Endocrinology*, **82**, 1005–1009.

Arai, Y. and Gorski, R. A. (1968b) The critical exposure time for androgenization of the developing hypothalamus in the female rat. *Endocrinology*, **82**, 1010–1014.

BEACH, F. A. (1971) Hormonal factors controlling the differentiation, development, and display of copulatory behavior in the ramstergig and related species. In *The Biopsychology of Development*, E. TOBACH, L. R. ARONSON AND E. SHAW (Eds.), Academic Press, New York, pp. 249–296.

CIACCIO, L. A. AND LISK, R. D. (1971) Estrogen effects on development and activation of neural systems mediating receptivity. In *Influence of Hormones on the Nervous System* (Proc. Int. Soc. Psychoneuroendocrinol., Brooklyn, 1970), Karger, Basel, pp. 441–450.

CLAYTON, R. B., KOGURA, J. AND KRAEMER, H. C. (1970) Sexual differentiation of the brain: effects of testosterone on brain RNA metabolism in newborn female rats. *Nature (Lond.)*, **226**, 810–812.

CLEMENS, L. G., HIROI, M. AND GORSKI, R. A. (1969) Induction and facilitation of female mating behavior in rats treated neonatally with low doses of testosterone propionate. *Endocrinology*, **84**, 1430–1438.

CLEMENS, L. G., SHRYNE, J. AND GORSKI, R. A. (1970) Androgen and development of progesterone responsiveness in male and female rats. *Physiol. Behav.*, **5**, 673–678.

DONOVAN, B. T. (1971) The extrahypothalamic control of gonadotrophin secretion. In *Control of Gonadal Steroid Secretion*, D. T. BAIRD AND J. A. STRONG. Edinburgh Univ. Press, Edinburgh, pp. 2–14.

DORNER, G. (1970) Neuro-endocrine pathogenesis, prevention and treatment of congenital sexual deviations. *German med. Monthly,* **15**, 108–113.

EVERETT, J. W. (1972) Brain, pituitary gland, and the ovarian cycle. *Biol. Reprod.*, **6**, 3–12.

GAY, V. L. AND REES MIDGLEY, JR., A. (1969) Response of the adult rat to orchidectomy and ovariectomy as determined by LH radioimmunoassay. *Endocrinology*, **84**, 1359–1364.

GORSKI, R. A. (1966) Localization and sexual differentiation of the nervous structures which regulate ovulation. *J. Reprod. Fertil.*, Suppl. **1**, 67–88.

GORSKI, R. A. (1968a) Influence of age on the response to paranatal administration of a low dose of androgen. *Endocrinology*, **82**, 1001–1004.

GORSKI, R. A. (1968b) The neural control of ovulation. In *Biology of Gestation, Vol. I, The Maternal Organism*, N. S. ASSALI (Ed.), Academic Press, New York, pp. 1–66.

GORSKI, R. A. (1970) Localization of hypothalamic regulation of pituitary function. *Amer. J. Anat.*, **129**, 219–222.

GORSKI, R. A. (1971a) Gonadal hormones and the perinatal development of neuroendocrine function. In *Frontiers in Neuroendocrinology, 1971*, L. MARTINI AND W. F. GANONG (Eds.), Oxford Univ. Press, New York, pp. 237–290.

GORSKI, R. A. (1971b) Steroid hormones and brain function: Progress, principles and problems In *Steroid Hormones and Brain Function* (UCLA Forum Med. Sci. No. 15), C. H. SAWYER AND R. A. GORSKI (Eds.), Univ. of California Press, Los Angeles, pp. 1–26.

GORSKI, R. A. (1971c) Sexual differentiation of the hypothalamus. In *The Neuroendocrinology of Human Reproduction*, H. C. MACK AND A. I. SHERMAN (Eds.), Thomas, Springfield, Ill., pp. 60–90.

GORSKI, R. A. AND SHRYNE, J. (1972) Intracerebral antibiotics and adrogenization of the neonatal female rat. *Neuroendocrinology*, **10**, 109–120.

GOY, R. W. AND PHOENIX, C. H. (1971) The effects of testosterone propionate administered before birth on the development of behavior in genetic female Rhesus monkeys. In *Steroid Hormones and Brain Function* (UCLA Forum Med. Sci. No. 15), C. H. SAWYER AND R. A. GORSKI (Eds.), Univ. of California Press, Los Angeles, pp. 193–202.

GRADY, K. L., PHOENIX, C. H. AND YOUNG, W. C. (1965) Role of the developing rat testis in differentiation of the neural tissues mediating mating behavior. *J. comp. physiol. Psychol.*, **59**, 176–182.

KAASJAGER, W. A., WOODBURY, D. M., VAN DIETEN, J. A. M. J. AND VAN REES, G. P. (1971) The role played by the preoptic region and the hypothalamus in spontaneous ovulation and ovulation induced by progesterone. *Neuroendocrinology*, **7**, 54–64.

KOBAYASHI, F. AND GORSKI, R. A. (1970) Effects of antibiotics on androgenization of the neonatal female rat. *Endocrinology*, **86**, 285–289.

KÖVES, K. AND HALÁSZ, B. (1970) Location of the neural structures triggering ovulation in the rat. *Neuroendocrinology*, **7**, 180–193.

LADOSKY, W. AND GAZIRI, L. C. J. (1970) Brain serotonin and sexual differentiation of the nervous system. *Neuroendocrinology*, **6**, 168–174.

LISK, R. D. (1967) Sexual behavior: hormonal control. In *Neuroendocrinology, Vol. II*, L. MARTINI AND W. F. GANONG (Eds.), Academic Press, New York, pp. 197–239.

LISK, R. D. (1971) The physiology of hormone receptors. *Amer. Zool.*, **11**, 755–767.

LOBL, R. T. (1972) Alterations in uptake of estrogen *in vitro* by cell nuclei of the anterior hypothalamus and uterus. *Excerpta Med. Int. Congr. Series No. 256*, 120.

MONEY, J. (1971) Clinical aspects of prenatal steroidal action on sexually dimorphic behavior. In *Steroid Hormones and Brain Function* (UCLA Forum Med. Sci. No. 15), C. H. SAWYER AND R. A. GORSKI (Eds.), Univ. of California Press, Los Angeles, pp. 325–338.

PAUP, D. C., CONIGLIO, L. P. AND CLEMENS, L. G. (1972) Masculinization of the female golden hamster by neonatal treatment with androgen or estrogen. *Hormones Behav.*, in press.

PFAFF, D. W. (1971) Steroid sex hormones in the rat brain: specificity of uptake and physiological effects. In *Steroid Hormones and Brain Function* (UCLA Forum Med. Sci. No. 15), C. H. SAWYER AND R. A. GORSKI (Eds.), Univ. of California Press, Los Angeles, pp. 103–112.

PFAFF, D. W. AND ZIGMOND, R. E. (1971) Neonatal androgen effects on sexual and non-sexual behavior of adult rats tested under various hormone regimes. *Neuroendocrinology*, **7**, 129–145.

PHOENIX, C. H., GOY, R. W., GERALL, A. A. AND YOUNG, W. C. (1959) Organizing action of prenatally administered testosterone propionate on the tissues mediating mating behavior in the female guinea pig. *Endocrinology*, **65**, 369–382.

QUADAGNO, D. M., SHRYNE, J., ANDERSON, C. AND GORSKI, R. A. (1972) Influence of gonadal hormones on social, sexual, emergence, and open field behaviour in the rat. *Rattus norvegicus. Animal Behav.*, in press.

RAISMAN, G. AND FIELD, P. M. (1971) Sexual dimorphism in the preoptic area of the rat. *Science*, **173**, 731–733.

RESKO, J. A., FEDER, H. H. AND GOY, R. W. (1968) Androgen concentrations in plasma and testis of developing rats. *J. Endocrinol.*, **40**, 485–491.

ROSS, J., CLAYBAUGH, C., CLEMENS, L. G. AND GORSKI, R. A. (1971) Short latency induction of estrous behavior with intracerebral gonadal hormones in ovariectomized rats. *Endocrinology*, **89**, 32–38.

SALAMAN, D. F. (1970) RNA synthesis in the rat anterior hypothalamus and pituitary: relation of neonatal androgen and the oestrous cycle. *J. Endrocrinol.*, **48**, 125–137.

SCHWARTZ, N. (1969) A model for the regulation of ovulation in the rat. *Rec. Progr. Hormone Res.*, **25**, 1–55.

SHIMADA, H. AND GORBMAN, A. (1970) Long lasting changes in RNA synthesis in the forebrains of female rats treated with testosterone soon after birth. *Biochem. biophys. res. Commun.*, **38**, 423–430.

STUMPF, W. E. (1971) Autoradiographic techniques and the localization of estrogen, androgen, and glucocorticoid in the pituitary and brain. *Amer. Zool.*, **11**, 725–739.

SUTHERLAND, S. D. AND GORSKI, R. A. (1972) An evaluation of the inhibition of androgenization of the neonatal female rat brain by barbiturate. *Neuroendrocrinology*, **10**, 94–108.

TALEISNIK, S., CALIGARIS, L. AND ASTRADA, J. J. (1971) Sex differences in hypothalamo-hypophyseal function. In *Steroid Hormones and Brain Function* (UCLA Forum Med. Sci. No. 15), C. H. SAWYER AND R. A. GORSKI (Eds.), Univ. of California Press, Los Angeles, pp. 171–184.

TALEISNIK, S. AND CARRER, H. F. (1972) Facilitatory and inhibitory mesencephalic influences on gonadotropin release. In *Proc. Second Congr. int. Soc. Psychoneuroendocrinol.*, Budapest, 1971, Akadémiai Kiadó, Budapest, in press.

VALE, J. R., RAY, D. AND VALE, C. A. (1972) The interaction of genotype and exogenous neonatal androgen: agonistic behavior in female mice. *Behav. Biol.*, **7**, 321–334.

VÉRTES, M. AND KING, R. J. B. (1971) The mechanism of oestradiol binding in rat hypothalamus: effect of androgenization. *J. Endocrinol.*, **51**, 271–282.

WADE, G. N. (1972) Gonadal hormones and behavioral regulation of body weight. *Physiol. Behav.*, **8**, 523–534.

WHALEN, R. E. (1968) Differentiation of the neural mechanisms which control gonadotropin secretion and sexual behavior. In *Perspectives in Reproduction and Sexual Behavior*, M. DIAMOND (Ed.), Indiana Univ. Press, Bloomington, Ind., pp. 303–340.

DISCUSSION

KITAY: I fully appreciate the precision with which you limited your conclusion about the use of antibiotics, but I am very curious to know whether you are aware of any experimental situations where implantation of very small amounts of protein inhibitors in circumscribed implants have affected protein synthesis in any way. Did you start out with the anticipation that you could have demonstrated a positive effect were one to be demonstrated?

GORSKI: No, I do not know of any experiments where anyone has implanted these antibiotics into the brain. We initially began this study by injecting actinomycin-D and puromycin subcutaneously along with androgen. Although we observed some competition, when we considered the interpretation of these results, we realized that we had no evidence to suggest that there was a specific interaction between these toxic agents and androgen in the preoptic area which is where we feel androgen is acting. In order to overcome this obstacle we put these potential inhibitors directly into this area of the brain. These agents do produce effects although we have not attempted to characterize these effects biochemically. In the adult female the intracerebral implantation of 0.18 μg actinomycin-D will kill the animal, so it does something! In the animals which survived neonatal implantation of antibiotics we usually do not see brain lesions. One animal which was not given androgen did develop sterility and that was an animal implanted with actinomycin (Table III). In this case we found that the preoptic area had been destroyed.

KITAY: Would it be fair to say then that the absence of a blocking effect doesn't prove anything? Had you come up with something it would have had meaning.

GORSKI: Yes, I would agree with that.

KORÁNYI: You demonstrated that barbiturates are able to inhibit androgenization. The barbiturates themselves have a long lasting effect on the central nervous system. After barbiturate administration, spindles can be recorded on the EEG for a day or more and paradoxical sleep cycles in the rat are altered for a week.

GORSKI: This effect of pentobarbital is intriguing because of its long action on other systems. I would like to mention some preliminary data obtained by Hayashi in our laboratory which might appear to contradict our results with barbiturates. From our work with pentobarbital, we conclude that the brain has to be exposed to androgen for only about 6 h. Hayashi has implanted crystalline testosterone fused to cannulae. After these cannulae were in the brain for a certain number of hours he removed them. He has found that the brain must be exposed to crystalline testosterone proprionate for about 72 h, not 6.

CARROLL: Could I draw you out Dr. Gorski on whether you think that the barbiturates have any effect in the organization of the normal male hypothalamus and if so, whether these might have any clinical significance?

GORSKI: In our laboratory we have shown and confirmed that barbiturates can prevent the action of androgen on the female rat brain. Since the normal male is exposed to his own androgen, theoretically one could prevent normal masculine differentiation by exposing the male to barbiturates, although we haven't studied this. In the clinical situation it is possible that pregnant women who are misusing barbiturates could be interfering with the psychosexual differentiation of their male offspring. Although there is no experimental evidence it is theoretically possible, for example, that the pregnant woman who misuses barbiturates might contribute to a predisposition toward homosexuality in her male child.

DICKEY: Progesterone, reserpine, chlorpromazine and phenobarbital all effect androgenization. This would seem to suggest that perhaps this isn't a question of a receptor but that transmission is involved in the action of androgen.

GORSKI: Let me review the data of Ladosky which may fit in with what you are suggesting. I quoted Ladosky as suggesting that serotonin metabolism might be involved in androgenization. He is able to block the effect of endogenous androgen which in our terms is over by the second or third day of life, as late as day 10 of life with chlorpromazine. Because the normal female and male have the same brain levels of serotonin until day 12, he believes the process of androgenization involves serotonin metabolism and, thus, maybe some transmission process. Our concept is that androgen by some mechanism initiates biochemical changes in the central nervous system which may take many weeks to express themselves, maybe not even until the time of puberty. Somewhere along the way certainly transmission may be involved. As to whether or not the initial event in androgenization involves steroid uptake, protein synthesis, or transmission, I really don't know.

Hypothalamic Monoamine Levels and Gonadotrophin Secretion Following Deafferentation of the Medial Basal Hypothalamus

RICHARD I. WEINER

Department of Anatomy, University of Southern California, School of Medicine, Los Angeles, Calif. 90033 (U.S.A.)

At the present time a voluminous literature suggests that brain monamines are putative neurotransmitters important in the regulation of luteinizing hormone (LH), follicle-stimulating hormone (FSH), and prolactin (see McCann *et al.*, 1972). Data obtained using the Falck-Hillarp formaldehyde fluorescence technique have shown the existence of at least three anatomically discrete populations of neurons containing the monoamines noradrenaline (NA), dopamine (DA), and serotonin (5-HT) which innervate the hypophysiotrophic region of the hypothalamus (see Hökfelt and Fuxe, 1972). A major impasse to our present understanding is the role these multiple monoaminergic systems play in the physiological regulation of gonadotrophin secretion. For example, there is evidence using various models which suggests that DA, NA, and adrenaline can stimulate the release of LH (Kamberi *et al.*, 1969; Kalra *et al.*, 1972; Rubinstein and Sawyer, 1970). Serotonin appears to inhibit LH release (Kordon *et al.*, 1968). However, there is incomplete information as to which monoaminergic system is important in the transfer of neural information resulting in the release of LH during various stages of the estrous cycle. As discussed below, recent studies performed in our laboratory which measured changes in the monoamine content of the deafferented medial basal hypothalamus (MBH) suggested that it might be possible to use the deafferented MBH as a model to study regulation of gonadotrophin secretion by dopamine-containing neurons in the absence of noradrenergic or serotoninergic influences.

CHANGES IN MONOAMINE LEVELS FOLLOWING DEAFFERENTATION

The medial basal hypothalami of mature Sprague-Dawley female rats were deafferented using the technique of Halász and Pupp (1965). The dimensions of the knife used were: height, 2.2 mm and rotational radius, 1.4–1.6 mm. All of the fibers entering or leaving the MBH were transected and this procedure is referred to as complete deafferentation. The deafferented island within the boundaries of the cut is coexistent with the hypophysiotrophic region. 3 to 5 weeks following deafferentation, the animals

References p. 169–170

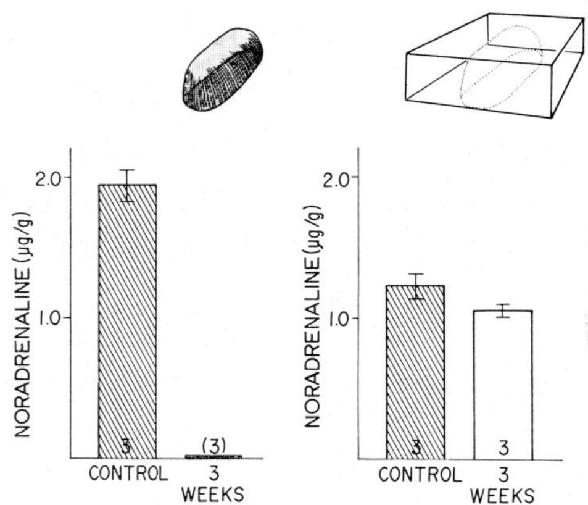

Fig. 1. Effect of complete deafferentation on the noradrenaline concentration of the deafferented island (left side) and the residual basal hypothalamic fragment (right side). Values are the mean ± the SEM of pools of tissue. The *n* for the mean is shown within each column. Redrawn from Weiner *et al.* (1972).

were sacrificed by decapitation and both the deafferented island and the residual basal hypothalamic tissue were dissected from the brain (Weiner *et al.*, 1972a). In the first series of studies, the deafferented island and residual basal hypothalamic fragment from 4–6 rats were pooled separately and analyzed for NA and DA. Controls were obtained from animals deafferented immediately before sacrifice. NA and DA levels were measured using a modification of the trihydroxindole fluorescence technique (Udenfriend and Zaltzman-Nirenberg, 1963). In a second series of studies the 5-HT content of the deafferented island was determined using the ninhydrin fluorescence technique (Snyder *et al.*, 1965). Since it was impossible to verify the completeness of the deafferentations by histological techniques, two other criteria were used: (*1*) visual observation of the boundaries of the deafferented island on the base of the brain under a dissecting microscope. (*2*) the occurrence of a persistently leukocytic vaginal smear for at least two weeks (Halász and Gorski, 1967).

NA was not detectable in the deafferented island 3 weeks after surgery (Fig. 1). The NA concentration of the residual hypothalamic fragment was not altered. The dopamine content of both the deafferented island and the residual basal hypothalamic fragment was not altered (Fig. 2). Confirming these findings in another study, in which the residual basal hypothalamic fragment and deafferented island were pooled, the DA concentration also was not found to decrease whereas the NA concentration decreased significantly (Weiner *et al.*, 1972a). The serotonin concentration of the deafferented island was found to be only 30% of its control level 4 weeks after deafferentation (Fig. 3). These data demonstrate that the vast majority of serotoninergic and noradrenergic terminals within the deafferented island degenerate. Only the dopaminergic terminals are left relatively intact. In the control animals the concentration of NA and DA in the deafferented island was almost double that of the residual basal hypothalamic fragment (Figs. 1 and 2). These data demonstrate that the NA- and DA-containing terminals are more concentrated in the medial basal hypothalamus

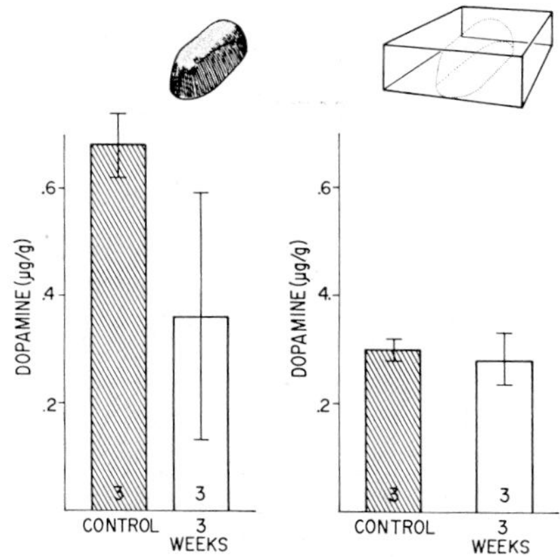

Fig. 2. Effect of complete deafferentation on the dopamine concentration of the deafferented island and the residual basal hypothalamic fragment. Values are the mean ± SEM of pools of tissue. The *n* for the mean is shown within each column. Redrawn from Weiner *et al.* (1972).

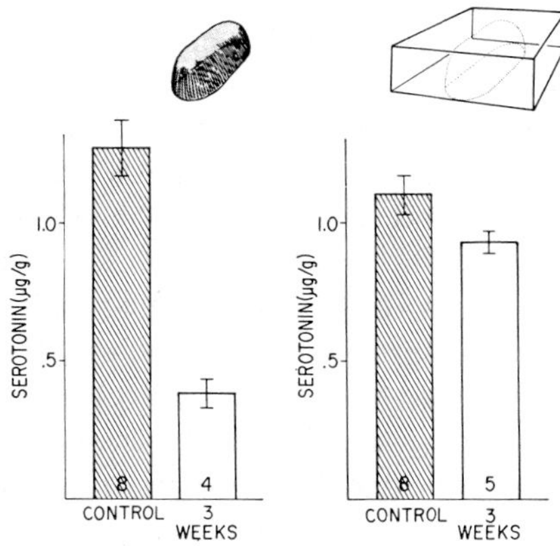

Fig. 3. Effect of complete deafferentation on the serotonin concentration of the deafferented island and the residual basal hypothalamic fragment. Values are the mean ± the SEM of pools of tissue. The *n* for the mean is shown within each column.

than in the surrounding hypothalamic tissue. The serotonin-containing terminals appear to be more evenly distributed throughout the hypothalamus (Fig. 3).

CHANGES IN GONADOTROPHIN SECRETION FOLLOWING DEAFFERENTATION

Following complete deafferentation of the MBH, the animals became persistently diestrous and the circulating levels of both LH and FSH were found to decrease when compared with normally cycling rats during diestrus I, estrus and proestrus (Weiner *et al.*, 1972b; Blake *et al.*, 1972a). Serum prolactin levels were not depressed following complete deafferentation (Blake *et al.*, 1972b). The ovulatory surge of all three hormones was absent in these animals. The data in the present study would indicate that the dopamine-containing neurons within the MBH (tubero-infundibular dopamine neurons) are intact following complete deafferentation. Other studies have demonstrated that the neurosecretory neurons which control pituitary, LH, FSH and prolactin secretion are functional within the deafferented island (Halász and Gorski, 1967). Therefore, dopaminergic and/or neurosecretory neurons within the deafferented island must have additional neural input in order to regulate the estrous cycle. The question then becomes whether dopaminergic neurons have any autonomous influence on hormone secretion in the absence of outside neural information.

Barraclough and Sawyer (1959) first demonstrated that depletion of brain amines results in prolactin release. More recent studies have demonstrated that the administration of alpha-methyl-*p*-tyrosine (α-MPT), a synthesis inhibitor of catecholamines, causes a rapid increase in the circulating levels of prolactin (Donoso *et al.*, 1971). We therefore tested whether α-MPT could stimulate prolactin release in the complete deafferented animal. Complete deafferented rats which had a persistently leukocytic vaginal smear for 2 weeks were injected with 250 mg/kg i.p. of α-MPT methylester and sacrificed 0.5 and 1 h later. Controls received either nothing or a placebo injection of water 0.5 h before sacrifice by decapitation. Serum prolactin levels were measured using the NIAMD radioimmunoassay. A 3- and 6-fold increase in serum prolactin levels were observed 0.5 and 1 h, respectively, after the injection of the drug (unpublished data). These data demonstrate that, in the absence of either noradrenergic or serotoninergic influences, the tubero-infundibular dopamine neurons tonically inhibit the secretion of prolactin, probably by stimulating the secretion of prolactin-inhibiting factor (PIF). Removal of this tonic action following α-MPT treatment resulted therefore in an increased prolactin release from the anterior pituitary. These results are in good agreement with work done on intact animals. Kamberi *et al.* (1971) demonstrated that the intraventricular injection of DA decreased the circulating levels of prolactin. Donoso *et al.* (1971), in experiments utilizing the systemic administration of multiple pharmacological agents, concluded that the stimulation of prolactin release in castrated rats by α-MPT was mediated *via* dopaminergic neurons.

The tubero-infundibular dopamine neurons appear to terminate in the external layer of the median eminence either axo-axonally or in immediate contact with the pericapillary space (Hökfelt and Fuxe, 1972). These neurons may influence the rate of secretion of neurosecretory neurons terminating in this region in a number of ways. One possibility is that the dopaminergic neurons may alter the firing rate of the neurosecretory neurons *via* axo-axonic endings. An alternate possibility is that DA is released in the region of the perivascular space of the portal vessels and reaches the endings of neurosecretory neurons *via* diffusion. Dopamine may stimulate the release of neurosecretory material without inducing a change in neural activity. Some indirect evidence for this hypothesis is that DA injected into the 3rd ventricle of female rats did not result in a change in neural activity in the median eminence (Weiner *et al.*, 1971). However, both NA and adrenaline caused dramatic changes in neural activity. Secondly, in the experiments of Schneider and McCann (1969), DA was capable of causing the release of neurosecretory material from a hypothalamic fragment *in vitro*.

The lability of the neural activity of brain tissue in response to anoxia is well established. Thirdly, DA injected into the 3rd ventricle caused morphological changes on the lining of the floor of the 3rd ventricle consistent with the induction of a secretory process (Schechter and Weiner, 1972).

Further studies are in progress using the complete deafferented rat as a model to study the role of dopaminergic neurons in the control of gonadotrophin secretion. Hopefully information obtained from this model will permit the integration of our present knowledge concerning the role of these multiple aminergic systems.

SUMMARY

Female Sprague-Dawley rats were deafferented by the Halász technique. Complete deafferentation of the medial basal hypothalamus resulted in the disappearance of most of the NA and serotonin from the circumscribed region. However, dopamine levels were not significantly affected. Administration of the catecholamine synthesis inhibitor alpha-methyl-*p*-tyrosine to these animals caused a 6-fold increase in serum prolactin levels. These data suggest that dopamine-containing neurons are involved in the alpha-methyl-*p*-tyrosine-induced release of prolactin.

REFERENCES

BARRACLOUGH, C. AND SAWYER, C. (1959) Induction of pseudopregnancy in the rat by reserpine and chlorpromazine. *Endocrinology*, **65**, 563–571.

BLAKE, C., WEINER, R., GORSKI, R. AND SAWYER, C. (1972a) Secretion of pituitary luteinizing hormone and follicle stimulating hormone in female rats made persistently estrous or diestrous by hypothalamic deafferentation. *Endocrinology*, **90**, 855–861.

BLAKE, C., WEINER, R. AND SAWYER, C. (1972b) Pituitary prolactin secretion in female rats made persistently estrous or diestrous by hypothalamic deafferentation. *Endocrinology*, **90**, 862–866.

DONOSO, A., BISHOP, W., FAWCETT, C., KRULICH, L. AND MCCANN, S. (1971) Effects of drugs that modify brain monoamine concentrations on plasma gonadotropin and prolactin levels in the rat. *Endocrinology*, **89**, 774–784.

HALÁSZ, B. AND PUPP, L. (1965) Hormone secretion of the anterior pituitary gland after partial or total interruption of neural afferents to the medial basal hypothalamus. *Endocrinology*, **77**, 553–562.

HALÁSZ, B. AND GORSKI, R. (1967) Gonadotrophic hormone secretion in female rats after partial or total interruption of neural afferents to the medial basal hypothalamus. *Endocrinology*, **80**, 608–622.

HÖKFELT, T. AND FUXE, K. (1972) On the morphology and the neuroendocrine role of the hypothalamic catecholamine neurons. In *Brain–Endocrine Interaction*, K. KNIGGE, D. SCOTT AND A. WEINDL (Eds.), Karger, München, pp. 181–223.

KALRA, P., KALRA, S., KRULICH, L., FAWCETT, C. AND MCCANN, S. (1972) Involvement of norepinephrine in transmission of the stimulatory influence of progesterone on gonadotropin release. *Endocrinology*, **90**, 1168–1776.

KAMBERI, I., MICAL, R. AND PORTER, J. (1969) Luteinizing hormone-releasing activity in hypophysial stalk blood and elevation by dopamine. *Science*, **166**, 388–390.

KAMBERI, I., MICAL, R. AND PORTER, J. (1971) Effect of anterior pituitary perfusion and intraventricular injection of catecholamines on prolactin release. *Endocrinology*, **88**, 1012–1020.

KORDON, C., JAVOY, F., VASSENT, G. AND GLOWINSKI, J. (1968) Blockade of superovulation in the immature rat by increased brain serotonin. *Europ. J. Pharmacol.*, **4**, 169–174.

MCCANN, S., KALRA, P., DONOSO, A., BISHOP, W., SCHNEIDER, H., FAWCETT, C. AND KRULICH, L. (1972) The role of monoamines in the control of gonadotropin and prolactin secretion. In *Brain–*

Endocrine Interaction, K. KNIGGE, D. SCOTT AND A. WEINDL (Eds.), Karger, München, pp. 224–235.

RUBINSTEIN, L. AND SAWYER, C. (1970) Role of catecholamines in stimulating the release of pituitary ovulating hormone(s) in rats. *Endocrinology*, **86**, 988–995.

SCHECHTER, J. AND WEINER, R. (1972) Ultrastructural changes in the ependymal lining of the median eminence following the intraventricular administration of catecholamine. *Anat. Rec.*, **172**, 643–650.

SCHNEIDER, H. AND MCCANN, S. (1969) Possible role of dopamine as transmitter to promote discharge of LH-releasing factor. *Endocrinology*, **85**, 121–132.

SNYDER, S., AXELROD, J. AND ZWEIG, M. (1965) A sensitive and specific fluorescence assay for tissue serotonin. *Biochem. Pharmacol.*, **14**, 831–835.

UDENFRIEND, S. AND ZALTZMAN-NIRENBERG, P. (1963) Norepinephrine and 3,4-dihydroxy-phenethylamine turnover in guinea pig brain *in vivo*. *Science*, **142**, 394–396.

WEINER, R., BLAKE, C., RUBINSTEIN, L. AND SAWYER, C. (1971) Electrical activity of the hypothalamus: effects of intraventricular catecholamines. *Science*, **171**, 411–412.

WEINER, R., SHRYNE, J., GORSKI, R. AND SAWYER, C. (1972a) Changes in the catecholamine content of the rat hypothalamus following deafferentation. *Endocrinology*, **90**, 867–873.

WEINER, R., GORSKI, R. AND SAWYER, C. (1972b) Hypothalamic catecholamines and pituitary gonadotropic function. In *Brain–Endocrine Interaction*, K. KNIGGE, D. SCOTT AND A. WEINDL (Eds.), Karger, München, pp. 236–244.

DISCUSSION

SCAPAGNINI: Dick, did you check the dopamine content 30 min or 1 h after α-MPT?

WEINER: No, we didn't. It is very difficult to measure dopamine content in complete-deafferented animals. In the studies in which I showed these measurement tissues from 5 or 6 animals were pooled for each determination.

SMELIK: In 1968, we reported that reserpine implants in the median eminence provoke pseudopregnancy indicative of increased prolactin secretion (Neuroendocrinol. 3, 177, 1968). I think that this is consistent with the kind of information you obtained.

WEINER: Yes, thank you for that comment.

MESS: You have shown that serotonin content of the deafferented hypothalamus is decreased. Have you investigated it following only frontal cuts, and have you investigated LH concentration following frontal deafferentation?

WEINER: Following frontal cuts, serum LH levels were increased. The levels were not tonically high but showed periodic increases throughout the day. In other studies Blake *et al.* (Endocrinology, 90, 855, 1972) found a significant increase in LH release in anterior deafferented rats. Studies designed to measure the hypothalamic serotonin content following anterior deafferentation are now being performed.

COLLU: I am glad to hear, Dick, that you found an increase in LH secretion in frontal deafferented rats because we have recently found that when prepubertal male rats are completely deafferented there is an inhibition in the development of puberty and the weights of their testes, prostate, and seminal vesicles are very low. In contrast, 25 days following frontal deafferentation the weights of these structures were much higher than those of the controls. This is in accord with your data on the effect of total or frontal deafferentation on plasma LH levels in adult female rats.

Role of Brain Noradrenaline in the Tonic Regulation of Hypothalamic Hypophyscal Adrenal Axis

UMBERTO SCAPAGNINI AND PAOLO PREZIOSI

Institute of Pharmacology, Faculty of Medicine, University of Naples, Via Pansini 5, 80131 Naples (Italy)

The role of the central nervous system in the regulation of the synthesis and release of corticotrophin (ACTH) has been generally recognized (Mangili *et al.*, 1966; McCann and Porter, 1969; Ganong, 1970, 1972). The neuronal pathways subserving this regulation are widespread, but finally they converge on the hypothalamus (Ganong, 1972).

The hypothalamus, moreover, contains peptidergic secretory neurons elaborating and releasing several "releasing factors" constituting a type of "final common pathway" by which the information is transmitted to the anterior pituitary. Although a corticotrophin-releasing factor (CRF) has not yet been chemically identified and synthesized, the neurovascular hypothesis of ACTH secretory cell regulation seems to be well founded (McCann and Porter, 1969). Since hypothalamic neurosecretory cells are located in a post-synaptic position with regard to the terminals of the central nervous pathways converging on the hypothalamus (Zambrano, 1968; Kobayashi and Matsui, 1969) and since many of the terminals contain monoamine granules (Zambrano, 1968; Fuxe and Hökfelt, 1969; Kobayashi and Matsui, 1969) one might assume that there is at that level a regulation by naturally occurring synaptic transmitters.

A possible role of brain catecholamines in the regulation of ACTH secretion has been considered by numerous investigators. These substances are not *per se* the hypothalamic CRFs (Guillemin and Rosenberg, 1955; Saffran and Schally, 1955; Martini *et al.*, 1960). Long (1952) suggested that adrenaline from the adrenal medulla is an important factor in the stimulation of ACTH secretion, but others have argued against the validity of this hypothesis (Ganong, 1963). Several groups of investigators have reported increased adrenal corticosteroid secretion after the injection of catecholamines directly into the brain (Endröczi *et al.*, 1963; Naumenko, 1968; Krieger and Krieger, 1965, 1970). On the other hand, numerous studies have failed to support an excitatory role of brain catecholamines in the regulation of ACTH secretion (Smelik, 1967; Carr and Moore, 1968; De Schaepdryver *et al.*, 1969).

A reappraisal of the literature suggests a different hypothesis as a basic one for an interaction between brain catecholamines and ACTH secretion.

Reserpine does not release active catecholamines (Kopin and Gordon, 1962, 1963). It produces depletion of brain catecholamines in association with increased secretion

References p. 181–183

of ACTH (Maickel *et al.*, 1961; Munson, 1963) and CRF (Bhattacharya and Marks, 1969a). Such an effect seems to be independent of the change in body temperature that may be produced by the drug (Bhattacharya and Marks, 1969a). Moreover, drugs interfering with the synthesis (Carr and Moore, 1968; Vernikos-Danellis, 1968; Bhattacharya and Marks, 1970) and with the site of action (De Wied, 1967; Bhattacharya and Marks, 1969a) of brain catecholamines increase the activity of the hypothalamic-pituitary-adrenal axis.

On the contrary, drugs such as amphetamine, which appears to release active catecholamines from nerve endings (Glowinski and Axelrod, 1966), and monoamine oxidase (MAO) inhibitors, which decrease catabolism of catecholamines, decrease ACTH secretion (Lorenzen and Ganong, 1967; Hirsch and Moore, 1968; Bhattacharya and Marks, 1969b).

Stresses such as electric shock, hemorrhage, and hypoglycemia are associated with decreased brain noradrenaline content (Bliss *et al.*, 1968; Thierry *et al.*, 1968) and increased ACTH secretion (Ganong and Lorenzen, 1967).

Moreover, the intravenous injection of L-3,4-dihydroxyphenylalanine (L-DOPA) a catecholamine precursor that crosses the blood brain barrier (Wurtman, 1966), is able to inhibit, in the dog, adrenocortical activation due to laparotomy stress, whereas systemically injected dopamine and noradrenaline, unable to cross the blood brain barrier, fail to do so. Pretreatment with drugs affecting the available stores of endogenous catecholamines modifies the amount of L-DOPA necessary to produce this inhibition (Van Loon *et al.*, 1971a).

The above-mentioned observations have led us to consider the possibility in the brain of an adrenergic system that inhibits ACTH secretion. This hypothesis was

TABLE I

DRUGS INJECTED INTO THE THIRD VENTRICLE IN SURGICALLY STRESSED DOGS

Data from Van Loon *et al.*, 1971b. Except in the case of L-DOPA (see text), the effective dose is the minimum dose producing consistent inhibition.

Produced inhibition of ACTH secretion	
	Effective total dose
L-DOPA	20 mg
Dopamine	4 mg
L-noradrenaline	5 mg
Tyramine	20 mg
α-Ethyltryptamine	8 mg
Produced no inhibition of ACTH secretion	
	Total dose
Saline	—
Acid saline, pH 4.2	—
Acid saline, pH 1.0	—
D-noradrenaline	5 mg
Vanylmandelic acid (VMA)	5 mg

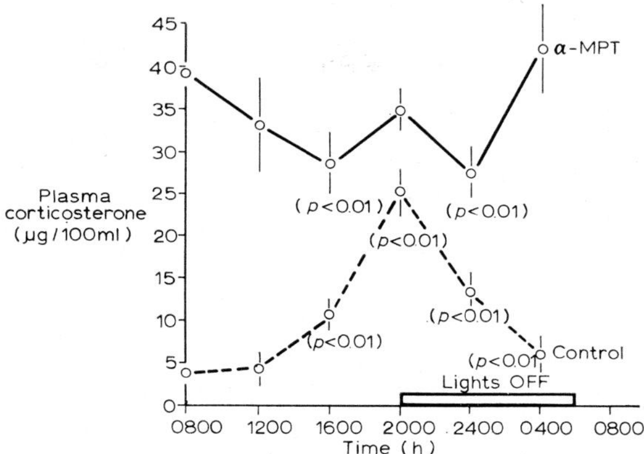

Fig. 1. Diurnal fluctuation of plasma corticosterone in control animals (dashed line) and animals treated with *α*-methyl-*p*-tyrosine (*α*-MPT) (solid line) 250 mg/kg, 9 h previously. The black bar represents the period of darkness (Data from Scapagnini *et al.*, 1970).

tested by our group by injecting catecholamines and related compounds directly into the third ventricle of the dog brain, near the median eminence (Van Loon *et al.*, 1971b). We found that catecholamine precursors, catecholamines and drugs that release or protect catecholamines from inactivation inhibit stress-induced ACTH secretion upon injection into the third ventricle. A metabolite (vanylmandelic acid) and a biologically less active isomer (*D*-noradrenaline) had no inhibitory effect (Table I).

However, we must emphasize that the amounts of drugs necessary to produce the inhibition were large compared with the levels of endogenous catecholamines present in the brain. This calls into question the physiological significance of the inhibition; it is possible to suggest that, in reality, the adrenocortical activation is reduced because the large amount of drugs injected gives a constriction of the portal vessels so that CRF cannot reach the anterior pituitary in a fair concentration. More experiments are required to settle this point.

The experiments in dogs mentioned above give only suggestions. It is in experiments in rats that we can show in a better way the existence of the central adrenergic mechanism inhibiting ACTH secretion. A first series of experiments (Scapagnini *et al.*, 1970) involved the intraperitoneal administration of α-methyl-*p*-tyrosine (α-MPT), a drug that inhibits catecholamine synthesis (Corrodi *et al.*, 1966), and the killing of the animals 9 h later, at which time we determined the hypothalamic catecholamine level and the plasma corticosterone level. The drug, no matter at what time of day it was injected, caused an increase in adrenocortical activity (Fig. 1). In our experiments we used the soluble form (methyl-ester) of the compound; in this way we avoided the possibility of interpreting the rise as due to local irritation, as did Carr and Moore (1968) who used the insoluble form.

Additional confirmation of the idea that α-MPT increases ACTH secretion *via* a mechanism involving decreased catecholamine synthesis, and thus probably decreases catecholamine release at synapses, was obtained by altering the effect of α-MPT by

TABLE II

INHIBITION BY L-DOPA OF THE EFFECT OF α-MPT ON PLASMA CORTICOSTERONE (μg/100 ml)

Values are means which have been compared using Duncan's multiple range test. Any two means underscored by the same continuous line are not significantly different. Any two means not underscored by the same continuous line are significantly different at $P < 0.05$. Data from Van Loon *et al.* (1971c).

Treatment	*α-MPT*[a] + L-*NA*[b]	*α-MPT*	*α-MPT* + L-*DOPA*[c]	L-*NA*	*Control*	L-*DOPA*
Number of animals	12	36	37	6	27	15
Mean	50.2	38.2	16.1	8.2	5.7	5.5

[a] α-Methyl-*p*-tyrosine, 250 mg/kg.
[b] L-noradrenaline, 0.5 mg/kg.
[c] L-DOPA, 100 mg/kg.

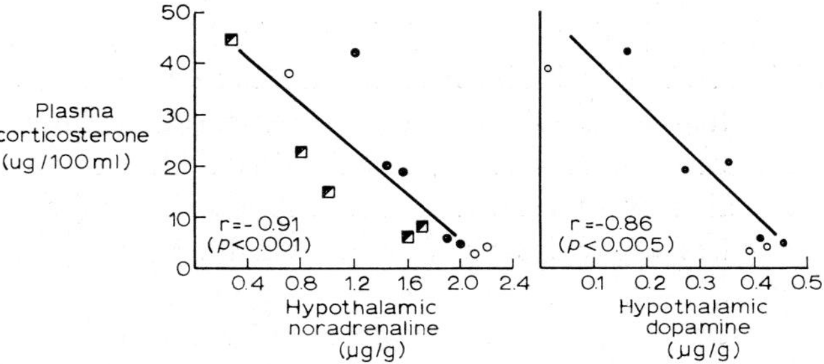

Fig. 2. Correlation between plasma corticosterone and hypothalamic noradrenaline and dopamine concentration after administration of α-MPT plus L-DOPA. The different symbols represent values obtained in experiments carried out on different days. (Data from Van Loon *et al.*, 1971b).

maintaining the availability of catecholamines in spite of tyrosine hydroxylase inhibition. We therefore administered L-DOPA to α-MPT-treated rats (Van Loon *et al.*, 1971c). The L-DOPA inhibited the mean increase in plasma corticosterone produced by α-MPT if administered simultaneously with it. On the other hand, administration of L-noradrenaline had no such effect (Table II). Moreover, a highly significant negative linear correlation was found between plasma corticosterone and hypothalamic concentrations of both noradrenaline and dopamine after α-MPT plus L-DOPA (Fig. 2).

The intraventricular administration of a systemically ineffective dose of α-MPT increased the plasma corticosterone concentration (Fig. 3). Even stronger evidence that the inhibitory system is a central one came from the use of guanethidine (Scapagnini *et al.*, 1971), a catecholamine depletor that does not cross the blood-brain barrier (Cox and Maickel, 1969). When the compound was administered systemically, it failed to increase plasma corticosterone and to deplete brain catecholamines; however, when guanethidine was injected into the third ventricle, it produced, 8 h later, an elevation of plasma corticosterone and a depletion of hypothalamic noradrenaline

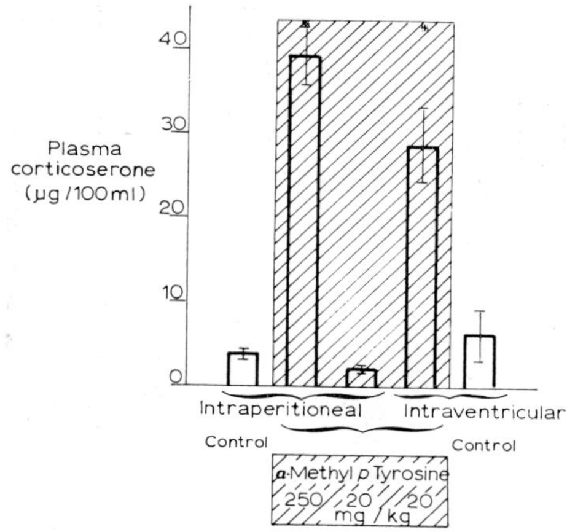

Fig. 3. Effects of intraventricular and i.p. administration of α-MPT on plasma corticosterone. The data are the pooled results of two experiments. *P* controls < 0.01. (Data from Van Loon *et al.* 1971b).

and dopamine (Table III). These results suggest that, in the rat, a central adrenergic system inhibits ACTH secretion.

To investigate whether dopamine or noradrenaline is the mediator of the inhibition, we used two pharmacological tools that gave us the possibility of a selective depletion of noradrenaline or dopamine (Scapagnini *et al.*, 1972). To deplete noradrenaline selectively we used the bis (4-methyl-1-homopiperazinylthiocarbonyl)-disulfide (FLA-63), an inhibitor of dopamine-β-oxidase. This drug, given at the dose of 10

TABLE III

CORRELATION BETWEEN PLASMA CORTICOSTERONE AND HYPOTHALAMIC CONTENTS OF NORADRENALINE AND DOPAMINE AFTER GUANETHIDINE

Treatment	*Number of animals*	*Plasma corticosterone (μg/100 ml)*	*Hypothalamic contents (μg/g)*	
			Noradrenaline	*Dopamine*
Guanethidine intraperitoneal (30 mg/kg)	12	4.7 ± 1.1[a]	1.86 ± 0.09	0.37 ± 0.02
Saline intraperitoneal	9	5.2 ± 1.0	1.90 ± 0.10	0.39 ± 0.08
Guanethidine intraventricular (1 mg/kg)	12	38.8 ± 3.2[b]	1.08 ± 0.10[b]	0.27 ± 0.06
Saline intraventricular	8	9.9 ± 4.0	1.91 ± 0.08	0.40 ± 0.12

[a]Values are means ± standard error.
[b]Significantly different from corresponding saline control at $P < 0.01$.

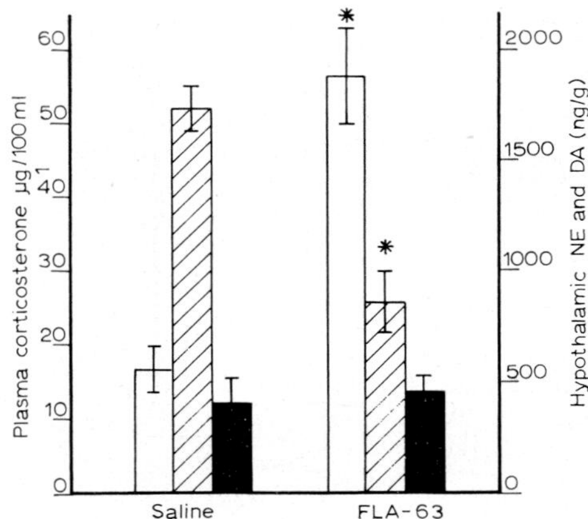

Fig. 4. Correlation among plasma corticosterone (open bars) and hypothalamic contents of noradrenaline (dashed bars) and dopamine (black bars) 4 h after administration of FLA-63, 10 mg/kg. Data from Scapagnini *et al.*, 1972).
* Significantly different from corresponding saline control at $P < 0.01$.

mg/kg, produced 4 h later a fall of brain noradrenaline without affecting dopamine. In these conditions a clearcut adrenocortical activation was present, stressing the importance of the role played by noradrenaline (Fig. 4); a highly significant negative linear correlation was found between plasma corticosterone and hypothalamic content of noradrenaline.

To deplete dopamine selectively we first depleted both noradrenaline and dopamine using α-MPT and then we repleted noradrenaline selectively with L-threo-dihydroxyphenylserine (DOPS). In this experiment we found that the adrenocortical activation usually occurring after α-MPT was strongly inhibited by administration of L-DOPS

TABLE IV

CORRELATION BETWEEN PLASMA CORTICOSTERONE AND HYPOTHALAMIC CONTENTS OF NORADRENALINE AND DOPAMINE AFTER α-MPT AND α-MPT PLUS L-DOPS

Treatment	*Number of animals*	*Plasma corticosterone (µg/100 ml)*	*Hypothalamic contents*	
			Noradrenaline	*Dopamine*
Saline	9	4.4 ± 0.8[d]	1.91 ± 0.09	0.37 ± 0.08
α-MPT (250 mg/kg)	12	41.2 ± 2.8[a]	0.62 ± 0.15[a]	0.10 ± 0.02[a]
α-MPT (250 mg/kg) + DOPS (200 mg/kg)	15	11.2 ± 2.4[b, c]	1.52 ± 0.08[b, c]	0.09 ± 0.07[a]

[a]Significantly different from saline-injected animals at $P < 0.01$.
[b]Significantly different from saline-injected animals at $P < 0.05$.
[c]Significantly different from α-MPT-injected animals at $P < 0.01$.
[d]Values are means ± standard error.

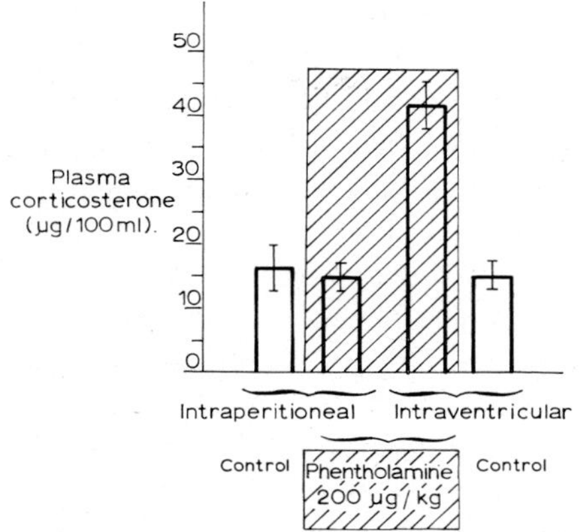

Fig. 5. Effect of i.p. and intraventricular administration of phentolamine 200 μg/kg, 1 h previously on plasma corticosterone level. (Data from Scapagnini and Preziosi, 1972).

(Table IV). These findings once more emphasize that fair amounts of hypothalamic noradrenaline are needed to control the activity of the hypothalamic-pituitary-adrenal axis. The nature of the adrenergic receptors involved in the ACTH inhibiting system was also considered in our study (Scapagnini and Preziosi, 1973).

In rats the systemic (intraperitoneal) administration of phentolamine, an α-blocking agent, is able to produce an increase of the plasma corticosterone level. The increase is found mainly 1 h after the administration and at the dose of 2 mg/kg. Because of the possible general effects produced by the systemic administration of the α-blocking agent—*e.g.* on the blood pressure—this result is not good evidence for specific adrenocortical activation due to a receptorial removal of the tonic noradrenergic inhibition. The administration of propranolol, a β-adrenergic blocking

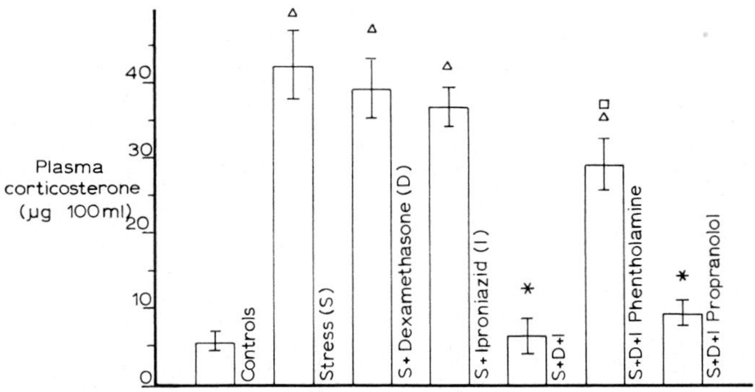

Fig. 6. Effects of i.p. injection of phentolamine or propranolol on the dexamethasone + iproniazid-induced block of adrenocortical activation provoked by laparotomy stress. Phentolamine (2 mg/kg) was given 45 min and propranolol (2 mg/kg) 30 min before the killing. Dexamethasone (1 mg/kg) was given 195 min and iproniazid (100 mg/kg) 17 h before the killing. △, P controls < 0.01; *, P stress < 0.01; □, P stress < 0.05. (Data from Scapagnini and Preziosi, 1972).

References p. 181–183

agent, at different doses did not produce any change in the plasma corticosterone level.

In an additional experiment, the injection into the third ventricle of the brain of a systemically ineffective dose of phentolamine (200 μg/kg) increased the plasma corticosterone concentration (Fig. 5). This is better evidence of the specificity of this mechanism.

Finally, further evidence favoring adrenergic α-mediation of the ACTH-inhibiting system is provided by the finding that, in laparotomized rats, phentolamine and not propranolol is able to remove in part the dexamethasone + iproniazid-induced inhibition of ACTH secretion (Fig. 6). This kind of inhibition has been reported by Dallman and Yates (1968), who found that the laparotomy-induced adrenocortical activation can be prevented by pretreatment with dexamethasone + iproniazid although either drug given alone is ineffective. Our results with the blocking agents indicate that, at least in part, this kind of inhibition is due to the increased levels of catecholamines since a block of the specific adrenergic receptor can remove it.

In another group of experiments we investigated the apparent discrepancy between the above hypothesis and the results obtained by several authors in long-term experiments. In fact, both after single (Maickel *et al.*, 1961; Carr and Moore, 1968) and repeated (Montanari and Stockham, 1962) injections of reserpine, in spite of the prolonged depletion of catecholamines, the adrenocortical activation lasted only a few hours. In our experiments, intraperitoneal (i.p.) administration in rats of reserpine (0.5 mg/kg for 9 days) strongly depleted hypothalamic noradrenaline, while the corticosteroid level, 18 h after the last injection, was not modified. The injection of α-MPT (i.p. 9 h before killing) into rats treated for 9 days with reserpine provoked adrenocortical activation and a further decrease of hypothalamic noradrenaline; on the other hand, the animals had a normal rise of plasma corticosterone level after exogenous ACTH (100 mU/kg/25 min before killing), revealing an unimpaired adrenocortical reactivity after prolonged treatment with reserpine (Fig. 7).

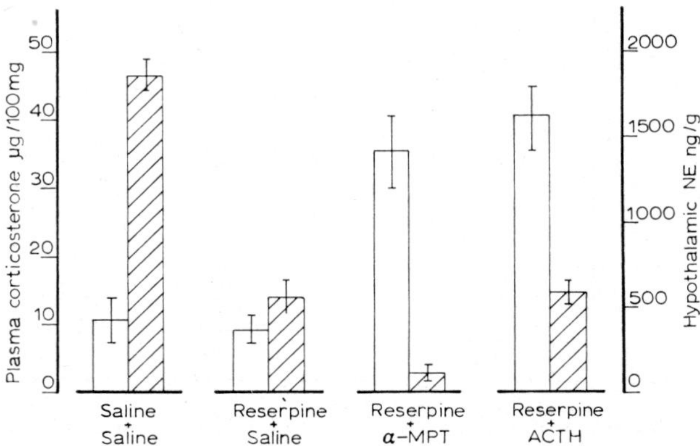

Fig. 7. Effect of α-MPT (250 mg/kg i.p. 9 h prior to sacrifice) and ACTH (100 mU/kg/25 min prior to the killing) on plasma corticosterone (open bars) and hypothalamic noradrenaline (dashed bars) in rats pretreated with reserpine (0.5 mg/kg i.p. for 9 days).

In peripheral studies, Kopin (1966) showed the presence of functionally active stores of noradrenaline maintained by synthesis after reserpine; more recently, Segal *et al.* (1971) found a significant increase of brain tyrosine hydroxylase activity after long-term treatment with low doses of reserpine. In view of these results, we suggest that the lack of adrenocortical activation in the presence of noradrenaline depletion after long-term treatment with reserpine is due to the presence of a small functionally active pool of noradrenaline available for the tonic inhibition of ACTH secretion.

In a similar series of experiments, long-lasting reduction in the brain concentration of catecholamines was obtained by using 6-hydroxydopamine (6-OHDA), a compound that causes a selective degeneration of nerve terminals that contain catecholamines (Bloom *et al.*, 1969). This drug, injected into the third or the lateral ventricle of the rat brain, caused after 3–15 and 30 days a significant decrease of hypothalamic noradrenaline while the corticosterone levels were unmodified (Table V). The injection of α-MPT (250 mg/kg/i.p. 9 h before the killing) into rats pretreated with 6-OHDA provoked adrenocortical activation (Fig. 8). Therefore, even after selective degeneration of catecholamine-containing terminals, there should still be present in the hypothalamus a pool of noradrenaline responsible for the inhibition of the hypothalamus-pituitary-adrenal axis. The availability of a sufficiently large pool could be due to the fact that those neurons containing noradrenaline that survive the degener-

TABLE V

CORRELATION BETWEEN PLASMA CORTICOSTERONE AND HYPOTHALAMIC CONTENTS OF NORADRENALINE AND DOPAMINE AFTER 6-HYDROXY-DOPAMINE (6-OHDA)

Treatment	*Place of injection*	*Number of animals*	*Days after injection*	*Plasma corticosterone (μg/100 ml)*	*Hypothalamic content (μg/g)*	
					Noradrenaline	*Dopamine*
6-OHDA 300 μg/		12	3	12.8±1.8[a]	1.36±0.08[b]	0.30±0.03
animal + 200	L.V.	15	15	3.2±2.2	1.01±0.12[b]	0.28±0.04[b]
μg/animal		12	30	4.2±3.0	0.82±0.07[b]	
after 72 h						
Saline 30 μl/		12	3	8.8±1.4	1.74±0.11	0.39±0.08
animal + 20	L.V.	12	15	7.9±2.0	1.84±0.09	0.41±0.03
μl/animal		9	30	9.2±1.5	1.87±0.10	0.41±0.11
after 72 h						
6-OHDA 50 μg/		15	3	14.8±2.1	1.26±0.10[b]	—
animal	III V.	15	15	7.3±2.0	1.06±0.07[b]	—
		12	30	6.6±1.8	0.99±0.06[b]	—
Saline 5 μl/		9	3	9.0±1.2	1.96±0.08	—
animal	III V.	9	15	8.1±1.3	1.88±0.10	—
		12	30	6.5±1.4	1.89±0.09	—

[a]Values are means ± standard error.
[b]Significantly different from corresponding saline control at $P < 0.01$.
L.V., lateral ventricle; III V., third ventricle.

References p. 181–183

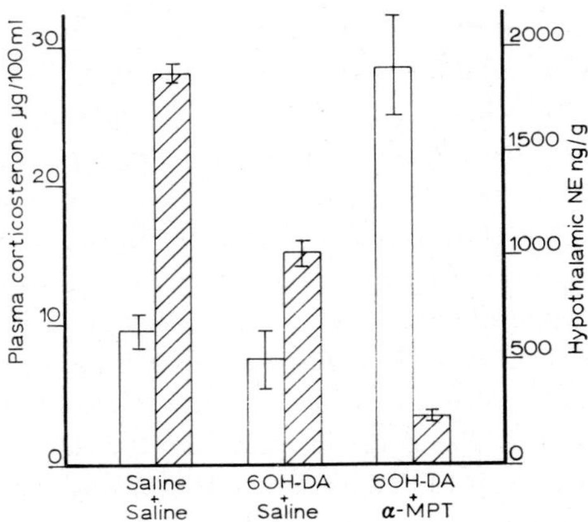

Fig. 8. Effect of α-MPT (250 mg/kg i.p. 9 h prior to the killing) on plasma corticosterone (open bars) and hypothalamic noradrenaline (dashed bars) in rats pretreated (30 days before with 6-OHDA 50 µg/animal into the third ventricle).

ative effects of 6-OHDA show an increase in their physiological state of activity to compensate for the loss of neuronal function after degeneration (Uretsky *et al.*, 1971).

In summary, there appears to be a central adrenergic system that tonically inhibits ACTH secretion. Although the physiological significance of this system, which seems to exist both in the rat and the dog, is not yet defined, our experiments indicate that noradrenaline rather than dopamine is the catecholamine involved. Preliminary results show that this adrenergic inhibitory tone is mediated *via* adrenergic α receptors. The long-term depletion experiments suggest the presence of a small, defined, functional pool of noradrenaline responsible for the tonic inhibition of ACTH secretion.

SUMMARY

The paper gives evidence in favour of a central noradrenergic system that tonically inhibits ACTH secretion *via* α-receptorial stimulation. In dogs, the injection into the third ventricle of catecholamine precursors, catecholamines and drugs that release or protect catecholamines from inactivation, inhibits stress-induced adrenocortical activation. In rats, drugs that decrease brain catecholamine levels provoke adrenocortical activation, also when injected directly into the third ventricle of systemically ineffective doses. Specific depletion of noradrenaline but not of dopamine is able to cause increase of plasma corticosterone. Blockade of α, but not of β receptors removes the tonic noradrenergic inhibition. Finally, experiments concerning long-term catecholamine depletion, suggest the presence of a small, defined, functional pool of noradrenaline responsible for the tonic inhibition of ACTH secretion.

ACKNOWLEDGMENTS

This paper includes the results of research supported in part from USPHS grant

AMO604 and from the Brooks Fund, and in part from the Consiglio Nazionale delle Richerche grant No. 71.00231.04.

The research was carried out primarily in the laboratory of W. F. Ganong by G. Moberg, U. Scapagnini and G. R. Van Loon (Department of Physiology, San Francisco Medical Center) and in the laboratory of P. Preziosi by L. Annunziato and U. Scapagnini.

REFERENCES

BHATTACHARYA, A. N. AND MARKS, B. H. (1969a) Reserpine and chlorpromazine-induced changes in hypothalamo-hypophyseal-adrenal system in rats in the presence and absence of hypothermia. *J. Pharmacol. exp. Ther.*, **165**, 108–116.

BHATTACHARYA, A. N. AND MARKS, B. H. (1969b) Effects of pargyline and amphetamine upon acute stress response in rats. *Proc. Soc. exp. biol. Med.*, **130**, 1194–1198.

BHATTACHARYA, A. N. AND MARKS, B. H. (1970) Effects of alpha-methyl-tyrosine and *p*-chlorophenylalanine on the regulation of ACTH secretion. *Neuroendocrinology*, **6**, 49–55.

BLISS, E. L., AILION, J. AND ZWANZIGER, J. (1968) Metabolism of norepinephrine, serotonin and dopamine in rat brain with stress. *J. Pharmacol. exp. Ther.*, **164**, 122–134.

BLOOM, F. E., ALGERI, S., GROPPETTI, A., REVELTA, A. AND COSTA, E. (1969) Lesion of central norepinephrine terminals with 6-hydroxydopamine: Biochemistry and fine structures. *Science*, **166**, 1284–1286.

CARR, L. A. AND MOORE, K. E. (1968) Effects of reserpine and α-methyltyrosine on brain catecholamines and the pituitary adrenal response to stress. *Neuroendocrinology*, **3**, 285–302.

CORRODI, H., FUXE, K. AND HÖKFELT, T. (1966) Refillment of the catecholamine stores with 3,4-dihydroxyphenylalanine after depletion induced by inhibition of tyrosine-hydroxylase, *Life Sci.*, **5**, 605–611.

COX, R. H. AND MAICKEL, R. P. (1969) Effects of guanethidine on rat brain serotonin and norepinephrine. *Life Sci.*, **8**, 1319–1324.

DALLMAN, M. F. AND YATES, F. E. (1968) Anatomical and functional mapping of central neural input and feedback pathways of the adrenocortical system. In *Memoirs of the Society for Endocrinology* (No. 17), V. H. T. JAMES AND J. LONDON (Eds.), Cambridge University Press, Cambridge, pp. 39–71.

DE SCHAEPDRYVER, A. F., PREZIOSI, P. AND SCAPAGNINI, U. (1969) Brain monoamines and stimulation or inhibition of ACTH release. *Arch. int. Pharmacodyn. Thér.*, **180**, 11–18.

DE WIED, D. (1967) Chlorpromazine and endocrine function. *Pharmacol. Rev.*, **19**, 251–288.

ENDRÖCZI, E., SCHREIBERG, G. AND LISSÁK, K. (1963) The role of central nervous activating and inhibitory structures in the control of pituitary-adrenocortical function. Effects of intracerebral cholinergic and adrenergic stimulation. *Acad. sci. hung.*, **24**, 211–221.

FUXE, K. AND HÖKFELT, T. (1969) Catecholamines in the hypothalamus and the pituitary gland. In *Frontiers in Neuroendocrinology 1969*, L. MARTINI AND W. F. GANONG (Eds.), Oxford University Press, New York, pp. 47–96.

GANONG, W. F. (1963) The central nervous system and the synthesis and release of adrenocorticotropic hormone. In *Advances in Neuroendocrinology*, A. V. NABALDOV (Ed.), University of Illinois Press, Urbana, Ill., pp. 92–149.

GANONG, W. F. AND LORENZEN, L. C. (1967) Brain neurohumors and endocrine function. In *Neuroendocrinology* (vol. 2), L. MARTINI AND W. F. GANONG (Eds.), Academic Press, New York, pp. 583–640.

GANONG, W. F. (1970) Control of ACTH and MSH secretion. In *The Hypothalamus*, F. FRASCHINI, M. MOTTA AND L. MARTINI (Eds.), Academic Press, New York, pp. 313–333.

GANONG, W. F. (1972) Evidence for a central noradrenergic system that inhibits ACTH secretion. In *Brain–Endocrine Interaction. Median Eminence: Structure and Function. Int. Symp. Munich, 1971*, Karger, Basel, pp. 254–266.

GLOWINSKI, J. AND AXELROD, J. (1966) Effects of drugs on the disposition of H^3-norepinephrine in the rat brain. *Pharmacol. Rev.*, **18**, 775–785.

GUILLEMIN, R. AND ROSENBERG, B. (1955) Humoral hypothalamic control of anterior pituitary: a study with combined tissue cultures. *Endocrinology*, **57**, 599–607.

HIRSCH, G. H. AND MOORE, K. E. (1968) Brain catecholamines and the reserpine-induced stimulation of the pituitary-adrenal-system. *Neuroendocrinology*, **3**, 398–405.

KOBAYASHI, H. AND MATSUI, T. (1969) Fine structure of the median eminence and its functional significance. In *Frontiers in Neuroendocrinology 1969*, W. F. GANONG AND L. MARTINI (Eds.), Oxford University Press, New York, pp. 3–46.

KOPIN, I. J. (1966) Metabolism and disposition of catecholamines in the central and peripheral nervous system. In *Endocrines and Central Nervous System*, R. LEVINE (Ed.), Williams and Wilkins, Baltimore, pp. 343–353.

KOPIN, I. J. AND GORDON, E. K. (1962) Metabolism of norepinephrine-H^3 released by tyramine and reserpine. *J. Pharmacol. exp. Ther.*, **138**, 351–359.

KOPIN, I. J. AND GORDON, E. K. (1963) Metabolism of administered and drug-released norepinephrine 7-H^3 in the rat. *J. Pharmacol. exp. Ther.*, **140**, 207–216.

KRIEGER, D. T. AND KRIEGER, H. P. (1965) The effect of intrahypothalamic injection of drugs on ACTH release in the cat. In *Proc. 2nd Int. Congr. Endocrinol., London 1964* (part 1), Excerpta Med., Amsterdam, pp. 640–645.

KRIEGER, H. P. AND KRIEGER, D. T. (1970) Chemical stimulation of the brain; effect of adrenal corticoid release. *Amer. J. Physiol.*, **218**, 1632–1641.

LONG, C. N. H. (1952) Regulation of ACTH secretion. *Recent Progr. Hormone Res.*, **7**, 75–97.

LORENZEN, L. C. AND GANONG, W. F. (1967) Effect of drugs related to α-ethyltryptamine on stress-induced ACTH secretion in the dog. *Endocrinology*, **80**, 889–892.

MAICKEL, R. P., WESTERMANN, E. O. AND BRODIE, B. B. (1961) Effects of reserpine and cold exposure on pituitary adrenocortical function in rats. *J. Pharmacol. exp. Ther.*, **134**, 167–175.

MANGILI, G., MOTTA, M. AND MARTINI, L. (1966) Control of adrenocorticotropic hormone secretion. In *Neuroendocrinology* (vol. 2), L. MARTINI AND W. F. GANONG (Eds.), Academic Press, New York, pp. 297–370.

MARTINI, L., PECILE, A., SAITO, S. AND TANI, F. (1960) The effect of midbrain transection on ACTH release. *Endocrinology*, **66**, 501–507.

MCCANN, S. M. AND PORTER, J. C. (1969) Hypothalamic pituitary stimulating and inhibiting hormones. *Physiol. Rev.*, **49**, 240–284.

MONTANARI, R. AND STOCKHAM, M. A. (1962) Effects of single and repeated doses of reserpine on the secretion of adrenocorticotrophic hormone. *Brit. J. Pharm.*, **18**, 337–345.

MUNSON, P. L. (1963) Pharmacology of neuroendocrine blocking agents. In *Advances in Neuroendocrinology*, A. V. NABALDOV (Ed.), University of Illinois Press, Urbana, Ill., pp. 427–444.

NAUMENKO, E. V. (1968) Hypothalamic chemoreactive structure and the regulation of pituitary-adrenal-function. Effects of local injection of norepinephrine, carbachol and serotonin into the brain of guinea pigs with intact brains and after mesencephalic transection. *Brain Res.*, **11**, 1–10.

SAFFRAN, M. AND SCHALLY, A. V. (1955) The release of corticotrophin by anterior pituitary tissue *in vitro*. *Canad. J. Biochem.*, **33**, 408–415.

SCAPAGNINI, U. AND PREZIOSI, P. (1973) Receptor involvement in the central noradrenergic inhibition of ACTH secretion in rat. *Neuropharmacology*, **12**, 57–62.

SCAPAGNINI, U., VAN LOON, G. R., MOBERG, G. P. AND GANONG, W. F. (1970) Effect α-methyl-p-tyrosine on the circadian variation of plasma corticosterone in rats. *Europ. J. Pharmacol.*, **11**, 266–270.

SCAPAGNINI, U., VAN LOON, G. R., MOBERG, G. P., PREZIOSI, P. AND GANONG, W. F. (1971) Evidence for a central adrenergic inhibition of ACTH secretion in rat. *Arch. Pharmakol.*, **269**, 408.

SCAPAGNINI, U., VAN LOON, G. R., MOBERG, G. P., PREZIOSI, P. AND GANONG, W. F. (1972) Evidence for a central norepinephrinergic inhibition of ACTH secretion in the rat. *Neuroendocrinology*, **10**, 155–160.

SEGAL, D. S., SULLIVAN, J. L., KUCRENSKI, R. T. AND MANDELL, A. J. (1971) Effects of long-term reserpine treatment on brain tyrosine-hydroxylase and behavioural activity. *Science*, **173**, 847–849.

SMELIK, P. G. (1967) ACTH secretion after depletion of hypothalamic monoamines by reserpine implants. *Neuroendocrinology*, **2**, 247–254.

THIERRY, A. M., JAVORY, F., GLOWINSKI, J. AND KETY, S. S. (1968) Effects of stress on the metabolism of norepinephrine, dopamine and serotonin in the central nervous system of the rat, I. Modification of norepinephrine turnover. *J. Pharmacol. exp. Ther.*, **163**, 163–171.

URETSKY, N. J., SIMMONDS, M. A. AND IVERSEN, L. L. (1971) Changes in the retention and metabolism of ^{3}H-1-norepinephrine in rat brain *in vivo* after 6-hydroxydopamine pretreatment. *J. Pharmacol. exp. Ther.*, **176**, 489–496.

VAN LOON, G. R., HILGER, A. B., KING, A. T., BORITZKA, A. T. AND GANONG, W. F. (1971a) Inhibitory effect of L-dihydroxyphenylalanine on the adrenal venous 17-hydroxycorticosteroid response to surgical stress in dogs. *Endocrinology*, **88**, 1404–1414.

VAN LOON, G. R., SCAPAGNINI, U., COHEN, R. AND GANONG, W. F. (1971b) Intraventricular administration of adrenergic drugs on the adrenal venous 17-hydroxycorticosteroid response to surgical stress in the dog. *Neuroendocrinology*, **8**, 257–272.

VAN LOON, G. R., SCAPAGNINI, U., MOBERG, G. P. AND GANONG, W. F. (1971c) Evidence for central adrenergic neural inhibition of ACTH secretion in the rat. *Endocrinology*, **89**, 1464–1469.

VERNIKOS-DANELLIS, J. (1968) The pharmacological approach to the study of the mechanisms regulating ACTH secretion. In *Pharmacology of Hormonal Polypeptides and Proteins*, N. BACK, L. MARTINI AND R. PAOLETTI (Eds.), Plenum, New York, pp. 175–189.

WURTMAN, R. J. (1966) Catecholamines, Little Brown, Boston.

ZAMBRANO, D. (1968) On the presence of neurons with granulated vesicles in the median eminence of rat and dog. *Neuroendocrinology*, **2**, 141–155.

DISCUSSION

DANELLIS: As you know, α-MPT is a rather unorthodox drug. You mentioned that after prolonged depletion of catecholamines corticosteroids returned to normal. I looked at early changes in plasma, corticosterone minutes after an intraperitoneal injection of α-MPT and found that at the time when brain noradrenaline was practically unchanged plasma corticosterone levels were the highest I have seen under any conditions (over 150 μg/100 ml). 6 to 9 h later when brain noradrenaline levels were lowest, the levels of plasma corticosterone were much lower.

SCAPAGNINI: We found that 1 h after injection of α-MPT some animals show high levels of ACTH and corticosteroids. We can explain this finding in two ways. One is that α-MPT alters the catecholamine pool in a matter of minutes causing impairment of adrenergic activity at the nerve endings responsible for inhibition of ACTH secretion. The other is that there may be individual or strain differences in the response to α-MPT.

DANELLIS: I think this is a very elegant approach from a pharmacological point of view but that we are stuck with the fact that drugs unfortunately do not do just one thing.

SMELIK: I would like to add to the confusion. We found that high doses of α-MPT cause depletion of brain noradrenaline and dopamine content and an increase in adrenal activity. However, giving a lower dose repeatedly you produce the same depletion without causing activation of the pituitary-adrenal system. Moreover, pituitary-adrenal activation was blocked by giving pentobarbital prior to high doses of α-MPT. Thus, we see a dissociation between the depletion of the catecholamines and the stimulation of the pituitary-adrenal system.

SCAPAGNINI: Using low doses of α-MPT I obtained results that are in agreement with yours. The thing that can be happening here is that we are not saturating tyrosine hydroxylase completely and a small functional pool remains available. Perhaps we should run these experiments measuring tyrosine hydroxylase activity as well as the turnover of the catecholamines. I see your point about the results with nembutal, but it can affect the sensitivity of the pituitary-adrenal system in spite of the fact that you are removing an inhibitory system with α-MPT; therefore, it doesn't mean too much to me because nembutal can be working at different levels.

DANELLIS: Most of the data in the literature concerning the influence of brain noradrenaline on pituitary-adrenal function has relied on the measurement of a change in resting plasma corticosterone levels. We looked at the effect of these drugs on the stress response and got opposite results. We could block the stress response with α-MPT and found that it was even more effective in the absence of steroids. We have come to the conclusion in trying to reconcile the results that in the presence of a high level of plasma corticosterone brain noradrenaline appears to be inhibitory but in the absence of circulating corticosteroids, brain noradrenaline is stimulatory. Thus we feel that circulating corticosterone levels may modulate the effect of noradrenaline on pituitary-adrenal function.

MARKS: Joan, you have anticipated some of my remarks—I couldn't agree with you more. Dr. Scapagnini, there appears to be an inhibitory adrenergic system as long as there are some circulating corticosteroids. Hall, Bhattacharya and I have done experiments suggesting this for the last 3 or 4 years. I have another comment to make, and that relates to the fact that the experiments usually involve only the measurement of plasma corticosterone. We, also, were bothered by the fact that catecholamines may remain depleted and plasma corticosteroids may return to relatively low levels; at those times animals don't respond to stress particularly well. I just wanted to remind you that Bhattacharya and I measured CRF under some of those circumstances and found a marked reduction of CRF content of the hypothalamus. I think that noradrenaline-dependent changes in CRF synthesis account for part of this problem.

CIARANELLO: I have a couple of questions. α-MPT at the dose you employed only partially blocks tyrosine hydroxylase. Blockade was rather transient in the experiments that Dr. Danellis described. We administered 250 mg/kg i.p. of either the methyl ester or straight drug and produced 70% inhibition of tyrosine hydroxylase which reached a maximum at 2 h. After that the fall off of noradrenaline and dopamine ceased. By 6 h after drug administration, levels began to rise suggesting that the tyrosine hydroxylase inhibition was overcome. Since tyrosine hydroxylase is under feedback control from noradrenaline and since newly synthesized noradrenaline appears to be preferentially utilized I wonder how much of the data could be explained by activation of tyrosine hydroxylase after inhibition? The second point is that I am somewhat skeptical about the data using dihydroxyphenylserine (DOPS). Using threo-DOPS, synthesized in our laboratory, we were unable to demonstrate any radioactive noradrenaline in the brain; this contradicts at least one published study. Furthermore, the result was not affected by administration of a peripheral decarboxylase inhibitor. Since DOPS will give a trihydroxyindole fluorescence and can be mistaken for noradrenaline, I would wonder if that might explain the rebound you described?

SCAPAGNINI: I agree that DOPS is a tricky drug to use. I agree also that DOPS can interfere with noradrenaline measurement. The only point on which we disagree is the possible meaning of results obtained using peripheral DOPA decarboxylase inhibitors. Since noradrenaline will not cross the blood-brain barrier and since DOPS can be decarboxylated in the brain to form noradrenaline, peripheral decarboxylation would not likely account for my results.

Involvement of Catecholamines in Feedback Mechanisms

PUSHPA S. KALRA* AND S. M. McCANN

Department of Physiology, University of Texas Southwestern Medical School, Dallas, Tex. (U.S.A.)

INTRODUCTION

Interest in the possible role of adrenergic mechanisms in the control of gonadotrophin release has been recently renewed. Catecholamine (CA)-containing neurons and terminals occur in discrete regions of the anterior hypothalamus and median-eminence arcuate areas. Fuxe and co-workers have demonstrated by fluorescence microscopy, the presence of two CA-containing neuron systems in the hypothalamus. These include the tuberoinfundibular-dopamine neurons, strategically located in arcuate nucleus with fiber systems extending to the median eminence, and afferent noradrenaline (NA) nerve terminals in the anterior hypothalamus and preoptic area which ascend from cell bodies located in mid-brain (for refs. Hökfelt and Fuxe, 1972). Unfortunately, due to conflicting reports from different laboratories of the specific role of each of the monoamines in control of gonadotrophin secretion, a clear picture has not yet emerged. Two opposing views exist regarding the specific role of dopamine (DA) in controlling release of gonadotrophins. Evidence, derived from variations in intensity of fluorescence and turnover rates of DA in neurons of medial basal hypothalamus of the rat during different phases of the reproductive cycle, led Fuxe *et al.* to believe that increased activity in DA neurons inhibits the release and/or synthesis of the gonadotrophin-releasing factors (luteinizing hormone-releasing factor, LRF, and follicle-stimulating hormone-releasing factor, FRF). On the other hand, Schneider and McCann (1969, 1970) and Kamberi *et al.* (1970, 1971) have provided evidence suggesting a stimulating effect of DA on LRF and FRF both *in vitro* and *in vivo*. Little is known about the role of NA in regulating the release of gonadotrophins. Sawyer *et al.* (1949) and Rubinstein and Sawyer (1970) have reported the ability of NA to induce ovulation in rabbit and rat. Furthermore, serotoninergic mechanisms in the hypothalamus may have an inhibitory effect on gonadotrophin secretion (Kordon and Glowinski, 1972).

The role of steroid hormones in regulating hypothalamic activity is well recognized. A direct interaction of ovarian steroids with the catecholaminergic neuronal system in the hypothalamus has not yet been clearly elucidated. Following removal of the

* Present address: Department of Dairy Science, IFAS, University of Florida, Gainesville, Fla. 32601 (U.S.A.).

References p. 196–197

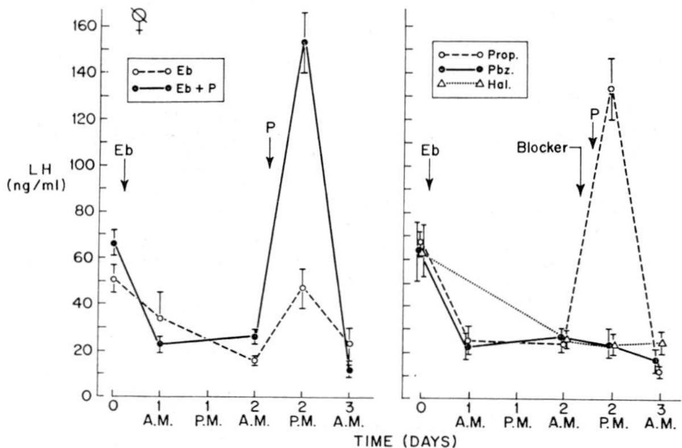

Fig. 1. Plasma LH of spayed rats treated with 5 μg of estradiol benzoate (Eb) followed by 1.5 mg progesterone (P) 48 h later. 1 h prior to administration of progesterone adrenergic blockers were injected. Prop., propranolol; Pbz., phenoxybenzamine; Hal., haloperidol.
In this and subsequent figures, vertical bars represent standard errors of the mean; figures in parentheses represent number of animals.

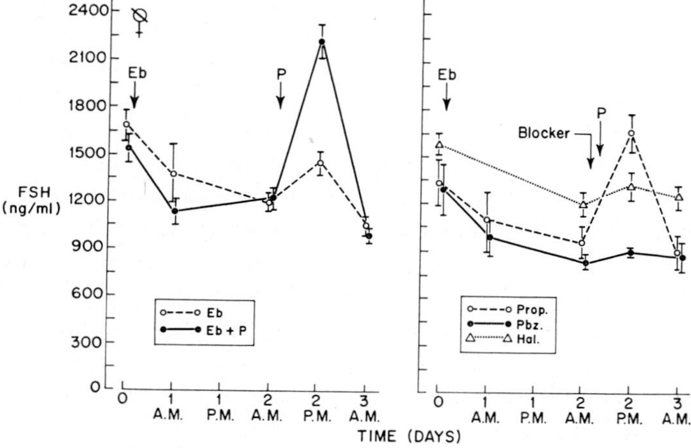

Fig. 2. Plasma FSH of Eb–P-treated rats; effects of adrenergic blockers administered as in Fig. 1. For abbreviations see text.

inhibitory effects of gonadal steroids by castration the rate of turnover of NA in the hypothalamus was accelerated (Anton-Tay and Wurtman, 1968; Coppola, 1968, Bapna *et al.*, 1971) while turnover of DA decreased (Fuxe and Hökfelt, 1969). Administration of gonadal steroids to castrate male and female rats was reported to influence DA and NA turnover in the hypothalamus. These studies, although inconclusive, suggest the involvement of CA's in mediating the feedback effects of steroids in the hypothalamus.

Caligaris *et al.* (1968) and Kalra *et al.* (1970, 1972) reported that injection of progesterone to spayed, estrogen pretreated rats resulted in a sharp rise of plasma luteinizing hormone (LH) and follicle-stimulating hormone (FSH) 6 h later (Figs. 1

TABLE I

EFFECTS OF ADRENERGIC RECEPTOR BLOCKERS ON THE STIMULATORY EFFECTS OF ESTRADIOL ON LH AND FSH RELEASE IN ESTROGEN-PRIMED SPAYED RATS

Blocker	*Dose (mg/kg)*	*Number of rats*	*Day 2*		*Day 3*	
			a.m.	*p.m.*	*a.m.*	*p.m.*
			Plasma levels of LH (ng/ml)			
Control	—	11	23.7 ± 4.3[a]	93.6 ± 22.8[b]	12.1 ± 1.1	85.2 ± 18.0[c]
Propranolol	20	8	9.1 ± 1.9	15.7 ± 4.6	7.2 ± 1.2	52.1 ± 13.2[b]
Phenoxybenzamine	20	8	10.2 ± 1.6	6.7 ± 0.8	5.2 ± 0.6	29.0 ± 17.7
Haloperidol	2	8	11.5 ± 2.6	7.5 ± 1.2	7.1 ± 2.5	44.4 ± 12.0[b]
			Plasma levels of FSH (ng/ml)			
Control	—	11	1136 ± 98	1261 ± 79	756 ± 54	1198 ± 113[b]
Propranolol	20	8	1564 ± 120	982 ± 62	651 ± 58	860 ± 88
Phenoxybenzamine	20	8	1128 ± 92	1292 ± 108	888 ± 112	808 ± 66
Haloperidol	2	8	1296 ± 95	1156 ± 94	943 ± 60	1167 ± 95

The receptor blockers were injected on the mornings of day 2 and day 3.

[a]Mean ± SEM.
[b]$p < 0.01$ *vs. a.m.* levels.
[c]$p < 0.001$ *vs. a.m.* levels.

and 2). Similarly, administration of estradiol benzoate to estrogen-primed spayed rats induced sharp peaks of plasma LH at 6 as well as 30 h (Caligaris *et al.*, 1971); plasma FSH was elevated only at 30 h (Kalra and McCann, 1972) (Table I). We have investigated these stimulatory effects of both estrogen and progesterone on the release of gonadotrophins to gain an insight into the possible involvement of CA's in mediating steroidal feedback effects.

MATERIALS AND METHODS

Adult female rats (230 g) of the Sherman strain were ovariectomized and used 3–5 weeks later for the study. Heparinized blood samples (1.0 ml) were drawn from the jugular vein of ether-anesthetized rats. Plasma LH was estimated by the radioimmunoassay (RIA) method developed by Niswender *et al.* (1968); values were expressed in terms of NIH-LH-SI. Plasma levels of FSH were measured by the RIA kit supplied by NIAMD and results were expressed in terms of the standards provided. The morning and afternoon levels of plasma LH and FSH in individual rats were analyzed by the paired "t" test.

Stimulatory effects of progesterone

Spayed rats were injected with five μg of estradiol benzoate on the morning of day 0.

References p. 196–197

48 h later on day 2, 1.5 mg progesterone was injected. Blood samples were drawn on day 0 and day 2 just prior to the injection of estradiol or progesterone and 6 h and 24 h after the injection of progesterone.

Effects of adrenergic receptor blockers

Adrenergic receptor blockers were injected 1 h prior to injection of 1.5 mg progesterone on day 2. Blockade of β-adrenergic receptors by treatment with propranolol (20 mg/kg) did not alter the progesterone-induced peaks of plasma LH and FSH; however, when α-adrenergic receptors were blocked by phenoxybenzamine (20 mg/kg) these peaks of plasma gonadotrophins were blocked completely (Figs. 1, 2). Release of LH and FSH was similarly blocked by treatment with haloperidol (2 mg/kg). Since recent studies have indicated that phenoxybenzamine and haloperidol block both central DA and NA receptors under different experimental conditions (Andén *et al.*, 1969) the blockade by these drugs was indicative only of the participation of an α-adrenergic component in the stimulatory effects of progesterone on gonadotrophin release.

Effects of inhibitors of CA synthesis

Biosynthesis of DA and NA from tyrosine in adrenergic neurons includes three enzymatic steps: tyrosine → dihydroxphenylalanine (DOPA) → DA → NA. This pathway can readily be disrupted at any of these three steps with certain specific drugs.

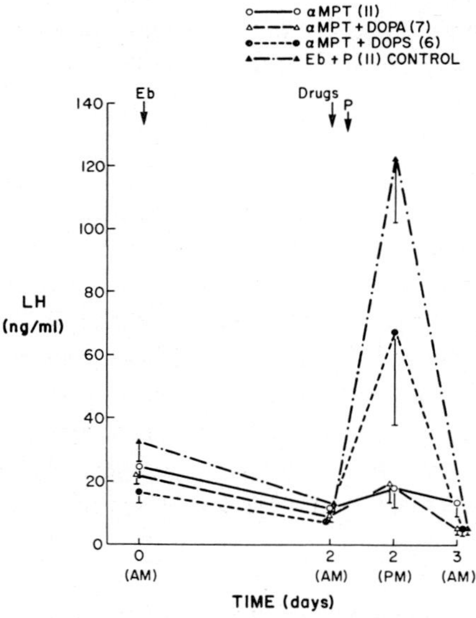

Fig. 3. The effect on plasma LH of blocking catecholamine synthesis by α-MPT (3 h prior to progesterone) in Eb–P-treated rats, and of restoring the synthesis of DA and NA by DOPA or NA alone by DOPS (from Kalra *et al.*, 1972). For abbreviations see text.

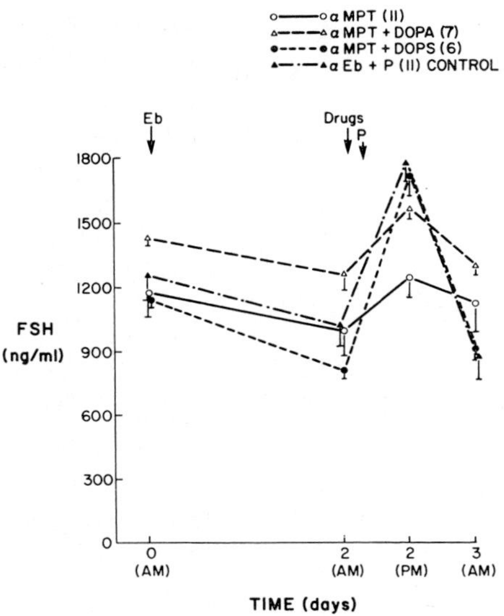

Fig. 4. Plasma FSH of rats treated as in Fig. 3 (from Kalra *et al.*, 1972). For abbreviations see text.

Tyrosine hydroxylase, which catalyses the conversion of tyrosine to DOPA, is a rate-limiting enzyme in the synthesis of CA. Consequently, levels of DA and NA decline markedly following inhibition of this enzyme by administration of α-methyl-*p*-tyrosine (α-MPT) (Spector *et al.*, 1965). This drug effectively blocked the progesterone-induced elevation of plasma LH and FSH only when administered 3 h prior to progesterone (Figs. 3, 4). Injection of α-MPT (200–250 mg/kg) at the same time as progesterone or 2 or 3 h later failed to modify the stimulatory action of progesterone. The ability of α-MPT to block the effects of progesterone was not unexpected in view of the earlier reports that it blocked ovulation in immature rats if administered during the critical period (Kordon and Glowinski, 1969). However, our results revealed certain interesting aspects of the temporal relationship between the administration of α-MPT and progesterone. Corrodi and Hanson (1966) reported that DA and NA levels decline markedly 2 h following the administration of α-MPT; maximum depletion occurred 16–20 h later. Since blockade of progesterone-induced effects was obtained only when α-MPT was administered 3 h before the injection of progesterone and was not observed at the other times, it appears that normal levels of CA in the brain are essential for progesterone to stimulate release of LH and FSH.

In addition, we have used two drugs, diethyldithiocarbamate (DDC) and 1-phenyl-3-(2-thiazolyl)-thiourea (U-14,624) to deplete levels of brain NA. These drugs block the conversion of DA to NA by inhibiting DA-β-oxidase thus resulting in reduced levels of brain NA, whereas the levels of DA either increased or remained unchanged (Goldstein and Nakajima, 1967; Johnson *et al.*, 1970).

U-14,624 was injected 18 h prior to progesterone at a dose of 200 mg/kg. DDC (400 mg/kg) was administered 40–90 min prior to progesterone. Following treatment with either of these drugs, there was a complete absence of the peaks of plasma LH

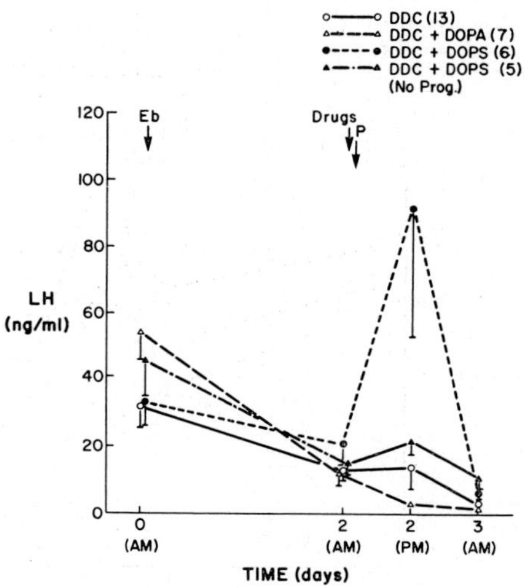

Fig. 5. The effect of blocking NA synthesis by DDC on plasma LH in Eb–P-treated rats; of restoring the synthesis of NA selectively by DOPS; or of elevating levels of DA by DOPA in DDC treated animals (from Kalra *et al.*, 1972). For abbreviations see text.

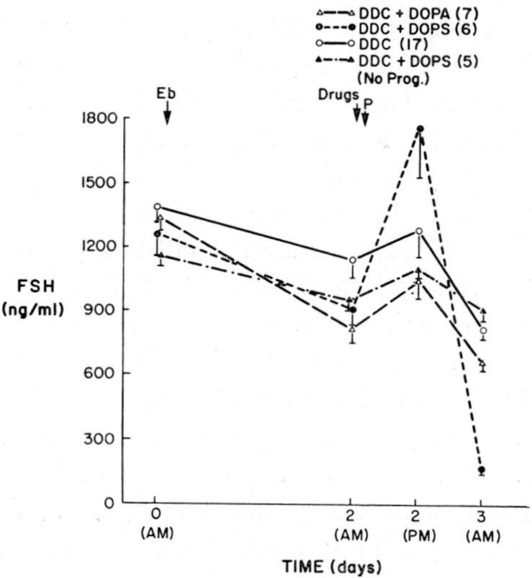

Fig. 6. Plasma FSH of rats treated as in Fig. 5 (from Kalra *et al.*, 1972). For abbreviations see text.

and FSH in response to the injection of progesterone (Figs. 5–7). These results implicate NA as the mediator which transmits the stimulatory effect of progesterone on the release of gonadotrophins.

This hypothesis was further tested by administering CA precursors in animals with drug-induced CA depletion.

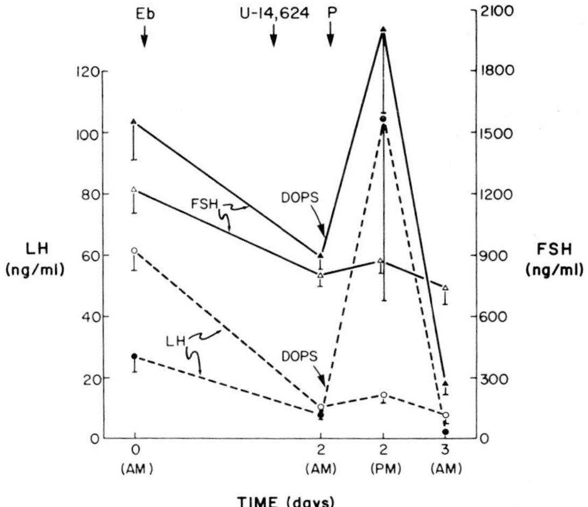

Fig. 7. The inhibition of plasma LH and FSH of Eb–P-treated rats by U-14,624 injected 18 h prior to P (open circle and triangles—10 rats); and recovery of the peaks by DOPS injected 1 h prior to P (solid circle and triangles—5 rats) (from Kalra *et al.*, 1972). For abbreviations see text.

Effects of selective re-synthesis of CA after inhibition of CA biosynthesis

Following blockage of endogenous DA and NA synthesis by administration of α-MPT, synthesis of DA and NA or NA alone was reinitiated by administration of the specific precursors, DOPA and dihydroxyphenylserine (DOPS), respectively (Creveling *et al.*, 1968). In animals treated with α-MPT to lower levels of both DA and NA, administration of DOPS (200 mg/kg, 30 min prior to progesterone) was effective in restoring the peak responses of both LH and FSH. However, treatment with L-DOPA (100 mg/kg, 45 min prior to progesterone), which might be expected to normalize first DA and later NA levels, failed to reverse the blockade of progesterone-induced LH release and only partially reversed the blockade in FSH release (Figs. 3 and 4).

Rats in which NA synthesis was blocked by DDC were injected with DOPA (100 mg/kg) to increase the endogenous levels of DA while conversion to NA was prevented. These rats having elevated levels of DA and subnormal levels of brain NA, did not exhibit increases in plasma LH and FSH in response to progesterone (Figs. 5 and 6). However, when DOPS (200 mg/kg) was administered to DDC- or U-14,624-blocked rats to restore brain NA levels, the peaks of LH and FSH were once again observed following progesterone injection (Figs. 5–7). Administration of DDC and DOPS to Eb-treated rats, which were not injected with progesterone, did not result in elevated levels of gonadotrophins on the afternoon of day 2 (Figs. 5 and 6).

Our data, therefore, support the hypothesis that NA mediates the progesterone-induced release of gonadotrophins. NA terminals have been demonstrated by fluorescence microscopy in the preoptic and anterior hypothalamic region. We have shown recently by implanting progesterone in various regions of the brain that the preoptic-anterior hypothalamic area is the site of stimulatory feedback of progesterone (Kalra and McCann, 1972). Further evidence of this was also obtained since progesterone was ineffective in rats with suprachiasmatic lesions (Bishop *et al.*, 1972) as well as in rats with knife cuts which severed the connection between the preoptic area and the hypothalamus (Taleisnik *et al.*, 1970). Although injection of DA into the third ventricle can induce LH and FSH release (Schneider and McCann, 1970 and Kamberi *et al.*, 1971), it appears that DA is not the mediator involved in progesterone-induced gonadotrophin release.

STIMULATORY EFFECTS OF ESTRADIOL

Estrogens play a predominant role in maintaining the estrous cycle in rats. Although it was believed initially that such a regulatory role was due to its inhibitory feedback effect on gonadotrophin release, Everett (1964) demonstrated that a single injection of estradiol was effective in inducing ovulation in pregnant rats and also of advancing ovulation in 5-day cycling rats. We have recently confirmed the stimulatory effects of estradiol during the estrous cycle; administration of estradiol on the day of estrus stimulated the release of LH and FSH (Kalra *et al.*, unpublished).

Administration of estradiol to estrogen-primed ovariectomized rats results in sharp increases of plasma LH at 6 and 29 h post-injection (Caligaris *et al.*, 1971). We observed these stimulatory effects on LH release at three dose levels of estradiol; plasma levels of FSH were significantly elevated only at 30 h (Table I).

The experimental design described above was used to investigate the involvement of adrenergic mechanisms in mediating the stimulatory effects of estradiol on gonadotrophin release. 5 μg of estradiol benzoate were injected to spayed rats on the morning of day 0 followed by a second injection (5 μg) 48 h later on day 2. Morning and afternoon blood samples of day 2 and day 3 were analysed by RIA for LH and FSH. Drugs were injected 1 h prior to estradiol on day 2 and again 24 h later on day 3.

Effects of adrenergic receptor blockers

Indications of the involvement of adrenergic mechanisms were obtained when blockage of LH and FSH release was observed following treatment with phenoxybenzamine, haloperidol as well as propranolol (Table I). These adrenergic receptor blockers were effective in inhibiting the peaks of LH at 6 h; phenoxybenzamine was also effective in blocking the rise of plasma LH and FSH on day 3 (30 h later).

Effects of inhibitors of CA synthesi

Reduction in brain CA levels achieved by treatment with α-MPT (3 h prior to estradiol) was effective in blocking the estrogen-induced release of LH and FSH at 6 and/or 30 h. Selective inhibition of NA synthesis was obtained by use of DDC and U-14,624 which block the activity of DA-β-oxidase. The stimulatory response of LH and FSH release to estradiol was completely inhibited by prior treatment with these drugs (Tables II and III).

These studies confirmed the involvement of CA in mediating the stimulatory effects of estradiol since adrenergic blockers as well as drugs, which inhibit the synthesis of DA and/or NA, were equally effective in blocking release of LH and FSH.

Effects of selective resynthesis of CA after inhibition of CA biosynthesis

Further attempts to identify the specific catecholaminergic mechanism involved the use of CA precursors described above. Restoration of brain DA and NA levels by DOPA in α-MPT-treated rats resulted in increased levels of plasma LH as well as FSH at 6 h. However, when conversion of administered DOPA to NA (*via* DA) was inhibited by DDC, the resulting higher levels of DA in the brain were not effective in restoring the peaks of LH and FSH at either time interval.

Selective resynthesis of NA alone by DOPS in rats treated with α-MPT or DDC was effective in elevating levels of plasma LH and FSH at 30 h to control levels. Rats treated with U-14,624 were injected with DOPS on day 2 only; peaks of plasma LH and FSH were observed 6 h later (Tables II and III).

TABLE II

EFFECTS OF MODIFICATION OF BRAIN CA LEVELS ON THE STIMULATORY EFFECT OF ESTRADIOL ON LH RELEASE IN ESTROGEN-PRIMED SPAYED RATS

Inhibitor (mg/kg)	*Precursor (mg/kg)*	*Number of rats*	*Plasma levels of LH (ng/ml)*			
			Day 2		*Day 3*	
			a.m.	*p.m.*	*a.m.*	*p.m.*
α-MPT (250)		8	7.6 ± 1.1[a]	22.2 ± 7.4	10.3 ± 4.1	37.7 ± 16.1
α-MPT (250)	DOPA (100)	8	9.5 ± 1.2	49.9 ± 14.2[b]	6.9 ± 0.7	17.9 ± 10.2
α-MPT (250)	DOPS (200)	11	8.6 ± 0.7	13.3 ± 2.4	11.1 ± 2.5	107.5 ± 43.0[b]
DDC (400)		7	9.3 ± 2.0	12.3 ± 5.1	3.4 ± 0.9	4.8 ± 1.1
DDC (400)	DOPA (100)	6	11.7 ± 1.8	5.3 ± 1.5	3.8 ± 0.5	28.3 ± 11.7
DDC (400)	DOPS (200)	8	8.3 ± 1.2	4.9 ± 0.6	3.0 ± 0.2	84.6 ± 15.3[c]
U-14,624 (200)		7	12.7 ± 2.5	20.3 ± 8.6	4.6 ± 1.0	3.1 ± 0.3
U-14,624 (200)	DOPS (200)	7	15.3 ± 4.5	65.1 ± 19.2[b]	8.1 ± 1.9	5.7 ± 0.7

The inhibitors and precursors were injected on the mornings of day 2 and day 3. U-14,624 was injected in the evening of day 1 and DOPS to these rats was injected only on day 2.

[a]Mean ± SEM.
[b]$p < 0.05$ *vs. a.m.* levels.
[c]$p < 0.001$ *vs. a.m.* levels.
For abbreviations see text.

References p. 196–197

TABLE III

EFFECTS OF MODIFICATION OF BRAIN CA LEVELS ON THE STIMULATORY EFFECT OF ESTRADIOL ON FSH RELEASE IN ESTROGEN-PRIMED SPAYED RATS

Inhibitor (mg/kg)	*Precursor (mg/kg)*	*Number of rats*	*Plasma level of FSH (ng/ml)*			
			Day 2		*Day 3*	
			a.m.	*p.m.*	*a.m.*	*p.m.*
α-MPT (250)		8	1535 ± 167[a]	1753 ± 106	1526 ± 138	1849 ± 342
α-MPT (250)	DOPA (100)	8	1489 ± 75	2123 ± 167[c]	1417 ± 104	1664 ± 204
α-MPT (250)	DOPS	11	1323 ± 78	1583 ± 76[b]	1386 ± 172	1914 ± 204[b]
DDC (400)		7	1321 ± 123	1284 ± 142	972 ± 48	1239 ± 174
DDC (400)	DOPA (100)	6	1330 ± 123	1318 ± 167	1082 ± 96	1230 ± 151
DDC (400)	DOPS (200)	8	1267 ± 139	1357 ± 57	1048 ± 40	1638 ± 79[d]
U-14,624 (200)		7	1425 ± 95	1494 ± 111	1255 ± 87	1015 ± 67
U-14,624 (200)	DOPS (200)	7	1332 ± 114	1815 ± 155[b]	1185 ± 52	1020 ± 84

The inhibitors and precursors were injected on the morning of day 2 and day 3. U-14,624 was injected in the evening of day 1 and DOPS to these rats was injected only on day 2.

[a]Mean ± SEM.
[b]$p < 0.05$ *vs. a.m.* levels.
[c]$p < 0.01$ *vs. a.m.* levels.
[d]$p < 0.001$ *vs. a.m.* levels.
For abbreviations see text.

Although these studies do not conclusively rule out dopaminergic involvement, they once again indicate that noradrenergic mechanisms have a predominant role in transmission of the stimulatory effects of estradiol on the release of gonadotrophins.

Since under certain circumstances DOPA (Karobath *et al.*, 1971) has been found to partially deplete brain serotonin stores, it appeared important to evaluate the role of serotonin in mediating the response of gonadotrophins to estrogen and progesterone. A drug, parachlorophenylalanine (PCPA), which blocks the activity of tryptophan hydroxylase thus inhibiting synthesis of serotonin (Koe and Weismann, 1966) was employed. Administration of PCPA on day 1 and day 2 (40–50 mg/kg) to estrogen-primed spayed rats failed to modify the stimulatory response of LH and FSH to progesterone or estradiol.

We have not investigated the role of adrenaline in progesterone- or estradiol-induced gonadotrophin release. Adrenaline and the enzyme which catalyses conversion of NA to adrenaline have recently been identified in the hypothalamus (Ciaranello *et al.*, 1969). The blockade of NA biosynthesis by the drugs used in the present study would also extend to adrenaline. Conversely, administration of DOPS would reinitiate adrenaline as well as NA biosynthesis.

At present it is known that the main site for feedback inhibition of gonadotrophin secretion by estrogen is probably in the medial basal hypothalamus (Davidson, 1969). Whereas other evidence derived from intracranial implantation of estrogen and progesterone (Kalra and McCann, 1972) as well as from electrophysiological studies show that the positive feedback centers for ovarian steroids are located in preoptic-anterior hypothalamic areas (Terasawa and Sawyer, 1970). Our results from these experiments would indicate that the interaction of estrogen or progesterone and the NA adrenergic system is integrated leading to impulse generation at the preoptic area-anterior hypothalamic level. It is also possible that NA synapses intervene further caudally during transmission of these stimulatory impulses to LRF and FRF secretory neurons.

Convincing evidence is thus available to demonstrate that the hypothalamic control of pituitary gonadotrophins is regulated by at least two important mechanisms namely steroid feedback and hypothalamic adrenergic systems. Both inhibitory and stimulatory monoaminergic systems represented by indoleamines and CA exist in the hypothalamus (Kordon and Glowinski, 1972). Although serotonin can suppress gonadotrophin release, there is no convincing evidence based on studies with inhibitors of serotonin synthesis that this occurs normally. It can be speculated likewise, that inhibitory and stimulatory feedback effects of ovarian steroids may be exerted by activation or modulation of one or both of the two monoaminergic systems.

SUMMARY

Administration of progesterone or estradiol to estrogen-pretreated spayed rats stimulated a dramatic increase in levels of LH and FSH. The involvement and nature of hypothalamic catecholamines mediating the transmission of these stimulatory effects has been investigated. Involvement of adrenergic receptors and catecholamines in transmission of the stimulatory stimuli was first established by use of the adrenergic receptor blockers propranolol, phenoxybenzamine and haloperidol. Drugs which modify brain catecholamine levels were used to identify the catecholamine involved in transmission of these stimuli. Blockade of DA and/or NA biosynthesis with α-MPT, diethyldithiocarbamate (DDC) or 1-phenyl-3-(2-thiazolyl)-2-thiourea (U-14,624) was effective in blocking the progesterone- or estradiol-induced stimulation of gonadotrophin release. Selective restoration of DA and/or NA levels in these animals was accomplished by treatment with specific precursors, DOPA and DOPS, respectively. Whereas DOPA was effective in restoring the progesterone- or estradiol-induced elevations of plasma gonadotrophins in α-MPT-treated rats, it was ineffective when conversion of DA to NA was blocked by DDC. On the other hand, selective resynthesis of NA by DOPS in rats in which DA and/or NA levels had been reduced was effective in reversing the blockage. These results indicate that NA plays a predominant role in transmission of the stimulatory effects of estradiol and progesterone on the release of LH and FSH.

References p. 196–197

ACKNOWLEDGEMENTS

Supported by Grant No. AM10073 from the USPHS, by a Ford Foundation Grant and by a grant from the Texas Population Crisis Foundation. Antiovine LH serum was provided through the courtesy of Drs. A. R. Midgley and Gordon Niswender (University of Michigan). Dr. Leo Reichert (Emory University) generously provided the purified ovine LH for radioiodination. Kit for the determination of FSH was provided through the NIAMD-NIH, Pituitary Hormones Program. We are indebted to Dr. G. A. Johnson of the Upjohn Company, Kalamazoo, Michigan, for supplies of U-14,624.

REFERENCES

Andén N.-E., Carlsson, A. and Haggendel, J. (1969) Adrenergic mechanisms. *Ann. Rev. Pharmacol.*, **9**, 119–134.

Anton-Tay, F. and Wurtman, R. J. (1968) Norepinephrine: turnover in rat brains after gonadectomy. *Science*, **159**, 1245.

Bapna, J., Neff, N. H. and Costa, E. (1971) A method for studying norepinephrine and serotonin metabolism in small regions of rat brain: Effect of ovariectomy on amine metabolism in anterior and posterior hypothalamus. *Endocrinology*, **89**, 1345–1349.

Bishop, W., Kalra, P. S., Fawcett, C. P., Krulich, L. and McCann, S. M. (1972) The effects of hypothalamic lesions on the release of gonadotropins and prolactin in response to estrogen and progesterone treatment in female rats. *Endocrinology*, **91**, 1404–1410.

Caligaris, L., Astrada, J. J. and Taleisnik, S. (1968) Stimulating and inhibiting effects of progesterone on the release of luteinizing hormone. *Acta endocrinol.*, **59**, 177–185.

Caligaris, L., Astrada, J. J. and Taleisnik, S. (1971) Release of luteinizing hormone induced by estrogen injection into ovariectomized rats. *Endocrinology*, **88**, 810–815.

Ciaranello, R. D., Barchas, R. E., Byers, G. S., Stemmie, D. W. and Barchase, J. D. (1969) Enzymatic synthesis of adrenaline in mammalian brain. *Nature (Lond.)*, **221**, 368–369.

Coppola, J. A. (1968) The apparent involvement of the sympathetic nervous system in the gonadotropin secretion of female rats. *J. Reprod. Fertil. Suppl.*, **4**, 35–45.

Corrodi, H. and Hanson, L. C. F. (1966) Central effects of an inhibitor of tyrosine hydroxylation. *Psychopharmacologia*, **10**, 116–125.

Creveling, C. R., Daly, J., Tokuyama, T. and Witkop, B. (1968) The combined use of α-methyltyrosine and threo-dihydroxyphenylserine—selective reduction of dopamine levels in the central nervous system. *Biochem. Pharmacol.*, **17**, 65–70.

Davidson, J. M. (1969) Feedback control of gonadotropin secretion. In *Frontiers in Neuroendocrinology* (Vol. I), W. F. Ganong and L. Martini (Eds.), Oxford Univ. Press, New York, pp. 343–388.

Everett, J. W. (1964) Central neural control of reproductive functions of the adenohypophysis. *Physiol. Rev.*, **44**, 373–431.

Fuxe, K. and Hökfelt, T. (1969) Catecholamines in the hypothalamus and pituitary gland. In *Frontiers in Neuroendocrinology* (Vol. I), W. F. Ganong and L. Martini (Eds.), Oxford Univ. Press, New York. pp. 47–96.

Goldstein, M. and Nakajima, K. (1967) The effect of disulfiram on catecholamine levels in the brain. *J. Pharmacol. exp. Ther.*, **157**, 96–102.

Hökfelt, T. and Fuxe, K. (1972) On the morphology and the neuroendocrine role of the hypothalamic catecholamine neurons. In *Brain–Endocrine Interaction Median Eminence: Structure and Function*, K. Knigge, D. Scott and A. Weindl (Eds.), Karger, Basel, pp. 181–223.

Johnson, G. A., Boukma, S. J. and Kim, E. G. (1970) *In vivo* inhibition of dopamine β-hydroxylase by 1-phenyl-3-(2-thiazolyl)-2-thiourea (U-14,624). *J. Pharmacol. exp. Ther.*, **171**, 80–87.

Kamberi, I. A., Schneider, H. P. G. and McCann, S. M. (1970) Action of dopamine to induce release of FSH-releasing factor (FRF) from hypothalamic tissue *in vitro*. *Endocrinology*, **86**, 278–284.

KAMBERI, I. A., MICAL, R. S. AND PORTER, J. C. (1971) Effect of anterior pituitary perfusion and intraventricular injection of catecholamines on FSH release. *Endocrinology*, **88**, 1003–1011.

KALRA, P. S. AND MCCANN, S. M. (1972) Effects of CNS implants of ovarian steroids on gonadotropin release. *IVth Int. Congr. Endocrinol., Washington, D.C.* (Abstr.).

KALRA, P. S., KRULICH, L., QUIJADA, M., KALRA, S. P., FAWCETT, C. P. AND MCCANN, S. M. (1970. Feedback of gonadal steroids on gonadotropins and prolactin in the rat. *Excerpta Med. Int. Congr) Ser.*, **219**, 708–715.

KALRA, P. S., KALRA, S. P., KRULICH, L., FAWCETT, C. P. AND MCCANN, S. M. (1972) Involvement of norepinephrine in transmission of the stimulatory influence of progesterone on gonadotropin release. *Endocrinology*, **90**, 1168–1176.

KAROBATH, M., DIAZ, J. L. AND HUTTENEN, M. O. (1971) The effect of L-DOPA on the concentrations of tryptophan, tyrosine and serotonin in rat brain. *European J. Pharm.*, **14**, 393–396.

KOE, B. K. AND WEISSMAN, A. (1966) *P*-chlorophenylalanine: A specific depleter of brain serotonin. *J. Pharm. exp. Ther.*, **154**, 499–516.

KORDON, C. AND GLOWINSKI, J. (1969) Selective inhibition of superovulation by blockade of dopamine synthesis during the "critical period" in the immature rat. *Endocrinology*, **85**, 924–931.

KORDON, C. AND GLOWINSKI, J. (1972) Role of hypothalamic monoaminergic neurones in the gonadotrophin release regulating mechanisms. *Neuropharmacology*, **11**, 153–162.

NISWENDER, G. D., MIDGLEY, A. R., MONROE, S. E. AND REICHERT, L. E. (1968) Radioimmunoassay for rat luteinizing hormone with anti-ovine LH serum and ovine LH-^{131}I. *Proc. Soc. exp. Biol. Med. (N.Y.)*, **128**, 807–811.

RUBINSTEIN, L. AND SAWYER, C. H. (1970) Role of catecholamine in stimulating release of pituitary ovulating hormone(s) in rats. *Endocrinology*, **86**, 988–995.

SAWYER, C. H., MARKEE, J. E. AND TOWNSEND, B. F. (1949) Cholinergic and adrenergic components in the neurohumoral control of the release of LH in the rabbit. *Endocrinology*, **44**, 18–37.

SCHNEIDER, H. P. G. AND MCCANN, S. M. (1969) Possible role of dopamine as transmitter to promote discharge of LH-releasing factor. *Endocrinology*, **85**, 121–132.

SCHNEIDER, H. P. G. AND MCCANN, S. M. (1970) Release of LH-releasing factor (LRF) into the peripheral circulation of hypophysectomized rats by dopamine and its blockage by estradiol. *Endocrinology*, **87**, 249–253.

SPECTOR, S., SJOERDSMA, A. AND UDENFRIEND, S. (1965) Blockade of endogenous norepinephrine synthesis by α-methyl-tyrosine, an inhibitor of tyrosine hydroxylase. *J. Pharmacol. exp. Ther.*, **147**, 86–95.

TALEISNIK, S., VELASCO, M. C. AND ASTRADA, J. J. (1970) Effect of hypothalamic deafferentation on the control of LH secretion. *J. Endocrinol.*, **46**, 1–7.

TERASAWA, E. AND SAWYER, C. H. (1970) Diurnal variation in the effects of progesterone on multiple unit activity in the rat hypothalamus. *Exp. Neurol.*, **27**, 359–374.

DISCUSSION

HYYPPÄ: Once again I raise the question about the specificity of drugs and their actions. Have you measured the catecholamines or indoleamines in brain or their metabolism there?

KALRA: In this particular study we did not measure the levels of catecholamines in the hypothalamus, however, Dr. Donoso in our laboratory has measured the hypothalamic content of noradrenaline following treatment with catecholamine depletors and precursors (Endocrinology 89, 774, 1971). α-MPT (200 mg/kg) depleted noradrenaline levels to 48% and diethyldithiocarbamate reduced noradrenaline levels to 40% of the levels in saline-injected control rats. Treatment with DOPA was effective in partial restoration of noradrenaline levels while DOPS restored the noradrenaline to control levels. We have not measured serotonin in our laboratory, however, we did not observe any effects of parachlorophenylalanine on the stimulatory effects of estradiol or progesterone.

SCAPAGNINI: You must be careful in your interpretation of results obtained in using the receptor blockers phenoxybenzamine and haloperidol. Phenoxybenzamine, as you know, can block the re-uptake of catecholamines and might therefore increase the available amount of catecholamines at some receptor site. On the other hand, haloperidol can increase catecholamine synthesis through a feedback mechanism and thereby also increase the amount of catecholamines at some receptor site.

KALRA: We may be increasing the amount of catecholamines but it seems to me that we are blocking the receptors at the time that we are injecting the stimulating steroid and transmission of that stimulus for a short period of time is blocked by blocking the receptors. We saw this very clearly today with the experiments with progesterone; but as you may have noticed with estradiol, where a longer time period is involved, we did not get any clear indication of whether alpha or beta receptors were involved.

JACOBY: Have you looked at the effects of DOPS on gonadotrophin release without prior adrenergic blockade?

KALRA: No, we have not. We have injected DOPS only after inhibiting either with α-MPT or with DDC or U-14,624. We have not given DOPS alone.

JACOBY: Then it's quite possible that the increase you see in gonadotrophins is due to DOPS which might be acting somewhere other than at an adrenergic site?

KALRA: We ran a control with α-MPT or blocker plus DOPS without steroid and got no stimulation. We are not just getting a non-specific or DOPS-induced stimulation in the absence of steroids.

Distribution of Biogenic Amines in the Pituitary Gland

DAVID M. JACOBOWITZ

Laboratory of Clinical Science, National Institute of Mental Health, Bethesda, Md. 20014 (U.S.A.)

The initial histochemical observation that there exists a remarkably dense accumulation of catecholamine-containing neurons in the median eminence, in addition to numerous monoaminergic fibers in the neurointermediate lobe of the pituitary, suggests a role for adrenergic mechanisms in the regulation of pituitary function (Carlsson *et al.*, 1962; Fuxe, 1964; Enemar and Falck, 1965). From these morphological observations, there has evolved considerable interest in the role of monoamines in the hypothalamous control of hormonal secretion from the three lobes of the pituitary. The purpose of this report is to survey the present status of our knowledge of the distribution of biogenic amines in the pituitary and its attachment to the base of the brain *via* the median eminence.

The methodology used involves the specific and sensitive catecholamine histochemical fluorescence technique of Falck and Hillarp (Falck, 1962; Falck *et al.*, 1962; Carlsson *et al.*, 1962; Falck and Owman, 1965). The catecholamine-containing nerve fibers have a green fluorescence while the serotonin neurons fluoresce yellow. The noradrenaline neurons can only be distinguished from the dopamine nerves by various drug manipulations (Dahlstrom and Fuxe, 1964; Fuxe and Hökfelt, 1969) and microspectrophotofluorimetric methods (Björklund *et al.*, 1970).

The tubero-infundibular (arcuato-hypophyseal) monoaminergic neurons constitute primarily dopamine-containing nerves whose cell bodies originate in the arcuate nucleus at the base of the medial hypothalamus with processes that course through the median eminence and terminate in the neurointermediate lobe of the pituitary. This neuronal system is relatively short in comparison with the noradrenergic system which dominates the hypothalamus (Fig. 1). Most of the noradrenergic cell bodies are contained in the pons-medulla region of the hindbrain (Dahlstrom and Fuxe, 1964; Fuxe and Hökfelt, 1969) and course through the reticular formation structures (Ungerstedt, 1971; Jacobowitz and Kostrzewa, 1971).

There are several groups of monoamine axons which enter the median eminence of the rat brain: (*1*) The major dopamine neurons originate from cell bodies in the arcuate nucleus and the ventral part of the anterior periventricular nucleus (Fig. 2) (Fuxe and Hökfelt, 1969; Björklund *et al.*, 1970). The arcuate nucleus cell bodies are mostly found in the anterior part of the nucleus. It has also been claimed that there are cell bodies in the dorsal part of the periventricular nucleus (Fuxe and Hökfelt, 1969). The dopamine nerves enter the median eminence close to the infundibular recess.

References p. 208–209

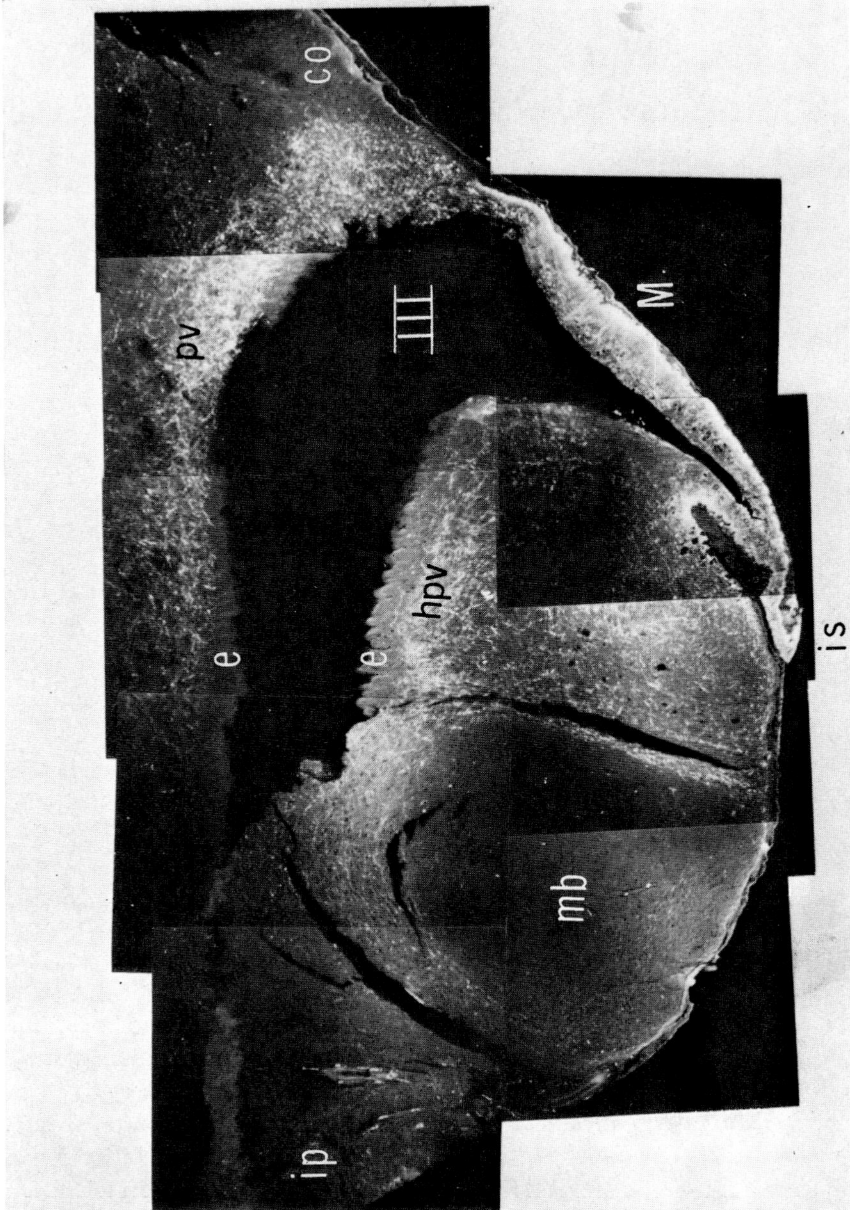

Fig. 1. Montage of a sagittal section of the rat hypothalamus-median eminence region. Noradrenergic nerve terminals are observed in the periventricular nucleus (hpv) and the paraventricular nucleus (pv). A dense accumulation of mostly dopamine-containing nerves is present in the external layer of the median eminence (M) which extends into the infundibular stem (is). Third ventricle (III); optic chiasm (CO); ependymal lining (e); mammillary body (mb); interpeduncular nucleus (ip). ($\times$ 28) (14 μ)

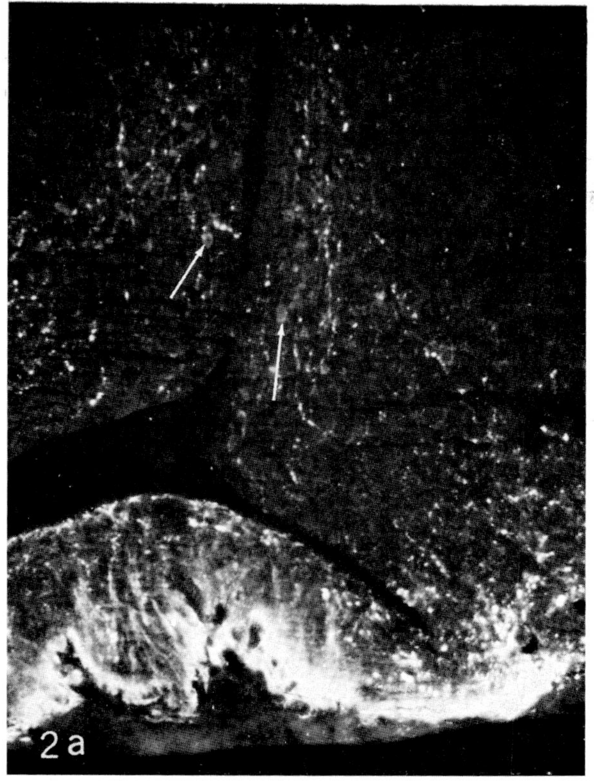

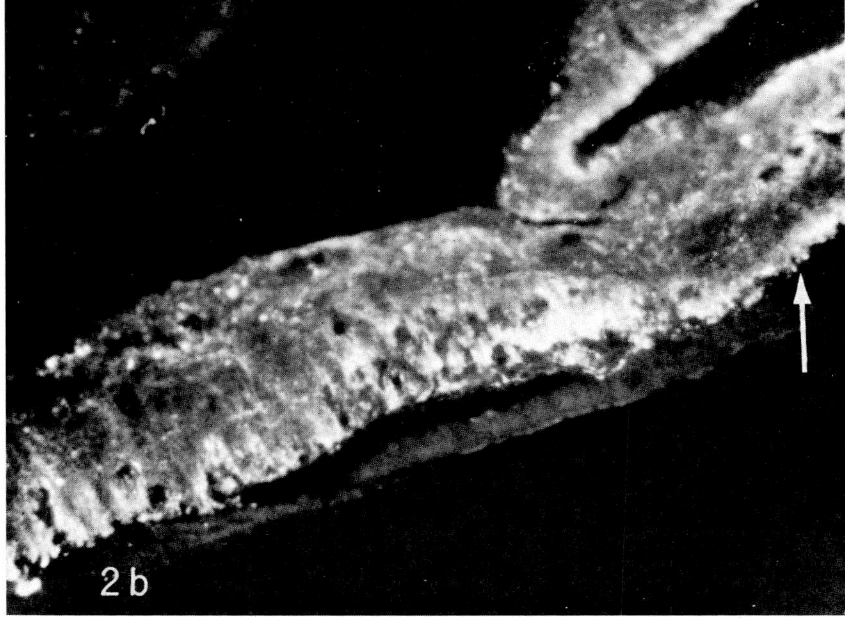

Fig. 2. (a) Transverse section through the hypothalamus-median eminence region. A dense accumulation of fluorescent nerves is observed in close proximity to the capillary plexus in the external layer. Fewer more discreet varicose fibers are observed in the internal layer of the median eminence. Low fluorescent arcuate nucleus cell bodies are present (arrows). (× 135)
(b) Median eminence, sagittal section. Posterior region where the infundibular stem (arrow) originates. (× 135) (14 μ)

References p. 208–209

The median eminence consists of an internal (subependymal) and external (palisade) layer. The external layer contains a dense aggregation of diffuse fluorescent fibers in close proximity to the primary plexus of the hypophyseal portal system (Figs. 1 and 2). These monoaminergic terminals probably also make synaptic contact with the neurons (peptidergic) which are responsible for the storage and release of the releasing and inhibiting factors that affect adenohypophyseal secretion. It is possible to distinguish fine varicose fibers in the external layer which are arranged perpendicular to the surface. Distinct fluorescent fasciculi can sometimes be followed into the external layer from the internal layer (Smith and Simpson, 1970). It is thought that these fasciculi represent preterminal axons which pass toward the external layer from sites of origin in the hypothalamus. Considerably fewer varicose terminals are observed to follow the capillary loops into the internal layer of the median eminence. Larger varicosities, thought to contain noradrenaline, are seen in the internal layer (Fuxe and Hökfelt, 1969). (*2*) Noradrenaline axons enter the median eminence from the lateral ventral surface of the brain and intermingle with the dopamine fibers in the internal and external layers (Björklund *et al.*, 1970). (*3*) Two minor groups of catecholamine axons have been reported (Björklund *et al.*, 1970). The identity of the monoamine is not certain. One group enters the median eminence from the anterior direction; the other can only be traced to the arcuate nucleus in a dorso-ventral direction along the third ventricle. (*4*) An unknown and rather obscure group of yellow fluorescent axons were observed in proximity to the median eminence only after lesions of the hypothalamus. Microspectrofluorimetric studies indicate that this system probably contains an indole derivative not identical to serotonin (Björklund *et al.*, 1970).

The infundibular stem (anatomical stem) is without an internal layer and is entirely surrounded by green fluorescent nerves with the same density seen in the upper median eminence (pars oralis and pars caudalis infundibuli) (Smith and Simpson, 1970). The fluorescence of the stem extends caudally to the pars nervosa (neural lobe) just beyond the most rostral portion of the pars intermedia where it terminates abruptly (Fig. 3). Two types of green fluorescent fibers are noted in the rat pars nervosa. An abundant number of fine varicose terminals which frequently appear to be more concentrated in the external layer (zone adjacent to the pars intermedia) (Fig. 4). Thick varicose fibers are observed around blood vessels mainly in the internal layer (central part of the lobe) (Odake, 1967; Björklund, 1968; Fuxe and Hökfelt, 1969). After superior cervical ganglionectomy, the fine fibers of the neurointermediate lobe are essentially normal but most of the larger varicose fibers around the blood vessels

---

Fig. 3. Sagittal section of a 10-day-old rat pituitary *in situ* at the base of the brain. The intense fluorescence (arrow) outlines the infundibular stem (IS) which extends caudally to the pars nervosa (PN). (× 85) (14 μ)

Fig. 4. Pituitary, pars nervosa (PN); pars intermedia (PI); pars distalis (PD). Fluorescent fibers in the PN and between the lobes of the PI. (× 180) (14 μ)

Fig. 5. Pars intermedia with fine fluorescent fibers surrounding lobules and individual cells. (× 450) (14 μ)

Fig. 6. Pars intermedia with a yellow fluorescent hue. Fine fibers enter the lobe from the densely innervated infundibular stem (arrow). (× 180) (14 μ)

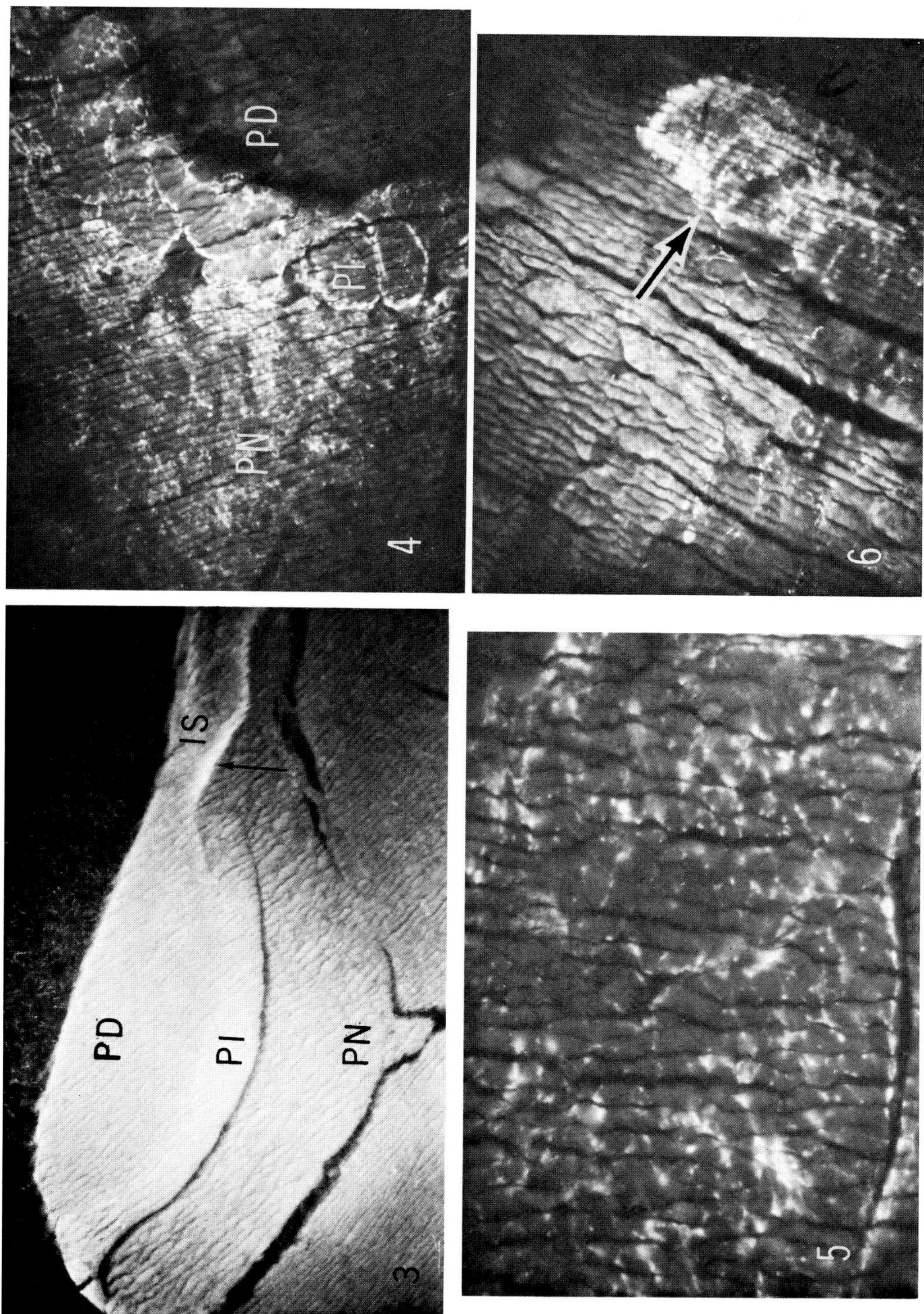

References p. 208–209

in the pars nervosa had disappeared (Fuxe, 1964; Björklund, 1968). The neural lobe is believed to be primarily innervated by dopamine-containing fibers (Björklund *et al.*, 1970). The pars intermedia innervation shows considerable variation between animals. Green fluorescent fibers are regularly seen between the lobes (Fig. 4), but the fine fibers between the lobules (Fig. 5) vary in number between individual rats. It would be of interest to learn whether a diurnal rhythm exists in the catecholamine content of this lobe. Current evidence appears to indicate that both dopamine and noradrenaline fibers are present in the pars intermedia (Björklund *et al.*, 1970). Further studies are needed to ascertain whether or not the dopaminergic fibers emanate from an area outside the arcuate-hypophyseal complex.

In addition to the monoaminergic fibers, the pars intermedia contains a specific yellow-green to yellow fluorescence (Dahlström and Fuxe, 1966; Björklund and Falck, 1968). The intensity of fluorescence and the particular hue observed appears to vary greatly from animal to animal (Fig. 6). The bright yellow fluorescent component fades quickly to ultraviolet irradiation while a dull yellow fluorescent hue remains and is more stable to irradiation. The quick-fading component is reminiscent of the yellow fluorescence observed in serotonergic nerves of the raphe region of the brain (Dahlström and Fuxe, 1964). It would seem that the quick-fading component is serotonin, particularly because it has been found in the pars intermedia in considerable quantities (0.25 μg/mg protein) (Piezzi and Wurtman, 1970). Björklund and Falck (1968) showed that the cells of the pars intermedia contain a fluorophore with the same microspectrofluorimetric characteristics of tryptamine. However, tryptamine has never been isolated from the rat pituitary (Saavedra and Axelrod, personal communication). It would be of great interest to determine if the more stable yellow fluorescence reflects the presence of a polypeptide with an N-terminal tryptophan or 5-hydroxytryptophan (Hakanson *et al.*, 1971).

Large green fluorescent masses or droplets up to 20 μ in diameter were observed in the internal layer of the median eminence, infundibular stem and pars nervosa. A more sparse number of fluorescent droplets are seen in the external layer of the median eminence and the pars intermedia (Fuxe, 1964; Odake, 1967; Björklund, 1968; Smith and Simpson, 1970). Electron-microscopic studies have indicated that the droplets are axonal swellings of spontaneously degenerating dopaminergic axons (Baumgarten *et al.*, 1972). The interesting suggestion was made that dopaminergic neural lobe fibers undergo continuous reorganization through degeneration–regeneration cycles.

Fig. 7 is a schematic representation of the foregoing observations of the monoaminergic innervation of the tubero-infundibular system. Dopamine neurons emanate from the arcuate nucleus, periventricular nucleus and possibly from an unknown source. They terminate in the median eminence, mostly the external layer, but also in the internal layers, pars nervosa and pars intermedia. Noradrenaline-containing fibers enter the median eminence from the ventral surface and reside in the internal and external layers of the median eminence and the pars intermedia. It is not yet established whether another group of neurons enters the median eminence along the third ventricle.

The pars distalis does not contain monoaminergic nerves. In the rat, only a small

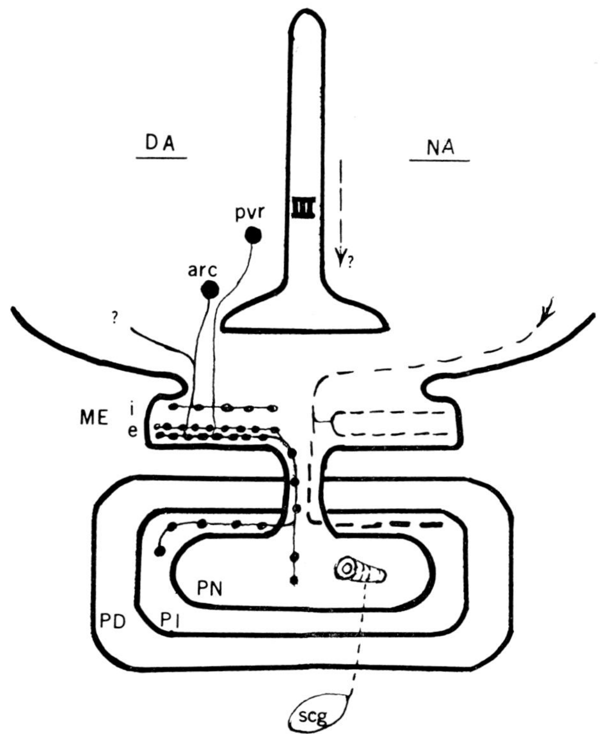

Fig. 7. Diagrammatic representation of the dopaminergic (DA) and noradrenergic (NA) innervation of the rat pituitary. DA neurons (–•–•–•–) emanate from the arcuate nucleus (arc) and periventricular nucleus (pvr); they are found in the external (e) and internal (i) layers of the median eminence (ME) and course through the infundibular stem to the pars nervosa (PN) and pars intermedia (PI). NA neurons (- - - -) from the ventral surface of the brain, and possibly along the third ventricle (III), enter the e and i layers of the ME and course through the infundibular stem to the PI. Blood vessels of the PN are innervated by NA neurons which emanate from the superior cervical ganglion (scg). No nerves are present in the pars distalis (PD).

number (if any) of the gland cells display a weak green to yellow-green fluorescence. However, in the cat, pig and dog, numerous cells are present with a moderate to strong green to yellow-green fluorescence (Dahlström and Fuxe, 1966; Fuxe and Hökfelt, 1969; Björklund and Falck, 1968). In contrast, the pars distalis of the newborn rat does contain moderate green fluorescent cells.

L-3,4-Dihydroxyphenylalanine (L-DOPA) causes an increase in the number and intensity of fluorescence of these cells which is blocked by a DOPA-decarboxylase inhibitor [NSD 1015 (Brocresine, Lederle Co.)]. A monoamine oxidase inhibitor (nialamide) in combination with dopamine causes a small increase in the number and intensity of fluorescence (Dahlström and Fuxe, 1966). In addition, administration of 5-hydroxytryptophan results in a small to medium number of weak to strong yellow fluorescent cells; this fluorescence is inhibited by a DOPA-decarboxylase inhibitor. The function of the fluorescent cells is obscure. No appreciable quantity of catecholamines has been reported in the anterior lobe of the adenohypophysis. The

References p. 208–209

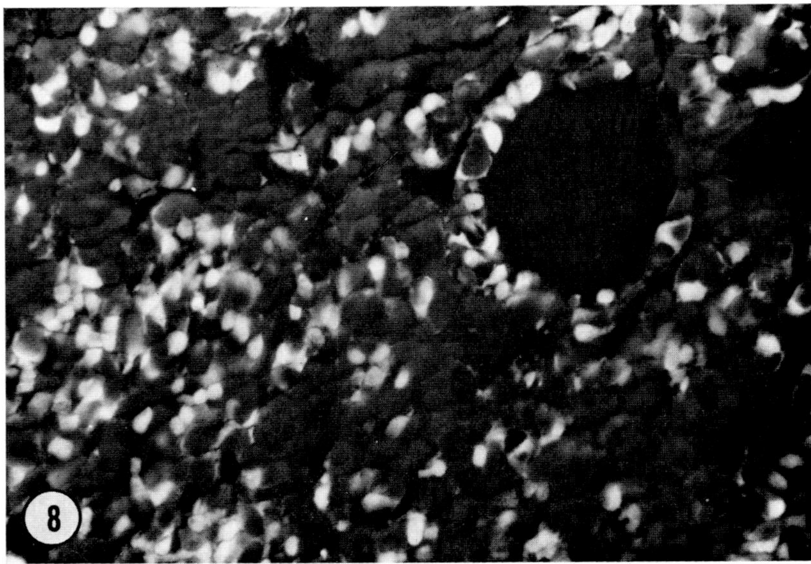

Fig. 8. Intense green fluorescent cells in the pars distalis of a rat treated with reserpine (5 mg/kg, 24 h) and tryptophan (400 mg/kg, 1.5 h). (× 215) (14 μ)

possibility that there is a specificity for uptake and decarboxylation of L-DOPA and 5-hydroxytryptophan exists, particularly in view of the work which suggest that monoaminergic mechanisms may be involved in the regulation of certain anterior pituitary hormones.

Work currently in progress has revealed that administration of tryptophan (400 mg/kg, 1.5 h) results in numerous, moderately intense, green fluorescent cells; the fluorescence is markedly enhanced if the rat is pretreated with a decarboxylase inhibitor (L-α-hydrazinemethyldihydroxyphenylalanine, MK 486) or reserpine (Fig. 8). Pretreatment with *para*-chlorophenylalanine, a tryptophan hydroxylase inhibitor, inhibits the formation of the fluorescence product. The possibility of the formation of large amounts of 5-hydroxytryptophan or a polypeptide with an N-terminal 5-hydroxytryptophan is under consideration.

The involvement of catecholamines in the regulation of release of pituitary hormones suggests that a possible common architectural feature of certain peptides with noradrenaline or dopamine may exist. Such a stereochemical, three-dimensional character of both types of molecules might provide an insight into the mechanism whereby pituitary hormones, inhibitory or releasing factors are influenced. Accordingly, with the use of molecular models, a comparison was made between noradrenaline and the first five amino acids of corticotrophin (ACTH) (Ser-Tyr-Ser-Met-Glu) which is identical with α-MSH (melanocyte-stimulating hormone) and α-CRF (corticotrophin-releasing factor) (Schally *et al.*, 1960). It was of great interest to note that there was a close apposition of the phenyl group of the second amino acid, tyrosine, with the serine end group (H_2N–CH–H_2COH) which made possible a juxtaposition of the noradrenaline molecule to the serine-tyrosine, three-dimensional, catecholamine-like

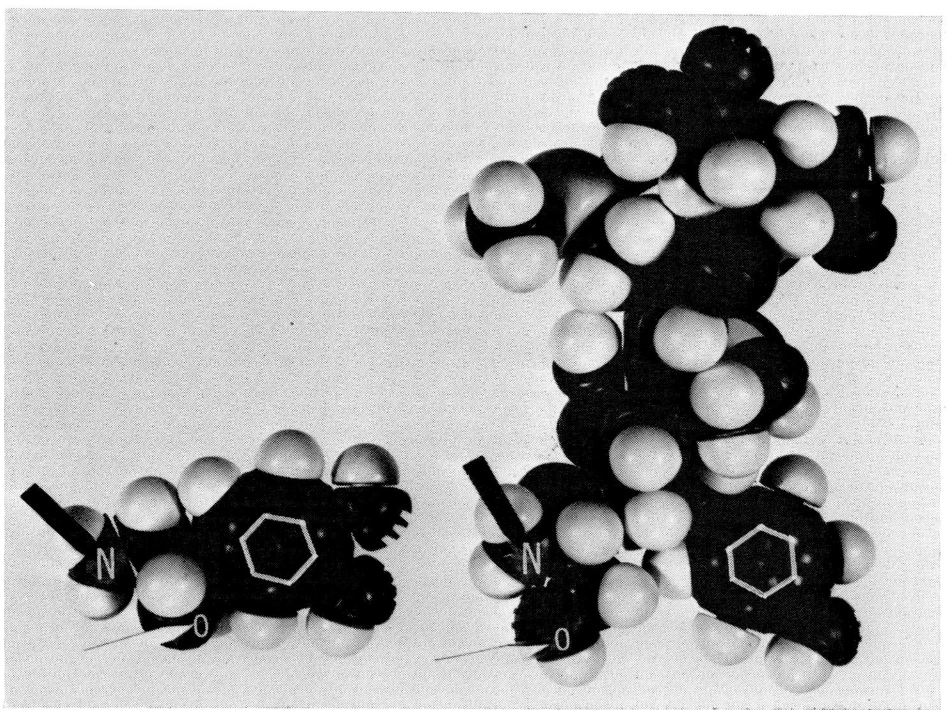

Fig. 9. Molecular models of the first five amino acids of ACTH (or α-MSH) (right) and noradrenaline (left). The phenyl group of the tyrosine moiety and the serine end group align to form a catecholamine-like configuration. Black arrow indicates the N atom of the -NH; white arrow indicates the O atom of the —OH group.

configuration (Fig. 9). This would suggest a competitive influence of the catecholamine molecule upon binding sites within peptidergic nerves or cells. It is of interest that the gonadotrophin-releasing factors (*e.g.* luteinizing hormone-releasing factor, LRF) contain a serine–tyrosine sequence in the third and fourth amino acid positions (Matsuo *et al.*, 1971; Burgus *et al.*, 1971). It remains for physiological and chemical studies to clarify whether the amines are involved in direct release of peptides or indirect release or inhibition *via* releasing or inhibiting factors.

SUMMARY

A survey was made of the distribution of monoaminergic nerves in the pituitary. Noradrenergic and dopaminergic neurons emanate from the brain and are distributed in the median eminence. These neurons course through the infundibular stem and terminate in the pars intermedia. In addition, dopaminergic neurons terminate in the pars nervosa. Noradrenergic neurons, which originate from the superior cervical ganglia, are present around blood vessels in the pars nervosa. The pars distalis contains a cell type that appears to have a specific uptake mechanism for tryptophan,

References p. 208–209

5-hydroxytryptophan and L-DOPA. The pars intermedia contains a variable yellow fluorescence which is probably partly serotonin.

A molecular configurational similarity between catecholamine and the end serine–tyrosine amino acids of ACTH is presented. A competitive mechanism between the catecholamine molecule and binding sites of certain peptides is suggested.

REFERENCES

BAUMGARTEN, H. G., BJÖRKLUND, A., HOLSTEIN, A. F. AND NOBIN, A. (1972) Organization and ultrastructural identification of the catecholamine nerve terminals in the neural lobe and pars intermedia of the rat pituitary. *Z. Zellforsch.*, **126**, 483–517.

BJÖRKLUND, A. (1968) Monoamine-containing fibres in the pituitary neuro-intermediate lobe of the pig and rat. *Z. Zellforsch.*, **89**, 573–589.

BJÖRKLUND, A. AND FALCK, B. (1968) An improvement of the histochemical fluorescence method for monoamines. Observations on varying extractability of fluorphores in different nerve fibers. *J. Histochem. Cytochem.*, **16**, 717–720.

BJÖRKLUND, A., FALCK, B., HROMEK, F., OWMAN, CH. AND WEST, K. (1970) Identification and terminal distribution of the tubero-hypophyseal monoamine fibre systems in the rat by means of stereotaxis and microspectrofluorimetric techniques. *Brain Res.*, **17**, 1–23.

BURGUS, R., BUTCHER, M., LING, N., MONAHAN, M., RIVIER, J., FELLOW, S. R., AMOSS, M., BLACKWELL, R., VALE, W. AND GUILLEMIN, R. (1971) Structure moléculaire du facteur hypothalamique (LRF) d'origine ovine contrôlant la secrétion de l'hormone gonadotrope hypophysaire de lutéinisation (LH). *Compt. rend. Acad. Sci.*, **273**, 1611–1613.

CARLSSON, A., FALCK, B. AND HILLARP, N.-A. (1962) Cellular localization of brain monoamines. *Acta physiol. scand.*, **56**, Suppl. 196.

DAHLSTRÖM, A. AND FUXE, K. (1964) Existence of monoamine-containing neurons in the central nervous system, I. Demonstration of monoamines in the cell-bodies of brain stem neurons. *Acta physiol. scand.*, **62**, Suppl. 232.

DAHLSTRÖM, A. AND FUXE, K. (1966) Monoamines and the pituitary gland. *Acta endocrinol.*, **51**, 301–314.

ENEMAR, A. AND FALCK, B. (1965) On the presence of adrenergic nerves in the pars intermedia of the frog, *Rana temporaria*. *Gen. comp. Endocrinol.*, **5**, 577–583.

FALCK, B. (1962) Observations on the possibilities for the cellular localization of monoamines with a fluorescence method. *Acta physiol. scand.*, **56**, Suppl. 197.

FALCK, B. AND OWMAN, D. (1965) A detailed methodological description of the fluorescence method for the cellular demonstration of biogenic monoamines. *Acta Univ. Lund,* Section II, No. **7**.

FALCK, B., HILLARP, N.-A., THIEME, G. AND TORP, A. (1962) Fluorescence of catecholamines and related compounds condensed with formaldehyde. *J. Histochem. Cytochem.*, **10**, 348–354.

FUXE, K. (1964) Cellular localization of monoamines in the median eminence of the infundibular stem of some mammals. *Z. Zellforsch.*, **61**, 710–724.

FUXE, K. AND HÖKFELT, T. (1969) Catecholamines in the hypothalamus and the pituitary gland. In *Frontiers in Neuroendocrinology*, W. F. GANONG AND L. MARTINI (Eds.), Oxford University Press, Oxford, pp. 61–83.

HÅKANSON, R., SJÖBERG, A.-K. AND SUNDLER, F. (1971) Formaldehyde-induced fluorescence of peptides with N-terminal 3,4-dihydroxyphenylalanine or 5-hydroxytryptophan. *Histochemie*, **28**, 367–371.

JACOBOWITZ, D. AND KOSTRZEWA, R. (1971) Selective action of 6-hydroxydopa on noradrenergic terminals: Mapping of preterminal axons of the brain. *Life Sci.*, **10**, 1329–1342.

MATSUO, H., BABA, K., NAIR, R. M. G., ARIMURA, A. AND SCHALLY, A. V. (1971) Structure of the porcine LH- and FSH-releasing hormone, I. The proposed amino acid sequence. *Biochem. biophys. res. Commun.*, **43**, 1334–1339.

ODAKE, G. (1967) Fluorescence microscopy of the catecholamine-containing neurons of the hypothalamohypophyseal system. *Z. Zellforsch.*, **82**, 46–64.

PIEZZI, R. S. AND WURTMAN, R. J. (1970) Pituitary serotonin content: Effects of melatonin or deprivation of water. *Science*, **169**, 285–286.

SCHALLY, A. V., ANDERSEN, R. N., LIPSCOMB, H. S., LONG, J. M. AND GUILLEMIN, R. (1960) Evidence for the existence of two corticotrophin-releasing factors, alpha and beta. *Nature*, **188**, 1192–1193.

SMITH, G. C. AND SIMPSON, R. W. (1970) Monoamine fluorescence in the median eminence of fetal, neonatal and adult rats. *Z. Zellforsch.*, **104**, 541–556.

UNGERSTEDT, U. (1971) Stereotaxic mapping of monoamine pathways in the rat brain. *Acta physiol. scand.*, Suppl. 367, 1–48.

Discussion on p. 222.

Biogenic Amines in the Pituitary Gland: What is Their Origin and Function? Pituitary Indolamines

MARKKU HYYPPÄ AND RICHARD J. WURTMAN

Laboratory of Neuroendocrine Regulation, Department of Nutrition and Food Science, Massachusetts Institute of Technology, Cambridge, Mass. (U.S.A.)

INTRODUCTION

With the histochemical fluorescence technique of Falck and Hillarp it has been revealed that endocrine cells of the mammalian adenohypophysis, as well as rich systems of nerve terminals in the intermediate and posterior lobes of the mammalian pituitary, exhibit formaldehyde-induced fluorescence (Pearse and McGregor, 1964, Dahlström and Fuxe, 1966; Odake, 1967; Björklund, 1968, Björklund and Falck, 1969a, b; Björklund *et al.*, 1968, 1970, 1973; Baumgarten *et al.*, 1972; Håkanson *et al.*, 1972). In this review we describe the occurrence of indole amines in the pituitary proper of mammals—excluding the median eminence region. The possible functional significance of local monoamines in the control of pituitary secretion is also discussed.

OCCURRENCE OF BIOGENIC AMINES IN THE PITUITARY GLAND

Notably high concentrations of what is apparently serotonin have been detected fluorometrically in the pituitaries of the cat (0.94 μg/g; Björklund and Falck, 1969a) and cow (Piezzi *et al.*, 1970). In the cow, the highest concentrations occurred in the neural lobe (5.4–6.7 μg/g), in the infundibular stem (5.3–6.0 μg/g), and in the pars intermedia (4.5–5.1 μg/g). Lower serotonin concentrations (1.7–1.9 μg/g) were found in the pars distalis (Piezzi *et al.*, 1970).

The identity of the assayed material as serotonin has not been fully established, and it seems possible that other indolamines could also be present (*cf.* Björklund *et al.*, 1970). Besides serotonin, low concentrations of tryptamine have been identified (about 0.05 μg/g) in extracts from steer pituitary (Martin *et al.*, 1971).

The pig pituitary contains high concentrations of dopamine in the pars intermedia and neural lobe (mean value 0.41 μg/g) and lower concentrations in the pars distalis (0.01 μg/g). Low concentrations of noradrenaline (0.01–0.04 μg/g) and serotonin (0.05–0.09 μg/g) are also present, equally distributed throughout the different lobes (Björklund *et al.*, 1967). In the rat (Björklund *et al.*, 1970), cat (Björklund and Falck,

References p. 214–215

1969a), horse (Iwata and Ishii, 1969) high concentrations of dopamine, and lower concentrations of noradrenaline are present in the neural lobe and pars intermedia. Adrenaline has not yet been detected in significant concentrations in any pituitary gland (Björklund and Falck, 1969a; Björklund *et al.*, 1970; Iwata and Ishii, 1969).

Besides catecholamines and indolamines, histamine is also present in the mammalian pituitary (Adam and Hye, 1966). Some of this histamine is located within mast cells. The remainder of this review will consider only pituitary indolamines.

DISTRIBUTION AND IDENTITY OF FORMALDEHYDE-INDUCED CELLULAR FLUORESCENCE IN THE MAMMALIAN ADENOHYPOPHYSIS

All cells in the mammalian pars intermedia and scattered cells in the mammalian pars distalis contain a substance which, after condensation with formaldehyde, forms a fluorescent compound (Dahlström and Fuxe, 1966; Björklund and Falck, 1969a, b). The nature of this fluorigenic substance has remained obscure. It was initially suggested that the compound was serotonin (Pearse and McGregor, 1964) or a primary catecholamine (Dahlström and Fuxe, 1966); however, later studies using micro-spectrofluorometric and chemical techniques suggested that the fluorigenic substance was not identical with either catecholamines or serotonin. The formaldehyde-induced fluorescence of the adenohypophyseal cells could be enhanced if the formaldehyde condensation was carried out in the presence of ozone or acid (Björklund and Falck, 1969a; Björklund *et al.*, 1972). In this respect, as well as in its spectral properties, the cellular fluorescence displayed the characteristics of the fluorophore of tryptamine (Björklund and Falck, 1969a, b). Since only very low concentrations of tryptamine have been isolated from mammalian pituitaries (Martin *et al.*, 1971; Håkanson *et al.*, 1972) it seems likely that at least a portion of the pituitary fluorescence derives from a compound other than tryptamine itself. Investigations undertaken to clarify this question showed that peptides with tryptophan in the NH_2-terminal position react in the formaldehyde-ozone procedure to give an intense fluorescence spectrally similar to that of tryptamine (Håkanson and Sundler, 1971a, b). It remains to be determined whether N-terminal tryptophyl peptides actually exist in the pituitary and whether they are responsible for the pituitary fluorescence.

The location of the serotonin in pituitary cells has not yet been established (Björklund *et al.*, 1967; Björklund and Falck, 1969a; Piezzi *et al.*, 1970; Piezzi and Wurtman, 1970). The relatively low fluorescence yield of serotonin, however, makes it more difficult than catecholamines to visualize with the Falck-Hillarp technique. Thus, it may be impossible to visualize serotonin's storage sites, especially if the serotonin has a more widespread distribution in the pituitary tissues. In the rat, the neuro-intermediate lobe contains serotonin-rich mast cells (Björklund *et al.*, 1973) which could be responsible for the chemically detectable serotonin in that species.

Most of the PAS-positive cells in the anterior pituitary can take exogenous L-3,4-dihydroxyphenylalanine (L-DOPA) from the blood and decarboxylate it to form dopamine (Dahlström and Fuxe, 1966). 1 h after i.p. administration of 100 mg/kg

L-DOPA, the amount of dopamine formed in the mouse pars distalis has fluorometrically been determined to be 2.5–5.4 ng/gland (Björklund and Nobin, unpublished). Similarly, some cells in the anterior pituitary take up exogenous 5-hydroxytryptophan (5-HTP) and decarboxylate it to serotonin, revealed as a yellow fluorescence after treatment with formaldehyde (Dahlström and Fuxe, 1966). The physiological significance of a cell's ability to make dopamine or serotonin from exogenous L-DOPA or L-5-HTP is not apparent. Both amino acids are taken up by the same membrane transport system that mediates the uptake of the aromatic amino acids which form proteins (*e.g.*, tyrosine, tryptophan); hence *all* cells can take them up. Moreover, the enzyme which catalyzes the decarboxylation of L-DOPA and L-5-HTP (aromatic amino acid decarboxylase) is present in most cells. Hence it does not appear that the accumulation of a monoamine in a cell following L-DOPA or L-5-HTP administration can be taken as evidence that the cell *normally* synthesizes dopamine or serotonin (Lytle *et al.*, 1972; Romero *et al.*, 1973).

POSSIBLE EFFECTS OF PITUITARY AMINES ON HORMONE SECRETION FROM PITUITARY CELLS

Indolamines and other biogenic amines could influence the hormone secretion of pituitary cells in one of three principal ways:

(*1*) Direct nervous control *via* monoaminergic neurons. The rich dopaminergic innervation of the neural lobe and pars intermedia, with its synapse-like contacts with neurosecretory axons and intermedia cells (Baumgarten *et al.*, 1972), suggests that dopamine, released from the nerve terminals, may directly influence the secretion of melanocyte-stimulating hormone (MSH), or possibly corticotrophin (ACTH), from intermedia cells, and of the octapeptides, oxytocin and vasopressin, from the neural lobe. In addition, noradrenaline released from vasomotor terminals in the neural lobe and at the border of the pars intermedia could influence their blood flow, thereby secondarily modifying the secretion of MSH or the octapeptides. So far, no direct experimental evidence is available that monoamines released from nerve terminals influence hormone secretion from the mammalian pituitary.

(*2*) Local, intracellular action. Amines stored within hormone-secreting cells could somehow influence the synthesis, storage, or release of these hormones. Biogenic amines, such as serotonin, dopamine, and histamine, have been demonstrated in many endocrine cell systems producing polypeptide hormones (for review, see Falck and Owman, 1968; Owman *et al.*, 1972). In certain cases, physiologic manipulations that cause the cells to secrete their hormone have been shown to modify their amine concentrations also. Administration of vitamin D_2, for example, depletes the cells of the chick ultimobranchial body of both thyrocalcitonin and dopamine (Melander *et al.*, 1971). At present there are no experimental data relating the piuitary stores of serotonin, tryptamine, or histamine to the secretion of pituitary hormones. However, the administration of melatonin, a pineal hormone which depletes the pituitary of MSH (Kastin and Schally, 1967), increases the serotonin content of the rat pars intermedia (Piezzi and Wurtman, 1970). It is not known in which cell structures

References p. 214–215

(*e.g.* intermedia cells or nerve terminals) this increase occurs, and the functional interpretation of this effect is therefore unclear. Water deprivation decreases the serotonin content of the anterior and posterior lobes of the rat pituitary (Piezzi and Wurtman, 1970), but since brain serotonin synthesis apparently depends upon plasma amino acid levels (Fernstrom and Wurtman, 1971, 1972), this decrease could result from the depressed food consumption that accompanies water deprivation.

(*3*) Effect *via* the circulation. Monoamines delivered to the pituitary by the circulation could influence the secretion of specific hormones. Parts of the pituitary receive blood from two circulations: systemic arterial blood, and blood from the hypothalamo-hypophyseal portal system. It is possible that the latter blood supply might deliver higher concentrations of catecholamines or serotonin (from nerve terminals in the median eminence) to the anterior pituitary; however, several attempts to demonstrate high concentrations in the portal blood have been unsuccessful (see Wurtman, 1971). The catecholamines in systemic arterial blood include noradrenaline liberated from peripheral sympathetic nerve terminals, and adrenaline secreted from the adrenal medulla. Exogenous circulating catecholamines increase the secretion of ACTH from the anterior lobe. These effects of circulating amines on pituitary function are discussed in detail elsewhere in this volume.

SUMMARY

Considerably high serotonin levels were found in the pituitaries of various mammalian species. The localization of the serotonin in pituitary cells has not yet been established, but a new fluorigenic substance, which was not identical with either catecholamines or serotonin, was recently found. This compound has some similarities to the fluorescence characteristics of peptides with tryptophan in the NH_2-terminal position.

The possible effects of pituitary indoleamines on hormone secretion from the pituitary cells is described in the present review from three different standpoints.

REFERENCES

Adam, H. M. and Hye, H. K. A. (1966) Concentration of histamine in different parts of brain and hypophysis of cat and its modification by drugs. *Brit. J. Pharmacol.*, **28**, 137–152.

Baumgarten, H. G., Björklund, A., Holstein, A. F. and Nobin, A. (1972) Organization and ultrastructural identification of the catecholamine nerve terminals in the neural lobe and pars intermedia of the rat pituitary. *Z. Zellforsch.*, **126**, 483–517.

Björklund, A. (1968) Monoamine-containing fibres in the neuro-intermediate lobe of the pig and rat. *Z. Zellforsch.*, **89**, 573–589.

Björklund, A., Falck, B. and Rosengren, E. (1967) Monoamines in the pituitary gland of the pig. *Life Sci.*, **6**, 2103–2110.

Björklund, A. and Falck, B. (1969a) Pituitary monoamines of the cat with special reference to the presence of an unidentified monoamine-like substance in the adenohypophysis. *Z. Zellforsch.*, **93**, 254–264.

Björklund, A. and Falck, B. (1969b) Histochemical characterization of a tryptamine-like substance stored in cells of the mammalian adenohypophysis. *Acta. physiol. scand.*, **77**, 475–489.

BJÖRKLUND, A., ENEMAR, A. AND FALCK, B. (1968) Monoamines in the hypothalamo-hypophysial system of the mouse with special reference to the ontogenetic aspect. *Z. Zellforsch.*, **89**, 590–607.

BJÖRKLUND, A., FALCK, B., HROMEK, F., OWMAN, CH. AND WEST, K. A. (1970) Identification and terminal distribution of the tubero-hypophyseal monoamine fibre systems in the rat by means of stereo-taxic and microspectrofluorimetric technique. *Brain. Res.*, **17**, 1–23.

BJÖRKLUND, A., MOORE, R. Y., NOBIN, A. AND STENEVI, U. (1973) The organization of tubero-hypophyseal and reticulo-infundibular catecholamine neuron systems in the rat brain. *Brain Res.*, in press.

BJÖRKLUND, A., NOBIN, A. AND STENEVI, U. (1972) Acid catalysis of the formaldehyde condensation reaction for a sensitive histochemical demonstration of tryptamines and 3-methoxylated phenylethylamines, 2. Characterization of amine fluorophores and application to tissues. *J. Histochem. Cytochem.*, **19**, 286–298.

DAHLSTRÖM, A. AND FUXE, K. (1966) Monoamines and the pituitary gland. *Acta endocrinol.*, **51**, 301–314.

FALCK, B. AND OWMAN, CH. (1968) 5-Hydroxytryptamine and related amines in endocrine cell systems. *Advanc. Pharmacol.*, **6A**, 211.

FERNSTROM, J. D. AND WURTMAN, R. J. (1971) Brain serotonin content: Increase following ingestion of carbohydrate diet. *Science*, **174**, 1023–1025.

FERNSTROM, J. D. AND WURTMAN, R. J. (1972) Brain serotonin content: Physiological regulation by plasma neutral amino acids. *Science*, **178**, 414.

HÅKANSON, R. AND SUNDLER, F. (1971a) Fluorometric determination of N-terminal tryptophan-peptides after formaldehyde condensation. *Biochem. Pharmacol.*, **20**, 3223–3225.

HÅKANSON, R. AND SUNDLER, F. (1971b) Formaldehyde-induced fluorescence of a tryptophyl tetrapeptide. *J. Histochem. Cytochem.*, **19**, 693–695.

HÅKANSON, R., LARSSON, L.-I., NOBIN, A. AND SUNDLER, F. (1972) Tryptamine or tryptophyl-peptides in endocrine cells of the mammalian adenohypophysis? *J. Histochem. Cytochem.*, in press.

IWATA, T. AND ISHII, S. (1969) Chemical isolation and determination of catecholamines in the median eminence and pars nervosa of the rat and horse. *Neuroendocrinology*, **5**, 140–148.

KASTIN, A. J. AND SCHALLY, A. V. (1967) Autoregulation of release of melanocyte stimulating hormone from the rat pituitary. *Nature (Lond.)*, **213**, 1238–1240.

LYTLE, L. D., HURKO, O., ROMERO, J. A., COTTMAN, K., LEEHEY, D. AND WURTMAN, R. J. (1972) The effects of 6-hydroxydopamine pretreatment on the accumulation of dopa and dopamine in brain and peripheral organs following L-dopa administration. *J. neural Transmission*, **33**, 63.

MARTIN, W. R., SLOAN, J. W. AND CHRISTIAN, S. T. (1971) Brain tryptamine. *Fed. Proc.*, **30**, 271.

MELANDER, A., OWMAN, CH. AND SUNDLER, F. (1971) Effect of vitamin D_2 stimulation on amine stores and secretory granules in the calcitonin cells of the mouse. *Histochemie*, **25**, 32.

ODAKE, G. (1967) Fluorescence microscopy of the catecholamine containing neurons of the hypothalamo-hypophyseal system. *Z. Zellforsch.*, **82**, 46–64.

OWMAN, CH., HÅKANSON, R. AND SUNDLER, F. (1973) Occurrence and function of amines in the polypeptide-hormone producing endocrine cells. *Fed. Proc.*, in press.

PEARSE, A. G. E. AND MCGREGOR, M. M. (1964) Functional cytology of the pituitary gland. *Ann. Rep. Brit. Emp. Cancer Camp.*, **2**, 665.

PIEZZI, R. S. AND WURTMAN, R. J. (1970) Pituitary serotonin content: Effects of melatonin and deprivation of water. *Science*, **169**, 285–286.

PIEZZI, R. S., LARIN, F. AND WURTMAN, R. J. (1970) Serotonin, 5-hydroxyindoleacetic acid (5-HIAA), and monoamine oxidase in bovine median eminence and pituitary gland. *Endocrinology*, **86**, 1460–1462.

ROMERO, J. A., LYTLE, L. D., ORDONEZ, L. A. AND WURTMAN, R. J. (1973) Effects of L-dopa administration on the concentrations of dopa, dopamine, and norepinephrine in various rat tissues. *J. Pharmacol. exp. Ther.*, **184**, 67.

WURTMAN, R. J. (Ed.) (1971) Brain monoamines and endocrine function. *Neurosci. Res. Program Bull.*, **9** (2).

Discussion on p. 222.

Catecholamines in the Pituitary: Origin and Fate

ROLAND D. CIARANELLO AND JACK D. BARCHAS

Section on Pharmacology, Laboratory of Clinical Science, National Institute of Mental Health, Bethesda, Md. and Department of Psychiatry, Stanford University School of Medicine Stanford, Calif. (U.S.A.)

Research on the subject of catecholamines and the pituitary has focused principally on (*1*) the regulation by the pituitary of catecholamine synthesis, metabolism and turnover in peripheral tissues and (*2*) regulation by central catecholamines of release of pituitary hormones. An extensive literature exists in both these areas, and we will make no attempt to review it here. Instead we would like to focus briefly on a less well-studied area, and discuss some aspects of catecholamines within the pituitary.

SYNTHESIS OF CATECHOLAMINES IN THE PITUITARY

Sadly, the pituitary seems to have been largely ignored when the classic catecholamine studies of the '50s and '60s were performed. There is currently no definitive evidence that the enzymatic machinery necessary for catecholamine biosynthesis is present in the pituitary. In our laboratory we have undertaken a search for tyrosine hydroxylase, the initial and rate-limiting enzyme in catecholamine biosynthesis, in the pituitary. Although a very low hydroxylase activity was seen, this could have been explained by the presence in pituitary extracts of high amounts of tryptophan hydroxylase. This enzyme, the initial step in serotonin biosynthesis, is present in appreciable amounts in the pituitary and has a slight affinity for tyrosine (Ichiyama *et al.*, 1970), the substrate used in the tyrosine hydroxylase assay. To establish the presence of tyrosine hydroxylase activity in the pituitary, it will be necessary to perform studies with specific inhibitors of the enzymes involved.

There is no data available which unequivocally establishes the presence of dopamine beta-hydroxylase in the pituitary. This very important enzyme is the last step in the formation of noradrenaline. It is released into the blood and is probably associated very closely with sympathetic nerve endings (Weinshilboum and Axelrod, 1971) Previous assays for this enzyme were relatively insensitive, and might not have detected low levels of activity. Recently, however, a new procedure (Molinoff *et al.*, 1971) has become available which is extremely sensitive, and might yield useful information when applied to the pituitary.

References p. 222

UPTAKE OF CATECHOLAMINES BY THE PITUITARY

The pituitary is capable of actively taking up substantial amounts of noradrenaline and adrenaline from the circulation. Axelrod *et al.* (1959) and Weil-Malherbe *et al.* (1959, 1961) demonstrated that the pituitary lay outside the blood-brain barrier for the catecholamines. This problem was further studied by Wilson *et al.* (1962) who showed that the pituitary actively took up adrenaline and concentrated it several-fold over plasma levels. They proposed a carrier-mediated saturable uptake system which obeyed Michaelis–Menten kinetics. The most recent uptake studies were performed by Steinman *et al.* (1969) and by Barchas *et al.* (1969). These studies confirmed the earlier findings that the pituitary avidly took up adrenaline against large plasma concentration gradients.

METABOLISM OF CATECHOLAMINES BY THE PITUITARY

The pituitary seems to possess the enzymatic machinery to inactivate catecholamines. The gland probably disposes of catecholamines by the same pathways as the brain, *i.e.*, deamination, *O*-methylation and conjugation. However, in the pituitary, clearance of unchanged catecholamine may be an important facet of metabolism, and the route of metabolism is in part determined by the concentration of catecholamine reaching the pituitary.

When [^{3}H]adrenaline is administered intravenously to rats, it is rapidly taken up

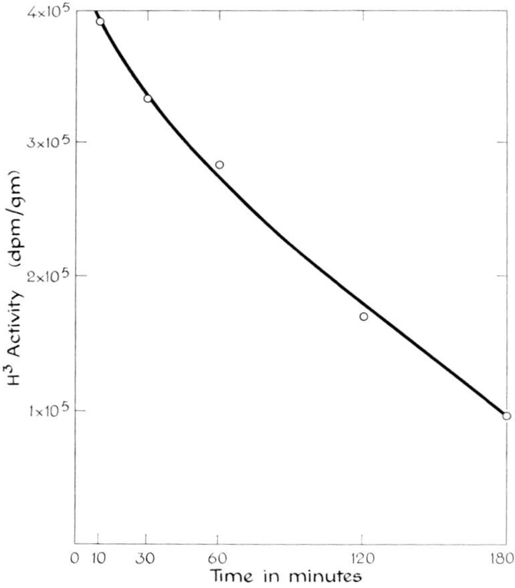

Fig. 1. [^{3}H]Adrenaline uptake and turnover in pituitary.
116 μCi [^{3}H]adrenaline (210 ng) was administered into the femoral vein of 3 rats. Each point represents the average of 3 animals.

TABLE I

PERCENTAGE OF ^{3}H METABOLITES IN PITUITARY FOLLOWING INTRAVENOUS [^{3}H] ADRENALINE ADMINISTRATION

116 μCi [^{3}H] adrenaline was administered into the femoral veins of three rats. The figures represent the percentages of the total activity present in the pituitary at each time point. Each value is the average of three animals.
Abbreviations: [^{3}H]A, [^{3}H]adrenaline, Conj., conjugated metabolites; Dm, deaminated metabolites; *O*-Me, *O*-methylated metabolite (metanephrine); *O*-Me-Dm, *O*-methylated-deaminated metabolite (vanylmandelic acid).

Time (min)	*[^{3}H]A*	*O-Me*	*O-Me-Dm*	*Conj.*	*Dm*
10	40.6	16.4	15.6	5.6	0.65
60	44.5	17.2	12.4	6.3	0.12
90	46.7	12.5	11.6	7.4	0.11
120	52.7	10.7	10.8	5.4	0.17
180	59.8	10.6	12.4	7.2	0.19

TABLE II

PERCENTAGE OF ^{3}H METABOLITES IN PITUITARY FOLLOWING INTRAVENTRICULAR [^{3}H]ADRENALINE ADMINISTRATION

2.43 μCi [3H]adrenaline was injected into the lateral ventricle of rats. Numbers represent the percentage of total activity present and are the average of three animals. For abbreviations see Table I.

Time (h)	*[^{3}H]A*	*O-Me*	*O-Me-Dm*	*Conj.*	*Dm*
1	32.4	10.6	9.8	26.7	12.6
16	42.4	12.4	13.7	19.9	8.6

by the pituitary. Fall-off from initial levels is very rapid (Fig. 1). Nonetheless, the bulk of the remaining radioactivity is present as unchanged adrenaline (Table I). The principal metabolites after intravenous administration are the *O*-methylated and *O*-methylated-deaminated metabolites. There are comparatively small amounts of conjugated or deaminated metabolites.

When the radiolabelled amine is administered into the lateral ventricles, however, a different metabolic profile is obtained (Table II). As before, unchanged adrenaline is the major radioactive compound. The *O*-methylated and *O*-methylated-deaminated derivatives are reduced somewhat in proportion to the rest of the radioactivity. The most notable feature after intraventricular administration is a substantial increase in the fraction of deaminated metabolites and in the amount of conjugated material. The conjugated fraction makes up the major metabolic component when the amine is administered intraventricularly.

These results may possibly be explained by the differences in the amount of adrenaline administered by each route. These data are summarized in Table III, where the absolute amounts of each fraction 60 min after isotope administration is shown. Between the two experiments, the ratios of each fraction are quite similar to the ratio of starting material, except for the conjugated and deaminated metabolites. The

References p. 222

TABLE III

COMPARISON OF ABSOLUTE AMOUNTS OF ADRENALINE AND METABOLITES REMAINING 1 h FOLLOWING ADMINISTRATION OF [^{3}H]ADRENALINE

Absolute amounts of adrenaline and its metabolites were calculated from the preceding tables. Numbers in parentheses are the proportions remaining of the starting radioactivity. *R* in the third column heading is the ratio of each compound in the two experiments. For abbreviations see Table I.

	Route of administration		
	Intravenous	*Intraventricular*	*R*
Initial amount (ng)	2104	44	48
Remaining at 1 h (ng)	1536	33	47
[^{3}H]A	685 (44.5%)	11.0 (32.4%)	62
O-Me	264 (17.2%)	3.4 (10.6%)	83
O-Me-Dm	191 (12.4%)	3.3 (9.8%)	58
Conj.	97 (6.3%)	8.5 (26.7%)	11
Dm	19 (0.12%)	4.1 (12.6%)	4.6

amounts of these compounds formed following intraventricular administration are considerably closer to the amounts formed after intravenous administration. These data might suggest that the amounts formed after intravenous injection reflect saturation values for the enzymes involved in conjugation and deamination. In the pituitary, conjugation might, then, be a first-line but low-capacity metabolic system. In the presence of low concentrations of catecholamines, conjugation is a preferred metabolic route. As this system begins to saturate with rising catecholamine concentration, other metabolic routes handle the overflow.

The ratio of the amount of deaminated metabolites to *O*-methylated-deaminated derivatives differs widely in the two experiments. Interpretation of this wide variation is complicated by the fact that the *O*-methylated-deaminated product may be arrived at by *O*-methylation followed by deamination, or *vice versa* (Fig. 2). At low exogenous adrenaline concentrations, the amounts of *O*-methylated, *O*-methylated-deaminated, and deaminated products are roughly similar. At high concentrations, *O*-methylation overwhelmingly predominates. These data might suggest that deamination is a relatively slow reaction in the pituitary compared to *O*-methylation. In the absence of further experimental data, these considerations must be considered speculative. Nonetheless, it would currently appear that the pattern of catecholamine metabolism

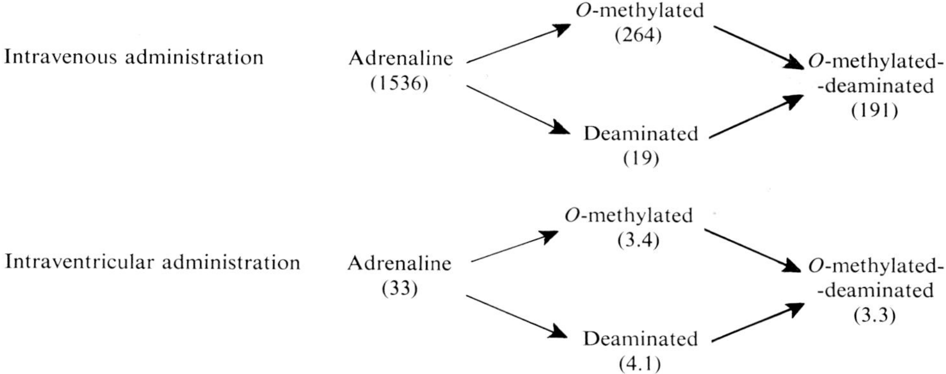

Fig. 2. Route of adrenaline metabolism in the pituitary.
Numbers in parentheses refer to the absolute amounts of each product remaining (in ng) 1 h after administration of [^{3}H]adrenaline.

in the pituitary is principally clearance of the unchanged catecholamine. Conjugation to sulfate and glucuronide may be an important route of metabolism when amine concentrations are low, but this system may saturate quick y. The preferred metabolic pathway when catecholamine concentrations are high appears to be *O*-methylation.

TURNOVER OF CATECHOLAMINES IN THE PITUITARY

The studies of Steinman *et al.* (1969) and Barchas *et al.* (1969) demonstrated a half-life of exogenously administered adrenaline of 3.5 h. This compared with a whole brain half-life of 2.5 h, as reported by the same investigators.

SUMMARY

There is no evidence that the enzymes involved in catecholamine biosynthesis are present in pituitary. The pituitary actively takes up catecholamines from the circulation; this seems to be mediated through a carrier-dependent saturable uptake system, The principal route of adrenaline metabolism in pituitary seems to be clearance of the unchanged catecholamine. On low concentrations of adrenaline, deamination and conjugation appear to be preferred routes of metabolism. These may saturate at higher concentrations, however, since *O*-methylation predominates in these circumstances. The half-life of adrenaline in the pituitary is 2.5 h.

ACKNOWLEDGMENT

The experiments described in this chapter were partially funded by ONR grant No. 101–715.

References p. 222

REFERENCES

AXELROD, J., WEIL-MALHERBE, H. AND TOMCHICK, R. (1959) The physiological disposition of H^3-epinephrine and its metabolite metanephrine. *J. Pharmacol. exp. Ther.*, **127**, 251.

BARCHAS, J. D., CIARANELLO, R. D. AND STEINMAN, A. M. (1969) Epinephrine formation and metabolism in mammalian brain. *Biol. Psychiat.*, **1**, 31–48.

ICHIYAMA, A., NAKAMURA, S., NISHIZUKA, Y. AND HAYAISHI, O. (1970) Enzymic studies on the biosynthesis of serotonin in mammalian brain. *J. biol. Chem.*, **245**, 1699–1709.

MOLINOFF, P. B., WEINSHILBOUM, R. AND AXELROD, J. (1971) A sensitive enzymatic assay for dopamine beta-hydroxylase. *J. Pharmacol. exp. Ther.*, **178**, 425–431.

STEINMAN, A. M., SMERIN, S. AND BARCHAS, J. (1969) Epinephrine metabolism in mammalian brain after intravenous and intraventricular administration. *Science*, **165**, 616.

WEIL-MALHERBE, H., AXELROD, J. AND TOMCHICK, R. (1959) Blood–brain barrier for adrenaline. *Science*, **129**, 1226–1227.

WEIL-MALHERBE, H., WHITBY, L. G. AND AXELROD, J. (1961) The uptake of circulating ^3H-norepinephrine by the pituitary gland and various areas of the brain. *Neurochem.*, **8**, 55–64.

WEINSHILBOUM, R. M. AND AXELROD, J. (1971) Serum dopamine beta-hydroxylase: decrease after chemical sympathectomy. *Science*, **173**, 931.

WILSON, C., MURRAY, A. AND TITUS, E. (1962) *J. Pharmacol.*, **135**, 1.

DISCUSSION

DANELLIS: A considerable amount of monoamine oxidase (MAO) has been demonstrated histochemically and biochemically in the anterior lobe. This pituitary MAO activity shows a pronounced diurnal rhythm. This rhythm of MAO activity is abolished and the activity practically disappears after adrenalectomy.

STUMPF: Cells like those in the anterior lobe of the pituitary that pick up dopamine are found also in other endocrine organs as has been mentioned by Dr. Hyyppä. These cells are designated by A. G. E. Pears as APUD cells, referring to amine precursor uptake decarboxylation. These cell types are found especially in the polypeptide hormone-producing glands in the intestinal lining and in endocrine organs derived from the intestine such as the C-cells in the thyroid, the enterochromaffin cells, and the alpha and beta cells of the pancreas. They are also seen in the juxtaglomerular apparatus. In the present context the question is are the cells that fluoresce in the brain also APUD cells? Are these also polypeptide producing cells?

JACOBOWITZ: Since the pituitary is so loaded with peptides it would seem that in all probability amines or their precursors are taken up in polypeptide-producing cells. Many of the cells in the periphery such as the beta cells of the pancreas and the C cells of the thyroid already possess catecholamines. The only analogy that pertains are cells in the intestine which avidly take up DOPA, particularly in the presence of an MAO inhibitor, and so there is precedence for this phenomenon. We don't know if there is a peptide in this particular type of intestinal cell which takes up the amine.

WEINER: In terms of the dopaminergic cells in the arcuate nucleus there appears to be a dichotomy between them and the cells which produce LRF. Dr. Krulich has demonstrated that LRF containing cells are distributed in the ventromedial hypothalamus and preoptic area, whereas the dopaminergic cells appear to be concentrated in the arcuate nucleus. Therefore there seems to be a separation between these catecholamine and peptide producing neurons.

DOUGLAS: In our electron microscopic studies where we have been looking particularly at the endings where the release of hormone occurs, we only rarely encounter endings containing the small granules with electron-dense cores that could possibly be aminergic endings and it is difficult for me to imagine that there is a general involvement of such endings in the release process. I would like to ask Dr. Hyyppä to expand on this to tell us particularly something of the density of neurons of this sort and their localization in the neural lobe.

HYYPPÄ: I would like to point to the recent work of Baumgarten *et al.* (Z. Zellforsch. 126, 483, 1972) in which they detected synapse-like contacts with the neurosecretory axons. However, there is no direct evidence available about the significance of this finding for the release of octapeptides.

KASTIN: Hopkins has reported that pretreatment of frogs with 6-hydroxydopamine does not change pituitary MSH content after exposure for at least one week to a light background (Mem. Soc. Endocr. 19, 823, 1971). He concluded that this constituted evidence against a role for catecholamines in the release of MSH.

SACHS: With respect to the role of the catecholamines in the release of vasopressin from neural lobes, some time ago, one of my former students, D. E. Haller, studied the effect of noradrenaline, adrenaline, histamine and a number of other transmitters on the release of vasopressin from isolated neural lobes under either basal conditions or in response to electrical stimulation. Under no circumstances did he ever find any significant effect on vasopressin release.

MEYERSON: I think a relationship between monoamines and endocrine function should be based upon the functional status of monoamine activity rather than on quantitative estimates of monoamines in certain brain areas. Assume an endocrine function is governed by a very high impulse rate in noradrenergic neurons. It seems reasonable then, that only a slight decrease of the noradrenaline synthesis will impair that function. Another system might not be influenced until a complete depletion has been achieved. The same reasoning might be valid if we have impaired a certain endocrine function, for instance the LH release, by α-MPT and then tried to reverse the effect by precursor amino acids. We then might not necessarily have to await a complete refilling of storage sites before an appropriate functional effect is present.

DANELLIS: I am intrigued by the suggestion that pituitary amines affect blood flow in the pituitary. This would be a very interesting role for the amines in the gland. In addition, Dr. Knigge yesterday mentioned that noradrenaline may increase the uptake of T_4 into the pituitary and many years ago it was shown by Saffran and Schally (1955) that noradrenaline increased the effect of CRF on the pituitary *in vitro*, thus providing further indications as to possible roles of the amines in the gland.

Biogenic Amines in the Hypothalamus: Effect of L-DOPA on Human Growth Hormone Levels in Patients with Huntington's Chorea*

STEPHEN PODOLSKY** AND NORMAN A. LEOPOLD***

***Assistant Professor of Medicine, Boston University School of Medicine; Chief, Intermediate Care Service and Clinical Metabolic Research Unit, Veterans Administration Hospital, Boston, Mass. and ***Resident in Neurology, Boston University School of Medicine, Boston, Mass. (U.S.A.)*

Huntington's chorea, transmitted as an autosomal dominant trait, is a progressively deteriorating disease of the central nervous system. Most of the important features were described in the original paper by Huntington (1872). It is characterized clinically, in general, by choreo-athetosis, progressive cachexia and varying degrees of dementia (Bruyn, 1968). The primary pathology is loss of small neurons and associated gliosis in the corpus striatum. There is also neuronal loss in the cerebral cortex as well as paraventricular, supraoptic and lateral tuberal hypothalamic nuclei (Bruyn, 1968) and dorsomedial nucleus of the hypothalamus (Facon *et al.*, 1957).

While certain vegetative symptoms of Huntington's disease, such as hyperhydrosis, hyperphagia and cachexia have been attributed to involvement of various portions of the hypothalamus (Bruyn, 1968; Facon *et al.*, 1957), biochemical evaluation of hypothalamic function has not been performed in this disease. Quite recently, hypersecretion of insulin was found in several patients with Huntington's disease (hereditary chorea), and the suggestion was made that hypothalamic function may be disturbed in patients with this disorder (Podolsky *et al.*, 1972a). Measurements of human growth hormone (HGH) levels are reported here which indicate that an abnormality of HGH secretion is a frequent hormonal disturbance in patients with Huntington's chorea, possibly related to hypersensitivity to intracerebral dopamine.

MATERIALS AND METHODS

Studies were carried out on 10 randomly selected unrelated hospitalized male patients with Huntington's disease. All had a progressive dementia of varying degree, choreiform movements, and a positive family history for the disease. None of the patients had the hypokinetic (Westphal) variant of Huntington's chorea. 5 lived at home with

* This study was supported in part by Veterans Administration Central Office Special Research Funds (Clinical Investigator Award of Dr. Podolsky).

References p. 232–234

their families and 5 were institutionalized at Veterans Administration chronic care facilities. The age range of the patients was 29–79 years with a mean age of 48.5 years. The average length of documented clinical signs was 6.6 years (range 3–17 years). All patients were non-obese, in good nutritional status, and off all medication for at least one week prior to the studies. In addition, 20 non-obese hospitalized patients without endocrine or metabolic disease were selected as controls (mean age of 40.8 years with a range of 21–64 years).

Each subject underwent a baseline standard 5-h oral glucose tolerance test (GTT) performed after an overnight fast, using 100 g of lemon-flavored glucose. In 9 of the patients with Huntington's chorea and 10 of the healthy controls a second GTT was done after 3 days of priming with 0.5 g L-3,4,dihydroxyphenylalanine (L-DOPA) p.o. T.I.D. plus 0.5 g L-DOPA administered 30 min prior to the repeat test. All subjects were supine, comfortable and free of stress during the GTTs. 10-ml blood samples were periodically withdrawn into heparinized Vacutainer tubes. The blood was kept chilled until being spun down in a refrigerated centrifuge at 4°. The plasma was then separated and stored in the frozen state until assay for growth hormone by a Dextran-coated charcoal modification of the radioimmunoassay (Lau *et al.*, 1966). All determinations were done in duplicate.

RESULTS

The mean fasting growth hormone level for the 20 normal control subjects was 1.3 ± 0.5 ng/ml (SEM). The mean fasting HGH level for the 10 patients with Huntington's chorea was slightly but not significantly higher than the controls. Control subjects demonstrated the expected suppression of HGH levels after oral glucose administration. In contrast, there were variable HGH responses in the patients with Huntington's disease, and all showed an elevation late in the course of the GTT to abnormally high levels. Some patients, with normal carbohydrate tolerance (labelled non-

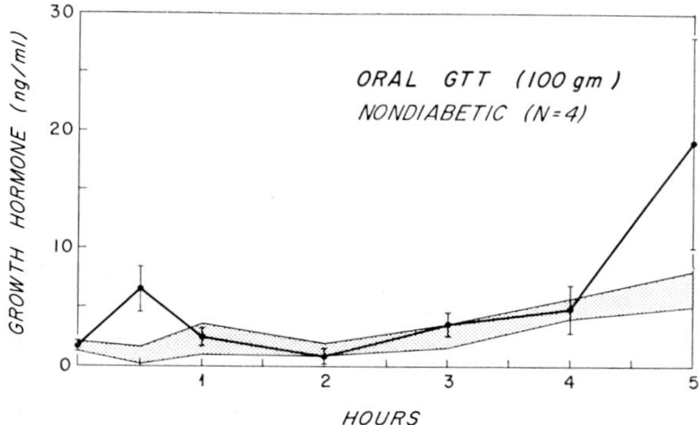

Fig. 1. Results of plasma HGH levels during oral GTT (100 g) in 4 patients with Huntington's chorea having non-diabetic glucose values. Shaded area represents the mean ± SEM for 20 normal controls.

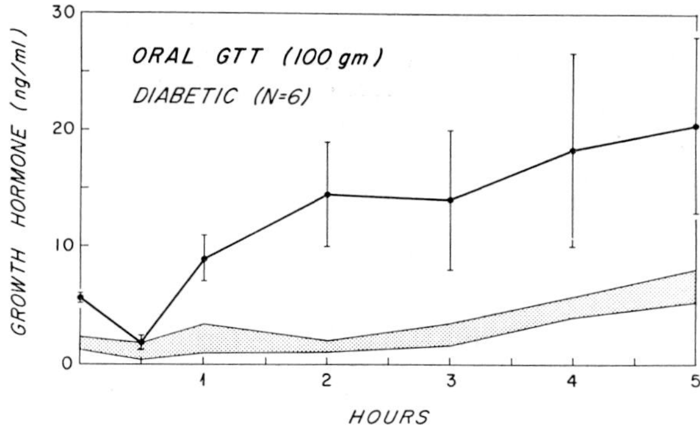

Fig. 2. Results of plasma HGH levels during oral GTT (100 g) in 6 patients with Huntington's chorea having diabetic glucose values. Shaded area represents the mean ± SEM for 20 normal controls.

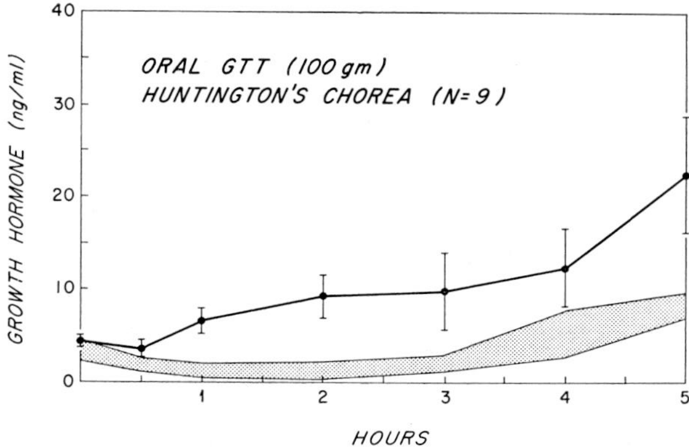

Fig. 3. Results of plasma HGH levels during oral GTT (100 g) for 9 of the patients with Huntington's chorea. Shaded area represents the mean ± SEM for 10 normal controls.

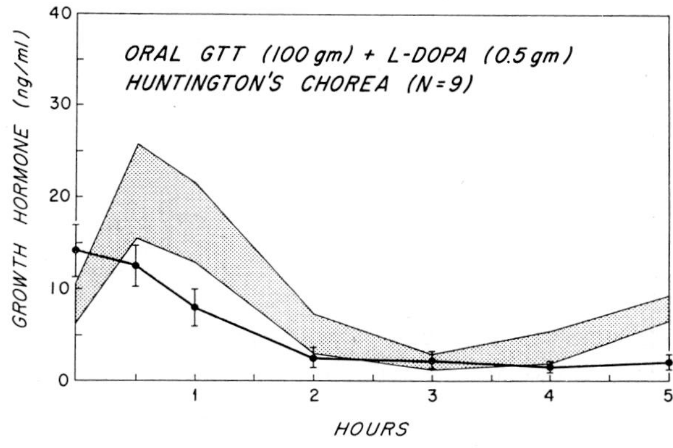

Fig. 4. Results of plasma HGH levels during oral GTT (100 g) modified by L-DOPA (0.5 g) priming for the same 9 patients with Huntington's chorea. Shaded area represents the mean ± SEM for the same 10 normal controls.

References p. 232–234

diabetic), showed a paradoxical rise of HGH 0.5 h after oral glucose (Fig. 1). Others, with impaired carbohydrate tolerance (labelled diabetic), had incomplete suppression of HGH levels after oral glucose, followed by a late rise to abnormal levels which were even higher (Fig. 2). When mean baseline HGH levels were plotted for the 9 patients with Huntington's chorea who were studied before and after L-DOPA administration, it was apparent that there was no suppression during the GTT (Fig. 3). Growth hormone levels actually rose significantly (Fig. 3).

When the GTT was repeated after 3 days of L-DOPA priming plus 0.5 g L-DOPA administered 30 min prior to the test, there were marked changes in the HGH responses in the 10 normal control individuals and also the patients with Huntington's disease (Fig. 4). Control patients no longer showed HGH suppression but instead had a sharp rise from 7.7 $\pm$ 1.7 ng/ml to 20.4 $\pm$ 5.4 ng/ml. In the patients with Huntington's chorea the mean fasting HGH level rose considerably after L-DOPA administration, with the value of 14.3 $\pm$ 2.7 ng/ml being in the acromegalic range. In contradistinction to the control patients, after oral glucose there was a dramatic and complete suppression of HGH levels in these L-DOPA primed neurological patients (Fig. 4). No clinical correlation could be made with the HGH results other than status of carbohydrate metabolism and duration of Huntington's disease.

DISCUSSION

Disturbances of carbohydrate metabolism occur frequently in Huntington's chorea, as they do in other hereditary neurological diseases, including Friedreich's ataxia (Podolsky *et al.*, 1964, 1970) and ataxia telangiectasia (Schalch *et al.*, 1970). The results reported here indicate that an abnormality in the release of human growth hormone is also present in all patients with Huntington's chorea that we studied.

Human growth hormone is known to be released from the anterior pituitary secondary to the release of growth hormone-releasing factor (GRF) from the tuberoinfundibular system of the hypothalamus (Halász, 1968). The stimuli for the release of GRF are not fully elucidated but may include hypoglycemia (Roth *et al.*, 1963), stress (Schalch and Reichlin, 1968), sleep (Takahashi *et al.*, 1968), various amino acids such as arginine (Podolsky and Sivaprasad, 1972), and biogenic amines such as L-DOPA (Boyd *et al.*, 1970; Eddy *et al.*, 1971), since these have all been associated with HGH rise in man. Furthermore, the tuberoinfundibular system can sustain the production and release of GRF even when it is totally deafferentated from the remainder of the hypothalamus (Halász, 1968).

Fluctuations in plasma glucose levels affect the release of HGH by a yet incompletely elucidated mechanism. Hypoglycemia induces the release of growth hormone while intrahypothalamic microinfusions of glucose block this response (Blanco *et al.*, 1966). Injection of glucose directly into the median eminence also inhibits the release of growth hormone but this is postulated to be, in part, due to diffusion of glucose into the surrounding hypothalamic regions (Schalch and Reichlin, 1968). More accurate localization of intrahypothalamic glucose effects were demonstrated by Chhina *et al.*

(1971) who delineated a medial hypothalamic "satiety" center and a lateral hypothalamic "feeding" center. The electrical activity of these neuronal groups reflected the level of circulating blood glucose.

Growth hormone response to an oral glucose load is one of the standard methods of evaluating the integrity of the hypothalamic-pituitary axis (Glick *et al.*, 1965). In previous reports we divided our patients with Huntington's disease into two groups, depending on their glucose tolerance (Podolsky *et al.*, 1972a; Leopold *et al.*, 1973). Both groups demonstrated growth hormone responses that deviate from the normal response to glucose in that there was no suppression but a slight paradoxical elevation of HGH, as in the patients with a non-diabetic GTT (Fig. 1), or incomplete suppression, followed by a rise to abnormally high levels, as in the patients with a diabetic GTT (Fig. 2). These types of abnormal HGH responses are seen in conditions associated with high circulating levels of HGH such as acromegaly (Hartog *et al.*, 1964), malnutrition (Alvarez *et al.*, 1972), and cirrhosis (Hernandez *et al.*, 1969; Podolsky *et al.*, 1970, 1971). A rise, rather than fall, of HGH level has also been reported during a GTT in a patient with polyostotic fibrous dysplasia and precocious puberty (Podolsky and Bryan, 1973).

Patients with cirrhosis having a normal total body potassium demonstrate elevated HGH levels and a paradoxical response of HGH levels after oral glucose (Podolsky *et al.*, 1970, 1973). While the mechanism of this has been partly attributed to an inability of the cirrhotic liver to metabolize circulating HGH, more recent evidence suggests that the elevated basal HGH levels in cirrhosis must be due to pituitary release, since HGH clearance by the cirrhotic liver is actually increased above normal (Taylor *et al.*, 1972). Cirrhotic patients with normal total body potassium stores also have increased insulin secretion in response to a glucose load (Podolsky *et al.*, 1970, 1973) when compared to that of normal and diabetic patients, and similar in type to that of patients with Huntington's disease (Podolsky *et al.*, 1972a; Leopold *et al.*, 1973). Hepatic function, however, has been reported to be normal in patients with hereditary chorea, and liver function tests were normal in our patients.

Emaciation, associated with a ravenous appetite, are frequent clinical features of patients with Huntington's disease, even when they are not malnourished (Bruyn, 1968). Only one of our patients, the oldest, had a body weight below his predicted normal weight. The diencephalic syndrome of childhood, associated with tumors of the anterior portion of third ventricle, is also characterized by emaciation, hyperkinesis and ravenous appetite (Gamstorp *et al.*, 1967). This group of patients also fail to suppress HGH in response to a glucose load (Pimstone *et al.*, 1970) and have an abnormal HGH response to insulin-induced hypoglycemia (Fishman and Peake, 1970). Whether the hyperkinesis evident in the diencephalic syndrome and Huntington's disease, alone, influences the release of HGH is not clear.

The emaciation of these patients with Huntington's chorea may be secondary to HGH mobilization of free fatty acids from fat stores. Disorders of excess growth hormone production are rarely characterized by the presence of much subcutaneous fat (Pimstone *et al.*, 1970). Furthermore, children with the congenital form of lipoatrophic diabetes have been reported to have gigantism as well as absence of subcutane-

References p. 232–234

ous fat (Podolsky, 1971). A unique lipid mobilizing hormone of pituitary origin has been isolated from the urine of some of these patients by Louis *et al.* (1963, 1968, 1972). Attempts to detect such a lipid mobilizing and diabetogenic hormone in patients with Huntington's chorea have not been done.

L-DOPA administration causes an acute increase of HGH levels in normal and Parkinsonian patients (Boyd *et al.*, 1970; Eddy *et al.*, 1971). This rise cannot be suppressed by glucose administration. The mechanism of action has been postulated to be due in part to elevated levels of dopamine in the tuberoinfundibular system of the hypothalamus which then stimulates the release of GRF by the median eminence (Boyd *et al.*, 1970). This hypothesis is supported by the presence of a dopamine-dependent pathway within the tuberoinfundibular system (Fuxe, 1963; Fuxe and Hökfelt, 1966). Phenothiazines block the excitatory actions of catecholamines and impair the release of HGH (Sherman *et al.*, 1971), as does phentolamine, an alpha adrenergic blocking agent. Propranolol, a beta adrenergic blocking agent, is associated with a transient rise of HGH levels as well as abnormalities of carbohydrate metabolism including both hypoglycemia (Kotler *et al.*, 1966) as well as hyperosmolar non-ketotic diabetic coma (Podolsky and Pattavina, 1973).

In our patients with Huntington's disease the HGH responses to an oral glucose load following L-DOPA administration were abnormal when compared to healthy control patients who had a marked rise in HGH. All patients with Huntington's chorea given this drug had a paradoxical complete suppression of their HGH levels. This response was similar to the expected HGH suppression seen in normal subjects after a glucose load without L-DOPA (Glick *et al.*, 1965). Potassium depletion is associated with low HGH levels (Podolsky *et al.*, 1972b), but this cannot explain our results because of the very high fasting HGH values after L-DOPA. A similar unusual HGH response was observed by Kansel *et al.* (1972) in Parkinsonian patients who received an insulin tolerance test while being treated with L-DOPA. Both insulin-induced hypoglycemia (Roth *et al.*, 1963) and L-DOPA administration (Boyd *et al.*, 1970; Eddy *et al.*, 1971) individually stimulate the release of HGH. However, when both stimuli were used together (Kansel *et al.*, 1972) there was an obvious and significant suppression of HGH analagous to what occurred in our patients. This suggests that excessive stimulation or hyperresponsiveness of the tuberoinfundibular system may lead to a suppression of the release of GRF, or the release of a growth hormone inhibiting factor (Krulich *et al.*, 1968). Recent experimentation in rats by Kamberi *et al.* (1971) has shown that the release of follicle-stimulating hormone (FSH) is stimulated by the injection of low doses of dopamine into the third ventricle and is suppressed by intraventricular injection of high doses of dopamine. Neither response occurred when dopamine was injected into the anterior pituitary (Kamberi *et al.*, 1971).

Increased sensitivity to intracerebral dopamine has been proposed by Klawans and Rubovitz (1972) as an explanation for the exacerbation of choreiform movements in patients with Huntington's disease after L-DOPA administration. Furthermore, Klawans *et al.* (1972) have recently reported that about 36% of unaffected family members of patients with Huntington's chorea develop chorea on doses of L-DOPA that produce no change in normal control subjects. The possibility of dopamine hypersensitivity being present in patients with Huntington's chorea is supported by the markedly elevated fasting HGH levels in our patients after L-DOPA priming, which did not occur in our control patients. There was, however, no detectable clinical deterioration in our patients at the dose of L-DOPA we employed.

An alternative explanation for the abnormal HGH response after L-DOPA loading in our patients with Huntington's disease is suggested by the dual response of caudate nuclei to dopamine iontophoresis. Dopamine acts as an inhibitory neurotransmitter for a majority of caudate nucleus neurons in animal studies, while in a significantly smaller number, as an excitatory neurotransmitter (McLennan and York, 1967). However, when York (1969) iontophoretically explored putamenal neurons the majority responded to dopamine by excitation. The population ratio of dopamine-responsive neurons in the human hypothalamus is not known. If one set of dopamine-dependent neurons is preferentially affected in Huntington's chorea, the normal physiologic responses of dopaminergic pathways, including the release of HGH, would be altered.

All of our patients with Huntington's disease had the paradoxical failure of HGH rise following the administration of L-DOPA plus glucose. While purely speculative at this time, the possible use of this biochemical alteration as a predictive test for those family members at risk to develop Huntington's disease is suggested by our results. This test for heterozygotes, while time-consuming, is at least psychologically preferable to one in which the end point is choreiform movements similar to the affected family member, as has been recently reported by Klawans *et al.* (1972). The dose schedule for L-DOPA as used in our theoretical test differs from that proposed by Klawens *et al.* (1972) and in no case caused worsening of the choreiform movements in the already symptomatic patients themselves. Of course, individuals with other disease states having altered HGH levels might also demonstrate this abnormal response to L-DOPA administration. This would not negate the significance of our test in unaffected Huntington's disease family members, but would necessitate the search for other pathology occurring concomitantly, such as cirrhosis.

SUMMARY

In previous studies we reported that an unusual form of diabetes mellitus with an abnormality of insulin secretion are commonly associated with Huntington's chorea. Further studies have been carried out on HGH levels in this patient population.

10 patients with documented Huntington's chorea had HGH levels measured during a 5-h oral glucose tolerance test. 9 of them had HGH levels measured during a repeat GTT which had been modified by a 3-day course of L-DOPA administration (1.5 g daily). The baseline test of non-diabetic patients with Huntington's disease did not show the normal suppression of HGH levels, but instead showed a paradoxical rise of HGH 0.5 h after oral glucose. The baseline test of the diabetic patients with Huntington's disease showed incomplete suppression of HGH levels after oral glucose, follow-

References p. 232–234

ed by a late rise to abnormally high levels, even higher than the former patients. Fasting growth hormone levels rose after L-DOPA priming in healthy control subjects and patients with Huntington's chorea, but much more so in the latter group. There was a sharp rise of HGH after the glucose load plus 0.5 g L-DOPA in control subjects, similar to the reports of others. In contrast, the patients with Huntington's chorea had a complete suppression of their elevated fasting HGH levels after glucose plus 0.5 g L-DOPA.

L-DOPA administration to patients with Huntington's disease has been reported to increase their choreic movements, although we did not observe such clinical deterioration. Nevertheless, the abnormalities in the release of HGH that we observed following L-DOPA loading could be interpreted to be in keeping with the concept that patients with Huntington's chorea have an increased sensitivity to intracerebral dopamine. Our findings could also be explained by pathologic involvement of the hypothalamus which is known to occur in these patients.

ACKNOWLEDGEMENT

Dr. Dean Squires, Staff Neurologist of the Brockton VA Hospital, referred two of the patients. Dr. Alfred E. Wilhelmi, Atlanta, Ga., supplied the highly purified human growth hormone (HS 1147) for radioimmunoassay standards, through the Endocrine Study Section, N.I.H. Miss Kay Pattavina provided superior technical assistance in the laboratory. The staff of the Intermediate Care Unit, Boston VA Hospital, provided outstanding and enthusiastic nursing care of the patients in this study.

REFERENCES

ALVAREZ, L. C., DIMAS, C. O., CASTRO, A., ROSSMAN, L. G., VANDERLAAN, E. F. AND VANDERLAAN, W. P. (1972) Growth hormone in malnutrition. *J. clin. Endocrinol.*, **34**, 400–409.

BLANCO, S., SCHALCH, D. S. AND REICHLIN, S. (1966) Control of GH secretion by glucoreceptors in the hypothalamic-pituitary unit. *Fed. Proc.*, **25**, 91.

BOYD, A. E., LEBOVITZ, H. E. AND PFEIFFER, J. B. (1970) Stimulation of human-growth-hormone secretion by L-DOPA. *New Eng. J. Med.*, **283**, 1425–1429.

BRUYN, G. W. (1968) Huntington's chorea. Historical, clinical and laboratory synopsis. In *Handbook of Clinical Neurology*, Vol. 6, P. J. VINKEN AND G. W. BRUYN (Eds.), North Holland, Amsterdam, pp. 298–378.

CHHINA, G. S., ANAND, B. K., SINGH, B. AND RAO, P. S. (1971) Effect of glucose on hypothalamic feeding centers in deafferented animals. *Amer. J. Physiol.*, **221**, 662–667.

EDDY, R. L., JONES, A. L., CHAKMAKJIAN, Z. H. AND SILVERTHORNE, M. C. (1971) Effect of levodopa (L-DOPA) on human hypophyseal trophic hormone release. *J. clin. Endocrinol.*, **33**, 709–712.

FACON, E., STERIADE, M., CORTEZ, P. AND VOINESCO, S. (1957) Contributions anatomocliniques à l'étude de la chorée de Huntington. *Acta neurol. belg.*, **57**, 898–912.

FISHMAN, M. A. AND PEAKE, G. T. (1970) Paradoxical growth in a patient with the diencephalic syndrome. *Pediatrics*, **45**, 973–982.

FUXE, K. (1963) Cellular localization of monamines in the median eminence and in the infundibular stem of some mammals. *Acta physiol. scand.*, **58**, 383–384.

FUXE, K. AND HÖKFELT, T. (1966) Further evidence for the existence of tuberoinfundibular dopamine neurons. *Acta physiol. scand.*, **66**, 245–246.

GAMSTORP, I., KJELLMAN, B. AND PALMGREN, B. (1967) Diencephalic syndromes of infancy. *J. Pediat.*, **70**, 383–390.

GLICK, S. M., ROTH, J., YALOW, R. S. AND BERSON, S. A. (1965) The regulation of growth hormone secretion. *Recent Progr. Hormone Res.*, **21**, 241–283.

HALÁSZ, B. (1968) The role of the hypothalamic hypophysiotrophic area in the control of growth hormone secretion. In *Growth Hormone*, A. PECILE AND E. E. MULLER (Eds.), Excerpta Med., Amsterdam, pp. 204–210.

HARTOG, M., GAAFAR, M. A., MEISSER, B. AND FRASER, R. (1964) Immunoassay of serum growth hormone in acromegalic patients. *Brit. med. J.*, **1**, 1229–1232.

HERNANDEZ, A., ZORRILLA, E. AND GERSHBERG, H. (1969) Decreased insulin production, elevated growth hormone levels and glucose intolerance in liver disease. *J. lab. clin. Med.*, **73**, 25–33.

HUNTINGTON, G. (1872) On chorea. *Med. surg. Reporter*, **26**, 317–321.

KAMBERI, I. A., MICAL, R. S. AND PORTER, J. C. (1971) Effect of anterior pituitary perfusion and intraventricular injection of catecholamines on FSH release. *Endocrinology*, **88**, 1003–1011.

KANSEL, P. C., BUSE, J., TALBERT, O. R. AND BUSE, M. G. (1972) The effect of L-DOPA on plasma growth hormone, insulin and thyroxine. *J. clin. Endocrinol.*, **34**, 99–105.

KLAWANS, H. L. AND RUBOVITS, R. (1972) Central cholinergic-anticholinergic antagonism in Huntington's chorea. *Neurology*, **22**, 107–116.

KLAWANS, H. L., JR., PAULSON, G. W., RINGEL, S. P. AND BARBEAU, A. (1972) Use of L-DOPA in the detection of presymptomatic Huntington's chorea. *New Eng. J. Med.*, **286**, 1332–1334.

KOTLER, M. N., BERMAN, L. AND RUBENSTEIN, A. H. (1966) Hypoglycemia precipitated by propranolol. *Lancet*, **2**, 1389–1390.

KRULICH, L., DHARIWAL, A. P. S. AND MCCANN, S. M. (1968) Stimulatory and inhibitory effects of purified hypothalamic extracts on growth hormone release from rat pituitary *in vivo*. *Endocrinology*, **83**, 783–790.

LAU, K. S., GOTTLIEB, C. W. AND HERBERT, V. (1966) Preliminary report on coated charcoal immunoassay of human chorionic "growth-hormone-prolactin" and growth hormone. *Proc. Soc. exp. biol. Med.*, **123**, 126–131.

LEOPOLD, N. A., SAX, D. S. AND PODOLSKY, S. (1973) Abnormal carbohydrate metabolism in Huntington's chorea. In *Proc. Centennial Symp. on Huntington's Chorea, Columbus, Ohio, 1972*, A. BARBEAU, T. J. CHASE AND G. W. PAULSON (Eds.), Raven, New York, pp. 571–580.

LOUIS, L. H. AND CONN, J. W. (1968) A diabetogenic polypeptide from hog and sheep adenohypophysis similar to that found in lipoatrophic diabetes. *Metabolism*, **17**, 475–484.

LOUIS, L. H. AND CONN, J. W. (1972) Diabetogenic polypeptide from human pituitaries similar to that excreted by proteinuric diabetic patients. *Metabolism*, **21**, 1-9.

LOUIS, L. H., CONN, J. W. AND MINNICK, M. C. (1963) Lipoatrophic diabetes: Isolation and characterization of an insulin antagonist from urine. *Metabolism*, **12**, 867–886.

MCLENNAN, H. AND YORK, D. H. (1967) Action of dopamine on neurons of the caudate nucleus. *J. Physiol.*, **189**, 393–402.

PIMSTONE, B. L., SOBEL, J., MEYER, E. AND EALE, D. (1970) Secretion of growth hormone in the diencephalic syndrome of childhood. *J. Pediat.*, **76**, 886–889.

PODOLSKY, S. (1971) Lipoatrophic diabetes and miscellaneous conditions related to diabetes mellitus. In *Joslin's Diabetes Mellitus*, 11th ed., *A.* MARBLE, P. WHITE, R. F. BRADLEY AND L. P. KRALL (Eds.), Lea and Febiger, Philadelphia, pp. 722–766.

PODOLSKY, S. AND BRYAN, R. S. (1973) Albright's syndrome (polyostotic fibrous dysplasia of bone) with sexual precocity, dermoid cyst of ovary, hyperthyroidism and insulin and growth hormone abnormalities. In *Clinical Aspects of Metabolic Bone Disease*, B. FRAME, A. M. PARFITT AND H. DUNCAN (Eds.), Excerpta Med., Amsterdam, pp. 484–486.

PODOLSKY, S. AND PATTAVINA, C. G. (1973) Hyperosmolar nonketotic diabetic coma. A complication of propranolol therapy. *Metabolism*, **22**, 685–694.

PODOLSKY, S. AND SHEREMATA, W. A. (1970) Insulin-dependent diabetes mellitus and Friedreich's ataxia in siblings. *Metabolism*, **19**, 555–561.

PODOLSKY, S. AND SIVAPRASAD, R. (1972) Assessment of growth hormone reserve: Comparison of arginine and glucagon stimulation tests. *J. clin. Endocrinol.*, **35**, 580–584.

PODOLSKY, S., POTHIER, A., JR. AND KRALL, L. P. (1964) Association of diabetes mellitus and Friedreich's ataxia. A study of two siblings. *Arch. int. Med.*, **114**, 533–537.

PODOLSKY, S., ZIMMERMAN, H. J. AND BURROWS, B. A. (1970) Relation between total body potassium and growth hormone and insulin response in cirrhosis. *J. clin. Invest.*, **49**, 75a–76a.

Podolsky, S., Gutman, R. A., Zimmerman, H. J. and Burrows, B. A. (1971) Effects of potassium on insulin, proinsulin and growth hormone release in diabetics with abnormal carbohydrate tolerance. *Diabetes*, **20**, 372–373.

Podolsky, S., Leopold, N. A. and Sax, D. S. (1972a) Increased frequency of diabetes mellitus in patients with Huntington's chorea. *Lancet*, **1**, 1356–1359.

Podolsky, S., Burrows, B. A., Zimmerman, H. J. and Pattavina, C. (1972b) Effect of chronic potassium depletion on growth hormone release in man. In *Growth and Growth Hormone*, A. Pecile and E. E. Muller (Eds.), Excerpta Med., Amsterdam, pp. 402–407.

Podolsky, S., Zimmerman, H. J., Burrows, B. A., Cardarelli, J. A. and Pattavina, C. G. (1973) Potassium depletion in hepatic cirrhosis: A reversible cause of impaired growth-hormone and insulin response to stimulation. *New Engl. J. Med.*, **288**, 644–648.

Roth, J., Glick, S. M., Yalow, R. S. and Berson, S. A. (1963) Hypoglycemia: A potent stimulus to secretion of growth hormone. *Science*, **140**, 987–988.

Schalch, D. S. and Reichlin, S. (1968) Stress and growth hormone release. In *Growth Hormone*, A. Pecile and E. E. Muller (Eds.), Excerpta Med., Amsterdam, pp. 211–225.

Schalch, D. S., McFarlin, D. E. and Barlow, M. H. (1970) An unusual form of diabetes mellitus in ataxia telangiectasia. *New Eng. J. Med.*, **282**, 1396–1402.

Sherman, L., Kim, S., Benjamin, F. and Kolodny, H. D. (1971) Effects of chlorpromazine on serum growth hormone concentration in man. *New Eng. J. Med.*, **284**, 72–74.

Takahashi, Y., Kipnis, D. M. and Daughaday, W. H. (1968) Growth hormone secretion during sleep. *J. clin. Invest.*, **47**, 2079–2090.

Taylor, A. L., Lipman, R. L., Salam, A. and Mintz, D. H. (1972) Hepatic clearance of human growth hormone. *J. clin. Endocrinol.*, **34**, 395–399.

York, D. H. (1969) Possible dopaminergic pathway from substantia nigra to putamen. *Brain Res.*, **20**, 233–249.

DISCUSSION

Taylor: How specific is this effect on endocrine systems? Have you looked at any other endocrine responses in these patients?

Leopold: This is the first time that hypothalamic function has been studied in any detail in patients with Huntington's chorea. They've had adrenal, thyroid, testicular and ovarian functions tested before and no abnormalities were found. As a matter of fact there have been no significant neuroendocrine abnormalities found by any of the methods of testing patients with Huntington's chorea prior to these growth hormone studies. Regarding other endocrine systems, we recently reported that 6 of 10 patients with Huntington's chorea had abnormally elevated glucose and insulin levels in response to the administration of glucose or arginine (Lancet **1**, 1356, 1972).

George (Jack): This is a very interesting phenomenon that you have described. My own guess though is that it's a general phenomenon and not specifically related to Huntington's chorea. We've been studying patients with cancer and they also have this paradoxical rise in growth hormone shortly after glucose. We got started on this because of isolated reports in the literature, and then as we started to look at our cancer patients more, we found that the sicker they were the more likely we were to get this paradoxical growth hormone response. Then when we compared them with sick patients without cancer rather than with normal controls we again found this paradoxical rise. This has also been reported after acute myocardial infarction, in the immediate post-operative period after surgery and in patients with kwashiorkor protein deficiency in Africa. It is our feeling now that this is a stress response involving the hypothalamus. I think your discussion of the L-DOPA effects and implications adds a new dimension to this and it certainly is interesting. My guess though would be that if you compared your Huntington's chorea patients to patients without Huntington's chorea but with similar degrees of malnutrition and other kinds of serious systemic disease that you would find that the same phenomena exist.

Podolsky: We are now in the midst of measuring growth hormone levels during GTT's before and after L-DOPA administration in patients with maturity onset diabetes mellitus and patients with Laennec's cirrhosis, to have other comparisons to the results in those with Huntington's disease.

Perhaps you missed the statement in our paper that patients with malnutrition and other conditions may have elevated fasting growth hormone levels and failure to suppress growth hormone levels after glucose administration. Endometrial carcinoma and porphyria should be added to your list of clinical disorders with this type of growth hormone response, including paradoxical growth hormone rises shortly after oral glucose. Furthermore, exercise *per se* is associated with such a growth hormone response and patients with Huntington's disease have marked chorea and hyperkinesis. However, none of our patients was malnourished or bedridden. All were ambulatory except one (the eldest) and were given adequate carbohydrate priming prior to the glucose tolerance tests and all were supine, comfortable and free from stress during the test. They were in as basal a state as is possible for patients with Huntington's chorea. It is important to note that the growth hormone level late in the course of the GTT rose to abnormally high levels in our neurological patients which is not typical of the aforementioned non-specific responses. Moreover, the unusual growth hormone responses in these patients after L-DOPA administration is further evidence that there may be altered hypothalamic function in Huntington's chorea.

Neuronal Control of Monoamines in Brain and Melatonin-Forming Systems in the Pineal

ALFRED HELLER, PAUL H. VOLKMAN AND RONALD A. BROWNING

Department of Pharmacology, The University of Chicago, Chicago, Ill. 60637 (U.S.A.)

The monoamines, noradrenaline, dopamine, serotonin and their derivatives, are believed to participate in a diverse array of biological functions. Evidence is available for participation of these compounds in a number of processes including synaptic transmission, carbohydrate and lipid metabolism, and neuroendocrine regulation. A large body of information is available on their biological activity, localization and mechanisms of biosynthesis and inactivation. It is the purpose of this paper to discuss the role of specific neuronal elements in the control of monoamine biosynthesis in brain, as well as the participation of central and peripheral neurons in the regulation of methoxyindole biosynthesis in pineal parenchymal cells.

In brain, the presence of monoamines can be shown to be the function of the integrity of a number of well defined neuronal systems. The medial forebrain bundle, a fiber system interconnecting the hypothalamus, the basal telencephalon, and the midbrain is essential for the biosynthesis of the monoamines, noradrenaline and serotonin, in widespread areas of brain (for review see Heller *et al.*, 1962; Heller and Moore, 1968, 1970; Moore, 1970; Heller, 1972). The presence of dopamine in the neostriatum is a function of a nigrostriatal projection. The neurons of this dopaminergic system have their cell bodies in the substantia nigra with axons passing *via* the internal capsule and lateral hypothalamus to innervate the caudate nucleus and putamen (Ehringer and Hornykiewicz, 1960; Poirier and Sourkes, 1965; Andén *et al.*, 1966; Moore *et al.*, 1971). Diencephalic lesions involving the lateral hypothalamus and medial portion of the internal capsule produce reductions of 80–90% in telencephalic levels of noradrenaline, serotonin and dopamine. The losses in brain monoamines are secondary to an effect on enzymatic activities essential for their bio-synthesis. Following such lesions, decreases are seen in tyrosine hydroxylase (Heller *et al.*, 1969; Heller, 1972) and 5-HTP/DOPA (5-hydroxytryptophan/3,4-dihydroxyphenylalanine) decarboxylase (Heller *et al.*, 1965, 1966b; Moore *et al.*, 1966, 1971). These effects result from destruction of the medial forebrain bundle and the nigrostriatal tract which lies at the diencephalic level within the medial forebrain bundle and medial internal capsule (Moore *et al.*, 1971).

The loss of striatal dopamine following lesions of the nigrostriatal tract appears to be secondary to section and degeneration of dopamine-containing neurons in a manner analogous to the loss of transmitter substances in the periphery following denervation.

References p. 247–249

Transection of the nigrostriatal pathway leads to a loss of dopamine in the area innervated, *i.e.*, the caudate nucleus, with a concomitant loss of enzymes essential for its biosynthesis. The mechanism of reduction in noradrenaline and serotonin by either diencephalic or mesencephalic lesions involving components of the medial forebrain bundle is not, however, as readily explicable. The medial forebrain bundle, while complex anatomically, is nevertheless a fiber pathway of fairly limited distribution. Ascending and descending components of this tract interconnect the hypothalamus, the midbrain and the basal telencephalon. By the use of lesions in the central nervous system (CNS) at the diencephalic level and silver impregnation techniques (Nauta, 1957), the medial forebrain bundle has been shown to innervate the lateral hypothalamus, the preoptic area, the anterior amygdala and the medial and lateral septal nuclei. There are a few fibers from this tract which pass rostral to the septum to innervate the hippocampal rudiment. A limited number of fibers also pass to the adjacent medial hypothalamus. There is, in addition, a substantial innervation which passes caudally to terminate in the midbrain reticular formation and periaqueductal gray matter. This distribution has been described in detail (Moore and Heller, 1967) and is in agreement with the results of other investigators. It should be noted, however, that a much more extensive projection of monoamine fibers within the medial forebrain bundle has been proposed on the basis of histochemical fluorescence studies (Andén *et al.*, 1966). The reason for discrepancy between silver impregnation and histochemical studies has been discussed extensively in previous publications (Heller and Moore, 1968, 1970; Moore, 1970; Moore and Heller, 1967).

The neurochemical consequences of lesions of the medial forebrain bundle are much more extensive than would be expected on the basis of anatomic considerations alone. If the decreases in monoamines were simply a function of section and degeneration of monoamine-producing neurons one would expect to see a reduction in noradrenaline and serotonin only in those areas innervated by the fiber tract. While the effects on monoamines are restricted to the side of the brain containing the lesions in agreement with the uncrossed distribution of medial forebrain bundle fibers (Harvey *et al.*, 1963; Heller *et al.*, 1966; Moore *et al.*, 1965), decreases are seen throughout the brain cranial to the lesion. Reductions in serotonin, noradrenaline and the biosynthetic enzymes occur in all telencephalic areas including amygdala, hippocampus, striatum, septal area, and neocortex, despite the fact that only a few of these areas are innervated by the fibers of this tract (Heller *et al.*, 1966a, 1969; Moore and Heller, 1967; Moore *et al.*, 1965; Heller *et al.*, 1966b). Although there is a large descending projection of axons from the medial forebrain bundle, no losses in monoamines are seen caudally, *i.e.*, in the brainstem.

A similar discrepancy between innervation and neurochemical effects is seen following lesions of the tegmentum. Ventrolateral placement of lesions at the level of the inferior colliculus produces a selective reduction in noradrenaline with no effect on brain serotonin or dopamine. Decreases in brain serotonin occur after medial placement of lesions in this area (Heller and Moore, 1965). The ventrolateral tegmental lesion destroys neurons which project to the diencephalon with a sparse innervation passing to the septal area *via* the medial forebrain bundle (Heller and Moore, 1968).

The loss of noradrenaline following such lesions occurs, however, in every area of the brain cranial to the lesion including diencephalon, amygdala, hippocampus, striatum, septal area and neocortex (Heller *et al.*, 1969).

The lack of correlation between the anatomic distribution of medial forebrain bundle components and the neurochemical consequences of their destruction has led to the conclusion that the effects of these lesions cannot be explained as a consequence simply of degeneration of monoamine-containing neurons as is the case with striatal dopamine following nigrostriatal lesions. The neurochemical effects of medial forebrain bundle lesions occur in areas directly innervated by neurons involved with this tract as well as in areas related to these cells across one or more synapses. Because of this, we have referred to these distant effects as "trans-synaptic neurochemical effects of central lesions". The trans-synaptic character of lesion effects has led to the suggestion that the neurons of the medial forebrain bundle play an essential role in the regulation of monoamine biosynthesis throughout the brain involving mediation of trophic influences over a widespread polyneuronal system. Since transneuronal degeneration is uncommon in the CNS outside of the sensory projections, it would seem likely that the losses in monoamines are occurring, at least in part, in intact cells. Central neurons receive afferent input from a great number of presynaptic elements and this input is, in part, believed to be a determinant of the biochemical status of the innervated cell. Lesions which disrupt the pathways over which afferent input is mediated result in an alteration or loss of information essential for the biochemical integrity of the cell. The loss of medial forebrain bundle neurons and the afferent influences they transmit from mesencephalic and diencephalic areas to the telencephalon results in a reduction in biosynthetic enzymes and secondarily, in cellular monoamine levels.

The evidence supporting this concept of neuronal control of monoamine biosynthesis by the medial forebrain bundle has been extensively discussed in previous publications (Heller and Moore, 1968, 1970; Moore, 1970; Heller, 1972). This evidence may be briefly summarized as follows: (*1*) The effects of medial forebrain bundle lesions on brain noradrenaline and serotonin as well as on enzymes essential for their biosynthesis occur in a much wider distribution than expected on the basis of the known anatomic distribution of this fiber tract. (*2*) The time course of loss of telencephalic noradrenaline and serotonin following medial forebrain bundle lesions is a fairly prolonged process. By three days noradrenaline, for example, has decreased by 16%, but the total fall of 80% requires some 12 days for completion. This is in contrast to the loss of dopamine from the striatum following nigrostriatal lesions which is believed to be secondary to section and degeneration of the dopaminergic system innervating this area. Following transection of the nigrostriatal tract either within the diencephalon or mesencephalon there is a 50% reduction in striatal dopamine by 2 days and a 70–80% reduction in 4–6 days, a time course of loss more in keeping with a direct denervation phenomena (Heller, 1972). (*3*) The effects of diencephalic lesions on carbohydrate metabolism in brain are region specific. Following diencephalic lesions producing reductions in telencephalic levels of noradrenaline, serotonin and dopamine there is an elevation in glycogen in only one area, namely,

References p. 247–249

the caudate nucleus. Other areas of telencephalon suffer a loss in catecholamines, but have normal glycogen values (Hoffmann *et al.*, 1973). This selective effect on glycogen may reflect the fact that the reduction in dopamine in the caudate is secondary to a direct denervation, while monoamine reductions in other telencephalic areas are believed to occur in otherwise intact neurons. (*4*) Lesions of the ventrolateral tegmentum reduce telencephalic levels of noradrenaline and tyrosine hydroxylase without influencing 5-HTP/DOPA decarboxylase (Heller *et al.*, 1969). If the effects on telencephalic noradrenaline were due simply to degeneration of monoamine-producing neurons arising in the area of the lesion, one would anticipate a reduction in all enzymatic activities involving catecholamine biosynthesis. The selective reduction in tyrosine hydroxylase following ventrolateral tegmental lesions is consistent with a lesion-induced change in the functional state of intact neurons resulting in the loss of a specific enzyme.

The concept of neuronal control of brain monoamine biosynthesis discussed above implies that the level of enzymes available for the biosynthesis of monoamines is, under normal circumstances, a function of afferent input arising in the tegmentum and reaching telencephalic monoamine-producing cells over a polysynaptic system involving the medial forebrain bundle. If this is correct, it should be possible to return enzyme levels toward normal following a lesion by appropriate manipulation of afferent input to the cells affected. While this has not been accomplished in brain, recent studies from our laboratory demonstrate that alterations in afferent input over the postganglionic sympathetic fibers to the pineal can produce marked changes in enzyme activities essential for the biosynthesis of melatonin.

The mammalian pineal is an active organ biochemically. It is capable of synthesizing and storing a number of physiologically active substances including serotonin, noradrenaline and histamine. It is unique in its ability to synthesize the antigonadal agent, melatonin (for review see Wurtman *et al.*, 1968). The biosynthesis of melatonin in the pineal begins with tryptophan. This amino acid is converted to 5-hydroxytryptophan which is then decarboxylated to form 5-hydroxytryptamine (serotonin). Serotonin is converted to its *N*-acetyl derivative in a reaction catalyzed by the enzyme, serotonin-*N*-acetyltransferase (NAcT) (Weissbach *et al.*, 1960). The last step in the synthesis involves the *O*-methylation of *N*-acetylserotonin to form *N*-acetyl-5-methoxytryptamine (melatonin). The first three reactions are not unique to the pineal, but the *O*-methylation step requires an enzyme, hydroxyindole-*O*-methyltransferase (HIOMT) which is found only in the pineal, retina and Harderian gland in mammals (Axelrod and Weissbach, 1960, 1961, Cardinal and Wurtman, 1972).

Hydroxyindole-*O*-methyltransferase activity is regulated by environmental lighting. The effects of light on pineal HIOMT are mediated across a polyneuronal pathway involving the retina, an accessory optic system and components of the sympathetic outflow passing *via* the superior cervical ganglia to innervate the pineal. Rats placed in continuous darkness show a higher level of enzyme activity than rats kept in continuous light (Wurtman *et al.*, 1963). The light–dark difference can be abolished by blinding or superior cervical ganglionectomy (Wurtman *et al.*, 1964). The central pathway involved in transmission of such lighting information to the autonomic nerves is distinct from the primary optic pathway subserving vision (Moore *et al.*, 1967, 1968). In the rat the axons of the retinal ganglion cells enter the optic nerve and separate at the chiasm into several components. The primary optic tract containing both crossed and uncrossed fibers from the retina innervates the lateral geniculate, the pretectal nuclei and the superior colliculus. In addition, there is an accessory optic system which undergoes complete decussation in the chiasm (Hayhow *et al.*, 1960, 1962). The inferior component of this system leaves the primary optic tract just beyond the optic chiasm and runs caudally as scattered fascicles lying ventrolaterally among the fibers of the medial forebrain bundle. The fibers terminate in the medial terminal nucleus of the accessory optic system within the midbrain tegmentum.

The differences in pineal HIOMT activity between animals kept in the light as compared to those in darkness can be abolished by bilateral ablation of the inferior accessory optic tract (Moore *et al.*, 1967). Such bilateral ablation can be accomplished by unilateral enucleation of an eye and an ipsilateral medial forebrain bundle lesion. Removal of one eye produces degeneration of the inferior accessory optic tract, contralateral to the orbital enucleation. The medial forebrain bundle lesion ipsilateral to the enucleation destroys the inferior accessory optic tract arising from the intact eye. Such animals show a normal behavioral response to visual stimuli (Chase *et al.*, 1969). Removal of this fiber tract, however, prevents the normal 2–3-fold difference in HIOMT activity between animals kept in continuous darkness as compared to animals kept in continuous light. This light–dark difference is, however, maintained in animals with unilateral orbital enucleation plus bilateral lesions of the caudal lateral thalamus at the level of the lateral geniculate nuclei. The latter procedure removes all light input to the lateral geniculate nuclei, the terminal nuclei of the primary optic tract. Following this lesion, one inferior accessory optic tract remains, *i.e.*, that arising from the intact eye. The animal though visually blind, shows a normal light–dark difference in HIOMT activity. This finding demonstrates that the integrity of the inferior accessory optic tract is essential for mediation of pineal HIOMT responses to environmental lighting and provides evidence for a central link in a polyneuronal pathway relaying environmental lighting information to the pineal.

While NAcT is not localized exclusively to the pineal, its activity in this organ, like HIOMT, is under regulation of environmental lighting. Pineal NAcT activity is 15 times higher during periods of darkness than during periods of light and exhibits a diurnal rhythm which is abolished by continuous light, but persists in continuous darkness or after blinding (Klein *et al.*, 1970; Klein and Weller, 1970). Synthesis of melatonin in the pineal is therefore a process modifiable by lighting conditions and involving transmission of this information to the pineal by components of the sympathetic division of the autonomic nervous system. HIOMT activity can be fixed at high levels by blinding or bilateral inferior accessory optic tract lesions, while NAcT activity can be suppressed by continuous exposure of rats to light. This ability to experimentally stabilize pineal HIOMT or NAcT activity is a very useful device for the study of the effects of alteration of afferent neuronal input on the activities of these enzymes. The feasibility of this approach was first demonstrated by studies on the effects of cervical sympathetic stimulation on pineal HIOMT activity in animals in

References p. 247–249

which the levels of this enzyme were elevated by bilateral inferior accessory optic tract lesions (Brownstein and Heller, 1968). In such animals the preganglionic sympathetic trunk leading to the superior cervical ganglion was cut and stimulated by use of a sleeve bipolar nichrome electrode. The superior cervical ganglion contralateral to the stimulation was also decentralized leading to a bilateral endophthalmos. Stimulation of the cervical trunk produces a prominent exophthalmos of the ipsilateral eye due to contraction of Müller's muscle, a sympathetically innervated strip of smooth muscle bridging the inferior orbital fissure. The production of exophthalmos was used to monitor thresholds of electrical stimulation and the maintenance of responses throughout the experimental period. Following superior cervical stimulation there was a linear, time-dependent reduction in HIOMT activity with a 56% decrease in 8 h of stimulation. These initial studies directly demonstrated that the activity of pineal HIOMT could be modified by alteration of the firing rates of sympathetic nerves innervating the pineal.

These studies have been continued and extended by an analysis of the effects of nerve stimulation and blinding on pineal NacT activity in intact animals exposed to continuous light, which suppresses the level of enzyme. For cervical stimulation studies, animals were placed in constant light for 8–12 h following which preganglionic electrical stimulation was applied. Such stimulation resulted in an approximate tripling of enzyme levels with 2 h of stimulation as compared to decentralized controls (Volkman and Heller, 1971). The pineal NAcT response to stimulation as well as to blinding, which produces a 9-fold increase in NAcT activity in 3 h (Table II), represents a convenient system in which to examine the details of the neural and mole-

TABLE I

EFFECT OF NORADRENALINE AND TYRAMINE ON PINEAL SEROTONIN *N*-ACETYLTRANSFERASE (NAcT) ACTIVITY *in vivo*[a]

Treatment[b]	*Ratio of treatment group to saline control group*[c]
Sham operated	0.8
Ganglionectomized	1.0
Pargyline	1.0
Sham operated, pargyline–noradrenaline	8.9
Ganglionectomized, pargyline–noradrenaline	24.3
Pargyline–tyramine	1.0

[a]Saline control NAcT activity = 71.2 picomoles serotonin *N*-acetylated/gland/h.

[b]Rats were operated 7 days prior to the treatment and underwent either bilateral removal of superior cervical ganglia or sham operation. On the treatment day all animals were housed in constant light (GE Chroma 75 fluorescent lamps) for 8–12 h. Pargyline (25 mg/kg) was administered 6 h before kill. DL-noradrenaline HCl, 1 mg/kg or tyramine DL-HCl, 1 mg/kg given 3 h before kill. All groups consisted of six rats.

[c]Mean NAcT activity of sham-operated pargyline–noradrenaline group greater than saline control $p < 0.02$.

Mean NAcT activity of ganglionectomized, pargyline–noradrenaline group greater than saline control and sham operated pargyline–noradrenaline animals $p < 0.02$.

TABLE II

EFFECT OF PHARMACOLOGIC AGENTS ON THE BLINDING-INDUCED INCREASE IN PINEAL SEROTONIN *N*-ACETYLTRANSFERASE (NAcT) ACTIVITY *in vivo*[a]

Treatment[b] *(animals blinded 3 h before kill)*	*Ratio of treatment group to non-blinded saline controls*[c]
Saline	9.4
Cycloheximide	0.7
Actinomycin D	3.4
Propranolol	0.9
Reserpine	5.5
L-α-methyl-*p*-tyrosine	5.2
p-Chlorophenylalanine	8.8
6-Hydroxydopamine	16.7
Bretylium	19.5
Atropine methylnitrate	5.8
Chlorpheniramine maleate	9.9

[a]Non-blinded saline control NAcT Activity = 67.6 pmoles [^{14}C]serotonin-*N*-acetylated/gland/h. 43 animals anesthetized with ether 3 h before kill.

[b]All rats blinded after 8 *p.m.* (during normal dark period) and killed 3 h later. Dosage schedules: cycloheximide, 2.5 mg/kg, 1 h before blinding and additional 2.5 mg/kg 1 h after blinding; actinomycin D, 1 mg/kg 1 h before blinding; propranolol, 10 mg/kg, 1 h before blinding and additional 10 mg/kg 1 h after blinding; reserpine 2.5 mg/kg 24 h before blinding; 125 mg/kg α-methyl-*p*-tyrosine 9 h before blinding and an additional 125 mg/kg α-methyl-*p*-tyrosine 3 h before blinding; *p*-chlorophenylalanine, 100 mg/kg once a day for 3 days, and sacrificed 12 h after last injection; 6-hydroxydopamine, 15 mg/kg free base *i.p.*, 36 h before kill; bretylium, 20 mg/kg 1 h before blinding; atropine methylnitrate, 2 mg/kg 0.5 h before blinding; chlorpheniramine maleate, 2.5 mg/kg 0.5 h before blinding.

Non-blinded rats treated with these doses of drug showed no change in pineal NAcT activity from non-blinded saline controls.

[c]For all groups other than cycloheximide, and propranolol, mean NAcT activity greater than non-blinded saline control, $p < 0.01$. Mean NAcT activity for actinomycin D less than saline-blinded group, $p < 0.01$. Mean NAcT activity for bretylium and 6-hydroxydopamine greater than saline-blinded group, $p < 0.02$.

cular events underlying a neuronally induced rise in enzyme activity in an innervated organ.

In vitro studies have already demonstrated that an increase in NAcT activity of isolated pineals can be produced by noradrenaline or dibutryl-cyclic AMP, but not by serotonin (Klein and Weller, 1970; Klein *et al.*, 1970). Noradrenaline also elevates pineal adenyl cyclase *in vitro* (Weiss and Costa, 1967, 1968). The noradrenaline-induced rise in NAcT is blocked by cycloheximide (Klein *et al.*, 1970; Klein and Berg, 1970). It would appear from these studies that the rise in NAcT activity *in vitro* is mediated by a noradrenaline-stimulated adenyl cyclase-cyclic AMP mechanism dependent on protein synthesis. Recent *in vivo* studies from our laboratory indicate that the rise in NAcT activity in the intact animals is likewise an adrenergic response dependent on protein synthesis. In rats with light-suppressed levels of pineal NAcT, noradrenaline after pargyline treatment produces an increase in enzyme by 3 h equivalent to the increase observed 3 h after blinding. The system demonstrates

References p. 247–249

TABLE III

EFFECT OF PHARMACOLOGIC AGENTS ON THE PREGANGLIONIC CERVICAL SYMPATHETIC STIMULATION-INDUCED INCREASE IN PINEAL SEROTONIN *N*-ACETYLTRANSFERASE (NAcT) ACTIVITY *in vivo*[a]

Treatment[b]	*Ratio of treatment stimulated group to saline non-stimulated decentralized controls*[c]
Saline	3.2
Cycloheximide	0.9
Propranolol	1.1
Bretylium	6.0

[a]Mean NAcT activity saline-treated decentralized non-stimulated controls = 97.8 pmoles/gland/h.
[b]Rats stimulated *via* a sleeve bipolar electrode on one preganglionic trunk for 2 h, 9 sec out of every 30 sec, 10 pulses per s, 10 ms duration, 0.5 to 4 volts. Current maintained at a level sufficient to produce vigorous exophthalmos in ipsilateral eye. Contralateral cervical trunk decentralized.

Drug dosage schedules: All drugs given i.p 2.5 h before kill

Cycloheximide	2.5 mg/kg
Propranolol	10 mg/kg
Bretylium	20 mg/kg

[c]Mean NAcT activity for saline and bretylium groups greater than saline non-stimulated decentralized controls, $p < 0.02$.

denervation supersensitivity in that the noradrenaline-induced rise is 2–3 times greater in animals subjected to bilateral superior cervical ganglionectomy than in sham-operated controls (Table I).

As can be seen in Tables II and III, the rise in NAcT activity produced by blinding or nerve stimulation is apparently secondary to initiation of protein synthesis, since these stimulatory procedures are completely or partially blocked by cycloheximide or actinomycin D. The adrenergic nature of the rise in enzyme activity is supported by the finding that the effects of nerve stimulation or blinding are blocked by propranolol, a beta-adrenergic blocking agent. Noradrenaline has also been shown to produce hyperpolarization of pinealocyte membrane potentials *in vitro*, an effect blocked by propranolol (Sakai and Marks, 1972).

These findings along with the *in vitro* studies all point to a rather straightforward neuronal mechanism for regulation of pineal NAcT. The pineal gland receives its sole innervation from the sympathetic division of the autonomic nervous system (Kappers, 1960, 1965). Postganglionic adrenergic fibers arising from the superior cervical ganglia presumably innervate pineal parenchymal cells (for review see Kappers, 1971) and when stimulated release noradrenaline thereby initiating a sequence of events leading to the synthesis of new enzyme. Examination of the effects of a series of agents which act on adrenergic nerve endings suggests, however, that the situation may be more complex. Administration of neuronal catecholamine depleting agents including reserpine and α-methyl *p*-tyrosine in doses shown to decrease noradrenaline in other adrenergically innervated tissues were without significant effect on the blinding-induced rise in pineal NAcT activity (Table II). 6-hydroxydopamine, an agent which selectively destroys noradrenergic nerve endings (Thoenen and Tranzer, 1968) enhanced rather than blocked the response to blinding. Similarly, an adrenergic neuron blocking agent, bretylium (Boura and Green, 1959) in doses which prevented the sympathetically induced exophthalmic response was without significant effect on the pineal NAcT response to nerve stimulation (Table III) and the response to blinding was greater in bretylium treated animals than in non-treated blinded controls (Table II). In addition, it was found that tyramine, an indirectly acting sympathomimetic amine, was without effect on pineal NAcT activity in animals kept in continuous light in contrast to the effects of noradrenaline (Table I). Atropine methylnitrate, a muscarinic blocking agent, chlorpheniramine maleate, an antihistaminic, and *p*-chlorophenylalanine which produced essentially complete depletion of pineal serotonin were without significant effect on the blinding-induced increase in NAcT activity (Table II).

The lack of effect of reserpine and α-methyl *p*-tyrosine might have been anticipated. Even with doses of reserpine which produce large reductions in noradrenaline, such as were used here (*i.e.*, a 95% reduction in salivary gland noradrenaline) some responses to adrenergic nerve stimulation persist (Wakade and Krusz, 1972). The dose of α-methyl *p*-tyrosine used in this study produced only a 50–60% reduction in brain and heart noradrenaline and may, for that reason, have been ineffective. With even higher doses of this tyrosine hydroxylase inhibitor, the response of the cat nictitating membrane to nerve stimulation is preserved (Thoenen *et al.*, 1966). The lack of effect of 6-hydroxydopamine and bretylium is less easily explained. The dose of 6-hydroxydopamine used in the present studies lowered salivary gland noradrenaline by 85%. Similar reductions in organ noradrenaline by chemical sympathectomy with 6-hydroxydopamine abolish responses to sympathetic nerve stimulation in cat nictitating membrane, isolated cat heart and mesenteric arteries of the rat (Haeusler *et al.*, 1969; Haeusler, 1971). As already noted (Table II), 6-hydroxydopamine, rather than blocking the effects of blinding actually produced an enhancement of the NAcT increase. Bretylium, a specific adrenergic blocking agent, likewise enhanced (rather than blocked) the effects of blinding on pineal NAcT activity (Table II). In the dose given, bretylium did block the adrenergic exophthalmic response during sympathetic nerve stimulation, but failed to block the rise in pineal NAcT activity induced by the same cervical sympathetic preganglionic stimulation (Table III).

The lack of effect on the NAcT increase by agents which act on adrenergic nerve endings is surprising in light of the *in vitro* and *in vivo* effects of noradrenaline on pineal enzyme synthesis. These results suggest that adrenergic endings in the pineal have unusual characteristics. It should be noted that the effects of these drugs on the pineal are similar to their actions on the adrenal medulla. 6-Hydroxydopamine does not reduce adrenal stores of catecholamines (Thoenen *et al.*, 1970), nor does it reduce the intense fluorescence of chromaffin cells within cholinergic ganglia of the atria (Goldman and Jacobowitz, 1971). Likewise, bretylium does not block the adrenal release of catecholamines either by nerve stimulation or dimethyl phenylpiperazine (Boura and Green, 1959; Aviado and Dil, 1960). Tyramine, an indirectly acting amine (*i.e.*, one which acts by releasing noradrenaline from nerve endings) was without effect on pineal NAcT activity in the light-treated animals while noradrenaline produced an approximately 9-fold increase in enzyme activity (Table I). Tyramine is without

References p. 247–249

effect on release of catecholamines (Strömblad, 1960; Stjärne, 1961) from the perfused adrenal. These pharmacologic studies, therefore, indicate that the storage-release mechanisms for catecholamines in the pineal bear a closer resemblance to the adrenal medulla than to the usual adrenergic nerve ending. It seems reasonable to suggest that consideration be given to a chromaffin-like mechanism for the storage and release of catecholamines in the pineal.

The pineal enzyme studies provide a convenient model for studying the role of the nervous system in the regulation of enzyme synthesis across polyneuronal systems. In the CNS, we have proposed that the neurons of the medial forebrain bundle regulate the synthesis of enzymes essential for noradrenaline and serotonin biosynthesis through mediation of afferent input across one or more synapses. Shifts in afferent input to the pineal have indeed been shown to affect enzyme activities in that structure. If the deficits in monoamine biosynthesis following medial forebrain bundle lesions are indeed occurring in intact neurons, as we have suggested, it may be possible as shown in the pineal experiments, to reverse the lesion-induced neurochemical deficits by appropriate manipulation of central afferent input.

SUMMARY

The presence of the monoamines, noradrenaline and serotonin, in brain is dependent on the integrity of the medial forebrain bundle. The nigrostriatal tract is responsible for the presence of dopamine in the caudate nucleus. Destruction of these fiber systems results in a loss in central monoamines. The reduction in dopamine is secondary to section and degeneration of the nigrostriatal pathway with resultant loss of catecholamine from the area innervated. Decreases in brain noradrenaline and serotonin following medial forebrain bundle lesions occur in a more widespread pattern than would be expected from the anatomic distribution of the axons of this system. This finding has led to the suggestion that the neurons of the medial forebrain bundle play an essential role in the mediation of trophic influences regulating monoamine biosynthesis throughout brain. Control of melatonin biosynthesis by environmental lighting is likewise mediated across a polyneuronal system, involving central neurons and autonomic fibers from the superior cervical ganglion which innervate the pineal. Alterations in afferent input to the gland by nerve stimulation or blinding can be shown to affect the levels of pineal enzyme activities essential for the biosynthesis of melatonin. These effects appear to be mediated by noradrenaline, but pharmacologic studies on this system indicate that the mechanisms for storage and release of catecholamines in the pineal bear a closer resemblance to chromaffin tissue than to most adrenergic nerve endings.

ACKNOWLEDGEMENTS

This work was supported in part by Research Grant MH-04954 from the National

Institute of Mental Health. A.H. is a recipient of a Research Scientist Development Award (K2-MH-21850) from the National Institute of Mental Health. P.H.V. is a predoctoral trainee, Medical Scientists Training Program Grant, PHS 5-TO5-GM-01939-03. R.A.B. is a postdoctoral fellow, USPHS MH-07083-12 from the National Institute of Mental Health.

REFERENCES

ANDÉN, N.-E., DAHLSTRÖM, A., FUXE, K., LARSSON, K., OLSON, L. AND UNGERSTEDT, U. (1966) Ascending monoamine neurons to the telencephalon and diencephalon. *Acta physiol. scand.*, **67**, 313–362.

AVIADO, D. M. AND DIL, A. H. (1960) The effects of a new sympathetic blocking drug (bretylium) on cardiovascular control. *J. Pharmacol. exp. Ther.*, **129**, 328–337.

AXELROD, J. AND WEISSBACH, H. (1960) Enzymatic O-methylation of N-acetylserotonin to melatonin. *Science*, **131**, 1312.

AXELROD, J. AND WEISSBACH, H. (1961) Purification and properties of hydroxyindole-*O*-methyltransferase. *J. biol. Chem.*, **236**, 211–213.

BOURA, A. L. A. AND GREEN, A. F. (1959) The actions of bretylium: Adrenergic neurone blocking and other effects. *Brit. J. Pharmacol.*, **14**, 536–548.

BROWNSTEIN, M. J. AND HELLER, A. (1968) Hydroxyindole-*O*-methyltransferase activity: Effect of a sympathetic nerve stimulation. *Science*, **162**, 367–368.

CARDINALI, D. P. AND WURTMAN, R. J. (1972) Hydroxyindole-*O*-methyl transferases in rat pineal, retina and Harderian gland. *Endocrinology*, **91**, 247–252.

CHASE, P. A., SEIDEN, L. S. AND MOORE, R. Y. (1969) Behavioral and neuroendocrine responses to light mediated by separate visual pathways in the rat. *Physiol. and Behav.*, **4**, 949–952.

EHRINGER, H. AND HORNYKIEWICZ, O. (1960) Verteilung von Noradrenalin und Dopamin (3-hydroxytyramin) im Gehirn des Menschen und ihr Verhalten bei Erkrankungen des extrapyramidalen Systems. *Klin. Wschr.*, **38**, 1236–1239.

GOLDMAN, H. AND JACOBOWITZ, D. (1971) Correlation of norepinephrine content with observations of adrenergic nerves after a single dose of 6-hydroxydopamine in the rat. *J. Pharmacol. exp. Ther.*, **176**, 119–133.

HAEUSLER, G. (1971) Early pre- and postjunctional effects of 6-hydroxydopamine. *J. Pharmacol. exp. Ther.*, **178**, 49–62.

HAEUSLER, G., HAEFELY, W. AND THOENEN, H. (1969) Chemical sympathectomy of the cat with 6-hydroxydopamine. *J. Pharmacol. exp. Ther.*, **170**, 50–61.

HARVEY, J. A., HELLER, A. AND MOORE, R. Y. (1963) The effect of unilateral and bilateral medial forebrain bundle lesions on brain serotonin. *J. Pharmacol. exp. Ther.*, **140**, 103–110.

HAYHOW, W. R., WEBB, C. AND JERVIE, A. (1960) The accessory optic fiber system in the rat. *J. comp. Neurol.*, **115**, 187–200.

HAYHOW, W. R., SEFTON, A. AND WEBB, C. (1962) Primary optic centers of the rat in relation to the terminal distribution of the crossed and uncrossed optic nerve fibers. *J. comp. Neurol.*, **118**, 295–322.

HELLER, A. (1972) Neuronal control of brain serotonin. *Fed. Proc.*, **31**, 81–90.

HELLER, A., HARVEY, J. A. AND MOORE, R. Y. (1962) A demonstration of a fall in brain serotonin following central nervous system lesions in the rat. *Biochem. Pharmacol.*, **11**, 859–866.

HELLER, A. AND MOORE, R. Y. (1965) Effect of central nervous system lesions on brain monoamines in the rat. *J. Pharmacol. exp. Ther.*, **150**, 1–9.

HELLER, A. AND MOORE, R. Y. (1968) Control of brain serotonin and norepinephrine by specific neural systems. In *Advances in Pharmacology, Vol. 6A*, E. COSTA AND M. SANDLER (Eds.), Academic Press, New York, pp. 191–206.

HELLER, A. AND MOORE, R. Y. (1970) Localization and neural control of brain monoamines. In *Biochemistry, Schizophrenia and Affective Illnesses*, H. E. HIMWICH (Ed.) Williams and Wilkins, New York, pp. 431–469.

HELLER, A., SEIDEN, L. S., PORCHER, W. AND MOORE, R. Y. (1965) 5-hydroxytryptophan decarboxylase in rat brain: Effect of hypothalamic lesions. *Science*, **147**, 887.

HELLER, A., SEIDEN, L. S. AND MOORE, R. Y. (1966a) Regional effects of lateral hypothalamic lesions on brain norepinephrine in the cat. *Int. J. Neuropharmacol.*, **5**, 91–101.

HELLER, A., SEIDEN, L. S., PORCHER, W. AND MOORE, R. Y. (1966b) Regional effects of lateral hypothalamic lesions on brain 5-hydroxytryptophan decarboxylase in the cat brain. *J. Neurochem.*, **13**, 967–974.

HELLER, A., BHATNAGAR, R. K. AND MOORE, R. Y. (1969) Selective neural control of telencephalic monoamines and enzymes involved in their biosynthesis. In *Progress in Neuro-Genetics*, (Proc. 2nd Int. Congr. Neuro-Genetics and Neuro-Ophthalmol., Montreal, Canada, September, 1967, Vol. 1), A. BARBEAU AND J. R. BRUNETTE (Eds.), Excerpta Med., Amsterdam, pp. 283–288.

HOFFMANN, P., TOON, R., KLEINMAN, J. AND HELLER, A. (1973) The association of lesion-induced reductions in brain monoamines with alterations in striatal carbohydrate metabolism. *J. Neurochem.*, **20**, 69–80.

KAPPERS, J. A. (1960) The development, topographical relations and innervation of the epiphysis cerebri in the albino rat. *Z. Zellforsch. mikroskop. Anat.*, **52**, 163–215.

KAPPERS, J. A. (1965) Survey of the innervation of the epiphysis cerebri and the accessory pineal organs of the vertebrates. *Progr. Brain Res.*, **10**, 87–153.

KAPPERS, J. A. (1971) *The Pineal Organ: An Introduction to the Pineal Gland* (Ciba Foundation Symposium), G. E. W. WOLSTENHOLME AND J. KNIGHT (Eds.), Livingstone, London.

KLEIN, D. C. AND BERG, G. R. (1970) Pineal gland: Stimulation of melatonin production by norepinephrine involves cyclic AMP mediated stimulation of N-acetyltransferase. *Advanc. Biochem. Psychopharmacol.*, **3**, 241–263.

KLEIN, D. C. AND WELLER, J. L. (1970) Indole metabolism in the pineal gland: A circadian rhythm in *N*-acetyltransferase. *Science*, **169**, 1093–1095.

KLEIN, D. C., BERG, G. R. AND WELLER, J. L. (1970) Melatonin synthesis: Adenosine 3′,5′-monophosphate and norepinephrine stimulate *N*-acetyltransferase. *Science*, **168**, 979–980.

MOORE, R. Y. (1970) Brain lesions and amine metabolism. *Int. Rev. Neurobiol.*, **13**, 67–91.

MOORE, R. Y. AND HELLER, A. (1967) Monoamine levels and neuronal degeneration in rat brain following lateral hypothalamic lesions. *J. Pharmacol. exp. Ther.*, **156**, 12–22.

MOORE, R. Y., WONG, S. R. AND HELLER, A. (1965) Regional effects of hypothalamic lesions on brain serotonin. *Arch. Neurol.*, **13**, 346–354.

MOORE, R. Y., BHATNAGAR, R. AND HELLER, A. (1966) Norepinephrine and DOPA decarboxylase in rat brain following hypothalamic lesions. *Int. J. Neuropharmacol.*, **5**, 287–291.

MOORE, R. Y., HELLER, A., WURTMAN, R. J. AND AXELROD, J. (1967) Visual pathway mediating pineal response to environmental light. *Science*, **155**, 220–223.

MOORE, R. Y., HELLER, A., BHATNAGAR, R. K., WURTMAN, R. J. AND AXELROD, J. (1968) Central control of the pineal gland: Visual pathways. *Arch. Neurol.*, **18**, 208–218.

MOORE, R. Y., BHATNAGAR, R. K. AND HELLER, A. (1971) Anatomical and chemical studies of a nigro-neostriatal projection in the cat. *Brain Res.*, **30**, 119–135.

NAUTA, W. J. H. (1957) Silver impregnation of degenerating axons. In *New Research Techniques of Neuroanatomy*, W. F. WINDLE (Ed.), Thomas, Springfield, Ill., pp. 17–26.

POIRIER, L. J. AND SOURKES, T. L. (1965) Influence of the substantia nigra on the catecholamine content of the striatum. *Brain*, **88**, 181–192.

SAKAI, K. AND MARKS, B. H. (1972) Adrenergic effects on pineal cell membrane potential. *Life Sci.*, **11**, 285–291.

STJÄRNE, L. (1961) Tyramine effects on catecholamine release. *Acta physiol. scand.*, **51**, 224–229.

STRÖMBLAD, B. C. R. (1960) Effect of denervation and of cocaine on the action of sympathomimetic amines. *Brit. J. Pharmacol.*, **15**, 328–332.

THOENEN, H. AND TRANZER, J. P. (1968) Chemical sympathectomy by selective destruction of adrenergic nerve endings with 6-hydroxydopamine. *Naunyn-Schmiedeberg's Arch. exp. Path. Pharmak.*, **261**, 271–288.

THOENEN, H., HAEFELY, W., GEY, K. F. AND HUERLIMANN, A. (1966) The effect of α-methyl-tyrosine in peripheral sympathetic transmission. *Life Sci.*, **5**, 723–730.

THOENEN, H., TRANZER, J. P. AND HAEUSLER, G. (1970) Chemical sympathectomy with 6-hydroxydopamine. In *New Aspects of Storage and Release Mechanisms of Catecholamines*, H. J. SCHUMANN AND G. KRONEBERG (Eds.), Springer, Heidelberg, pp. 130–142.

VOLKMAN, P. H. AND HELLER, A. (1971) Pineal *N*-acetyltransferase activity: Effect of sympathetic stimulation. *Science*, **173**, 839–840.

WAKADE, A. R. AND KRUSZ, J. (1972) Effect of reserpine, phenoxybenzamine and cocaine on neuro-

muscular transmission in the vas deferens of the guinea pig. *J. Pharmacol. exp. Ther.*, **181**, 310–317.
WEISS, B. AND COSTA, E. (1967) Adenyl cyclase activity in rat pineal gland: Effects of chronic denervation and norepinephrine. *Science*, **156**, 1750–1752.
WEISS, B. AND COSTA, E. (1968) Selective stimulation of adenyl cyclase of rat pineal gland by pharmacologically active catecholamines. *J. Pharmacol. exp. Ther.*, **161**, 310–319.
WEISSBACH, H., REDFIELD, B. G. AND AXELROD, J. (1960) Biosynthesis of melatonin: Enzymic conversion of serotonin to *N*-acetylserotonin. *Biochim. biophys. acta*, **43**, 352–353.
WURTMAN, R. J., AXELROD, J. AND CHU, E. W. (1963) Melatonin, a pineal substance: Effect on the rat ovary. *Science*, **141**, 277–278.
WURTMAN, R. J., AXELROD, J. AND FISCHER, J. E. (1964) Melatonin synthesis in the pineal gland: Effect of light mediated by the sympathetic nervous system. *Science*, **143**, 1328–1330.
WURTMAN, R. J., AXELROD, J. AND KELLY, D. E. (1968) *The Pineal*, Academic Press, New York, pp. 58–59.

DISCUSSION

GOLDMAN: As you know, we have been looking at blood flow in the pineal for a long time and one of the things that always puzzled us is that the pineal has a very large blood flow; on a weight basis it's greater than that of kidney. One of the things that has always troubled us was when it is denervated, presumably totally deafferented by superior cervical ganglionectomy, its blood flow drops by about a third and there is slight atrophy. However, even under these circumstances the blood flow is still greater than that of any endocrine organ in the body. I wonder why a structure whose primary information source is gone requires that kind of perfusion? What kind of business is it transacting?

DOUGLAS: The pharmacology of this system is very very puzzling. I know that there is plenty of evidence that there are noradrenergic or catecholamine elements there, but could you tell me the evidence that fibers innervating the pineal are really not cholinergic and that there may be an intercollated adrenergic element there? What do ganglion-blocking substances do?

HELLER: That is precisely what we are beginning to wonder. The answer to your question is very complicated in part because the histology and anatomy of this system is not well understood. There are in some species intrapineal ganglion cells, but they have never been seen in the rat. However, there are cells in the rat which conceivably could be intrapineal nerve cells. There are certainly adrenergic neurones coming to the gland. Whether they are the neurones that transmit information is an interesting question. Very few of them come close to the pinealocytes; most appear around the pericapillary spaces. It is possible that there is a cholinergic connection and perhaps the preganglionic sympathetic fiber itself comes all the way through and innervates the pineal. We recently started a number of experiments using blocking agents. They are not easy to do because it is necessary to give the blocking agent intracisternally in order to avoid blocking the superior cervical ganglion. Interestingly, pentolinium did not block the response to stimulation but it did raise the enzyme level in the nonstimulated animal suggesting that perhaps this was an agonist effect. We just started looking at cholinergic agonists in this system. I would not be surprised if we find a cholinergic link here.

DOUGLAS: If I might add to that when one stimulates the cervical sympathetic ganglion, one is stimulating predominately cholinergic preganglionic fibers and there are always fibers that are transversing various ganglia. These well could be cholinergic fibers going up towards the pineal. You might have there the same sort of system that obtains in the guinea pig and rabbit where you have intercollated dopaminergic neurones. Is the pineal inside or outside of the blood brain barrier?

HELLER: It's outside.

DOUGLAS: Well if it's outside, you should block very cheerfully with conventional things like hexamethonium if you stimulate the postganglionic fibers.

HELLER: Unfortunately the postganglionic elements are nearly impossible to reach anatomically. The ganglion is too high in the neck.

HYYPPA: We have some data which show that sex hormones can regulate enzyme activity in the pineal. We chemically sympathectomized newborn rats with different doses of 6-OH dopamine. 30 days later we assayed pineal and retinal HIOMT activity. Surprisingly, chemical sympathectomy increased pineal HIOMT activity but only in males. This elevation in enzyme activity is androgen-dependent as tested in several models. We think that neonatal androgens can block inhibitory sympathetic transmission to the pineal enzyme system, probably at the level of the anterior hypothalamus where we find a very marked decrease of noradrenaline.

REITER: Histochemically it is well known that the pineal has relatively extensive cholinergic innervation, apparently from the superior cervical ganglion. We have been unable to inactivate the pineal gland with chemical sympathectomy whereas if we surgically sympathectomize animals we invariably render the pineal gland nonfunctional. Therefore, if you chemically sympathectomize an animal it is important to do the appropriate studies to insure that it has in fact been done.

HELLER: There are neurons containing cholinesterase and one must be very careful with equating cholinesterase with cholinergic.

JACOBOWITZ: Histochemical studies of the rat pineal for cholinergic nerves using the Koelle method demonstrated cholinergic nerves around blood vessels mostly outside of the gland and cholinergic nerves within the pineal are extremely sparse. There is some recent evidence by Eränko that there is some cholinesterase in the pineal. This cholinesterase is interpreted to be on the outside membrane of adrenergic nerves, thus supporting the existence of a cholinergic link.

TAYLOR: With respect to cholinergic influences on the pineal, I should like to add that a few years ago together with Dr. Steven Wartman in my laboratory and in collaboration with Dr. Robert George (Life Sci., 8, 1263, 1969) we presented evidence for a cholinergic action on the rat pineal. In these studies atropine methyl bromide was found to inhibit the response of HIOMT to darkness, *i.e.* HIOMT activity was not elevated. This effect was reversed by the cholinomimetic, oxotremorine. The action of light to lower HIOMT levels was not affected by atropine. So we consider this to be direct evidence for cholinergic influences on the pineal. Since the question of the innervation of the pineal has been raised, I should like to add that our experiments in which the electrical activity of the pineal was recorded in the rat would indicate that there must be another route of innervation besides the superior cervical ganglion. In these experiments the electrical activity of the pineal was shown to be directly responsive to photic stimulation (Experientia 26, 267, 1970). The effects of light on pineal electrical activity were not affected by superior cervical ganglionectomy or by preganglionic denervation of the superior cervical ganglion. Although the ganglionic blocking agent, hexamethonium chloride, appeared to abolish the response this effect was probably secondary to the lowered blood pressure (and pineal blood flow) resulting from this drug. Thus, there must be another pathway by which photic information is transmitted to the pineal, perhaps directly from the brainstem *via* the pineal stalk.

HELLER: I think one has to distinguish between the possibility of other pathways to the pineal and the pathways which have been demonstrated to be specific for certain effects on biochemical events. There seems to be little doubt that the inferior accessory optic system and the peripheral autonomic pathway are essential for the light-dark differences in HIOMT in light- *vs.* dark-treated animals. It is important not to confuse input to the pineal with input subserving specific biochemical functions.

MARKS: I wonder if the pineal and gonadotrophin specialists here can tell us about the current status of non-melatonin antigonadotrophin of the pineal?

REITER: I would like to see Dr. Taylor's studies repeated under the following experimental conditions. First, in animals in which the pineal stalk has been sectioned. This is a very simple surgical procedure and would tell us if fibers enter the pineal by way of the stalk. Secondly, because of the proximity of the pineal gland to the visual cortex, I would like to see those studies repeated in animals which have their lateral geniculate bodies lesioned. I think it ostensibly could be easy to be recording from the pineal gland when, in fact, you would be recording from the visual cortex. In reply to Dr. Mark's question about potent antigonadotrophic polypeptide, it has a molecular weight apparently of 500–1000. It is more potent than melatonin on an equivalent weight basis. It has antigonadotrophic activity in the Swiss Wistar mouse when the compensatory hypertrophic response is studied. This information has recently been published by Benson *et al.* (Acta endocr., 69, 257, 1972) and, of course, Moszkowska and Ebels (J. neuro-visc. Rel., Suppl. X, 160, 1971).

The role of Pineal Principles in Ovulation

B. MESS*, L. TIMA* AND G. P. TRENTINI**

*Department of Anatomy, University Medical School, Szigeti ut 12, Pecs (Hungary) and **Department of Pathology, University of Modena, Via Berengario 4, 41100 Modena (Italy)

INTRODUCTION

In 1968 we reported with Fraschini and Martini that pinealectomy increases the synthesis and mobilization of luteinizing hormone (LH) in the adult male rat. In addition, implantation of a pineal gland or of purified melatonin into the median eminence of the hypothalamus, or into the reticular formation of the mesencephalon, caused a significant decrease in the elevated pituitary LH content of castrated male rats (Fraschini *et al.*, 1968a and b). These results furnished evidence supporting the hypothesis that the pineal body has an inhibitory effect on LH secretion by the anterior pituitary.

The previous consideration led us to the idea of trying to elicit the formation of corpora lutea and of ovulation by pinealectomy in permanent-estrous anovulatory rats. This latter syndrome was induced by frontal deafferentation of the anterior hypothalamus. As was reported at the Ciba Symposium in London, devoted to the pineal gland, formation of corpora lutea, as well as tubal ova, were found in permanent-estrous anovulatory rats after pinealectomy (Mess *et al.*, 1971). These findings confirmed our assumption that pinealectomy causes an increase in pituitary LH secretion by decreasing circulating levels of the melatonin. This elevation of LH level is sufficient to induce ovulation in the polyfollicular ovaries of rats suffering from the anovulatory syndrome.

Wurtman *et al.* (1964a and b) and Axelrod *et al.* (1965) found that extirpation of the superior sympathetic cervical ganglia led to a complete functional inactivity of the pineal gland; therefore, these authors equated bilateral superior cervical ganglionectomy to "functional pinealectomy". These findings gave rise to the question whether the ovulation-inducing effect of pinealectomy in the frontally deafferented animal could similarly be reproduced by superior cervical ganglionectomy.

Two further thoughts remained. Firstly, whether pinealectomy or ganglionectomy provokes only a single ovulation causing an acute, transitory increase in LH mobilization, or whether there is a long lasting, permanent elevation of pituitary LH secretion, resulting in repeated ovulation. The second unsolved problem was whether the ova, released by the originally polyfollicular ovaries as a result of either pinealectomy or sympathetic cervical ganglionectomy, are physiologically competent,

References p. 257–258

capable of being fertilized and producing normal embryos, or whether these are only unripe, infertile, biologically debilitated cells.

In the present study we have attempted to answer these questions, which seem to be fundamental in the consideration of the role of the pineal gland in the control of ovulation.

MATERIAL AND METHODS

Frontal deafferentation, *i.e.* transection of the neural connections between the preoptic area and the hypothalamus, was performed by the technique described by Halász and Pupp (1965). Starting 1 month after operation, vaginal smears were recorded daily for a period of 4 weeks. Animals showing permanent vaginal estrus were laparotomized and ovaries were carefully inspected, and those in which only a single corpus luteum was detected were discarded. Only rats with undoubtedly polyfollicular ovaries were used for further experiments.

In rats selected as above, pinealectomy was performed by the technique of Grant *et al.* (1966) as modified in our laboratory. In another group of rats the superior sympathetic cervical ganglia were removed bilaterally (no pinealectomy). The recording of vaginal smears was continued after either pinealectomy or ganglionectomy.

The ganglionectomized animals and one series of pinealectomized rats were exposed to fertile males 3 days after each operation. Copulation was verified by detection of sperm in the vaginal smears. Length of pregnancies, deliveries, number of litters and physical state of the newborn were carefully registered over a period of about 5 months.

In another series of experiments, 72 days after pinealectomy, animals were killed and the histology of the ovaries was investigated regarding formation of corpora lutea. In the subsequent experiment the oviduct on one side was dissected on the second estrous day following the first diestrous phase post-pinealectomy, and the number of tubal ova was counted. The ovary of the same side was also removed for histological investigation. Again on the second estrous day following the next diestrous phase, the remaining oviduct was dissected and tubal ova were sought.

The second ovary was also preserved for histological evaluation.

Ovaries were fixed in 10% neutral formalin, and the frozen sections were stained with Sarlach-R-haematoxylin stain.

The exact site of the frontal cut and the completeness of the frontal deafferentation of the hypothalamus was checked by histological examination of serial sections of the brain stained with haematoxylin and eosin.

RESULTS

(1) Effect of bilateral removal of the superior sympathetic cervical ganglia of rats bearing frontal brain cuts and polyfollicular ovaries on the frequency of ovulation and fertility

The permanent vaginal cornification changed immediately after ganglionectomy,

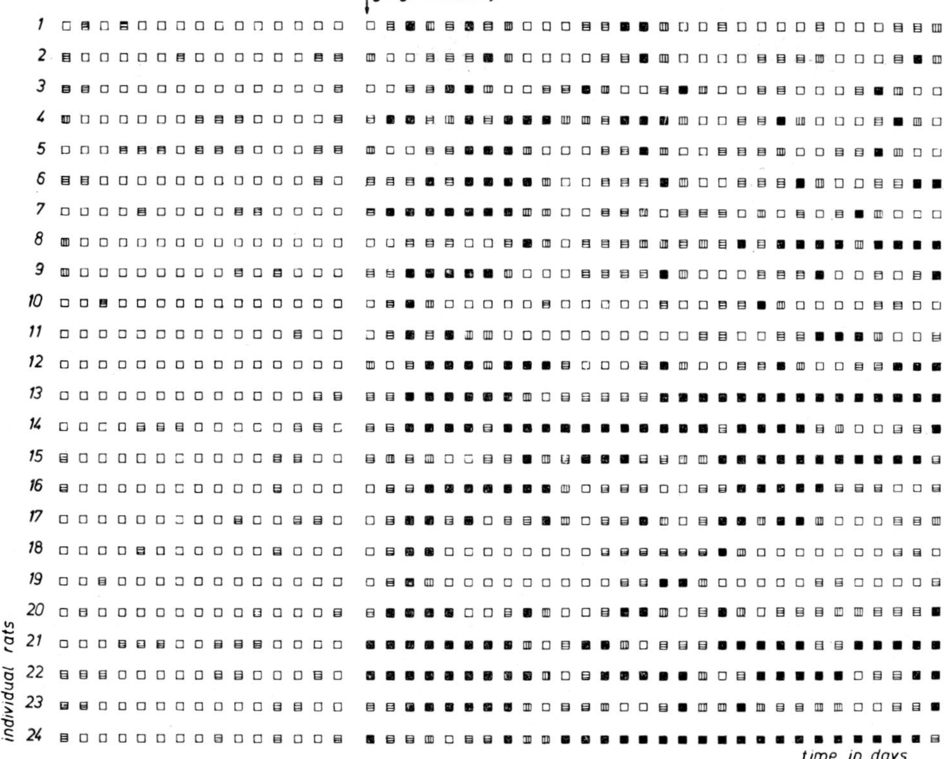

Fig. 1. Changes in vaginal smears after bilateral removal of the superior sympathetic cervical ganglia in rats with frontal deafferentation of the hypothalamus. The first recorded day is the 30th day after hypothalamic deafferentation. ▥, proestrus; □, estrus, ▤, metaestrus; ■, diestrus.

which was similar to that seen after pinealectomy (Mess *et al.*, 1971). The cycles were not as regular as in the intact females, but irregular, though cycle-like changes in the vaginal smears were evident (Fig. 1).

TABLE I

OCCURRENCE OF LUTEINIZATION AND OF PREGNANCIES FOLLOWING PINEALECTOMY OR BILATERAL REMOVAL OF THE SUPERIOR SYMPATHETIC CERVICAL GANGLIA IN ANOVULATORY RATS WITH FRONTAL HYPOTHALAMIC DEAFFERENTATION

Experimental group	*Number of animals*	*Occurrence of corpora lutea*		*Single pregnancy*		*Two pregnancies*		*Three or more pregnancies*	
		Number	*%*	*Number*	*%*	*Number*	*%*	*Number*	*%*
Ganglionectomy	24	16	66.6	11	45.8	8	33.3	7	29.1
Pinealectomy	14	6	42.9	5	35.7	2	14.3	Not investigated	

As Table I shows, 11 of 24 (46%) rats became pregnant and bore young; of the 11 fertile rats 8 became pregnant twice (33.3%) and 7 three or more times (29.1%). The number of pups delivered varied between 7 and 12, which is within the normal range in our strain of rats. The length of pregnancy appeared somewhat longer (23.6 days) than normal. This aspect will be discussed further on.

The ovaries of the 13 infertile ganglionectomized rats showed viable corpora lutea in 5 cases (20.8% of the total) and only in 8 rats (33.3% of the total) were polyfollicular ovaries found. This means that luteinization occurred in 16 of the 24 animals (66.6%), which represents the same proportion of luteinization, as was previously found after pinealectomy. The occurrence of gravidity was also in the same range as we found tubal ova in the pinealectomized animals (Mess *et al.*, 1971).

(2) *Effect of pinealectomy on the frequency of ovulation and fertility of rats bearing frontal brain cuts and polyfollicular ovaries*

Initial indirect evidence for the prolonged effect of pinealectomy is seen by the finding that 72 days after pinealectomy the percentage occurrence and histological character of the corpora lutea were the same as when investigated a few days after pineal removal.

In the next series of experiments we tried to obtain more direct evidence that rats bearing the anovulatory syndrome also ovulate at least twice after pinealectomy. The main results of these latter experiments are summarized in Table II. Unfortunately, there was only a single case to be reported where tubal ova were found in both oviducts but 22 days apart. This is direct evidence that rats possessing the anovulatory syndrome are able to ovulate repeatedly after pinealectomy.

In 7 additional rats, tubal ova were present 2 days after the first postoperative diestrous period, whereas somewhat later, when the oviduct of the remaining side was dissected, no tubal ova were found; but there were two generations of well-defined corpora lutea. The new generation of corpora lutea still contained a central hollow, a residuum of the follicular cavity, the lipoid deposition in the luteal cells being very scarce (Fig. 2a). In the previous generation of corpora lutea, luteal cells were filled with rough lipoid droplets (Fig. 2b). Further evidence is presented in the 5 cases where no ova were found in the oviduct at the first examination, but well developed fresh corpora lutea were present in the ovaries; whereas later, on the other side, tubal ova were also detected.

The incidence of single and repeated pregnancies was somewhat lower in the pinealectomized than in the ganglionectomized group (Table I). Although the number of animals in the pinealectomized group was fairly limited, the similar character of the results obtained in these two experimental groups seems to be appreciable: of a total of 14 pinealectomized rats, 5 became pregnant (35.7%); and of the 5 fertile animals, 2 mated twice (14.3%). The number of fetuses per litter was also completely normal. In one infertile pinealectomized rat fresh corpora lutea were found in the ovaries, whereas the ovaries of 8 animals remained in the original polyfollicular state (57.1%).

TABLE II

OCCURRENCE OF OVULATION AND OF LUTEINIZATION SEPARATELY INVESTIGATED IN THE LEFT AND RIGHT TUBO-OVARIAN COMPLEX DURING DIFFERENT INTERVALS FOLLOWING PINEALECTOMY IN THE ANOVULATORY RAT BEARING FRONTAL DEAFFERENTATION OF THE HYPOTHALAMUS

Rat No.	*Left side*			*Right side*		
	Days after pinealec-tomy	*Number of tubal ova*	*Ovarian histology*	*Days after pinealec-tomy*	*Number of tubal ova*	*Ovarian histology*
1	15	1	2 genera-tions of corp. lut.	37	6	2 genera-tions of corp. lut.
2	6	3	3 corp. lut.	16	—	2 gen. corp. luteum
3	7	4	5 corp. lut.	15	—	2 gen. corp. luteum
4	11	2	3 corp. lut.	17	—	2 gen. corp. luteum
5	13	6	2 gen. corp. lut.	18	—	2 gen. corp. luteum
6	14	3	7 corp. lut.	18	—	2 gen. corp. luteum
7	30	2	5 corp. lut.	51	—	2 gen. corp. luteum
8	32	3	3 corp. lut.	44	—	2 gen. corp. luteum
9	9	—	5 corp. lut.	36	7	7 corp. lut.
10	13	—	6 corp. lut.	18	8	2 gen. corp. luteum
11	13	—	2 corp. lut.	31	8	8 corp. lut.
12	18	—	7 corp. lut.	22	8	7 corp. lut.
13	18	—	3 corp. lut.	23	8	2 gen. corp. luteum

DISCUSSION

From the data presented the following conclusions might be drawn initially.

(*a*) Bilateral removal of the superior cervical ganglia has the same effect in inducing ovulation and luteinization in the polyfollicular ovaries of the frontal-deafferented rats, as has been seen previously after pinealectomy. Ganglionectomy may be considered in synonymous relation to ovulation control with "functional pinealectomy".

(*b*) Pinealectomized, as well as ganglionectomized rats, bearing an anovulatory syndrome, are able to produce repeated multiple ovulations.

(*c*) The number of ova released by pinealectomy, or ganglionectomy, is within the range of a physiological ovulation observed in intact rats.

(*d*) Nearly 50% of the pinealectomized or ganglionectomized rats are fertile, showing that the ova released by these surgical manipulations are viable.

The problem of the mechanism of this ovulation-inducing effect of pinealectomy

References p. 257–258

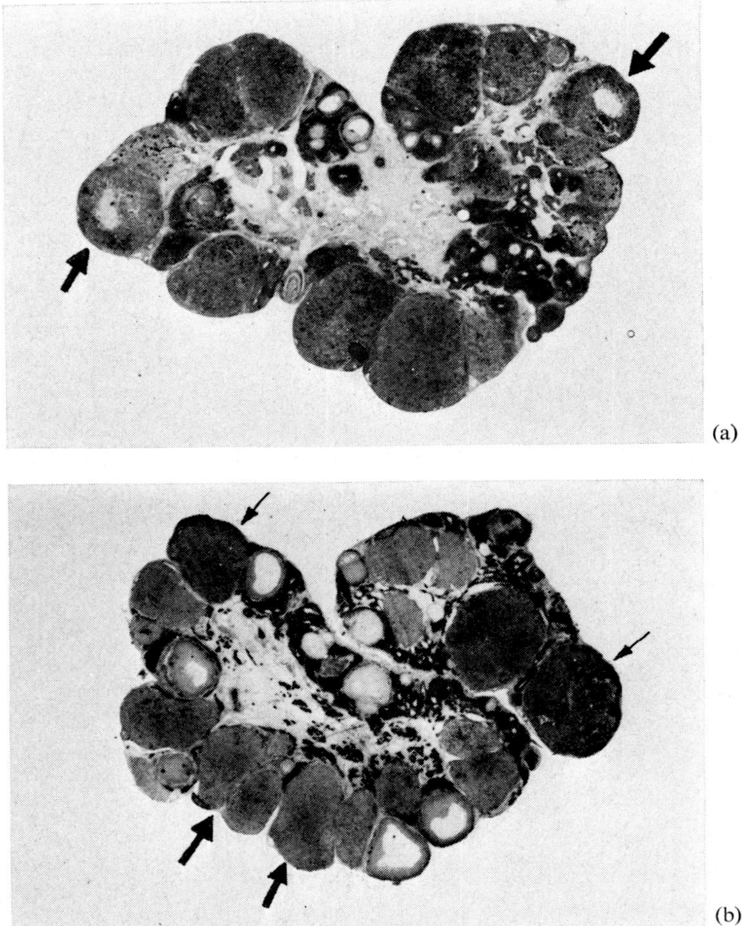

Fig. 2. Two generations of corpora lutea induced by pinealectomy in the ovaries of anovulatory rats bearing frontal deafferentation. (a) New generation (developing) corpora lutea containing a central hollow (thick arrows). (b) New generation of corpora lutea (thick arrows) and previous generation of corpora lutea (thin arrows).

and of ganglionectomy is relatively complicated. On the basis of our investigations, performed in Milan with Fraschini and Martini (1968a and b), it is suggested that these interventions elevate pituitary LH secretion. Furthermore, we have convincing evidence (Fraschini *et al.*, 1968a and b), confirmed by Anton-Tay (1971), that pineal principles act through the central nervous system. The problem, however, is far from being solved.

Labhsetwar (1971) reported that a single subcutaneous injection of serotonin (50 mg/kg), given during the so-called critical period before ovulation, interfered with ovulation in the normal adult rat. Chronic administration of serotonin (1 mg/kg body weight) normalized the alterations of the vaginal cycle caused by pinealectomy (Albertazzi *et al.*, 1966). Infusion of serotonin into the third ventricle decreased the release of LH (Schneider and McCann, 1970). On the other hand, the biochemical investigations of Anton-Tay (1971) showed that serotonin concentration increases in the midbrain and also, but less significantly, in the hypothalamus 1 h after the administration of 50 μg of melatonin. A critical review of these data led us to the assumption that pinealectomy and ganglionectomy might act through the serotoninergic system of the hypothalamus and/or of the midbrain. Pinealectomy might decrease the serotonin level of the brain, and since serotonin inhibits LH mobilization (Schneider and McCann, 1970) and prevents ovulation (Labhsetwar, 1971), the decreased serotonin level might be responsible for an increase in LH mobilization and consequently for inducing ovulation. If this speculation is correct, serotonin administration should counteract the effect of pinealectomy in our frontally deafferented rats bearing polyfollicular ovaries.

To verify our hypothesis, we injected 20 anovulatory pinealectomized rats with a daily dose of serotonin either at 1 mg/kg or 10 mg/kg. After 30 days of chronic serotonin administration only 2 pinealectomized rats (1 in each dose group) showed corpora lutea; the ovaries of the other 18 animals remained in the original polyfollicular state.

These latter findings lend support to our assumption that the effect of pinealectomy acts through the serotoninergic system of the central nervous system; at least the LH-mobilizing effect of pinealectomy might be elicited in this fashion.

Investigations concerning the possible interplay of the other brain amines and pineal indoleamines are in progress in our laboratory.

SUMMARY

The influence of pinealectomy and of superior sympathetic cervical ganglionectomy in the control of ovulation was investigated. An anovulatory syndrome with permanent vaginal cornification and polyfollicular ovaries was provoked by frontal deafferentation of the hypothalamus. Pinealectomy, as well as bilateral removal of the superior sympathetic cervical ganglia, elicited ovulation and formation of corpora lutea in these anovulatory rats. Nearly 50% of the pinealectomized or ganglionectomized rats became pregnant, and about one-third of the operated animals were able to be remated. The effect of pinealectomy and of ganglionectomy was counteracted by chronic administration of serotonin. The mechanism whereby the pineal body exerts its influence on the LH mobilization of the anterior pituitary is discussed briefly.

REFERENCES

ALBERTAZZI, E., BARBANTI-SILVA, C., TRENTINI, G. P. AND BOTTICELLI, A. (1966) Influence de l'épiphysectomie sur le cycle oestral de la ratte albinos. *Ann. Endocrinol. (Paris)*, **27**, 93–100.

ANTÓN-TAY, F. (1971) Pineal–brain relationships. In *Ciba Foundation Symposium on "The Pineal Gland"*, G. E. W. WOLSTENHOLME AND J. KNIGHT (Eds.), Churchill, London, pp. 213–227.

AXELROD, J., WURTMAN, R. J. AND SNYDER, S. H. (1965) Control of hydroxy-indole-*O*-methyl transferase activity in the rat pineal by environmental lighting. *J. biol. Chem.*, **240**, 949–954.

FRASCHINI, F., MESS, B. AND MARTINI, L. (1968a) Pineal gland, melatonin and the control of luteinizing hormone secretion. *Endocrinology*, **82**, 919–924.
FRASCHINI, F., MESS, B., PIVA, F. AND MARTINI, L. (1968b) Brain receptors sensitive to indole compounds: function in control of luteinizing hormone secretion. *Science*, **159**, 1104–1105.
GRANT, L., JENNER, F. A. AND WILLY, B. (1966) Pinealectomy in the rat. *J. Physiol.*, **182**, 24.
HALÁSZ, B. AND PUPP, L. (1965) Hormone secretion of the anterior pituitary gland after physical interruption of all nervous pathways to the hypophysiotrophic area. *Endocrinology*, **77**, 553–562.
LABHSETWAR, A. P. (1971) Effect of serotonin on spontaneous ovulation in rats. *Nature (Lond.)*, **229**, 203–204.
MESS, B., HEIZER, A., TÓTH, A. AND TIMA, L. (1971) Luteinization induced by pinealectomy in the polyfollicular ovaries of rats bearing anterior hypothalamic lesions. In *Ciba Foundation Symposium on "The Pineal Gland"*, G. E. W. WOLSTENHOLME AND J. KNIGHT (Eds.), Churchill, London, pp. 229–240.
SCHNEIDER, H. P. G. AND MCCANN, I. M. (1970) Mono- and indoleamines and control of LH-secretion. *Endocrinology*, **86**, 1127–1133.
WURTMAN, R. J., AXELROD, J. AND FISCHER, J. E. (1964a) Melatonin synthesis in the pineal gland: Effect of light mediated by the sympathetic nervous system. *Science*, **143**, 1328–1330.
WURTMAN, R. J., AXELROD, J., CHU, E. W. AND FISCHER, J. E. (1964b) Mediation of some effects of illumination on the rat estrous cycle by the sympathetic nervous system. *Endocrinology*, **75**, 266–272.

DISCUSSION

SHASKAN: I think your findings are very interesting. One comment, however, may clarify some of your findings. Serotonin in the concentrations which you used doesn't cross the blood-brain barrier. However, the median eminence is outside of the blood-brain barrier, so that the serotonin that you administered i.p. has access to and may be acting at these loci.

MESS: It's possible, but there are published data (Labhsetwar, Nature (Lond.), 229, 203, 1971 and Albertazzi *et al.*, Ann. Endocrinol., 27, 93, 1966) showing that serotonin administration was effective in regulating LH secretion. I have no positive data and can only speculate about this.

WEINER: When we inserted cannulas into the right atria of anterior deafferented rats which had shown constant vaginal cornification for approximately 2 weeks the animals became diestrous. In some animals diestrous vaginal smears were observed for 10 to 12 days. However, in most animals diestrous smears were observed for only 3 to 5 days followed by constant vaginal cornification. I was wondering whether you did any sham operations to see if just the stress of the surgical procedure could induce ovulation in anterior deafferented animals.

MESS: Yes, sham operations involving opening the skull, blood loss, and cortical injury never produced ovulation or luteinization (Mess *et al.*, Ciba Found. Symp., "The Pineal Gland", London, 1971).

STUMPF: Our autoradiographic data support the possible involvement of the pineal in the feedback of estradiol. We find a small population of pineal cells labeled with estradiol but don't know what type of cells they are.

MESS: Together with Dr. Kordon and Madame Gogan in Paris, we also found pineal uptake of tritium-labeled estradiol. What its significance might be I don't know, but I hardly believe that the estradiol uptake capacity of the pineal body would be directly related to the effect reported here. This is, of course, only an opinion.

DE WIED: It has been reported that pinealectomy affects water metabolism in such a way that reduction in the release of ADH would occur. Have you seen any effects on water metabolism in the pinealectomized animals?

MESS: We have not investigated directly the water metabolism in our rats, but Dr. Lengvary, in our laboratory obtained data suggesting the subcommissural organ and the habenular region, but not the pineal body are related to water metabolism through the mineralocorticoid system of the adrenal cortex.

REITER: Of course, De Vries (Neuroendocrinology, 9, 244, 1972) has shown that the pineal gland is involved with ADH and water metabolism.

SHASKAN: Using the Reiter paradigm again, this time using a blinded hamster, I tried to test whether the antigonadotrophic effect of blinding could be reversed using either D- or L-amphetamine. D- or L-amphetamine was put into the drinking water beginning 1 day after blinding at 25 days after birth. Once a week, to be certain that the hamsters received 10 mg/kg D- or L-amphetamine, they were individually weighed and injected with D- or L-amphetamine (10 mg/kg) intraperitoneally. 6 weeks after blinding no reversal of the atrophy of testes or seminal vesicle weights was observed. However, changes in body weight showed a paradoxical relationship to D-amphetamine when blinded *vs.* seeing hamsters were compared. In both the blinded and the seeing animals receiving plain drinking water and weakly i.p. saline injections, the rate of increase of growth was not significantly different. In seeing animals treated with D-amphetamine there was an initial anorectic response which displayed tolerance. In blinded hamsters receiving D-amphetamine a significant increase in body weight as compared to controls was observed, and the rate of increase was greater than that in the control blinded or seeing hamsters. Thus, blinding paradoxically alters the anorectic response to D-amphetamine in hamsters. Water consumption in all experimental groups was comparable. However, food consumption and basal metabolic rate were not measured. It is concluded that blinding, possibly *via* activation of the pineal gland, alters the anorectic response to D-amphetamine, possibly in those hypothalamic areas concerned with food intake, TSH control, or growth hormone control.

The Role of Brain Monoamines and Pineal Indoles in the Secretion of Gonadotrophins and Gonadotrophin-Releasing Factors

I. A. KAMBERI

Department of Obstetrics and Gynecology, UCLA School of Medicine, Harbor General Hospital Campus, Division of Reproductive Biology, Torrance, Calif. 90509 (U.S.A.)

INTRODUCTION

Hypothalamic hypophysiotrophic hormones (HHH) constitute the final signals which mediate hypothalamic control of the anterior pituitary gland (Harris, 1970). In recent years, considerable attention has been focused on the possible involvement of pineal indoles and brain monoamines in neurohumoral control of pituitary function (Martini *et al.*, 1968; Wurtman *et al.*, 1968; Reiter and Fraschini, 1969; Hökfelt and Fuxe, 1972; McCann *et al.*, 1972; Porter *et al.*, 1972; Weiner *et al.*, 1972; Ganong, 1972). The first evidence that catecholamines participate in regulation of gonadotrophin secretion was obtained by Sawyer and his associates (1947), who showed that ovulation can be blocked by dibenamine. Much later, Sawyer and his co-workers (Sawyer, 1964) demonstrated that reserpine, an agent which depletes brain catecholamines, would block ovulation, induce pseudopregnancy and lactation. More recently, Coppola and his associates (1971) reported that pseudopregnancy could also be induced by other catecholamine depletors, such as L-methyl-DOPA or tetrabenazine and that this effect could be counteracted by treatment with L-3,4-dihydroxyphenylalanine (L-DOPA) or monoamine oxidase inhibitors.

Of particular interest are the findings of Fuxe and Hökfelt (1969) using fluorescence microscopy. They have shown the presence of catecholaminergic and serotoninergic neurons in the hypothalamus. A role for these particular neurons in control of gonadotrophin secretion is suggested by the alterations in their content of dopamine in situations associated with altered gonadotrophin secretion (Fuxe *et al.*, 1967). Kordon and his associates blocked the superovulation of pregnant mare serum (PMS)-primed immature rats by increasing hypothalamic serotonin content and also by inhibiting dopamine synthesis during the critical period of the immature rat (Kordon and Glowinski, 1970).

Additional evidence supporting the view that monoamines play a role in the regulation of gonadotrophin secretion could be found in the experiments which have demonstrated the alteration in hypothalamic catecholamine content and turnover

References p. 276–279

(Donoso *et al.*, 1967; Anton-Tay and Wurtman, 1971) and monoamine oxidase activity (Kato and Minaguchi, 1964; Zolovick *et al.*, 1966; Kamberi and Danhof, 1968; Kamberi and Kobayashi, 1970) with the stage of the estrous cycle or following alteration in the levels of gonadal steroids.

These findings and other indirect evidence (Everett, 1964) suggest a number of hypothetical questions as to the role of hypothalamic monoamines in the regulation of gonadotrophin secretion. For example, are monoamines themselves HHH? Do these monoamines and HHH potentiate each other at the pituitary level? Or, do the monoamines act as synaptic transmitters to stimulate or inhibit the release of HHH from neurosecretory elements of the hypothalamus? To answer these questions, a variety of experimental approaches under *in vitro* and *in vivo* conditions have been applied to the problem. Follicle-stimulating hormone (FSH), luteinizing hormone (LH) and prolactin were measured in most of the studies by radioimmunoassay or as otherwise explained.

I. BRAIN MAO ACTIVITY AND ESTROUS CYCLE

The activity of monoamine oxidase (MAO) was measured in the entire hypothalamus (Ht) and different Ht regions, in the amygdala (Am), brain cortex of male and female rats (Fig. 1–3), using radioisotopic methods (Kamberi and Danhof, 1968; Kamberi and Kobayashi, 1970). 4-day cycling rats were autopsied at 10 *a.m.* (P_1), 3 *p.m.* (P_2) and 6 to 7 *p.m.* (P_3) of the day of proestrus. Female rats in estrus (E), metestrus (M)

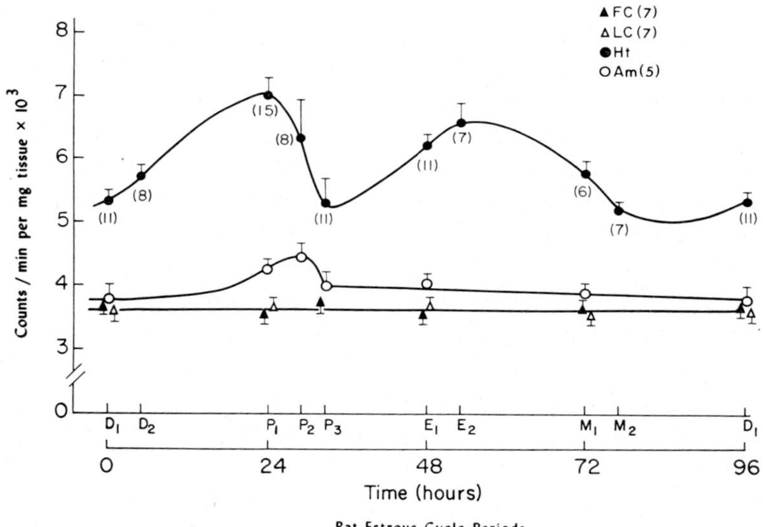

Fig. 1. Activity of MAO in tissues of rat brain during the estrous cycle. The number of animals is in brackets; each point represents the mean value and the vertical line at each point represents the magnitude of the SEM. See text for explanation of the various periods of the estrous cycle, and abbreviations (from Kamberi and Kobayashi, 1970).

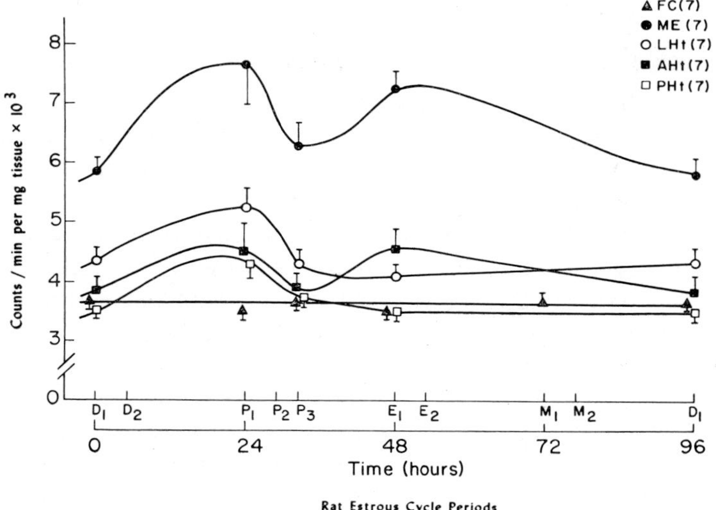

Fig. 2. Activity of MAO in various portions of the Ht and FC of the rat during the estrous cycle. For further explanation see Fig. 1 and text (from Kamberi and Kobayashi, 1970).

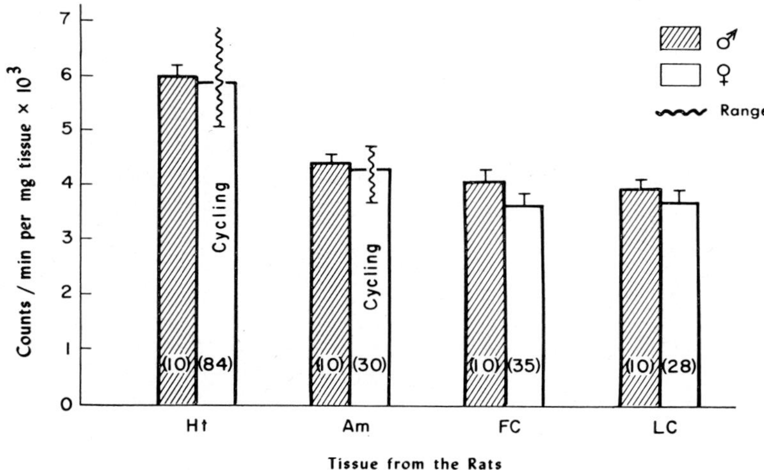

Fig. 3. Activity of MAO in some regions of the brain of the male and female rats. The height of each bar represents the mean value and the vertical line atop each bar represents the magnitude of the SEM value (or the range of values, as indicated). Cycling indicates that all determinations for whole hypothalamus and amygdala made during the estrous cycle (Fig. 1) were averaged. For further explanation see Fig. 1 and text (from Kamberi and Kobayashi, 1970).

and diestrus (D) and male rats were autopsied at 10 *a.m.* (E_1, M_1, D_1) and 3 *p.m.* (E_2, M_2, D_2).

As shown in Fig. 1, MAO showed cyclic changes during the estrous cycle. The extract of whole hypothalamus shows a peak of activity at P_1 of the day of proestrus, followed by a smaller peak on the day of estrus. Lowest levels occurred at P_3, D_1 and

References p. 276–279

M_2. A dramatic fall in MAO activity occurred in the afternoon of the day of proestrus (P_2, P_3) which is coincidental with the occurrence of gonadotrophin surge. The amygdala also showed some cyclic activity that followed the hypothalamic pattern during proestrus, but not thereafter. MAO in amygdala was much less marked with an increase at P_1 and peaking at P_2 on the day of proestrus (Fig. 1). Frontal (FC) and lateral cortex (LC) of the brain possessed much lower levels of MAO activity and showed no cyclic changes.

Cyclic changes were found when the various hypothalamic zones were dissected and measured individually (Fig. 2). The median eminence (ME) showed the highest activity throughout the cycle, which is similar to MAO activity of whole hypothalamus. The anterior hypothalamus (AHt) shows a biphasic change in MAO activity mirroring the levels in the median eminence. The lateral (LHt) and posterior hypothalamic (PHt) areas show a single elevation coincident with P_1 of the day of proestrus with an absence of a peak during the remaining phases of the estrous cycle. In comparison with the MAO activity in the median eminence, the hypothalamic zone concentrations show considerably lower activities. These latter show MAO activities which are substantially higher than that seen in the brain cortex (Fig. 2).

While MAO activities vary with the zone of brain tissue (Fig. 2), there are no significant differences between males and cycling females of any particular zone (Fig. 3). The MAO activity of the hypothalamus is substantially higher than that in amygdala, frontal or lateral cortex, the latter three showing no significant differences among these areas apart from the cyclic elevation in the amygdala previously noted during the proestrus. Changes in MAO activity observed in the entire hypothalamus, hypothalamic zones and amygdala during the day of proestrus appear to be related to the gonadotrophin and prolactin surge which is known to take place in the afternoon of the day of proestus. This suggests an involvement of MAO in gonadotrophin-releasing mechanism(s).

II. BIOGENIC AMINES AND RELEASE OF FSH, LH AND PROLACTIN FROM PITUITARIES INCUBATED *in vitro*

White *et al.* (1968) reported that some polyamines were very effective in depleting pituitary FSH *in vivo*. These workers isolated from hog hypothalamic extract, five biogenic amines (histamine, putrescine, spermine, spermidine and lysine, ranging 1–10 ng/hypothalamic fragment) which depleted pituitary FSH to varying degrees. From their results, it appears that putrescine had the highest biological potency, and it alone could account for most of the activity of the crude hypothalamic extract. These investigators have speculated that (*a*) the combined activities of these amines might account for most if not all of the FSH-depleting properties of hypothalamic extract, and (*b*) the FSH-releasing factor (FRF) is itself an amine.

In an attempt to elucidate the relationship between amines and releasing factors, we (Kamberi and McCann, 1969) found that a variety of amines and even basic peptides can alter FSH release (as measured by bioassay) from anterior pituitary

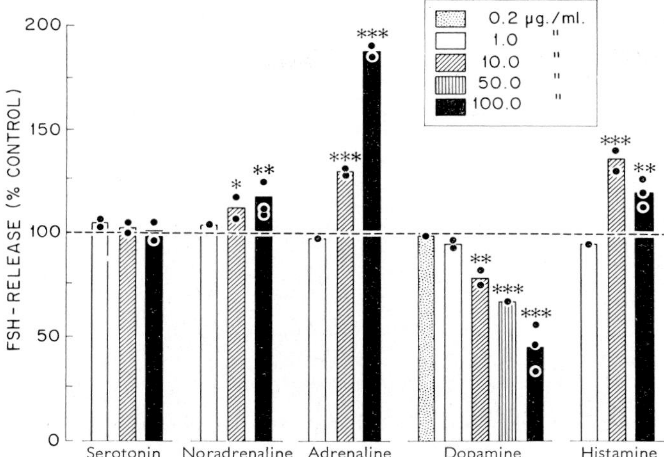

Fig. 4. Effect of some monoamines (MA) on the release of FSH by AP incubated *in vitro*. The values are illustrated as percent of control release, that is, resting release in the absence of MA. Each point shown on the graph represents data from 7 rats/assay (from Kamberi and McCann, 1969). *$p <$ 0.05; ** $p < 0.01$; *** $p < 0.001$.

halves incubated *in vitro*, if used in sufficient amounts (Fig. 4). It is probable that the concentrations of amines used were pharmacological rather than physiological. As is shown in Fig. 4, serotonin, an indolamine, has no effect on FSH release from the pituitary. The catecholamines, adrenaline and noradrenaline at a dose level over 10 μg/ml incubation medium, were capable of stimulating the release of FSH. Dopamine in small doses (0.2–1 μg/ml) was without effect, whereas, in large dose levels (10–100 μg/ml) had an inhibitory effect on FSH release from the pituitary (Kamberi and McCann, 1969) or changed the molecular structure (destruction) of LH, FSH or prolactin (Kamberi, 1972a). As we can see in the latter portion of this presentation, the small doses of dopamine (approx. 1 μg) have been of particular interest, since they have been capable of inducing the discharge of FRF, LH-releasing factor (LRF) and prolactin-inhibiting factor (PIF) from the neurosecretory elements of the hypothalamus. Similar results on the effect of some of these amines on LH and prolactin release from anterior pituitaries incubated *in vitro* have been reported by McCann *et al.* (1972).

III. MONOAMINE DISCHARGE OF HHH FROM HYPOTHALAMIC FRAGMENTS INCUBATED *in vitro*

Contrary to the destruction effect of relatively large doses of dopamine on FSH, LH and prolactin *in vitro*, the dopamine in relatively small doses (1–5 μg/ml) had a stimulatory effect on FSH release from anterior pituitaries co-incubated in presence of ventral hypothalamic fragments. Hypothalamic fragments included the median eminence, arcuate nucleus plus adjacent hypothalamic tissue (Kamberi *et al.*, 1970e). The response was dose-related, up to a dose of 2.5 μg/ml. The control studies revealed

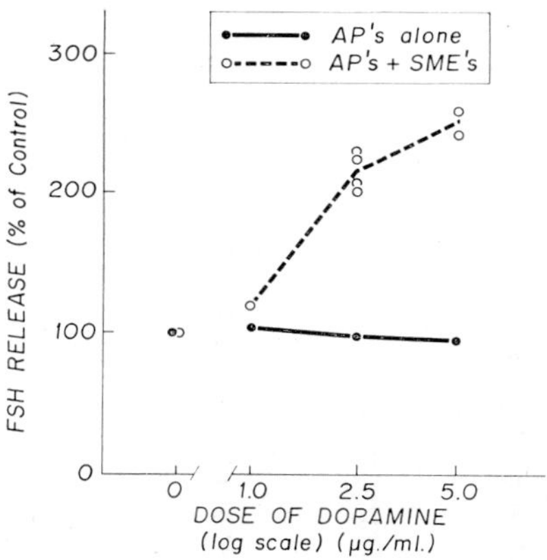

Fig. 5. Effect of dopamine on release of FSH from anterior pituitaries (AP) incubated alone or together with stalk median eminence (SME) fragments. Each point shown on the graph represents data from 7 rats/assay (from Kamberi *et al.*, 1970e).

that dopamine failed to stimulate the release of FSH from anterior pituitaries (AP) incubated alone (Fig. 5). In addition, there was no indication of a potentiating action of dopamine with partially purified FRF, since it did not increase FSH release from pituitaries incubated in the presence of partially purified FRF. Therefore, the increase of FSH release provoked by dopamine in the co-incubation system, appears to be due to a release of FRF from hypothalamic fragments (Kamberi *et al.*, 1970e). Dopamine was reported also to provoke a release of LRF and PIF from the hypothalamic fragments incubated *in vitro* (McCann *et al.*, 1972). This interpretation is further supported by the ability of the α-adrenergic blocking agents (phentolamine, phenoxybenzamine) to prevent the effect of dopamine to induce discharge of HHH from neurosecretory elements of the hypothalamus, whereas pronethalol, a β-blocking agent, had no effect on dopamine-induced alterations of LH, FSH and prolactin (Kamberi *et al.*, 1970d, e)

IV. INTRAVENTRICULAR OR SYSTEMIC INJECTION OF MONOAMINES AND LH, FSH OR PROLACTIN RELEASE

1. Catecholamines

To further clarify the role of catecholamines in the release of anterior pituitary hormones, we decided that the *in vitro* results would have to be supplemented by *in vivo* experiments, before the role of catecholamines as synaptic transmitters to induce discharge of HHH could be considered established. Because of a possible impediment as a result of the blood–brain barrier, metabolism, *etc.*, we elected to inject in most cases the test substances into the third ventricle of the brain rather than a peripheral blood vessel.

Intraventricular injection of 2.5–5 μl of saline in anesthetized male rats had no effect

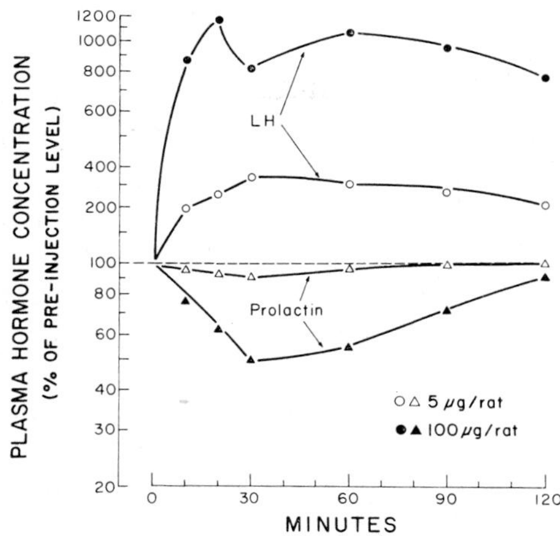

Fig. 6. Effect of 5 μg (open symbols) and 100 μg (solid symbols) noradrenaline bitartrate injected into the third ventricle at 0 min on release of LH (circles) and prolactin (triangles). The values are expressed in terms of the response of those animals given saline alone, which was taken as 100%. Each point represents a mean value of 8–10 rats/group. The values are plotted on a logarithmic scale (from Kamberi *et al.*, 1970a; 1971b).

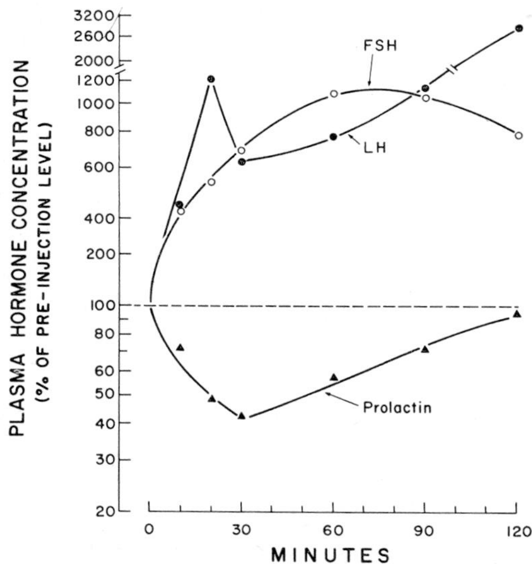

Fig. 7. Effect of dopamine hydrochloride (1.25 μg) injected into the third ventricle at 0 min on the release of LH (closed circles), FSH (open circles) and prolactin (triangles). For further explanation see Fig. 6 and text (from Kamberi *et al.*, 1970a; 1971a, b).

on the release of LH, FSH and prolactin. Intraventricular administration of small doses (1–5 μg) of adrenaline bitartrate or noradrenaline bitartrate had slight effect on LH, FSH or prolactin release as determined by radioimmunoassays. However, in large dose levels (100 μg), both catecholamines caused a dramatic release of LH (Kamberi

References p. 276–279

et al., 1970a) and FSH (Kamberi *et al.*, 1971a) and an inhibition of prolactin (Kamberi *et al.*, 1971b) release in peripheral blood circulation.

As shown in Fig. 6, a dose of 5 μg of noradrenaline had very little effect on the stimulation of LH release or the inhibition of prolactin. However, a 100-μg dose caused a significant increase in LH release with simultaneous decrease in prolactin release. Comparative doses of dopamine to those of adrenaline and noradrenaline had a reverse effect. It was found that dopamine in relatively lower doses (Fig. 7), soon after intraventricular injection has a dramatic effect in the release of LH (Kamberi *et al.*, 1970a), FSH (Kamberi *et al.*, 1971a) and a suppression of prolactin release (Kamberi *et al.*, 1971b), whereas high doses (10–100 μg) were without effect. As illustrated in Fig. 8, 20 min after the intraventricular injection of 1.25 μg dopamine-HCl, the concentration of LH and FSH are 7.5- and 6.5-fold greater than the control levels respectively, whereas the plasma prolactin levels were only one-third that of control. It is interesting to note that with an increase in the dose of dopamine, the effect decreases, namely, the extent in the increase of LH and FSH release and inhibition of prolactin release is inversely related to the dose of intraventricularly injected dopamine (Fig. 8).

Recently, by sequential intra-arterial injections of 10–20 mg/rat of L-DOPA, a catecholamine precursor capable of crossing the blood–brain barrier, we observed in ovariectomized estrogen-progesterone-primed rats a stimulation of LH and FSH release

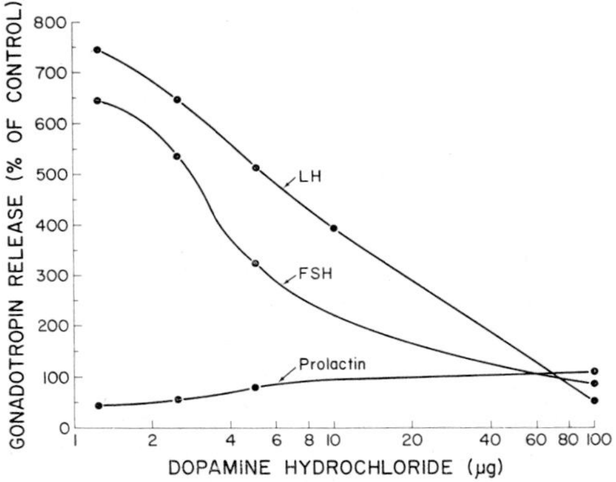

Fig. 8. The concentration of LH, FSH and prolactin in plasma of male rats 20 min after the injection of saline or dopamine hydrochloride into the third ventricle of the brain. For further explanation see Fig. 6 and text (from Kamberi *et al.*, 1970a, 1971a, b).

in peripheral circulation and an early decrease in prolactin during the first 30 min, with an increase thereafter (Kamberi, 1972b).

2. *Indolamines*

The intraventricular injection of serotonin, or its metabolic product melatonin in dose levels of 1, 5 or 50 μg/rat, in anesthetized male rats, appears to have an opposite effect

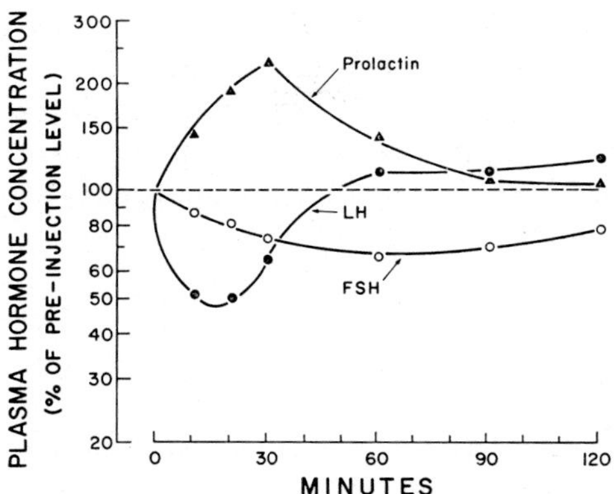

Fig. 9. Effect of serotonin (5 μg) injected into the third ventricle at 0 min on the release of prolactin (triangles), LH (closed circles) and FSH (open circles). For further explanation see Fig. 6 and text (from Kamberi *et al.*, 1970a; 1971c).

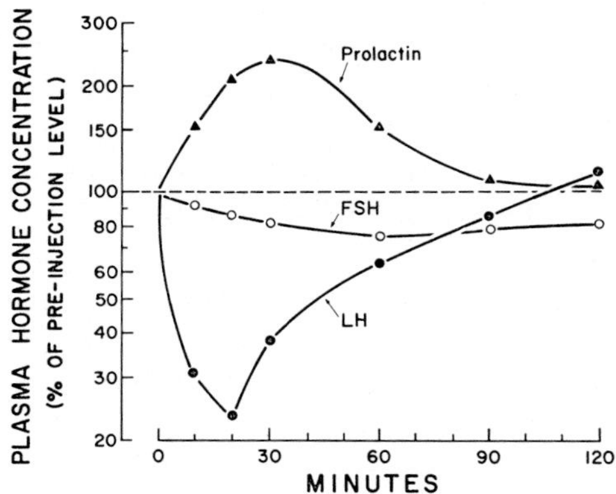

Fig. 10. Effect of melatonin (5 μg) injected into the third ventricle at 0 min on the release of prolactin (triangles), LH (closed circles) and FSH (open circles). For further explanation see Fig. 6 and text (from Kamberi *et al.*, 1970a; 1971c).

than that seen with small doses of dopamine or large doses of noradrenaline or adrenaline. Either agent, serotonin (Fig. 9) or melatonin (Fig. 10), suppressed the release of LH and FSH with simultaneous increase in prolactin release. The degree of inhibition of gonadotrophins or stimulation of prolactin was dose-related, *i.e.* with the increase of the dose, the effect was more pronounced (Kamberi *et al.*, 1970a; Kamberi *et al.*, 1971c).

We also observed a suppression of LH and FSH release with concomitant increase in prolactin release in castrated male and female rats, after intraperitoneal injection (20–30 mg/rat) of 5-hydroxytryptophan, a precursor of serotonin (Kamberi, 1973). More recently, using unanesthetized cyclic female rats, in which a cannula had previously been implanted into the third ventricle, we observed that intraventricular injection of melatonin or serotonin (1–5 μg/rat) between 13:00–14:00 h on the day of proestrus, suppressed proestrous surge of LH and FSH and inhibited ovulation

References p. 276–279

(Kamberi, 1972b). The blood samples were taken at various time intervals during the afternoon of the day of proestrus, *via* the carotid artery, previously cannulated and attached through tygon tubing to a peristaltic pump. In addition, multiple intracardiac injections of melatonin or 5-hydroxytryptophan, but not serotonin (1–5 mg/rat) between 13:00–14:00 h on the day of proestrus, also inhibited ovulation and proestrous gonadotrophin surge (Kamberi, 1972b).

V. ANTERIOR PITUITARY PERFUSION OF MONOAMINES

The results of intraventricular administration of monoamines suggest two possibilities concerning the action of these monoamines on LH, FSH and prolactin release. First, the monoamines may have stimulated or inhibited the release of LRF, FRF or PIF from the neurosecretory elements, which is reflected in the alteration of the release of LH, FSH or prolactin. Second, these monoamines may have reached the anterior pituitary and exercised their effect by a direct action on the pituitary. To clarify these questions, we infused dopamine into anterior pituitary *via* a cannulated portal vessel by the method previously described (Porter *et al.*, 1970). Infusion of dopamine at the rate of 2, 20, 200 or 2000 ng/min for 30 min, did not alter the release of LH, FSH or prolactin in peripheral blood. The infusion of adrenaline, noradrenaline, serotonin or melatonin also was without effect (Kamberi *et al.*, 1970a; Kamberi *et al.*, 1971a, b, c). This indicates that these monoamines did not cause alteration of gonadotrophin and prolactin release by direct action on the pituitary. These conclusions seem justified in view of the findings, that an acidic extract of rat hypothalamus tissue, neutralized to pH 7.2, stimulated the release of LH or FSH and inhibited prolactin when infused into hypophysial portal vessels for 30 min (Kamberi *et al.*, 1971d). The degree of

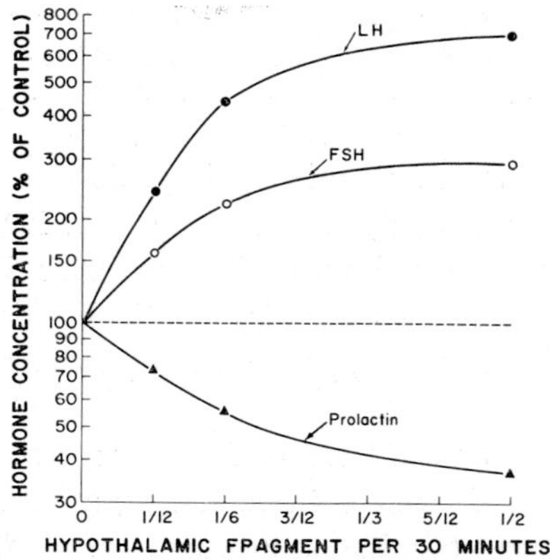

Fig. 11. Effect of pituitary portal vessel infusion of hypothalamic extract for 30 min on the release of plasma LH, FSH and prolactin. The values are plotted against the amount of tissue injected shown on a logarithmic scale. All values are expressed in terms of the response of the animals which were infused with an extract of cerebral cortex as a control of 100%. For further explanation see text and Fig. 6 (from Kamberi *et al.*, 1971d).

stimulation or inhibition was directly related to the concentration of the hypothalamic extract (Fig. 11). A cortical extract had no effect on LH, FSH or prolactin release.

VI. RELEASE OF HHH INTO PORTAL BLOOD

To ascertain if the HHH are altered into hypophysial portal blood, we have undertaken *in vivo* and *in vitro* experiments. In the *in vivo* experiments, we have collected

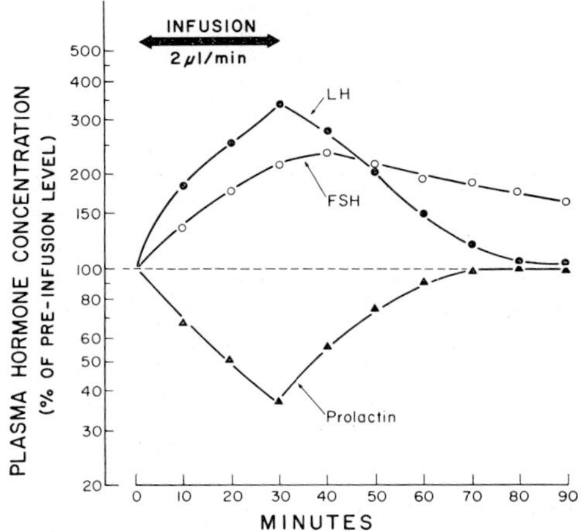

Fig. 12. Effect of pituitary portal vessel infusion of femoral artery plasma or pituitary stalk plasma from dopamine-treated donors and the release of LH, FSH or prolactin. The symbols represent mean responses. The values are expressed in terms of the response observed in recipient rats infused with plasma from femoral artery blood from dopamine-treated donors, which was taken as 100%. Each point represents a mean value of 8–10 rats/group. For further explanation see text and Fig. 6 (from Kamberi *et al.*, 1971e).

simultaneously femoral artery blood and portal blood from pituitary stalk (Porter *et al.*, 1971) of male rats (donors) untreated (saline injected) or dopamine-treated (dopamine injected into the third ventricle). Plasma from femoral artery blood or stalk blood was then infused back into the anterior pituitary, *via* a cannulated portal vessel of the pituitary stalk of another group of untreated male rats (recipients) at the rate of 2 μl/min for 30 min by the method previously described (Porter *et al.*, 1970). In Fig. 12, one can observe that infusion of pituitary stalk plasma from dopamine-treated donors causes an increase in the plasma concentration of LH and FSH and a decrease in the prolactin levels in peripheral circulation of the recipient animals. On cessation of infusion the release of LH and FSH and inhibition of prolactin stopped. We have observed the corresponding activities LRF, FRF and PIF activity in the pituitary stalk plasma of untreated donor rats, but these activities were less pronounced. Infusion of femoral artery plasma from dopamine-treated or untreated donors was without effect (Kamberi *et al.*, 1971e).

We have also observed LRF, FRF and PIF activities under *in vitro* conditions

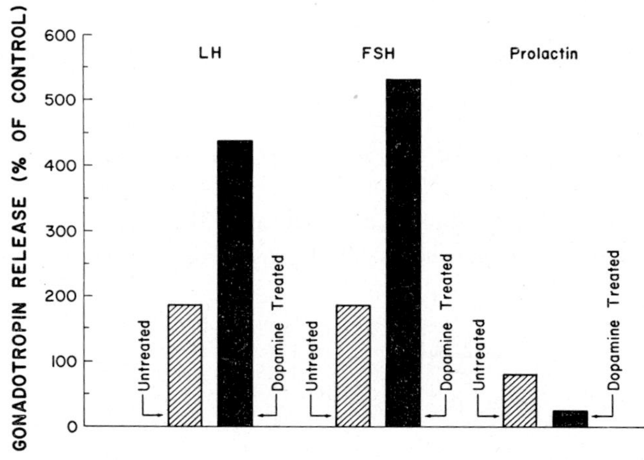

Fig. 13. Release of LH, FSH and prolactin from hemipituitaries incubated *in vitro* in plasma from femoral artery, which served as a control, and from the contralateral halves incubated in stalk plasma The values are expressed in terms of the response of the hemipituitaries incubated in femoral artery plasma, which was taken as 100%. Each bar represents a mean value of 10 rats/group. For further explanation see text (from Kamberi *et al.*, 1969; 1970b, c).

(Kamberi *et al.*, 1969; Kamberi *et al.*, 1970b, c). Anterior pituitary halves of intact male rats were incubated in the presence of femoral artery or pituitary stalk plasma obtained from untreated or dopamine-treated male rats. As illustrated in Fig. 13, anterior pituitary halves incubated in pituitary stalk plasma from untreated donor rats released significantly more LH and FSH, and less prolactin than did the contralateral halves incubated in femoral artery plasma. Furthermore, anterior pituitary halves incubated in pituitary stalk plasma from rats receiving 2.5 μg dopamine-HCl *via* the third ventricle released over 4 times as much LH and over 5 times as much FSH as the controls, which were incubated in femoral artery plasma. Prolactin release by anterior pituitary halves incubated in pituitary stalk plasma from dopamine-treated rats was 4 times less than the controls.

VII. DELAY OF PUBERTY, SUPPRESSION OF OVULATION AND PROESTROUS SURGE OF GONADOTROPHINS BY PINEAL EXTRACT OR INDOLES

An imposing array of evidence indicates that sexual maturation and gonadal function may be influenced by the pineal gland (Kamberi, 1965; Wurtman *et al.*, 1968; Reiter and Fraschini, 1969; Collu and Martini, 1973; Mess, 1973). The antigonadotrophic effect of the pineal gland seems to be mediated through a number of substances known to be secreted by the pineal gland (Wurtman *et al.*, 1968).

We have investigated earlier (Kamberi, 1965) the effect of pineal extract on sexual maturation, and more recently (Kamberi, 1972; and unpublished data) the effect of indoles on the phenomenon of ovulation and gonadotrophin release (Tables I, II). Injection of pineal extract to the immature rats (27–28 days old at the beginning of the first injection and continued for 15 or 20 days) at the higher dose level used (Table I)

TABLE I

EFFECT OF PINEAL, ANTERIOR (AP), POSTERIOR PITUITARY (PP), CEREBRAL CORTEX AND HYPOTHALAMIC (Ht) EXTRACT FROM CASTRATED FEMALE RATS ON PRECOCIOUS PUBERTY

Type of extract	*Daily dose*	*Days of treatment*	*Rats per group*	*Opening of vagina Mean ± SEM (days from birth)*	*First cornified smear Mean ± SEM (days from birth)*
Saline	1 ml	20	20	41.1 ± 0.56	47.8 ± 0.66
Pineal	1 gland	15	10	42.0 ± 0.88	48.2 ± 0.73
Pineal	4 glands	20	8	46.5 ± 0.80[a]	53.9 ± 1.34[a]
AP	0.5 gland	5	10	30.0 ± 0.30[b]	30.0 ± 0.30[b]
PP	1 gland	10	9	40.9 ± 0.89	47.4 ± 0.85
Cortex	1 fragm.	10	8	41.4 ± 0.88	48.4 ± 0.82
Ht	1 fragm.	10	12	33.6 ± 0.34[b]	33.6 ± 0.34[b]

[a]$p < 0.05$ *vs.* control (saline).
[b]$p < .01$ *vs.* control.
(From Kamberi, 1965; and unpublished data.)

delayed the vaginal opening and the appearance of the estrous rhythm, *i.e.* first cornified smear. Contrary to these inhibitory effects with pineal extract, extracts from hypothalamic tissue or anterior pituitary gland had stimulatory effects on the opening of the vagina, immediately followed by cornified smear. The extract from cerebral cortex or posterior pituitary was without effect (Table I). The stimulatory effect of hypothalamic extract was attributed to the presence of FSH-releasing activity in the hypothalamic tissue, *i.e.* FRF, which in turn induced the release of FSH from pituitary (Kamberi, 1965).

TABLE II

EFFECT OF INDOLAMINES ON OVULATION IN RAT

Groups	*Total dose*	*Incidence of ovulation* Number	%	*Average number of ova mean ± SEM*
Intraventricular				
Saline	20 μl	8/8	100.0	10.2 ± 0.72
Melatonin	1 μg	4/7	57.1[a]	5.0 ± 1.07[a]
Melatonin	10 μg	3/10	30.0[b]	3.25 ± 0.59[b]
Melatonin	100 μg	1/6	16.7[b]	
5-HT	10 μg	1/7	14.3[b]	
Intracardiac				
Saline	1 ml	6/6	100.0	11.6 ± 0.98
Melatonin	1–5 mg	3/9	33.4[b]	4.3 ± 0.80[b]
5-HT	5 mg	5/5	100.0	10.6 ± 0.89
5-HTP	20 mg	2/9	22.2[b]	
Melatonin + LH	5 mg + 10 μg	7/7	100.0	9.7 ± 0.64
Melatonin + Ht	5 mg + 2 fragm.	4/5	80.0	10.6 ± 0.88

[a]$p < 0.01$ *vs.* control (saline); [b]$p < 0.001$ *vs.* control.
(From Kamberi, 1972b; 1973; and unpublished data.)

References p. 276–279

Our recent results (obtained in unanesthetized cyclic female rats, in which a cannula had previously been implanted into the third ventricle or carotid artery) indicate that pineal indoles have an inhibitory effect on the release of plasma LH and FSH (Kamberi *et al.*, 1970a; Kamberi *et al.*, 1971c; Kamberi, 1972b, 1973). This confirms our previous finding (Table I), that pineal extract delays precocious puberty as a result of inhibition of LH and FSH release. We also found recently (Table II) that multiple intraventricular or intracardiac injections of melatonin (beginning at 12:00–14:00 h aliquots of the total dose are injected every 60 min, with the last injection at 17:00–19:00 h) on day of proestrus, inhibited ovulation in rats examined for ova in the morning of the day of estrus. The inhibitory effect was dose-related. Multiple intraventricular injections of serotonin (5-HT), was also followed by inhibition of ovulation, but cardiac injection failed to do so. Intracardiac injection of 5-hydroxytryptophan (5-HTP), a precursor of serotonin, was very effective in inhibiting ovulation (Table II). The blockade of ovulation was in all cases preceeded by inhibition of proestrous surge of gonadotrophins in peripheral circulation (Kamberi, 1972b; 1973 and unpublished data). The inhibition of ovulation was overcome by administration of LH or hypothalamic extract (Table II).

VIII. SUPPRESSION OF OVULATION AND PROESTROUS SURGE OF GONADOTROPHIN BY ATROPINE

Everett *et al.* (1949) reported that atropine, an anticholinergic drug, was capable of blocking ovulation and suggested that cholinergic synapses were involved in neural control of gonadotrophin secretion. More recently, Kato and Minaguchi (1964) reported changes into choline acetylase activity in states of altered gonadotrophin secretion. In view of these findings, we injected atropine-sulfate subcutaneously (600–700 mg/kg) or into the third ventricle (200–300 μg/rat) in female rats, between 12:00–13:00 h on the day of proestrus. Injection of atropine by either route suppressed the proestrous surge of LH and FSH. Furthermore, some of these rats examined for ova on the day of estrus, showed no evidence of ovulation. The inhibition of ovulation can be overcome by intravenous injection of 10 μg LH or crude hypothalamic extract, which excludes the possibility that atropine acts directly on the ovarian or pituitary levels (Kamberi, 1972b).

DISCUSSION

From these studies, it is clear that catecholaminergic, cholinergic and indolaminergic pathways are involved in the control of gonadotrophin and prolactin secretions. It appears that catecholaminergic and cholinergic systems have a stimulatory effect on the release of HHH from neurosecretory elements of hypothalamus and the indolaminergic system has the opposite effect on the release of HHH. Furthermore, these systems are modulated by changes in the levels of gonadal steroids. The precise origin of aminergic pathways relevant for neuroendocrine regulations is not well defined. We suggest that monoaminergic neurons may have axons which run parallel to those of HHH neurosecretory neurons and may establish axo-axonal contacts with them. Thus, release of monoamines may depolarize the axon of HHH-containing neurons and produce the discharge of HHH. Alternatively, HHH-containing vesicles may be present in the axons of monoaminergic neurons. Indeed, vesicles of the two different sizes have been described in neurons in this locus. Release of monoamines would then provoke release of HHH from the same neuron. Presumably, specificity of different HHH is obtained by the fact that any given neuron synthesizes and releases only one HHH and is affected by monoaminergic neurons linked to the controlling mechanism(s) for that HHH.

The results of a number of other investigators (Schwartz and McCormack, 1972), support our view that indolamines have an inhibitory effect on the release of LRF, FRF and PIF. It can be suggested that cerebrospinal fluid of the brain ventricles serve as a transmittal route of the melatonin and other pineal indoles to the hypothalamus. This is compatible with the anatomic relationships existing between the pineal gland and the neuroglial cells as noted by Sheridan *et al.* (1969). Furthermore, it appears that the effect of indolamines is linked to the serotoninergic neurons known to be present in the hypothalamus (Fuxe and Hökfelt, 1969). This view is in agreement with the finding that systemic injection of melatonin increases the hypothalamic stores of serotonin (Anton-Tay and Wurtman, 1971), and that the blockade of ovulation induced by the administration of monoamine oxidase inhibitors is specifically linked to increased brain serotonin levels (Kordon and Glowinski, 1970).

However, discrepancies exist as to which of the catecholamines are involved in the release mechanism(s) of LRF, FRF and PIF. From our data it appears that dopamine in relatively low doses and noradrenaline and adrenaline in high doses can provoke discharge of LRF, FRF and PIF. In agreement with this view are data reported by Kordon and Glowinski (1970) who found that the phenomenon of superovulation in PMS primed immature rats can be prevented by inhibiting the dopamine synthesis. In support of our view are also recent results by Saffran (1972), that incubation of anterior pituitaries in the presence of hypothalamic fragments and dopamine, stimulate the release of corticotrophin (ACTH). Also, Reichlin *et al.* (1973), in the *in vitro* studies, observed that dopamine and noradrenaline markedly increased thyrotrophin-releasing activity of the hypothalamus. Results that dopamine, adrenaline and noradrenaline play a role in the release of GH have been also reported (Müller *et al.*, 1968). On the other hand, Rubinstein and Sawyer (1970) found that adrenaline is the most potent drug in inducing ovulation, whereas noradrenaline and dopamine failed to do so. Fuxe and Hökfelt (1969) on the basis of their fluorescence-microscopic data suggest that dopamine has an inhibitory effect on LRF and FRF release and a stimulatory effect on PIF. More recently, Fuxe and his associates (Corrodi *et al.*, 1971), have reported that 7-(2′-pyrimidyl)-4-piperonylpiperazine (ET-495), an active monoamine metabolite, is the new dopamine receptor stimulating agent.

Obviously there is a discrepancy which has to be resolved. Specific and highly sensitive assays (radioimmunoassay) for dopamine, noradrenaline, adrenaline,

References p. 276–279

serotonin and other monoamines or metabolites of monoamines, will be of great help in the answering of these puzzling questions.

SUMMARY

The evidence for involvement of monoamines in the regulation of release of anterior pituitary hormones is beyond question. In both *in vitro* and *in vivo* experiments, relatively small doses of dopamine and large doses of noradrenaline and adrenaline induced the release of LH and FSH and inhibited prolactin, secondary to the discharge of LRF, FRF and PIF. Contrary to this stimulatory effect of catecholamines, other monoamines, serotonin and melatonin, had an opposite effect, *i.e.* inhibited the release of LH and FSH and stimulated the release of prolactin, secondary to the inhibition of the release of LRF, FRF and PIF. For at least one monoamine, dopamine, the stimulating effect on HHH release seems to be mediated by an α-adrenergic mechanism.

ACKNOWLEDGEMENTS

The author wishes to thank Miss Patrice de Vilmorin, Miss Lisa Bacleon and Mrs. M. A. Kamberi for their generous assistance in the preparation of this manuscript. Supported by Attending Staff Association GRS Grant 1389 from NIH.

REFERENCES

ANTON-TAY, F. AND WURTMAN, R. J. (1971) Brain monoamines and endocrine function. In *Frontiers in Neuroendocrinology*, L. MARTINI AND W. F. GANONG (Eds.), Oxford University Press, New York, pp. 45–66.

COLLU, R., FRASCHINI, F. AND MARTINI, L. (1973) Role of indoleamines and catecholamines in the control of gonadotrophin and growth hormone secretion. In *Drug Effects on Neuroendocrine Regulation* (Progr. Brain Res., Vol. 39), E. ZIMMERMANN, W. H. GISPEN, B. H. MARKS AND D. DE WIED (Eds.), Elsevier, Amsterdam, pp. 289–299.

COPPOLA, J. A. (1971) Brain catecholamines and gonadotrophin secretion. In *Frontiers in Neuroendocrinology*, L. MARTINI AND W. F. GANONG (Eds.), Oxford University Press, New York, pp. 129–143.

CORRODI, H., FUXE, K. AND UNGERSTEDT, U. (1971) Evidence for a new type of dopamine receptor stimulating agent. *J. Pharm. Pharmacol.*, **23**, 989–991.

DONOSO, A. O., STEFANO, F. J. E., BISCARDI, A. M. AND CUKIER, J. (1967) Effects of castration on hypothalamic catecholamines. *Amer. J. Physiol.*, **212**, 737–739.

EVERETT, J. W. (1964) Central neural control of reproductive functions of the adenohypophysis. *Physiol. Rev.*, **44**, 373–431.

EVERETT, J. W., SAWYER, C. H. AND MARKEE, J. E. (1949) A neurogenic timing factor in control of the ovulatory discharge of luteinizing hormone in the cyclic rat. *Endocrinology*, **44**, 234–250.

FUXE, K. AND HÖKFELT, T. (1969) Catecholamines in the hypothalamus and pituitary gland. In *Frontiers in Neuroendocrinology*, W. F. GANONG AND L. MARTINI (Eds.), Oxford University Press, New York, pp. 47–96.

FUXE, K., HÖKFELT, T. AND NILSSON, O. (1967) Activity changes in tubero-infundibular DA neurons of the rat during various states of the reproductive cycle. *Life Sci.*, **6**, 2057–2061.

GANONG, W. F. (1972) Evidence for a central noradrenergic system that inhibits ACTH secretion. In *Brain–Endocrine Interaction. Median Eminence: Structure and Function*, K. M. KNIGGE, D. E. SCOTT AND A. WEINDL (Eds.), Karger, Basel, pp. 254–266.

HARRIS, G. W. (1970) Unsolved problems in the portal vessel-chemotransmitter hypothesis. In *Hypophysiotropic Hormones of the Hypothalamus*, J. MEITES (Ed.), Williams and Wilkins, Baltimore, pp. 1–20.

HÖKFELT, T. AND FUXE, K. (1972) On the morphology and the neuroendocrine role of the hypothalamic catecholamine neurons. In *Brain–Endocrine Interaction. Median Eminence: Structure and Function*, K. M. KNIGGE, D. E. SCOTT AND A. WEINDL (Eds.), Karger, Basel, pp. 181–223.

KAMBERI, I. A. (1965) Neuroendocrine regulation of the sexual activity. *Ph.D. Thesis*, University of Belgrade, Belgrade, p. 240.

KAMBERI, I. A. (1972a) Discussion to the presentation of S. Reichlin. *Recent Progr. Hormone Res.*, **28**, 280–283.

KAMBERI, I. A. (1972b) Suppression of ovulation and the proestrous surge of LH and FSH by atropine or melatonin. *Physiologist*, **15**, 187.

KAMBERI, I. A. (1973) Biogenic amines and neurohumoral control of gonadotrophin and prolactin secretion. In *Proceedings of the IVth International Congress of Endocrinology*, R. O. SCOW (Ed.), Excerpta Med., Amsterdam, In press.

KAMBERI, I. A. AND DANHOF, I. E. (1968) Monoamine oxidase activity in hypothalamus, amygdala and cerebral cortex during the estrous cycle. *Fed. Proc.*, **27**, 388.

KAMBERI, I. A. AND MCCANN, S. M. (1969) Effect of biogenic amines, FSH-releasing factor (FRF) and other substances on the release of FSH by pituitaries incubated *in vitro*. *Endocrinology*, **85**, 815–824.

KAMBERI, I. A. AND KOBAYASHI, Y. (1970) Monoamine oxidase activity in the hypothalamus and various other brain areas and in some endocrine glands of the rat during the estrous cycle. *J. Neurochem.*, **17**, 261–268.

KAMBERI, I. A., MICAL, R. S. AND PORTER, J. C. (1969) Luteinizing hormone-releasing activity in hypophysial stalk blood and elevation by dopamine. *Science*, **166**, 388–390.

KAMBERI, I. A., MICAL, R. S. AND PORTER, J. C. (1970a) Effect of anterior pituitary perfusion and intraventricular injection of catecholamines and indoleamines on LH release. *Endocrinology*, **87**, 1–12.

KAMBERI, I. A., MICAL, R. S. AND PORTER, J. C. (1970b) Follicle stimulating hormone releasing activity in hypophysial portal blood and elevation by dopamine. *Nature (Lond.)*, **227**, 714–715.

KAMBERI, I. A., MICAL, R. S. AND PORTER, J. C. (1970c) Prolactin-inhibiting activity in hypophysial stalk blood and elevation by dopamine. *Experientia*, **26**, 1150–1151.

KAMBERI, I. A., MICAL, R. S. AND PORTER, J. C. (1970d) Possible role of α-adrenergic receptors in mediating the response of the hypothalamus to dopamine. *Physiologist*, **13**, 239.

KAMBERI, I. A., SCHNEIDER, H. P. G. AND MCCANN, S. M. (1970e) Action of dopamine to induce release of FSH-releasing factor (FRF) from hypothalamic tissue *in vitro*. *Endocrinology* **86**, 278–284.

KAMBERI, I. A., MICAL, R. S. AND PORTER, J. C. (1971a) Effect of anterior pituitary perfusion and intraventricular injection of catecholamines on FSH release. *Endocrinology*, **88**, 1003–1011.

KAMBERI, I. A., MICAL, R. S. AND PORTER, J. C. (1971b) Effect of anterior pituitary perfusion and intraventricular injection of catecholamines on prolactin release. *Endocrinology*, **88**, 1012–1020.

KAMBERI, I. A., MICAL, R. S. AND PORTER, J. C. (1971c) Effects of melatonin and serotonin on the release of FSH and prolactin. *Endocrinology*, **88**, 1288–1293.

KAMBERI, I. A., MICAL, R. S. AND PORTER, J. C. (1971d) Pituitary portal vessel infusion of hypothalamic extract and release of LH, FSH, and prolactin. *Endocrinology*, **88**, 1294–1299.

KAMBERI, I. A., MICAL, R. S. AND PORTER, J. C. (1971e) Hypophysial portal vessel infusion: *In vivo* demonstration of LRF, FRF and PIF in pituitary stalk plasma. *Endocrinology*, **89**, 1042–1046.

KATO, J. AND MINAGUCHI, H. (1964) Cholinergic and adrenergic mechanisms in the female rat hypothalamus with special reference to reproductive functions. In *Neurosecretion and Neural Control of Internal Secretion* (Gunma Symp. Endocrinol., Vol. 1), K. KUROSUMI (Ed.), Gunma University Press, Maebashi (Japan), pp. 269–281.

KORDON, C. AND GLOWINSKI, J. (1970) Role of brain catecholamines in the control of anterior pituitary functions. In *Neurochemical Aspects of Hypothalamic Function*, L. MARTINI AND J. MEITES (Eds.), Academic Press, New York, pp. 85–100.

MARTINI, L., FRASCHINI, F. AND MOTTA, M. (1968) Neural control of anterior pituitary functions. *Recent Progr. Hormone Res.*, **24**, 439–485.

MCCANN, S. M., KALRA, P. S., DONOSO, A. O., BISHOP, W., SCHNEIDER, H. P. G., FAWCETT, C. P. AND KRULICH, L. (1972) Role of monoamines in control of gonadotrophin and prolactin secretion. In *Brain–Endocrine Interaction. Median Eminence: Structure and Function*, K. M. KNIGGE, D. E. SCOTT AND A. WEINDL (Eds.), Karger, Basel, pp. 224–235.

MESS, B., TIMA, L. AND TRENTINI, G. P. (1973) The role of pineal principles in ovulation. In *Drug Effects on Neuroendocrine Regulation* (Progr. Brain Res., Vol. 39), B. H. MARKS AND D. DE WIED (Eds.), Elsevier, Amsterdam, pp. 000. In press.

MÜLLER, E. E., PRA, D. P. AND PECILE, A. (1968) Influence of brain neurohumors injected into the lateral ventricle of the rat on growth hormone release. *Endocrinology*, **83**, 893–896.

PORTER, J. C., MICAL, R. S., KAMBERI, I. A. AND GRAZIA, Y. R. (1970) A procedure for the cannulation of a pituitary stalk portal vessel and perfusion of the pars distalis in the rat. *Endocrinology*, **87**, 197–201.

PORTER, J. C., KAMBERI, I. A. AND GRAZIA, Y. R. (1971) Pituitary blood flow and portal vessels. In *Frontiers in Neuroendocrinology*, L. MARTINI AND W. F. GANONG (Eds.), Oxford University Press, New York, pp. 145–175.

PORTER, J. C., KAMBERI, I. A. AND ONDO, J. G. (1972) Role of biogenic amines and cerebrospinal fluid in the neurovascular transmittal of hypophysiotropic substances. In *Brain–Endocrine Interaction. Median Eminence: Structure and Function*, K. M. KNIGGE, D. E. SCOTT AND A. WEINDL (Eds.), Karger, Basel, pp. 245–253.

REICHLIN, S., MITNICK, M. A. AND GRIMM, Y. (1973) Hypothalamus and pituitary. In *Proceedings of the IVth International Congress of Endocrinology*, R. O. SCOW (Ed.), Excerpta Med., Amsterdam, In press.

REITER, R. J. AND FRASCHINI, F. (1969) Endocrine aspects of the mammalian pineal gland: A review. *Neuroendocrinology*, **5**, 219–255.

RUBINSTEIN, L. AND SAWYER, C. H. (1970) Role of catecholamines in stimulating the release of pituitary ovulating hormone(s) in rats. *Endocrinology*, **86**, 988–995.

SAFFRAN, M. (1972) Problems of identifying hypothalamic releasing factors. Nature of CRF. *UCLA BIS Conference Rept*, **22**, 4–6.

SAWYER, C. H. (1964) Control of secretion of gonadotropins. In *Gonadotropins*, H. H. COLE (Ed.), Freeman, San Francisco, pp. 113–159.

SAWYER, C. H., MARKEE, J. E. AND HOLLINSHEAD, W. H. (1947) Inhibition of ovulation in the rabbit by the adrenergic-blocking agent dibenamine. *Endocrinology*, **41**, 395–402.

SCHWARTZ, N. B. AND MCCORMACK, C. E. (1972) Reproduction: Gonadal function and its regulation. *Ann. Rev. physiol.*, **34**, 425–472.

SHERIDAN, M. N., REITER, R. J. AND JACOBS, J. J. (1969) An interesting anatomical relationship between the hamster pineal gland and the ventricular system of the brain. *J. Endocrinol.*, **45**, 131–132.

WEINER, R. I., GORSKI, R. A. AND SAWYER, C. H. (1972) Hypothalamic catecholamines and pituitary gonadotropic function. In *Brain–Endocrine Interaction. Median Eminence: Structure and Function*, K. M. KNIGGE, D. E. SCOTT AND A. WEINDL (Eds.), Karger, Basel, pp. 236–244.

WHITE, W. F., COHEN, A. I., RIPPEL, R. H., STORY, J. C. AND SCHALLY, A. V. (1968) Some hypothalamic polyamines that deplete pituitary follicle stimulating hormone. *Endocrinology*, **82**, 742–752.

WURTMAN, R. J., AXELROD, J. AND KELLY, D. E. (1968) *The Pineal*, Academic Press, New York, p. 199.

ZOLOVICK, A. J., PEARSE, R., BOEHLKE, K. W. AND ELEFTHERIOU, B. E. (1966) Monoamine oxidase activity in various parts of the rat brain during the estrous cycle. *Science*, **154**, 649.

DISCUSSION

REITER: Dr. Kamberi, in your original publication you reported that intraventricular injection of melatonin depressed peripheral levels of FSH by about 50%. In the slide you just showed, the intraventricular injection of melatonin depressed FSH levels by about 20%. Do you think that represents a significant depression of FSH and what is your current opinion about the anti-FSH activity of melatonin?

KAMBERI: We previously observed a drop in FSH to about 50% of its control value after intraventricular injection of 50 μg of melatonin. For lack of time and only for purposes of comparison, I chose here to show the effect of 5 μg melatonin, since this dose was most often used in experiments with other drugs. As you noted on the slide, intraventricular injection of 5 μg melatonin had a clear effect on LH and prolactin levels in peripheral circulation. The suppression of FSH release was about 20–25%, which is of borderline significance. Since our experimental procedure is limited to about 2 h, and since the half life of FSH is relatively long (about 2 h), it is difficult to say at present if this effect is of any significance.

MEYERSON: You seem to consider the change of monoamine oxidase activity primary to the LH surge. Is it possible that the LH surge or subsequent endocrine events instead influenced the monoamine oxidase activity? Have you tested, for instance the effect of LH and LRF on monoamine oxidase activity?

KAMBERI: This is a very good question. We have not tested the effect of LH and LRF on monoamine oxidase activity. We plan to undertake these experiments.

SHASKAN: I recently began some work on pineal regulation of serotonin synthesis in brain in relation to gonadotrophin secretion. Tryptophan hydroxylase was measured in brain regions of rats which had been blinded at 25 days after birth and sacrificed at 72 days. Both testes and seminal vesicle weights of blinded animals were significantly decreased as compared to controls, confirming earlier work from Dr. Reiter's laboratory. A highly significant ($p < 0.001$) decrease in seminal vesicle weight correlated with an increase in tryptophan hydroxylase activity in three brain regions but especially in the diencephalon and hippocampus. Treatment with two i.p. injections of *p*-chlorophenylalanine methylester (PCPA, 500 mg/kg) at 26 days (1 day after blinding) or at 68 days (4 days prior to sacrifice) resulted in no effect on seminal vesicle or testicular weights of blinded or control animals. The early PCPA treatment, however, inhibited the observed increase in brain tryptophan hydroxylase of blinded rats at 72 days. The late PCPA treatment (4 days before sacrifice) inhibited diencephalic, hippocampal and midbrain tryptophan hydroxylase in the blinded animals significantly more than in seeing animals. This observation suggests that tryptophan hydroxylase in blinded rats at this time is turning over at a more rapid rate than in seeing animals. Testosterone proprionate injections (0.5 mg subcutaneously, 5 injections every other day for 10 days before sacrifice) increased seminal vesicle weights and tryptophan hydroxylase activity returned to control levels in all three brain regions studied.

KAMBERI: Thank you for your interesting results and comments, which are in support of our view that melatonin and serotonin as well suppress gonadotrophin release.

TABAKOFF: What substrate did you use to assay for your monoamine oxidase activity? We found at least two different sites in hypothalamic tissue, one that metabolizes primarily phenylethylamines and one for indoleamines.

KAMBERI: The substrate used was [^{14}C]tyramine. The method used was that introduced by Otsuka and Kobayashi (Biochem. Pharmacol., 13, 995, 1964).

KNIGGE: I hope my question doesn't illustrate my ignorance of catecholamine pharmacology, but it relates to what may happen to the dopamine in your intraventricular injections. Our *in vitro* studies suggest that nerve terminals in the median eminence have a vigorous re-uptake mechanism for both dopamine and noradrenaline. My question concerns the possibility that the intraventricularly administered dopamine is taken up by noradrenergic terminals, contributes to synthesis and release of greater than normal amounts of endogenous noradrenaline and that the effects you witness may be due to this noradrenaline rather than to the original dopamine.

KAMBERI: It could be. Dopamine after intraventricular injections, certainly is taken up from surrounding hypothalamic tissue and re-released as dopamine or some other monoamine form. It could be speculated that dopamine can enter the intercellular pool, and could then be taken up into adrenergic nerve endings, where it is transformed into noradrenaline, adrenaline or some other active monoamine or metabolic product of monoamines. Because of lack of tools, we have not been able to measure these changes.

McCANN: I might just mention one piece of evidence that would possibly support the idea that dopamine is taken up by the hypothalamus and then re-released. In experiments done some time ago with Schneider, we found that addition of reserpine to the *in vitro* co-incubation system with hypothalami plus pituitaries blocked the response to dopamine. This would fit in with the possibility that reserpine might inhibit entry of dopamine into cells.

Involvement of Pineal Indoles and Polypeptides with the Neuroendocrine Axis*

RUSSEL J. REITER**

Department of Anatomy, The University of Texas Medical School at San Antonio, San Antonio, Tex. 78229 (U.S.A.)

The number of endocrine organs that the pineal gland influences is truly remarkable. Most, if not all, of the hormones derived from the anterior pituitary gland are modulated by pineal secretions (Wurtman *et al.*, 1968; Reiter and Fraschini, 1969). Furthermore, many of the extra-pituitary regulated endocrine glands are also under control of this multipotent epithalamic structure (Moreau, 1964; Quay, 1969). Virtually every organ tested, endocrine or otherwise, has been shown to be directly or indirectly influenced by the pineal or its constituents.

Because of its profuse blood supply, several investigators predicted an endocrine role for the pineal gland at a time during which it was unpopular to do so (for reviews see Moreau, 1964; Kappers, 1967). Later, the elucidation of several secretory products convinced other workers of the pineal's legitimacy as an endocrine structure (Wurtman *et al.*, 1968; Moszkowska *et al.*, 1971). Finally, detailed biochemical studies of pineal tissue emphasize its secretory nature since it has been shown to exhibit an active hexomonophosphate pathway for the oxidation of glucose (Krass *et al.*, 1971). This is a characteristic criterion of secretory cells and is a universal feature of endocrine organs.

COMPOUNDS THAT MAY BE PINEAL HORMONES

Two schools of thought concerning the structural nature of the active pineal substances have clearly emerged. Since the isolation of *N*-acetyl-5-methoxytryptamine (melatonin) from bovine pineal tissue (Lerner *et al.*, 1958), a great deal of effort has been expended investigating the endocrine properties of this compound. In fact, melatonin is the prototype of a family of pineal indoles, several of which have gained the status of hormones (Wurtman *et al.*, 1968; Fraschini and Martini, 1970). The second category of compounds that have received a great deal of interest are the polypeptides. Although not all of these have been structurally identified, these potential hormones are recruiting progressively more attention (Moszkowska and Ebels, 1971;

* Work by the author was supported by NIH grants HD-02937 and HD-06523.

** U.S.P.H.S. Career Development Awardee.

References p. 285–286

Thieblot and Menigot, 1971). The two schools are not mutually exclusive nor do investigators in either area necessarily deny the existence of the other category of alleged hormones.

(*1*) *Indolic compounds*

Fig. 1 illustrates the partial metabolism of indoles within the pineal gland. The majority of these have been examined as to their inhibitory activity on pituitary gonadotrophins. Many of them have been isolated from pineal tissue (McIsaac *et al.*, 1965; Sellei and Frauchiger, 1968). Undoubtedly, the most widely investigated of the pineal indoles is melatonin. Its synthesis within the pineal gland has been thoroughly studied (Shapiro and Kejl, 1967; Axelrod, 1970; Klein and Berg, 1970). The concentration of this indoleamine in the pineal gland of experimental animals varies with the photoperiod (Lynch, 1971), with locomotor activity (Ralph *et al.*, 1971; Reiter *et al.*, 1971), and possibly, in female rats, with the stage of the estrous cycle (Wurtman *et al.*, 1965).

Whereas most investigators acknowledge that melatonin has an inhibitory effect on sexual physiology (Shapiro and Kejl, 1967; Wurtman *et al.*, 1968; Reiter and Fraschini, 1969), some workers strenuously deny that it is the pineal hormone (Thieblot *et al.*, 1966a). When administered peripherally, by means of daily injections (Quay, 1969; Vaughan *et al.*, 1971) or by means of subcutaneously implanted pellets (Rust and Meyer, 1969; Sorrentino *et al.*, 1971), melatonin usually restricts the growth of the gonads and their adnexae. The intraperitoneal injection of melatonin at the anticipated time of luteinizing hormone (LH) release from the pituitary of female rats also prevents ovulation (Longenecker and Gallo, 1971) and the associated rise in plasma LH levels (Reiter and Sorrentino, 1971) (Fig. 2). The implantation of depots of melatonin into the brain (Fraschini and Martini, 1970) or its injection directly into

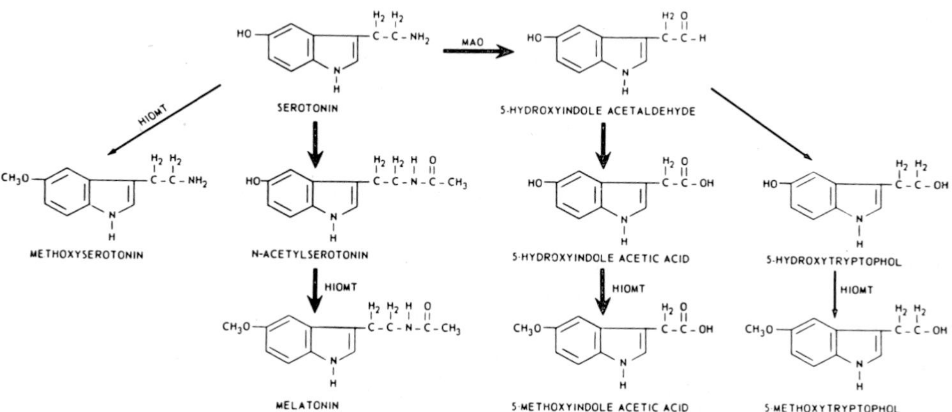

Fig. 1. Metabolism of some of the pineal indoles. Several of these compounds (*N*-acetylserotonin, melatonin, 5-hydroxytryptophol, 5-methyoxytryptophol) exhibit antigonadotrophic activity in mammals. HIOMT, hydroxyindole-*O*-methyltransferase; MAO, monoamine oxidase.

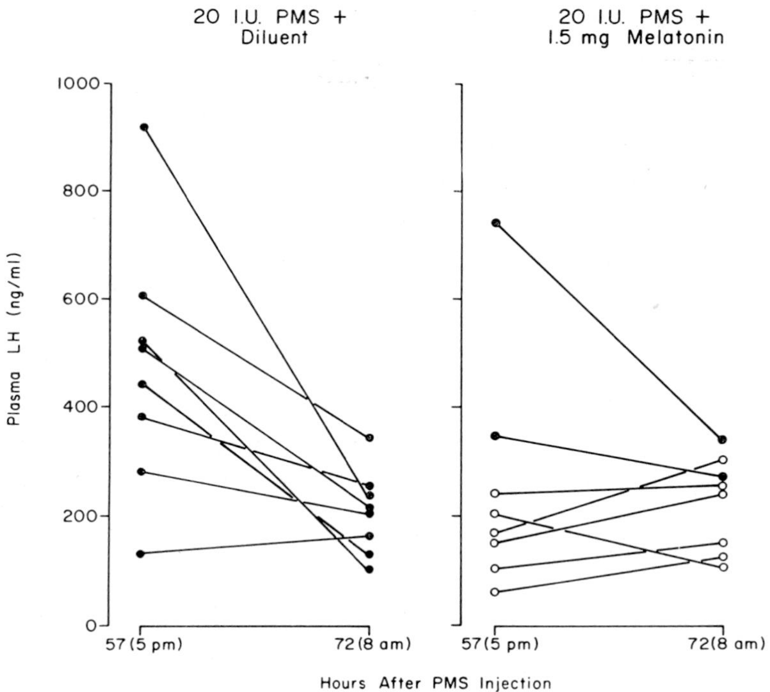

Fig. 2. Radioimmunoassayable plasma LH levels and ovulatory responses of immature rats after the injection of pregnant mare's serum (PMS). PMS was injected subcutaneously at 8.00 *a.m.* when the rats were 28 days old. Melatonin was administered subcutaneously in three 500-μg doses at 54, 55 and 56 h after PMS injection. The 57-h blood sample was collected by jugular vein puncture with the animals anesthesized with ether. The final blood sample (72 h) was taken after the animals were decapitated. Solid points represent rats that ovulated; hollow points indicate animals that did not ovulate.

the cerebrospinal fluid (Kamberi *et al.*, 1971) also influences the secretion of gonadotrophins from the anterior pituitary.

Another product of pineal hydroxyindole-*O*-methyltransferase activity, 5-methoxytryptophol (Otani *et al.*, 1969), has also been implicated in the control of the anterior pituitary. In fact, McIsaac *et al.*, (1964) claimed it had greater antigonadotrophic activity than melatonin while Vaughan and colleagues (1972) found that it was at least as potent as melatonin in restricting compensatory ovarian hypertrophy in mice. The immediate precursor of 5-methoxytryptophol, namely 5-hydroxytryptophol, also curtails ovarian enlargement after unilateral ovariectomy in mice (Vaughan *et al.*, 1972) and reportedly inhibits pituitary LH by a mechanism which involves specific receptors within the median eminence (Fraschini and Martini, 1970). 5-Hydroxytryptamine (serotonin), a compound that is abundant in the pineal gland, has been proposed as a pineal hormone by some workers (Albertazzi *et al.*, 1966) but has been found to be inactive under other experimental conditions (Vaughan *et al.*, 1972). In view of the rather ubiquitous nature of serotonin, it is difficult to envisage how it could be an essential pineal hormone. The only other pineal indole which has been

References p. 285–286

found to possess antigonadotrophic activity is *N*-acetylserotonin. On a comparative basis, it has about the same degree of antagonistic action on the reproductive system as the previously discussed pineal indoles (Vaughan *et al.*, 1972).

(2) *Peptidic compounds*

The second category of potential pineal hormones, the polypeptides, have obtained somewhat less publicity than have the indoles. About a decade ago, Milcu *et al.* (1963) and Pavel (1963) isolated from acetone-dried powder of bovine pineal tissue a polypeptide with pressor and oxytocic activity. After attempted characterization, they concluded that the active constituent was probably arginine vasotocin. Although Ebels *et al.* (1965) were unable to recover this peptide from sheep and bovine pineal glands, Cheesman (1970) claimed to have isolated and, by mass spectroscopic analysis, to have characterized a gonadotrophin-inhibiting substance of pineal origin which is identical to 8-arginine vasotocin. The antigonadotrophic action of arginine vasotocin had previously been verified by experiments from two separate laboratories. Pavel and Petrescu (1966) and Moszkowska and Ebels (1968) observed that a synthetic arginine vasotocin was an effective inhibitor of gonadal growth. The results of these studies indicated that the peptide interfered with the action of the gonadotrophin or gonadal hormones at a peripheral level but a central level of action was not precluded. Usually the pineal indoles are believed to act at the level of the neuroendocrine axis.

Perhaps the most persistent advocates of the idea that the pineal hormones are peptides rather than indoles are Thieblot and colleagues (Thieblot *et al.*, 1966b; Thieblot and Menigot, 1971). This group of workers admits to the presence of melatonin in pineal extracts, but finds it to be progonadotrophic rather than antigonadotrophic. Conversely, another pineal fraction, which has a low molecular weight and reportedly contains 5 peptides, is found to possess antigonadotrophic activity. This compound, when administered in daily 50-μg doses, suppressed pituitary gonadotrophin levels and prevented gonadal growth which was a consequence of pinealectomy.

Several other, yet unidentified, hormonally active fractions have been separated from pineal tissue. After gel filtration on Sephadex G-25, Moszkowska, Ebels and colleagues (Ebels *et al.*, 1970; Moszkowska and Ebels, 1971; Moszkowska *et al.*, 1971) successfully isolated several constituents from bovine pineal powder which exhibited activity when it was incubated with rat anterior pituitary glands. At least 2 of these fractions modulated follicle-stimulating hormone (FSH) release, one (F_2) acting in a stimulatory manner and the other being inhibitory (F_3). Unfortunately, purification and identification of these fractions has proven difficult and their exact chemical nature remains unknown.

Using a sensitive bioassay system in which to test the gonad-inhibiting ability of pineal extracts, Benson and colleagues (Matthews *et al.*, 1971; Benson *et al.*, 1972) concluded that a small polypeptide (MW 500–1000) is the envoy which accounts for the suppressive effects of the pineal on ovarian growth. How or whether this material has any relationship to arginine vasotocin is unknown. Benson *et al.* (1972) found the polypeptidic fraction to be 60–70 times more potent than melatonin in blocking compensatory ovarian hypertrophy in mice.

CONCLUDING REMARKS

It seems that neither the pineal indoles nor the pineal polypeptides consistently yield unequivocal results in reference to their gonadotrophin-inhibiting ability. The question of the specific pineal substance(s) responsible for the gonad-regulating capability of the pineal obviously remains unanswered. As noted earlier, however, the two possibilities are not mutually exclusive. Perhaps both the indoles and the polypeptides are secreted by the pineal gland and act through different mechanisms on the neuroendocrine-gonadal system. The indoles may act on the brain where they modify monoamine or catecholamine metabolism while the polypeptides may act on the anterior pituitary in a manner similar to the action of other polypeptides, the hypothalamic releasing factors.

REFERENCES

ALBERTAZZI, E., BARBANTI-SILVA, C., TRENTINI, G. P. AND BOTTICELLI, A. (1966) Influence de l'épiphysectomie et du traitement avec la 5-hydroxytryptamine sur le cycle oestral de la ratte albinos. *Ann. d'Endocr.*, **27**, 93–100.

AXELROD, J. (1970) Comparative biochemistry of the pineal gland. *Amer. Zool.*, **10**, 259–267.

BENSON, B., MATTHEWS, M. J. AND RODIN, A. E. (1972) Studies on a non-melatonin pineal antigonadotrophin. *Acta endocrinol.*, **69**, 257–266.

CHEESMAN, D. W. (1970) Structural elucidation of a gonadotrophin-inhibiting substance from the bovine pineal gland. *Biochim. biophys. acta*, **207**, 247–253.

EBELS, I., VERSTEEG, D. H. G. AND VLIEGENTHART, J. F. G. (1965) An attempt to isolate arginine vasotocin from sheep and bovine pineal body. *Proc. koninkl. nederl. Akad. Wetensch. Amsterdam*, Series B, **68**, 127–130.

EBELS, I., MOSZKOWSKA, A. AND SCÉMAMA, A. (1970) An attempt to separate a sheep pineal extract fraction showing antigonadotropic activity. *J. neuro-visc. Rel.*, **32**, 1–10.

FRASCHINI, F. AND MARTINI, L. (1970) Rhythmic phenomena and pineal principles. In *The Hypothalamus*, L. MARTINI, F. FRASCHINI AND M. MOTTA (Eds.), Academic Press, New York, pp. 529–549.

KAMBERI, I. A., MICAL, R. S. AND PORTER, J. C. (1971) Effects of melatonin and serotonin on the release of FSH and prolactin. *Endocrinology*, **88**, 1288–1293.

KAPPERS, J. A. (1967) The mammalian epiphysis cerebri as a center of neurovegetative regulation. *Acta neuroveg.*, **30**, 190–200.

KLEIN, D. C. AND BERG, G. R. (1970) Pineal gland: stimulation of melatonin production by norepinephrine involves AMP-mediated stimulation of *N*-acetyltransferase. *Advanc. Biochem. Psychopharmacol.*, **3**, 241–263.

KRASS, M. E., LABELLA, F. S., SHIN, S. H. AND MINNICK, J. (1971) Biochemical features of the pineal gland compared with other endocrine and nervous tissues. In *Subcellular Organization and Function in Endocrine Tissues*. H. HELLER AND K. LEDERIS (Eds.), Cambridge University Press, Cambridge, pp. 49–76.

LERNER, A. B., CASE, J. D., TAKAHASHI, Y., LEE, T. H. AND MORI, W. (1958) Isolation of melatonin, the pineal factor that lightens melanocytes. *J. Amer. chem. Soc.*, **80**, 2587.

LONGENECKER, D. E. AND GALLO, D. G. (1971) The inhibition of PMSG-induced ovulation in immature rats by melatonin. *Proc. Soc. exp. biol. Med.*, **137**, 623–625.

LYNCH, H. J. (1971) Diurnal oscillation in pineal melatonin content. *Life Sci.*, **10**, 791–795.

MATTHEWS, M. J., BENSON, B. AND RODIN, A. E. (1971) Antigonadotropic activity in a melatonin-free extract of human pineal glands. *Life Sci.*, **10**, 1375–1379.

McISAAC, W. M., TABORSKY, R. G. AND FARRELL, G. (1964) 5-methoxytryptophol: effect on estrus and ovarian weight. *Science*, **145**, 63–64.

McISAAC, W. M., FARRELL, G., TABORSKY, R. G. AND TAYLOR, A. N. (1965) Indole compounds: isolation from pineal tissue. *Science,* **148**, 102–103.

MILCU, S. M., PAVEL, S. AND NEACSU, C. (1963) Biological and chromatographic characterization of a polypeptide with pressor and oxytocic activities isolated from bovine pineal gland. *Endocrinology*, **72**, 563–566.

MOREAU, N. (1964) Contribution à l'étude de certaines correlations endocriniennes de l'épiphyse. *Ann. sci. l'Univ. Besançon*, **10**, 1–185.

MOSZKOWSKA, A. AND EBELS, I. (1968) A study of the antigonadotrophic action of synthetic arginine vasotocin. *Experientia*, **24**, 610–611.

MOSZKOWSKA, A. AND EBELS, I. (1971) The influence of the pineal body on the gonadotrophic function of the hypophysis. *J. neuro-visc. Rel.*, **Suppl. X**, 160–176.

MOSZKOWSKA, A., KORDON, C. AND EBELS, I. (1971) Biochemical fractions and mechanisms involved in the pineal modulation of pituitary gonadotropin release. In *The Pineal Gland*, G. E. W. WOLSTENHOLME AND J. KNIGHT (Eds.), Churchill, London, pp. 241–258.

OTANI, T., CREAVEN, P. J., FARRELL, G. AND McISAAC, W. M. (1969) Studies on the biosynthesis of 5-methoxytryptophol in the pineal. *Biochim. biophys. acta*, **184**, 184–190.

PAVEL, S. (1963) Cercetări asupra unui nou hormon pineal cu structură peptidică. *Stud. Cercet. Endocr.*, **14**, 665–668.

PAVEL, S. AND PETRESCU, S. (1966) Inhibition of gonadotrophin by a highly purified pineal peptide and by the synthetic arginine vasotocin. *Nature (Lond.)*, **212**, 1054.

QUAY, W. B. (1969) The role of the pineal gland in environmental adaptation. In *Physiology and Pathology of Adaptation Mechanisms*, E. BAJUSZ (Ed.), Pergamon, New York, pp. 508–550.

RALPH, C. L., MULL, D., LYNCH, H. J. AND HEDLUND, L. (1971) A melatonin rhythm persists in rat pineals in darkness. *Endocrinology*, **89**, 1361–1366.

REITER, R. J. AND FRASCHINI, F. (1969) Endocrine aspects of the mammalian pineal gland: a review. *Neuroendocrinology*, **5**, 219–255.

REITER, R. J. AND SORRENTINO, S. JR. (1971) Inhibition of luteinizing hormone release and ovulation in PSM-treated rats by peripherally administered melatonin. *Contraception*, **4**, 385–392.

REITER, R. J., SORRENTINO, S. JR., RALPH, C. L., LYNCH, H. J., MULL, D. AND JARROW, E. (1971) Some endocrine effects of blinding and anosmia in adult male rats with observations on pineal melatonin. *Endocrinology*, **89**, 895–900.

RUST, C. C. AND MEYER, R. K. (1969) Hair color, molt, and testis size in male, short-tailed weasels treated with melatonin. *Science*, **165**, 921–922.

SELLEI, K. AND FRAUCHIGER, E. (1968) Melatonin und Serotonin in der Glandula pinealis bei einigen Tierarten. *Sch. Arch. Tierheil.*, **110**, 395–398.

SHAPIRO, H. A. AND KEJL, C. P. (1967) Melatonin. *Prob. endokr. Hormonter.*, **13**, 110–116.

SORRENTINO, S., JR., REITER, R. J. AND SCHALCH, P. S. (1971) Hypotrophic reproductive organs and normal growth in male rats treated with melatonin. *J. Endocrinol.*, **51**, 213–214.

THIEBLOT, L. AND MENIGOT, M. (1971) Acquisitions récentes sur le facteur antigonadotrope de la glande pinéale. *J. neuro-visc. Rel.*, **Suppl. X**, 153–159.

THIEBLOT, L., ALASSIMARE, A. AND BLAISE, S. (1966a) Étude chromatographique et électrophorétique du facteur antigonadotrope de la glande pinéale. *Ann. d'Endocr.*, **27**, 861–866.

THIEBLOT, L., BERTHELAY, J. AND BLAISE, S. (1966b) Action de la mélatonine sur la sécrétion gonadotrope du rat. *C. R. Soc. Biol.*, **160**, 2306–2309.

VAUGHAN, M. K., BENSON, B., NORRIS, J. T. AND VAUGHAN, G. M. (1971) Inhibition of compensatory ovarian hypertrophy in mice by melatonin, 5-hydroxytryptamine and pineal powder. *J. Endocrinol.*, **50**, 171–175.

VAUGHAN, M. K., REITER, R. J., VAUGHAN, G. M., BIGELOW, L. AND ALTSCHULE, M. D. (1972) Inhibition of compensatory ovarian hypertrophy in the mouse and vole: a comparison of Altschule's pineal extract, pineal indoles, vasopressin, and oxytocin. *Gen. comp. Endocrinol.*, **18**, 372–377.

WURTMAN, R. J., AXELROD, J., SNYDER, S. H. AND CHU, E. W. (1965) Changes in the enzymatic synthesis of melatonin in the pineal during the estrous cycle. *Endocrinology*, **76**, 798–800.

WURTMAN, R. J., AXELROD, J. AND KELLY, D. E. (1968) In *The Pineal*, Academic Press, New York.

DISCUSSION

KASTIN: That was a great slide, Russ, but there was a serious grave error in it. It neglected to indicate that the pineal also influences one of the more important hormones, and I won't even name it.

Reiter: I did not mean that these are the only hormones that the pineal controls. Undoubtedly, the pineal controls MSH as shown by your work and furthermore, it regulates several other hormones not mentioned on this slide.

Marks: I think that this is a very interesting paper, Dr. Reiter. We have been looking at estrogen receptors in the various parts of the brain and for some reason we had not found data in the literature about soluble cytoplasmic estrogen receptor activity in the pineal. When we measured it we were surprised to find that it had enormous soluble protein estrogen receptor activity approximately equalling that of the pituitary gland. It is much greater than in any other part of the brain.

Reiter: Interestingly, estrogen has a feedback apparently on pineal biosynthetic activity as evidenced by the fact that it changes cyclic AMP activity within the gland. The pineal also concentrates a number of other compounds from the blood-vascular system; in particular, thyroxine and TSH are avidly taken up by the pineal.

Lott: During the past several years, there have been numerous reports which indicate that the pineal gland does play a significant role in mammalian physiology—yet, in most of the current texts in physiology and even endocrinology, the role of the pineal is still neglected. How would you account for this state and what do you think could be done to correct the apparent wrong to this small gland?

Reiter: I have several recommendations but no solutions for rectifying the situation. You're right though, characteristically textbooks lag considerably behind symposia publications in terms of the state of the art.

Kitay: As you may know, through the ages the pineal has been assigned a variety of imaginative functions which have obscured its role in mammalian physiology. Some of the sixteenth century anatomists referred to the pineal as the penis of the brain and perhaps that accounts for so many fallacious discussions that have been presented since then.

Reiter: Would you please spell fallacious?

Role of Indoleamines and Catecholamines in the Control of Gonadotrophin and Growth Hormone Secretion

R. COLLU, F. FRASCHINI AND L. MARTINI

Department of Pediatrics, University of Montreal (Canada) and Department of Pharmacology, University of Milan (Italy)

INTRODUCTION

The elucidation of the chemical structure of various releasing factors has recently given a new dimension to the field of neuroendocrinology. However, the mechanism that modulates the secretion of these factors is rather obscure, although the role of the central autonomic nervous system seems to be fundamental in this respect.

Early and more recent papers have shown that central indoleaminergic and catecholaminergic nervous pathways exert a mutually antagonistic influence on the secretion of gonatrophins (GTH). An inhibitory influence is exerted on the reproductive system by indoleaminergic neurons through such neurohumors as serotonin (5-HT) and melatonin. In effect, the administration of *p*-chlorophenylalanine, a specific inhibitor of the synthesis of 5-HT (Koe and Weissman, 1966), stimulates sex behavior in male rats and rabbits (Tagliamonte *et al.*, 1969). Pinealectomy, which suppresses an abundant source of indoleamines, also liberates the reproductive system from an inhibitory influence, inducing in female rats an acceleration of puberty and ovarian hypertrophy (Kitay and Altschule, 1954; Wurtman *et al.*, 1959) and, in males, an increase in accessory organ weights as well as an increment in pituitary content of GTH (Fraschini and Martini, 1970). On the other hand, the administration of indoleamines, either by direct implantation into the median eminence (Fraschini, 1969) or by injection into the brain's ventricles, inhibits GTH secretion (Kamberi *et al.*, 1970; 1971a). Catecholaminergic neurons have, on the contrary, a stimulatory influence. Early evidence of this was obtained by Sawyer et al. (1947), who demonstrated that dibenamine, an adrenergic blocker, suppressed ovulation. This drug is able to prevent the reflex release of luteinizing hormone (LH) in rabbits (Markee *et al.*, 1948) and the spontaneous release of LH in rats (Everett, 1961). Reserpine, a catecholamine depletor, can also block ovulation (Barraclough and Sawyer, 1957). Specific depletion of brain catecholamines with the drug α-methyl-*p*-tyrosine, during the "critical period", inhibits superovulation in the immature rat (Kordon and Glowinski, 1969). The intraventricular administration of catecholamines, on the contrary, stimulates the secretion of GTH (Schneider and McCann, 1970; Kamberi *et al.*,

References p. 297–299

1971b). Recently, biochemical and histochemical studies of hypothalamic catecholamines have brought additional, although somewhat contradictory, evidence of their role in the control of GTH secretion. (For reviews see Hökfelt and Fuxe, 1972; McCann *et al.*, 1972.)

Numerous papers have also reported the existence of a catecholaminergic regulation of growth hormone (GH) secretion in man, baboon, sheep and rat. Contradictory data exist, however, on the mode of action of the monoamines, and species differences have been reported (Blackard and Heidingsfelder, 1968; Imura *et al.*, 1968; Boyd *et al.*, 1970; Werrbach *et al.*, 1970; Toivola and Gale, 1970; Hertelendy *et al.*, 1969; Müller *et al.*, 1968).

The purpose of our work was to investigate two hypotheses. The first was that the administration of indoleamines, through the consequent inhibition of GTH, could modify two GTH-dependent phenomena: puberty and ovulation. The second was that the secretion of GH could also be under the antagonistic influence of catecholaminergic and indoleaminergic nervous pathways. In all these studies we have used the same method of injecting monoamines into a lateral ventricle of the brain through a permanent cannula. This approach was chosen to bypass the blood-brain barrier, which is impermeable to these substances (Axelrod *et al.*, 1959), and also to avoid the peripheral effects of systemically administered monoamines.

RESULTS

Effects of indoleamines on puberty

Previous experiments performed in Dr. Martini's laboratory have shown that a specific inhibitory effect is exerted by two methoxyindoles on pituitary GTH, *i.e.* melatonin inhibits LH, and 5-methoxytryptophol inhibits follicle-stimulating hormone

TABLE I

EFFECTS OF INTRAVENTRICULAR INJECTIONS OF MELATONIN AND OF 5-METHOXYTRYPTOPHOL ON THE TIME OF VAGINAL OPENING

Groups	*Number of rats*	*Days*
Untreated controls	65	36.0 ± 0.44[a]
Saline	36	37.0 ± 0.98
Melatonin 80 μg/rat/day[e]	15	40.7 ± 1.30[b, c]
5-Methoxytryptophol 80 μg/rat/day[e]	14	40.3 ± 1.00[b, d]

[a]Values are means ± S.E.M.
[b]$P < 0.0005$ *vs.* untreated control.
[c]$P < 0.025$ *vs.* saline.
[d]$P < 0.05$ *vs.* saline.
[e]Treatment begun on day 25 of age.

(From: Collu *et al.*, 1971a).

(FSH) (Fraschini, 1969). The effect—on the time of vaginal opening—of the intraventricular administration of either of these indoles to immature rats is shown in Table I. The animals were injected from the 25th day of age till canalization of the vagina. There was a statistically significant difference between the vaginal opening time of methoxyindole-treated animals and that of the two groups of controls (untreated and treated with the vehicle, 6% methanol in saline). These results indicate that both melatonin and 5-methoxytryptophol, when administered intraventricularly, can delay sexual maturation. The delaying effect of melatonin has already been reported by Wurtman *et al.* (1963) and by Motta *et al.* (1967). These authors, however, used a peripheral route of administration and higher dosages. On the contrary, 5-methoxytryptophol has been found inactive, in this respect, by McIsaac *et al.* (1964) who injected the compound subcutaneously.

The observation that both methoxyindoles, when given independently, may delay the appearance of puberty, leads one to suggest that a balanced secretion of LH and FSH is necessary to induce the onset of sexual maturation.

Effect of indoleamines on ovulation

The property of melatonin of specifically inhibiting LH (which is probably the major ovulatory GTH in the rat) led us to investigate the effect of this indole on the ovulation of normal adult rats. For this purpose, melatonin was injected intraventricularly on the day of proestrus every hour for 4 h, beginning 1 h before the "critical period", which in our strain of rats, and with the lighting conditions of our animal quarters, lasts from 2 *p.m.* to 4 *p.m.* Adult females, showing at least two regular 4-day estrous cycles, were used, and the injections were performed without anesthesia. Four injections were given because the half-life of melatonin is only 30 min (Kopin *et al.*, 1961), whereas the "critical period", during which ovulatory amounts of LH are

TABLE II

EFFECTS ON OVULATION OF INTRAVENTRICULAR AND SUBCUTANEOUS INJECTIONS OF MELATONIN DURING THE "CRITICAL PERIOD" IN MATURE RATS

Groups	*Number of rats treated*	*Number of rats ovulating*	*Percent of rats ovulating*	*Average of ova per rat*	*Number of rats not ovulating*
Saline (i.v.t.)	8	8	100	11.7 ± 0.09[a]	0
Melatonin (i.v.t.) 100–500 μg/rat	19	12	63	5.0 ± 0.70[b]	7
Melatonin (s.c.) 800–1200 μg/rat	11	11	100	10.1 ± 0.90	0

[a]Means ± S.E.M.
[b]$P < 0.0005$ *vs.* saline.
i.v.t., intraventricular; s.c., subcutaneous.

(From: Collu *et al.*, 1971b).

References p. 297–299

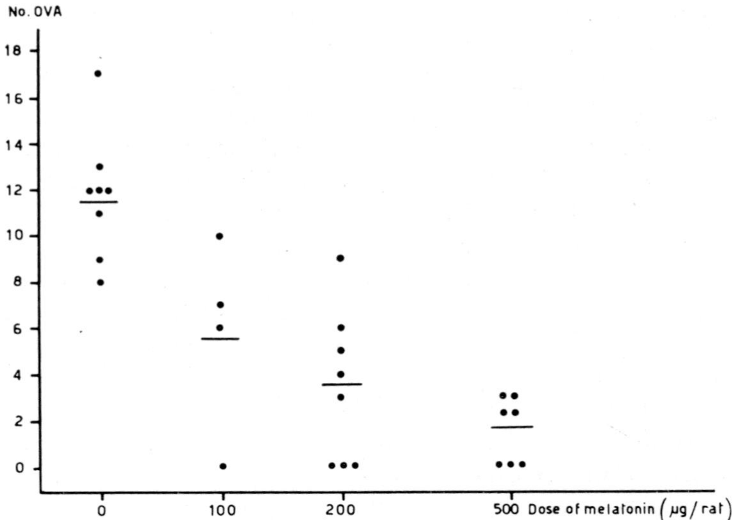

Fig. 1. Number of ova found in Fallopian tubes of normal adult rats after intraventricular injection of increasing amounts of melatonin during the "critical period" of the day of proestrus. (From: Collu *et al.*, 1971b)

released (Everett *et al.*, 1949; Monroe *et al.*, 1969), lasts about 2 h. The animals were killed next day, and the ova counted in the Fallopian tubes under a microscope. The results are shown in Table II. 19 rats received a total amount of melatonin varying from 100 to 500 μg per rat. In 7 rats, ovulation was completely blocked, while in the other 12, a mean number of only 5 ova was found. All the 8 rats treated with saline ovulated a mean number of 11.7 ova. When injected subcutaneously around the "critical period", even in higher amounts, melatonin was unable to block ovulation. Fig. 1 shows that an inverse relationship seems to exist between the amounts of melatonin injected intraventricularly and the mean number of ova recovered in the tubes.

These results show that melatonin can block ovulation when injected intraventricularly. This effect can be explained by the fact that this compound specifically inhibits the LH secretion, probably by altering the discharge of the releasing factor. It is also possible that the effect is due to the central nervous system depressant activity of melatonin (Marczynski *et al.*, 1964; Barchas *et al.*, 1967), in which case the mode of action of this indole would be similar to that of barbiturates and other sedatives (Everett *et al.*, 1949).

Effect of monoamines on GH secretion

The existence of an antagonistic role between catecholamines and indoleamines for the control of GTH induced us to investigate the existence of a similar role for the control of GH secretion in the rat. An α-adrenergic stimulatory and a β-adrenergic inhibitory control of GH secretion has been described in man (Blackard and Heidingsfelder, 1968; Imura *et al.*, 1968; Parra *et al.*, 1970) and sheep (Hertelendy *et al.*, 1969). In baboons, the intraventricular administration of dopamine (DA) has an inhibitory effect (Toivola and Gale, 1970). In rats, Müller *et al.* (1968) have described a stimulatory effect of catecholamines, but these authors only studied the effects on pituitary GH content, using a bioassay and the controversial pituitary depletion method.

The utilization of radioimmunological methods for the study of GH secretion in rats has been marred by the existence of a large spread of base-line plasma GH values

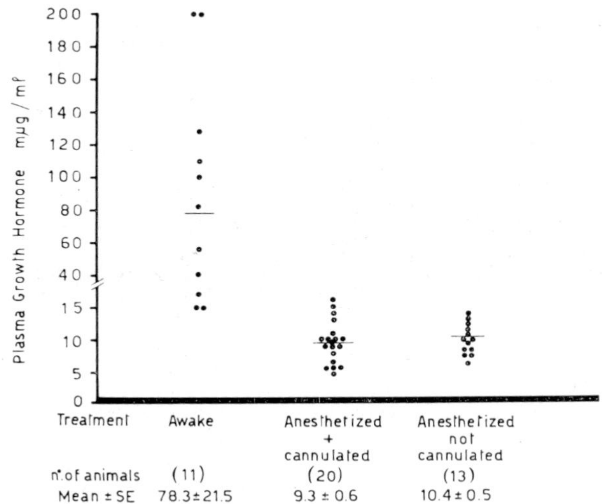

Fig. 2. Plasma GH levels found in samples obtained, in adult male rats, either by decapitation while awake, or after 2 h of urethane anesthesia. (From: Collu *et al.*, 1972)

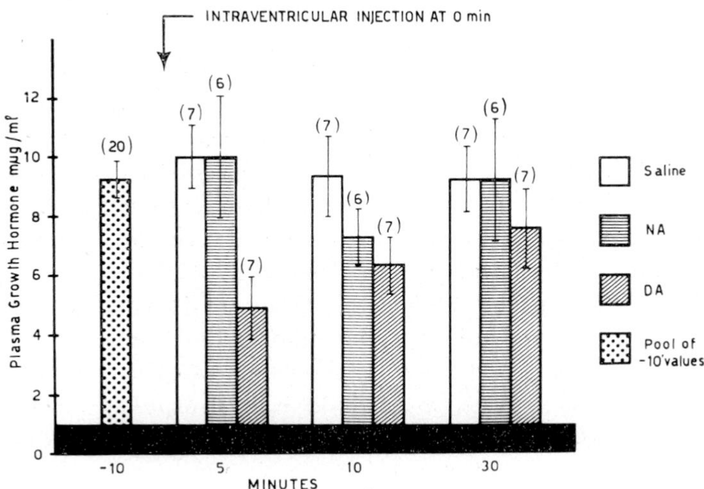

Fig. 3. Plasma GH levels after intraventricular injection at 0 min of either 1.0 μg of noradrenaline (NA), or 1.0 μg of dopamine (DA). The preinjection values of all experimental groups were pooled together because they were not statistically different. (From: Collu *et al.*, 1972)

References p. 297–299

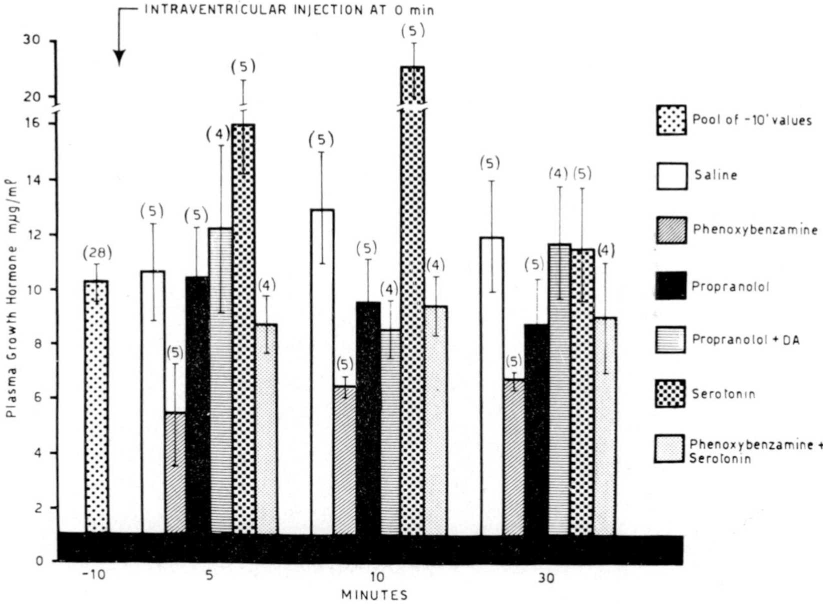

Fig. 4. Plasma GH levels after intraventricular injections at 0 min of either 50 μg of phenoxybenzamine, or 50 μg of propranolol, or 1.0 μg of serotonin (5-HT), and after either the intraventricular injection at −10 min of 50 μg of propranolol followed by the intraventricular injection at 0 min of dopamine (DA), or the intraventricular injection at −10 min of 50 μg of phenoxybenzamine followed by the intraventricular injection at 0 min of 1.0 μg of 5-HT. The pre-injection values of GH of all experimental groups were pooled together because they were not statistically different. (From: Collu *et al.*, 1972)

(Schalch and Reichlin, 1966). However, in adult male rats anesthetized for 2 h with urethane, plasma GH values are strikingly uniform (Collu *et al.*, 1971c), and this type of preparation was utilized in our experiments (Fig. 2).

Fig. 3 shows the effects on plasma GH levels of the intraventricular administration of noradrenaline (NA) or DA. The injection of 1.0 μg of NA induced a small decrease of GH 10 min later; the injection of 1.0 μg of DA was immediately followed by a significant decrease of plasma GH levels, which returned to base-line values at 30 min.

Fig. 4 shows the effects of the intraventricular administration of adrenergic blockers and of 5-HT on plasma GH levels. Phenoxybenzamine, an α-adrenergic blocker, induced a prompt, highly significant and persistent inhibition. On the contrary, propranolol, a β-adrenergic blocker, had no effect on GH. However, when DA was injected 10 min after propranolol, no inhibition of GH secretion was observed. The injection of 1.0 μg of 5-HT was followed by a rapid increase of plasma GH values which, at 10 min, reached a maximum equivalent to 2.5 times the base-line values. GH levels returned to base-line at 30 min. When 5-HT was injected 10 min after phenoxybenzamine, GH levels remained unchanged.

These results indicate the existence, in the rat, of an antagonistic role between sympathetic and parasympathetic systems for the control of GH secretion analogous, although acting in the opposite way, to the one existing for GTH.

TABLE III

HYPOTHALAMIC MECHANISMS OF ACTION OF DOPAMINE (DA), 5-HYDROXYTRYPTAMINE (5-HT) AND ADRENERGIC BLOCKERS, AND EFFECTS ON PLASMA GH VALUES OF URETHANE-ANESTHETIZED ADULT MALE RATS

Effects	*DA*	*5-HT*	*Phenoxy-benzamine*	*Propranolol*	*Propranolol + DA*	*Phenoxy-benzamine + 5-HT*
On hypothalamic receptors						
α-Adrenergic	+	0	−	+	+	−
β-Adrenergic	+	0	+	−	−	+
Tryptaminergic	0	+	−	0	0	−
On plasma GH	↓	↑	↓	→	→	→

0 or → means no effect; ↑ or + means stimulation; ↓ or − means inhibition.

(From: Collu *et al.*, 1972).

The hypothetical mechanism of action of DA and 5-HT, based on the interpretation of the experimental data obtained with these two monoamines and the two adrenergic blockers, is illustrated in Table III. DA inhibits GH secretion apparently by acting on central β-adrenergic receptors, since propranolol, a specific β-adrenergic blocker, abolishes this effect.

Serotonin stimulates GH release by acting through central tryptaminergic receptors. This effect is abolished by phenoxybenzamine, a drug able to block α-adrenergic, tryptaminergic, histaminergic and cholinergic receptors (Goodman and Gilman, 1970). The strong inhibitory action of this drug is probably due to the summation of a dual effect: blockade of the stimulatory serotoninergic tone, and activation of the inhibitory β-adrenergic receptor (Andén *et al.*, 1966; Persson, 1970). α-Adrenergic receptors do not seem to stimulate the secretion of GH in the rat, as shown by the observation that plasma levels remained unchanged after the administration of propranolol alone or with DA.

The dopaminergic inhibitory and serotoninergic stimulatory effects could be exerted by respectively inhibiting and stimulating the release of a GH-releasing factor, although it is also possible that the same results are obtained through respectively stimulating and inhibiting the release of a GH-inhibiting factor. Since both a GH-releasing and a GH-inhibiting factor probably exist, changes in plasma GH are possibly modulated by various interactions of all four neurohumors.

The different response of man and rat to the same stimuli, [*e.g.* stress, which is known to increase the turnover of brain catecholamines (Thierry *et al.*, 1968), stimulates human, but inhibits rat, GH secretion (Schalch and Reichlin, 1968; Collu *et al.*, 1973)], could be explained by the existence of a completely different monoaminergic mechanism of control. However, some recent data seem to indicate that serotoninergic pathways may also stimulate the secretion of *human* GH. In effect, the recently

References p. 297–299

described nocturnal surge of human GH (Sassin *et al.*, 1969; Honda *et al.*, 1969; Van der Laan *et al.*, 1970) occurs during the slow-wave or serotoninergic (Jouvet, 1969) part of the sleep cycle. In addition, Imura (1972) has recently described a stimulating effect of 5-hydroxytryptophan (a precursor of 5-HT) on the secretion of human GH. These observations led us to theorize that the mechanisms of control of GH secretion are not basically different in man and rat, but that, in man, evolutionary changes have brought a measure of additional sophistication to an already complex system.

CONCLUSIONS

Our experimental work seems to indicate that GTH-dependent physiological phenomena, such as puberty and ovulation, can be inhibited by two pineal indoles, 5-methoxytryptophol and/or melatonin. This effect is probably exerted through a depression of pituitary GTH secretion; it confirms the existence of a general inhibitory influence of indoleaminergic nervous pathways on the reproductive system.

Our results show that a mutually antagonistic role is also played by catecholaminergic and indoleaminergic nervous pathways for the control of GH secretion in the rat. In effect, DA inhibits, through β-adrenergic receptors, while 5-HT stimulates, GH secretion.

SUMMARY

Immature female rats injected intraventricularly with either melatonin or 5-methoxytryptophol showed a delay in the time of opening of the vagina. Melatonin, injected intraventricularly into adult female rats around the "critical period" of the day of proestrus, was able to block ovulation. These results confirm the existence of an inhibitory influence of indoleaminergic nervous pathways on the reproductive system.

The secretion of GH in adult male rats was inhibited by the intraventricular injection of DA (1.0 μg), and stimulated by the intraventricular injection of 5-HT (1.0 μg). Phenoxybenzamine also inhibited the secretion of GH, and was able to block the stimulating effect of 5-HT. Propranolol had no direct effect on GH, but was able to block the inhibitory effect of DA. These results indicate the existence of a mutually antagonistic role of catecholaminergic and indoleaminergic nervous pathways also for the control of GH secretion.

ACKNOWLEDGEMENTS

The experimental work was performed during the tenure, by R. Collu, of a Research Fellowship of the Medical Research Council of Canada, and was supported in part by a Ford Foundation grant No. 67-530.

REFERENCES

ANDÉN, N. E., FUXE, K. AND HÖKFELT, T. (1966) The importance of the nervous impulse flow for the depletion of the monoamines from central neurons by some drugs. *J. Pharm. Pharmacol.*, **18**, 630–632.

AXELROD, J., WEIL-MALHERBE, H. AND TOMCHICK, R. (1959) The physiological disposition of H^3 epinephrine and its metabolite metanephrine. *J. Pharmacol. exp. Ther.*, **127**, 251–256.

BARCHAS, J., DA COSTA, F. AND SPECTOR, S. (1967) Acute pharmacology of melatonin. *Nature (Lond.)*, **214**, 919–920.

BARRACLOUGH, C. A. AND SAWYER, C. H. (1957) Blockade of the release of pituitary ovulating hormone in the rat by chlorpromazine and reserpine: possible mechanisms of action. *Endocrinology*, **61**, 341–351.

BLACKARD, W. G. AND HEIDINGSFELDER, S. A. (1968) Adrenergic receptor control mechanism for growth hormone secretion. *J. clin. Invest.*, **47**, 1407–1414.

BOYD, A. E., LEBOVITZ, H. E. AND PFEIFFER, J. B. (1970) Stimulation of human-growth-hormone secretion by L-DOPA, *New Engl. J. Med.*, **283**, 1425–1429.

COLLU, R., FRASCHINI, F. AND MARTINI, L. (1971a) The effect of methoxyindoles on vaginal opening time. *J. Endocrinol.*, **50**, 679–683.

COLLU, R., FRASCHINI, F. AND MARTINI, L. (1971b) Blockade of ovulation by melatonin. *Experientia*, **27**, 844–845.

COLLU, R., VISCONTI, P., FRASCHINI, F. AND MARTINI, L. (1971c) Growth hormone (GH) secretion in the urethane-anesthetized rat. Proc. 2nd Int. Symp. Growth Hormone, *Excerpta med.*, **236**, abstract 64.

COLLU, R., FRASCHINI, F., VISCONTI, P. AND MARTINI, L. (1972) Adrenergic and serotoninergic control of growth hormone secretion in adult male rats. *Endocrinology*, **90**, 1231–1237.

COLLU, R., JÉQUIER, J.-C., LETARTE, J., LEBOEUF, G. AND DUCHARME, J. R. (1973) Effect of stress and hypothalamic deafferentation on the secretion of growth hormone in the rat. *Neuroendocrinology*, **11**, 183–190.

EVERETT, J. W. (1961) The mammalian female reproductive cycle and its controlling mechanisms. In *Sex and Internal Secretions*, 3rd ed., W. C. YOUNG (Ed.), Williams and Wilkins, Baltimore, pp. 497–555.

EVERETT, J. W., SAWYER, C. H. AND MARKEE, J. E. (1949) A neurogenic timing factor in control of the ovulatory discharge of luteinizing hormone in the cyclic rat. *Endocrinology*, **44**, 234–250.

FRASCHINI, F. (1969) The pineal gland and the control of LH and FSH secretion. In *Progress in Endocrinology*, C. GUAL (Ed.), Excerpta Medica, Amsterdam, pp. 637–644.

FRASCHINI, F. AND MARTINI, L. (1970) Rhythmic phenomena and pineal principles. In *The Hypothalamus*, L. MARTINI, M. MOTTA AND F. FRASCHINI (Eds.), Academic Press, New York, pp. 529–549.

GOODMAN, L. S. AND GILMAN, A. (1970) *The Pharmacological Basis of Therapeutics*, 4th ed., Mac-Millan, London, p. 552.

HERTELENDY, F., MACHLIN, L. AND KIPNIS, D. H. (1969) Further studies on the regulation of insulin and growth hormone secretion in the sheep. *Endocrinology*, **84**, 192–199.

HÖKFELT, T. AND FUXE, K. (1972) On the morphology and the neuroendocrine role of the hypothalamic catecholamine neurons. In *Brain–Endocrine Interaction. Median Eminence: Structure and Function*, K. M. KNIGGE, D. E. SCOTT AND A. WEINDL (Eds.), Karger, Basel, pp. 181–223.

HONDA, Y., TAKAHASHI, K., TAKAHASHI, S., AZUMI, K., IRIE, M., SAKUMA, M., TSUSHIMA, T. AND SHIZUME, K. (1969) Growth hormone secretion during nocturnal sleep in normal subjects. *J. clin. Endocrinol.*, **29**, 20–29.

IMURA, H. (1972) Effect of adrenergic agents on growth hormone and ACTH secretion. *Program of the IVth International Congress of Endocrinology, Washington, June 18–24*, p. 51.

IMURA, H., KATO, Y., IKEDA, M., MORIMOTO, M., YAWATA, M. AND FUKASE, M. (1968) Increased plasma levels of growth hormone during infusion of propranolol. *J. clin. Endocrinol.*, **28**, 1079–1081.

JOUVET, M. (1969) Biogenic amines and the states of sleep. *Science*, **163**, 32–41.

KAMBERI, I. A., MICAL, R. S. AND PORTER, J. C. (1970) Effect of anterior pituitary perfusion and intraventricular injection of catecholamines and indoleamines on LH release. *Endocrinology*, **87**, 1–12.

KAMBERI, I. A., MICAL, R. S. AND PORTER, J. C. (1971a) Effects of melatonin and serotonin on the release of FSH and prolactin. *Endocrinology*, **88**, 1288–1293.

KAMBERI, I. A., MICAL, R. S. AND PORTER, J. C. (1971b) Effects of anterior pituitary perfusion and intraventricular injection of catecholamines on FSH release. *Endocrinology*, **88**, 1003–1011.

KITAY, J. I. AND ALTCHULE, M. D. (1954) *The Pineal Gland*. Harvard University Press, Cambridge.

KOE, B. K. AND WEISSMAN, A. (1966) *P*-chlorophenylalanine: A specific depletor of brain serotonin. *J. Pharmacol. exp. Ther.*, **154**, 499–516.

KOPIN, I. J., PARE, C. M. B., AXELROD, J. AND WEISSBACH, H. (1961) The fate of melatonin in animals. *J. biol. Chem.*, **236**, 3072–3075.

KORDON, C. AND GLOWINSKI, J. (1969) Selective inhibition of superovulation by blockade of dopamine synthesis during the "critical period" in the immature rat. *Endocrinology*, **85**, 924–931.

MARCZYNSKI, T. J., YAMAGUCHI, N., LING, G. M. AND GRODZINSKA, L. (1964) Sleep induced by the administration of melatonin (5-methoxy-*N*-acetyl-tryptamine) to the hypothalamus of unrestrained rats. *Experientia*, **20**, 435–437.

MARKEE, J. E., SAWYER, C. H. AND HOLLINGSHEAD, W. H. (1948) Adrenergic control of the release of luteinizing hormone from the hypophysis of the rabbit. *Recent Progr. Hormone Res.*, **2**, 117–131.

MCCANN, S. M., KALRA, P. S., DONOSO, A. O., BISHOP, W., SCHNEIDER, H. P. G., FAWCETT, C. P. AND KRULICH, L. (1972) The role of monoamines in the control of gonadotropin and prolactin secretion. In *Brain–Endocrine Interaction. Median Eminence: Structure and Function*, K. M. KNIGGE, D. E. SCOTT AND A. WEINDL (Eds.), Karger, Basel, pp. 223–235.

MCISAAC, W. M., TABORSKY, R. G. AND FARREL, G. (1964) 5-Methoxy-tryptophol: effect on estrous and ovarian weight. *Science*, **145**, 63–64.

MONROE, S. E., REBAR, R. W., GAY, V. L. AND MIDGLEY, A. R. JR. (1969) Radioimmunoassay determination of luteinizing hormone during the estrous cycle of the rat. *Endocrinology*, **85**, 720–724.

MOTTA, M., FRASCHINI, F. AND MARTINI, L. (1967) Endocrine effects of pineal gland and of melatonin. *Proc. Soc. exp. biol. Med.*, **126**, 431–435.

MÜLLER, E. E., DALPRA, P. AND PECILE, A. (1968) Influence of brain neurohumors injected into the lateral ventricle of the rat on growth hormone release. *Endocrinology*, **83**, 893–896.

PARRA, A., SCHULTZ, R. B., FOLEY, T. P. JR. AND BLIZZARD, R. M. (1970) Influence of epinephrine-propranolol infusions on growth hormone release in normal and hypopituitary subjects. *J. clin. Endocrinol.*, **30**, 124–137.

PERSSON, T. (1970) Catecholamine turnover in central nervous system. In *Scandinavian University Books*, Elanders Boktryckeri, Gothenburg, p. 33.

SASSIN, J. F., PARKER, D. C., MACE, J. W., GOTLIN, R. W., JOHNSON, L. C. AND ROSSMAN, L. G. (1969) Human growth hormone release: relation to slow-wave sleep and sleep–waking cycles. *Science*, **165**, 513–515.

SAWYER, C. H., MARKEE, J. E. AND HOLLINGSHEAD, W. H. (1947) Inhibition of ovulation in the rabbit by the adrenergic-blocking agent Dibenamine. *Endocrinology*, **41**, 395–402.

SCHALCH, D. S. AND REICHLIN, S. (1966) Plasma growth hormone concentration in the rat determined by radioimmunoassay: Influence of sex, pregnancy, lactation, anesthesia, hypophysectomy and extrasellar pituitary transplants. *Endocrinology*, **79**, 275–280.

SCHALCH, D. S. AND REICHLIN, S. (1968) Stress and growth hormone release. In *Growth Hormone*, A. PECILE AND E. MÜLLER (Eds.), Excerpta Medica, Amsterdam, pp. 211–225.

SCHNEIDER, H. P. G. AND MCCANN, S. M. (1970) Dopaminergic pathways and gonadotropin releasing factors. In *Aspects of Neuroendocrinology*. W. BARGMANN AND B. SCHARRER (Eds.), Springer, Berlin, pp. 177–191.

TAGLIAMONTE, A., TAGLIAMONTE, P., GESSA, G. L. AND BRODIE, B. B. (1969) Compulsive sexual activity induced by *p*-chlorophenylalanine in normal and pinealectomized male rats. *Science*, **166**, 1433–1435.

THIERRY, A.-M., JAVOY, F., GLOWINSKI, J. AND KETY, S. S. (1968) Effects of stress on the metabolism of norepinephrine, dopamine and serotonin in the central nervous system of the rat, I. Modifications of norepinephrine turnover. *J. Pharmacol. exp. Ther.*, **163**, 163–171.

TOIVOLA, P. AND GALE, C. C. (1970) Effect on temperature of biogenic amine infusion into hypothalamus of baboon. *Neuroendocrinology*, **6**, 210–219.

VAN DER LAAN, W. P., PARKER, D. C., ROSSMAN, L. G. AND VAN DER LAAN, E. F. (1970) Implications of growth hormone release in sleep. *Metabolism*, **19**, 891–897.

WERRBACH, J. H., GALE, C. C., GOODNER, C. J. AND CONWAY, M. J. (1970) Effects of autonomic blocking agents on growth hormone, insulin, free fatty acids and glucose in baboons. *Endocrinology*, **86**, 77–82.

WURTMAN, R. J., ALTSCHULE, M. D. AND HOLMGREN, U. (1959) Effects of pinealectomy and of a bovine pineal extract in rats. *Amer. J. Physiol.*, **197**, 108–110.
WURTMAN, R. J., AXELROD, J. AND CHU, E. W. (1963) Melatonin, a pineal substance: effect on the rat ovary. *Science*, **141**, 277–278.

DISCUSSION

GORSKI: When Dr. Halász was at UCLA we studied the influence of various deafferentations on growth hormone and found that plasma growth hormone levels were more or less normal over a 7 week period. Later, Mitchell *et al.* (Neuroendocrinology, 10, 31–45, 1972) restudied this problem and found that beginning at about 7 weeks after deafferentation animals actually grew significantly more than controls. In your data, at least after the frontal cut you had what looked like significantly elevated growth hormone levels. I would like to know if you studied the growth of these animals and, secondly, do you have any explanation for the very low growth hormone levels after the incomplete deafferentation?

COLLU: We didn't actually measure the bodily growth of the rats but my impression is that they grow at a normal rate. In answer to your second question, there is probably an inhibitory pathway which travels along the stria terminalis and enters the medial basal hypothalamus through an anterior route and the inhibitory stimulus originates in the corticomedial nucleus of the amygdala. In the group of incompletely deafferented rats, which were anesthetized with pentobarbital, plasma growth hormone levels were not significantly different from those of controls. This finding supports the suggestion that low "base-line" values of growth hormone in incompletely deafferented rats are due to an inhibitory nervous influence which can be suppressed by a central nervous system depressant such as pentobarbital.

DICKEY: We have had some very good discussions about indoleamines and catecholamines but not very much about cholinergic mechanisms. In work done with Dr. Marks several years ago we gave carbachol and found no effect on FSH or LH release, but later using intact male rats we gave atropine and saw a decrease in both FSH and in LH. We then gave hexamethonium intraventricularly and saw a rather marked increase in FSH but no change in LH. This would suggest that, as you found using catecholamines and serotonin, we were dealing with dual inputs in a cholinergic system where both stimulation and perhaps inhibition are possible. We think this area need further investigation.

COLLU: I have some very preliminary data which seem to indicate that acetylcholine is able to stimulate growth hormone release in the rat. I think that there are also *in vitro* data in the literature which show the same phenomenon.

MCCANN: We have been looking at possible cholinergic control of gonadotrophin secretion in our laboratory and Dr. Libertun presented our findings at the recent meeting in East Lansing. Atropine given subcutaneously can block ovulation and, of course, this is accompanied by suppression of the plasma FSH and LH peaks. This confirms the observations of Sawyer and Everett some years ago. Intraventricular atropine in much smaller doses can also block gonadotrophin release during pro-estrus. Furthermore, atropine, either subcutaneously or intraventricularly, can either prevent the post-castration rise in gonadotrophins or lower already elevated gonadotrophins in castrates. Thus, I would like to reinforce what Dr. Dickey said that there may well be a cholinergic control here.

SCAPAGNINI: Your inhibition of serotonin stimulation with phenoxybenzamine could be interpreted as a blockade of the alpha receptor and an inhibition of dopamine reuptake, thus, you may have a balance between effects of dopamine inhibition and serotonin stimulation. This could explain why you find a decrease of serotonergic excitation.

Brain Serotonin and Pituitary-Adrenal Function

JOAN VERNIKOS-DANELLIS, P. BERGER AND J. D. BARCHAS

Biomedical Research Division, Ames Research Center, NASA, Moffett Field, California and Department of Psychiatry, Stanford University Medical School, Stanford, Calif. (U.S.A.)

Several reports in the literature have indicated that there is an important relationship between corticosteroids and serotonin (5-HT) in the rat brain. The work of Azmitia and McEwen (1969) though not corroborated by others (Lovenberg, 1972; Barchas, 1972) has shown that tryptophan hydroxylase which is believed to be the rate-limiting enzyme in the conversion of tryptophan to 5-HT (Lovenberg *et al.*, 1968) is sensitive to corticosteroid variations. Adrenalectomy was shown to decrease the activity of this enzyme and to decrease the conversion of labelled tryptophan to 5-HT in the midbrain. On the other hand corticosterone administration or stress increased the activity of tryptophan hydroxylase in the midbrain and the conversion of tryptophan to 5-HT (Millard *et al.*, 1972).

In addition, there appears to be a correlation between the daily rhythm of 5-HT content in the limbic system and that of circulating corticosterone. Scapagnini *et al.* (1971) reported that treatment with *para*chlorophenylalanine (PCPA) abolished the diurnal variation of plasma corticosterone at an intermediate level in the rat, and Krieger and Rizzo (1969) reported that drugs that affect the metabolism or action of 5-HT abolished the daily rise in plasma 17-hydroxycorticosteroids (17-OHCS) in the cat but did not block the response to stress. These findings led Scapagnini *et al.* (1971) to suggest that the frontal cortex, hippocampus and amygdala, that are rich in 5-HT-containing nerve fibers (Fuxe *et al.*, 1968), are part of a serotoninergic functional unit that plays a modulatory role in the regulation of corticotrophin (ACTH) secretion. Their general conclusion was that brain 5-HT was involved in the regulation of the diurnal rhythm of the pituitary-adrenal system but not in the stress response.

We decided to investigate this further by evaluating the effects of altering brain 5-HT levels on the daily fluctuation of plasma corticosterone and on the response of the pituitary-adrenal system to a stressful or noxious stimulus in the rat. Our approach was to either inhibit brain 5-HT synthesis with PCPA or to try and raise its level with precursors such as tryptophan or 5-hydroxytryptophan (5-HTP). In these experiments male Sprague-Dawley rats (150–200 g) were used. They were kept in a 12L:12D environment (lights on at 07.00) and given food and water *ad libitum*. The animals were injected intraperitoneally (i.p.) with pyrogen-free saline or PCPA in saline at a dose of 300 mg/kg/day. Daily injections of PCPA for 2 or 4 days raised the morning low and prevented the evening rise in plasma corticosterone only if the

References p. 308–309

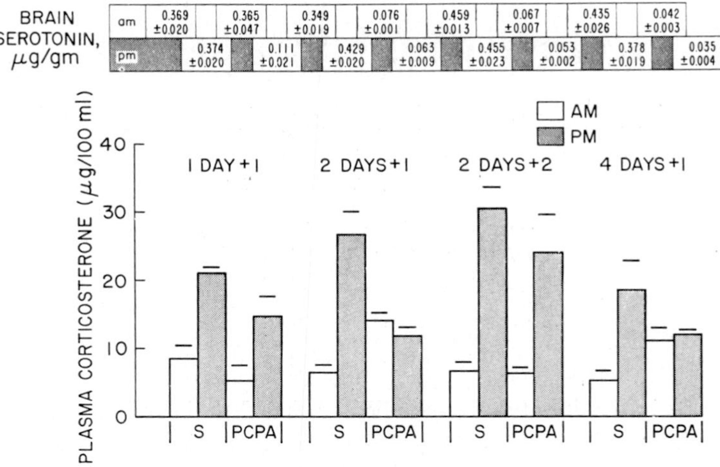

Fig. 1. Effect of PCPA pretreatment (300 mg/kg/day i.p.) on 8:00 *a.m.* and 8:00 *p.m.* levels of plasma corticosterone in rats. Rats were killed 24 h after one, two or four daily injections or 48 h after two daily injections. Horizontal bars denote S.E.M. ($n = 7$). S, saline.

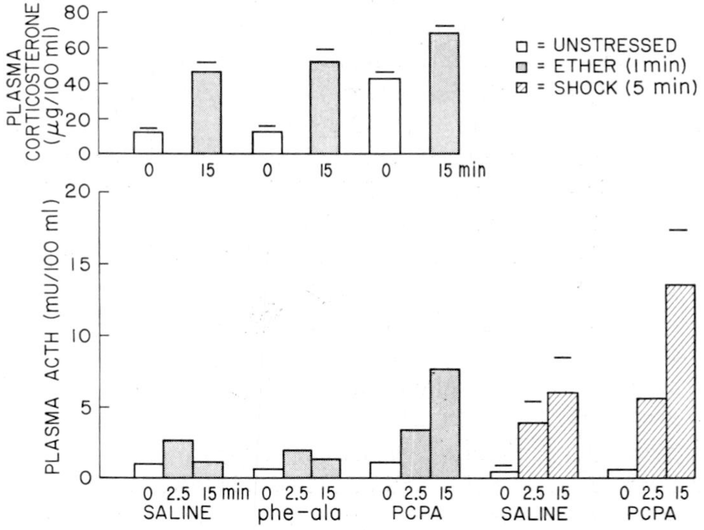

Fig. 2. Effect of PCPA on the corticosterone and ACTH concentrations in response to ether (1 min) or shock (4.5 min) stress. Horizontal bars denote S.E.M.

animals were killed within 24 h after the last injection (Fig. 1). If sacrificed 48 h after the last injection normal diurnal rhythmicity was restored. In order to evaluate the effect of PCPA on the stress-induced secretion of ACTH, rats were injected with daily doses of PCPA (300 mg/kg i.p.) for 4 days. At 10:00 *a.m.* on the day following the last injection they received 4.5 min electric shock (90 shocks per 4.5 min session) or 1 min of ether. The effects were compared to controls receiving an equal dose of phenylalanine or saline. Fig. 2 shows that PCPA elevated basal plasma corticosterone levels.

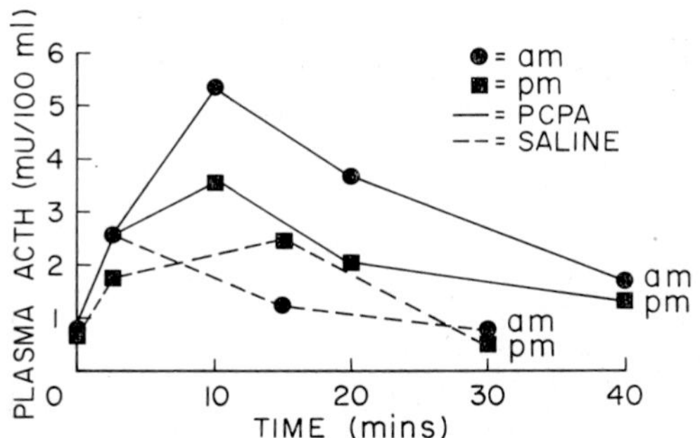

Fig. 3. Effect of PCPA on the time course of changes in circulating ACTH in response to ether stress.

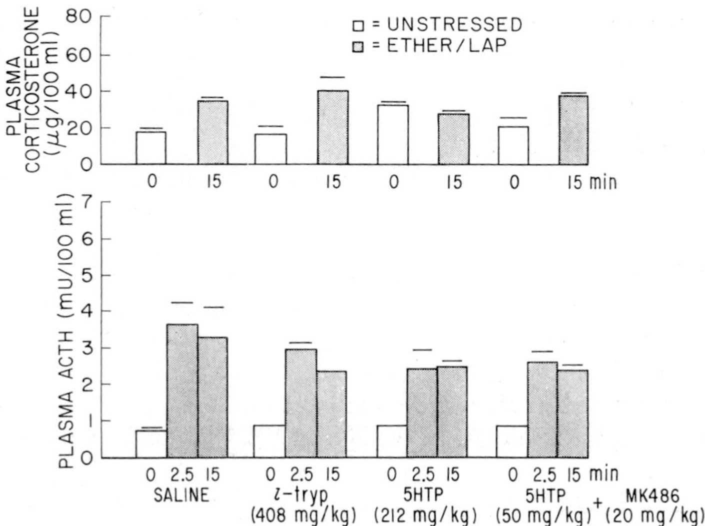

Fig. 4. Effect of L-tryptophan, 5-HTP or 5-HTP with MK 486 on the pituitary-adrenal response to the stress of ether and laparotomy (LAP). Horizontal bars denote S.E.M.

This was reflected in the changes in plasma ACTH concentrations where the responses to both shock and ether were greatly enhanced and sustained. Pretreatment with PCPA also resulted in a 50% increase in anterior pituitary ACTH concentration (9.34 ± 0.51 mU./mg in control rats to 13.97 ± 1.89 mU./mg pituitary tissue in PCPA-treated animals).

In order to assess whether this sustained response was due to the effect of PCPA on the diurnal variation in the rate of secretion of ACTH in response to stress, the time course of this response to ether stress was determined at 8:00 *a.m.* or 8:00 *p.m.*

Fig. 3 shows that whereas in the controls blood ACTH levels after stress peaked at 2.5 min in the morning and at about 15 min in the afternoon, depletion of 5-HT greatly altered the rhythm in the response to ether stress; maximum stress responses occurred at 10 min both in the morning and in the afternoon. Thus, inhibition of brain

References p. 308–309

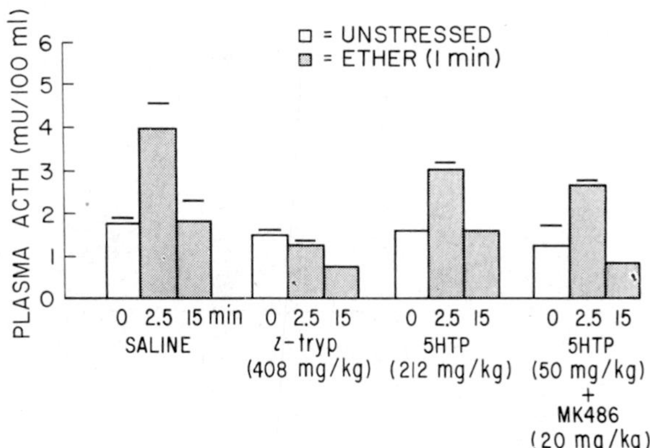

Fig. 5. Effect of L-tryptophan, 5-HTP or 5-HTP with MK 486 on the pituitary-adrenal response to the stress of ether (1 min) in rats adrenalectomized 24 h previously. Horizontal bars denote S.E.M.

5-HT synthesis enhanced the stress response in addition to altering the diurnal pattern of the pituitary-adrenal system.

Our alternate approach in the study of the role of brain 5-HT in the regulation of pituitary-adrenal function was to attempt to raise brain 5-HT by the use of precursors. L-tryptophan (408 mg/kg) or 5-HTP alone (212 mg/kg) or 5-HTP (50 mg/kg) with the peripheral decarboxylase inhibitor, L-α-hydrazinomethyldihydroxyphenylalanine (MK 486; 20 mg/kg), were injected i.p. into groups of rats. The animals were then studied 2 h later when brain 5-HT had been reported at maximal levels after injection of precursors in a similar study (Graham-Smith, 1971) and when plasma corticosterone levels have usually returned to normal in control animals after the stress of an injection. The animals were decapitated and bled 2.5 or 15 min after the stress of ether and laparotomy.

L-tryptophan did not affect the resting level of corticosterone though 5-HTP raised it. The response to the stress of ether and laparotomy was somewhat suppressed by tryptophan as it was in the 5-HTP-treated animals.

An identical experiment was performed in rats 24 h after bilateral adrenalectomy with the exception that ether alone was used as the stress stimulus. In the adrenalectomized animal tryptophan completely abolished the stress-induced secretion of ACTH. 5-HTP alone or in combination with MK 486 reduced the stress response in both intact and adrenalectomized animals significantly ($P < 0.05$). Hence, these precursors of 5-HT tended to decrease or inhibit the pituitary-adrenal response to stress. This inhibition was more evident in the absence of the adrenals.

In order to evaluate the implications to man of the 5-HT/pituitary-adrenal relationship that we observed in these experiments in the rat, urinary 17-OHCS response was determined to oral ingestion of MK 486 and 5-HTP in four normal human volunteers. Fig. 6 shows the results of this preliminary test in one of the four subjects, where 24-h urinary 17-OHCS excretion was measured daily for 12 days. After 2 days of control collections the subjects were given placebo capsules containing lactose for 2 days. This was followed by 2 days of MK 486 (50 mg, 4 times a day) with placebo (for 5-HTP),

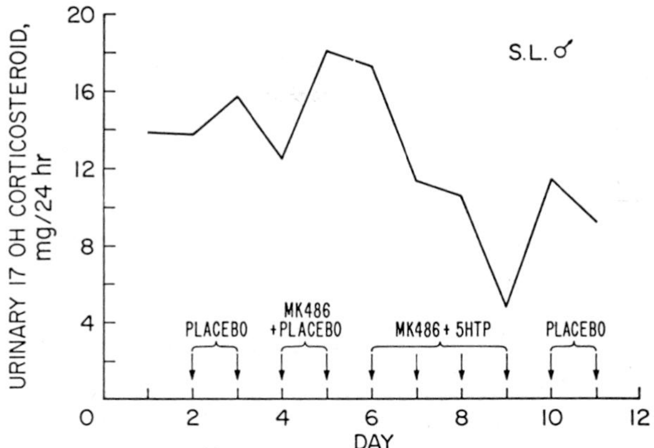

Fig. 6. Effect of 5-HTP and MK 486 on 24 h urinary excretion of 17-OHCS in a normal human subject.

to control for possible MK 486 effects on the steroid excretion, an additional 4 days of MK 486 (50 mg, 4 times a day) with increasing doses of 5-HTP (100, 200, 300 and 400 mg/day, respectively) and finally 2 days of placebo only. MK 486 raised 17-OHCS excretion. The combination of MK 486 and 5-HTP produced nausea and vomiting. In spite of this, they caused a prompt drop in 17-OHCS excretion with a return to baseline levels when the treatment was discontinued. Although it is evident that the MK 486/5-HTP combination is not acceptable, at least in this dose, for human use, nevertheless the results provide additional evidence that 5-HT precursors suppress pituitary-adrenal secretion in both experimental animals and in man.

It is now reasonably well accepted that the pituitary-adrenal system functions as a closed loop system. In this system the positive vector or "driving force" corresponds to environmental stimuli activating *via* hypothalamic neurohumoral pathways (Harris, 1948) and the negative vector corresponds to the level of corticosteroids (Sayers and Sayers, 1947).

Although it was originally assumed that the pituitary was the primary site of corticoid feedback inhibition (Rose and Nelson, 1956; Ganong and Hume, 1955), the bulk of more recent evidence has suggested that the hypothalamus and its ACTH-releasing activity are the primary targets of this inhibition rather than the pituitary gland itself.

Most of this evidence has been obtained in animals where hypothalamic implants of corticosteroids have been shown to suppress adrenocortical activity. Smelik and Sawyer (1962) in fact, using implants of hydrocortisone in various diencephalic and mesencephalic areas and into the adenohypophysis itself, were able to show that the greatest inhibition of stress-induced blood corticoid levels was obtained with implants in the median eminence and postoptic region. This region of maximum inhibition by corticoids coincides with the area of rat hypothalamus showing the greatest ACTH-releasing activity (Vernikos-Danellis, 1964). Furthermore pretreatment with hydrocortisone in a single dose that blocked the stress response but had no effect on pituitary

References p. 308–309

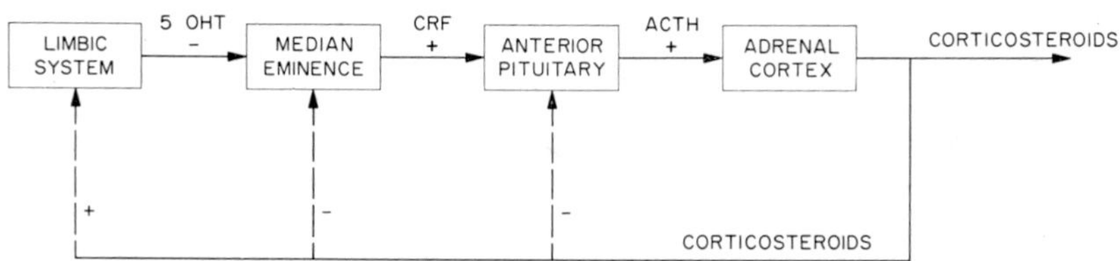

Fig. 7. Negative feedback regulation of ACTH secretion. 5-OHT, hydrocortisone; CRF, corticotrophin-releasing factor.

ACTH content, led within 4 h to an almost complete disappearance of the ACTH-releasing activity of the median eminence (Vernikos-Danellis, 1965) thus supporting the view that inhibition by corticoids occurs at a site distal to the pituitary.

Nevertheless, this appears to be a dose-dependent phenomenon and very large doses of hydrocortisone have been shown to inhibit the responsiveness of the pituitary gland itself (Vernikos-Danellis, 1964).

On the other hand there have been several pieces of evidence through the years suggesting the existence of extra-hypothalamic neural mechanisms or loci that inhibit ACTH secretion. Most of the work supports the theory of an inhibitory center in the region of the hippocampus. Stimulation of the hippocampus prevented the adrenocortical responses to stress (Porter, 1954; Endroczi *et al.*, 1959) or subsequent stimulation of the infundibulum (Mason, 1958). On the other hand lesions in this area have been shown to result in high plasma corticosterone levels in rats (Knigge, 1960; 1961). Lesion experiments and electrical stimulation through chronically implanted electrodes have indicated that the hippocampus, septum, midbrain reticular formation and amygdala are all involved in the regulation of ACTH secretion *via* pathways which feed into the hypothalamus (Mangili *et al.*, 1966).

More recently the work of McEwen and his associates (1969) has focused on the hippocampus as the site of specific uptake and binding of corticosterone in the rat and suggested this region as the site of negative feedback control of pituitary-adrenal function. The septum, amygdala and midbrain also contain smaller amounts of corticosterone binding factors. The high content of 5-HT in this region, our findings of an enhancement of the stress response by inhibition of 5-HT synthesis, and indications of a reduction of the stress response by serotonin precursors, suggested that serotonin may mediate this negative feedback mechanism regulating pituitary-adrenal function.

In this scheme of things it could be proposed that the absence of corticosterone after adrenalectomy results in a decreased brain 5-HT synthesis and secretion, thus allowing greater ACTH synthesis and secretion, and an increased sensitivity of the hypothalamic-pituitary unit to stress. In contrast, increased levels of corticoids stimulate brain 5-HT synthesis (by activating tryptophan hydroxylase) which in turn exerts an inhibitory effect on the hypothalamic-pituitary unit. If this hypothesis were correct then the inhibitory effectiveness of corticosteroids would be expected to be reduced in animals in which brain 5-HT was depleted, and enhanced when brain 5-HT synthesis was increased. Fig. 8 illustrates the results of an experiment which compares

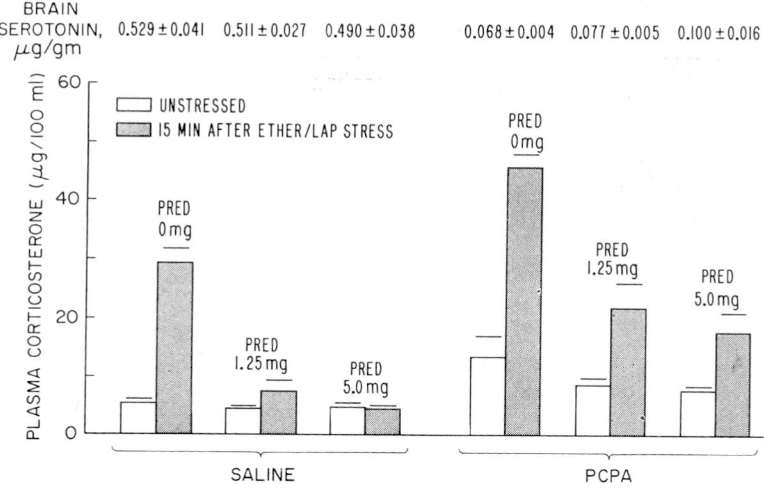

Fig. 8. Stress-inhibiting effects of prednisolone (PRED) in control or 5-HT-depleted rats. Rats were stressed 24 h after two daily injections of PCPA (300 mg/kg/day i.p.) or saline and 4 h after injection of the steroid.

the stress-inhibiting properties of two doses of prednisolone in control rats and in animals whose brain 5-HT content was markedly reduced by pretreatment with PCPA. Rats were stressed 24 h after two daily injections of PCPA (300 mg/kg/day i.p.) or saline and 4 h after the injection of the steroid (1.25 mg or 5.0 mg/100 g body weight s.c.).

Both doses of the steroid inhibited effectively the response to the stress of ether and laparotomy in the control animals. In 5-HT depleted animals neither dose was capable of blocking the stress response.

Additional evidence for the possible participation of brain 5-HT in the corticosteroid negative feedback mechanism regulating ACTH secretion can be found in clinical reports. Biochemical observations of severe depression have pointed to changes in 5-HT metabolism as evidenced by decreased cerebrospinal fluid 5-hydroxyindolacetic acid and alterations in pituitary adrenal function (Ashcroft and Sharman, 1960; Board *et al.*, 1957; Gibbons and McHugh, 1962) reflected by increased 17-OHCS excretion.

In addition attention has been brought recently to the analogies that exist between some forms of depressive illness and Cushing's disease. Both are characterized by chronically elevated plasma cortisol levels, an abnormal diurnal cortisol rhythm and an inability to suppress this parameter with dexamethasone (Carroll, 1971). These characteristics apparently are restored to normal in the depressed after appropriate therapy.

The elegant work of James *et al.* (1968) showed that in addition, Cushing's patients had an impaired adrenal response to pyrogen, although their response to ACTH, lysine vasopressin and metyrapone was normal or in fact, enhanced. They proposed that these findings implied an abnormality of "hypothalamic or cerebral control and not a primary defect of pituitary function as proposed originally by Harvey Cushing".

References p. 308–309

These facts and our studies lead us to speculate that what Cushing and some depressed patients may have in common is a defect in serotoninergic neuronal transmission that impairs pituitary-adrenal feedback mechanisms. Thus we reasoned that 5-HT precursors may be useful as a diagnostic test to differentiate those cases of Cushing's disease where the dysfunction is of cerebral rather than of pituitary or adrenal origin. Similarly, the dexamethasone suppression test may identify those depressed patients that would respond to 5-HT precursor therapy. We are presently investigating these possibilities.

SUMMARY

The effects of altering brain 5-HT synthesis on the diurnal rhythm of plasma corticosterone and on the pituitary adrenal response to stress was studied in rats and man. PCPA for 2 or 4 days abolished the diurnal rhythm in plasma corticosterone, enhanced the response to electric shock or ether stress and raised pituitary ACTH content. PCPA also prevented the stress-inhibiting properties of prednisolone. The hypothesis is proposed that 5-HT mediates the corticosteroid negative feedback mechanism that regulates ACTH secretion and that the primary site of this feedback is extra-hypothalamic. In contrast, pretreatment with l-tryptophan, 5-HTP alone or 5-HTP and MK 486 reduced slightly the stress response in intact rats and 5-HTP with MK 486 reduced 24 h urinary 17-OHCS excretion in humans. In 24 h adrenalectomized rats l-tryptophan completely abolished the response to stress.

ACKNOWLEDGEMENTS

These studies were supported in part by a grant from the Grant Foundation and NIHM 13-259, the technical assistance of Miss Anne Goodwin, Mrs. Pam Angwin, and Humberto Garcia are gratefully acknowledged. We also wish to thank Doctors S. Levine and R. Conner for their participation in the shock-stress experiment, and Dr. H. K. H. Brodie for his participation in the human clinical studies.

REFERENCES

ASHCROFT, G. W. AND SHARMAN, D. (1960) 5-Hydroxyindoles in human cerebrospinal fluids. *Nature (Lond.)*, **186**, 1050–1051.

AZMITIA, E. C. AND MCEWEN, B. S. (1969) Corticosterone regulation of tryptophan hydroxylase in midbrain of the rat. *Science*, **166**, 1274–1276.

BARCHAS, J. D. (1972) Unpublished observations.

BOARD, F., WADESON, R. AND PERSKY, H. (1957) Depressive affect and endocrinal functions. *Arch. Neurol. Psychiat.*, **78**, 612–620.

CARROLL, B. J. (1971) *Metabolic Studies in Depressive Illness*. Ph.D. Thesis, University of Melbourne.

ENDRÖCZI, E., LISSÁK, D., BOHUS, B. AND KOVÁCS, S. (1959) The inhibitory influence of archicortical structures on pituitary-adrenal function. *Acta physiol. acad. sci. hung.*, **16**, 17–22.

FUXE, K., HÖKFELT, T. AND UNGERSTEDT, V. (1968) Localization of indolealkylamines. *Advanc. Pharmacol.*, **6A**, 235–251.

GANONG, W. F. AND HUME, D. M. (1955) Effect of hypothalamic lesions on steroid-induced atrophy of adrenal cortex in dog. *Proc. Soc. exp. Biol. Med.*, **88**, 528–533.

GIBBONS, J. L. AND MCHUGH, P. R. (1962) Plasma cortisol in depressive illness. *J. psychiat. Res.*, **1**, 162–171.

GRAHAME-SMITH, D. G. (1971) Studies *in vivo* on the relationship between brain tryptophan, brain 5-HT synthesis and hyperactivity in rats treated with a monoamine oxidase inhibitor and L-tryptophan. *J. Neurochem.*, **18**, 1053–1066.

HARRIS, G. W. (1948) Neural control of the pituitary gland. *Physiol. Rev.*, **28**, 139–179.

JAMES, V. H. T., LANDON, J., WYNN, V. AND GREENWOOD, F. C. (1968) A fundamental defect of adrenocortical control in Cushing's disease. *J. Endocrinol.*, **40**, 15–28.

KNIGGE, K. M. (1960) Neuroendocrine mechanisms influencing ACTH and TSH secretion and their role in cold acclimation. *Fed. Proc.*, **19**, 45–51.

KNIGGE, K. M. (1961) Adrenocortical response to immobilization in rats with lesions in hippocampus and amygdala. *Fed. Proc.*, **20**, 185.

KRIEGER, D. T. AND RIZZO, F. (1969) Serotonin mediation of circadian periodicity of plasma 17-hydroxycorticosteroids. *Amer. J. Physiol.*, **217**, 1703–1707.

LOVENBERG, W. (1972) Serotonin synthesis in the brain. *Fifth int. pharmacol. Congr., San Francisco*, pp. 250–251.

LOVENBERG, W., JEQUIER, E. AND SJOERDSMA, A. (1968) Tryptophan hydroxylase in mammalian systems. *Advanc. Pharmacol.*, **6A**, 21–36.

MANGILI, C., MOTTA, M. AND MARTINI, L. (1966) Control of adrenocorticotrophic hormone secretion. In *Neuroendocrinology*, Vol. I, L. MARTINI AND W. G. GANONG (Eds.), Academic Press, New York, pp. 297–370.

MASON, J. W. (1958) The central nervous regulation of ACTH secretion. In *Reticular Formation of the Brain.* H. H. JASPER, L. D. PROCTOR, R. S. KNIGHTON, W. C. NOSHAY AND R. T. COSTELLO (Eds.), Little, Brown, Boston, pp. 645–662.

MCEWEN, B. S., WEISS, J. M. AND SCHWARTZ, L. S. (1969) Uptake of corticosterone by rat brain and its concentration by certain limbic structures. *Brain Res.*, **16**, 227–241.

MILLARD, S.A., COSTA, E. AND GAL, E. M. (1972) On the control of brain serotonin turnover rate by end product inhibition. *Brain Res.*, **40**, 545–551.

PORTER, R. W. (1954) The central nervous system and stress-induced eosinopenia. *Recent Progr. Hormone Res.*, **10**, 1–27.

ROSE, S. AND NELSON, J. (1956) Possible humoral mediators for release of ACTH in stress. *Austral. J. exp. Biol. med. Sci.*, **34**, 205–210.

SAYERS, G. AND SAYERS, M. A. (1947) Regulation of pituitary adrenocorticotrophic activity during response of rat to acute stress. *Endocrinology*, **40**, 265–273.

SCAPAGNINI, U., MOBERG, G. F., VAN LOON, G. R., DE GROOT, J. AND GANONG, W. F. (1971) Relation of brain 5-hydroxytryptamine content to the diurnal variation in plasma corticosterone in the rat. *Neuroendocrinology*, **7**, 90–96.

SMELIK, P. G. AND SAWYER, C. H. (1962) Effects of implantation of cortisol into the brain stem or pituitary gland on the adrenal response to stress in the rabbit. *Acta endocrinol.*, **41**, 561–570.

VERNIKOS-DANELLIS, J. (1964) Estimation of corticotropin-releasing activity of rat hypothalamus and neurohypophysis, before and after stress. *Endocrinology*, **75**, 514–520.

VERNIKOS-DANELLIS, J. (1965) The effect of stress, adrenalectomy, hypophysectomy and hydrocortisone on the corticotropin releasing activity of rat median eminence. *Endocrinology*, **76**, 122–126.

DISCUSSION

SCAPAGNINI: First of all I was delighted that you could replicate our results. I should point out, however, that our conclusion that serotonin may be responsible for the circadian regulation was based on a variety of different experiments, including the PCPA experiment. We lesioned the fornix and found the same result that we got with PCPA. Later, I obtained similar results after lesioning the raphe nuclei. Furthermore, circadian variation of serotonin was observed mainly in the hippocampus, less in the amygdala, and not at all in the hypothalamus. In the light of these results we felt that serotonin in the hippocampus might be responsible for modulation of the pituitary-adrenal rhythm. I would like to know how you reconcile your hypothesis of corticosteroid stimulation of serotonin synthesis with published reports that corticosteroid injection results in a sharp fall in serotonin content to 50% of the original level.

DANELLIS: I wonder if Dr. McEwen would like to respond to that question.

MCEWEN: I would like to comment on the relationship between glucocorticoids and serotonin biosynthesis. The work in our laboratory is incomplete but is continuing. Stimulated by our original observations, recent studies by my colleague Efrain Azmitia (Science, 169, 201, 1970) and by Millard, Gal and Costa (Brain Res., 40, 545–551, 1972) support the notion that increased glucocorticoid secretion increases *in vivo* conversion of tryptophan to serotonin in brain, while decreased glucocorticoid levels (by adrenalectomy) decrease this conversion. The time course of the effects is short compared with recent data showing slow turnover and slow axonal transport of tryptophan hydroxylase (Meck and Hopp, J. Neurochem. 19, 1519, 1972) suggesting that alterations of tryptophan hydroxylase itself may not be involved in these effects. Rather it may be that other regulatory factors, controlling tryptophan hydroxylase activity or other steps in uptake and conversion of tryptophan to serotonin, may be regulated by glucocorticoids. These factors remain to be discovered.

DANELLIS: I would like to thank Dr. McEwen for his comment. My suggestion is strictly a hypothesis based partly on the information from the literature and I would concede some steps in the pathway involved as new information becomes available.

MARKS: Regardless of the mechanisms involved, these are terribly interesting results. I have just a couple of technical questions. First, did you give serotonin alone to human volunteers and, second, what doses of serotonin do you use?

DANELLIS: Let me answer your second question first. We used 50 mg per day of MK 486 and increasing doses of 5-HTP. (100, 200, 300 and 400 mg per day, respectively, over the four days). We did not give 5-HTP. alone, unfortunately, and I am hoping that this summer when we will continue this work we will test 5-HTP. alone as well as tryptophan alone.

HYYPPÄ: I want to comment on the use of tryptophan. Tryptophan hydroxylase is theoretically the rate-limiting enzyme in serotonin synthesis but it is the availability of tryptophan that is the most important factor, determining brain serotonin levels. In addition, serotonin is taken up by all cells in brain and may replace catecholamines in their storage sites, such as alpha-DOPA does for serotonin. Tryptophan enhancement of brain serotonin is more valid and physiological because it does not act as a false transmitter.

CARROLL: Relations between serotonin and adrenal function in humans may not be the same in pathological states as in normals. In patients with Cushing's disease the serotonin receptor blocking drug, cinanserine, lowered urinary free cortisol excretion and potentiated the suppressive effect of dexamethasone. These results are, I think, in the opposite direction than we would expect with your tryptophan-serotonin results.

BOHUS: Your presentation may help explain previous findings about the hippocampal inhibitory mechanism. However, I was puzzled by one thing. You regarded the pituitary as possible site of feedback action of steroids especially at high pharmacological doses. But after brain serotonin depletion you couldn't show a block of ACTH release even with a very high dose of 5 mg of prednisolone. Do you have any explanation for this?

DANELLIS: Doses of steroid that affect the responsiveness of the pituitary gland to CRF are on the order of 150 to 300 mg/kg in the rat. We have shown previously that at the dose levels used here (12,5–50 mg/kg) we can block effectively the stress response without affecting the responsiveness of the pituitary gland to CRF or median eminence extracts.

DE WIED: Since you started to say, in order to wake us up, that hypothalamic CRF is serotonin, I would like to recall just for the record that Peter Smelik and I many years ago (Experientia, XIV, 17, 1958) showed that in animals with lesions which blocked ACTH release, serotonin injection had no effect on the release of ACTH.

Catecholamines and The Control of Prolactin Secretion in Humans

ANDREW G. FRANTZ

Department of Medicine, Columbia University College of Physicians and Surgeons, 630 West 168th Street, New York, N.Y. 10032 (U.S.A.)

The existence of prolactin in human blood, for so long a matter of speculation, has been firmly established within the last three years by the development of bioassay systems sensitive enough to be applied to unextracted human plasma, and the demonstration that the material so measured is immunologically distinct from growth hormone (Frantz and Kleinberg, 1970; Loewenstein *et al.*, 1971). The subsequent isolation of the human hormone from pituitary glands (Lewis *et al.*, 1971; Hwang *et al.*, 1972) has permitted the development of a homologous radioimmunoassay (Hwang *et al.*, 1971). It has also been shown that a heterologous radioimmunoassay, in which labeled porcine prolactin is incubated with anti-ovine prolactin, can be used to measure the hormone in human plasma (Jacobs *et al.*, 1972). The present paper will briefly review some of the recently gathered data from this and other laboratories regarding the normal physiology of prolactin secretion in humans, after which the action of pharmacological agents will be discussed. The role of catecholamines will be discussed in terms of studies with agents that deplete or antagonize cerebral catecholamines, such as phenothiazines, as well as studies with L-3,4-dihydroxyphenylalanine (L-DOPA).

MATERIALS AND METHODS

Plasma prolactin measurements in this laboratory were all carried out either by the mouse breast bioassay (Frantz and Kleinberg, 1970; Kleinberg and Frantz, 1971) or by a homologous radioimmunoassay similar to that of Hwang *et al.* (1971), using human prolactin standards supplied by Dr. Henry Friesen and rabbit anti-human prolactin antibody. The human prolactin preparation HPr-71-9-4, had a potency in the mouse breast bioassay of 30.5 I.U./mg [95% confidence limits: 23.8 to 37.2 I.U./mg (Frantz *et al.*, 1972a)]. A standard curve of the radioimmunoassay is shown in Fig. 1. Sensitivity is adequate to measure prolactin in virtually all human plasma specimens. Human growth hormone (HGH) produces no significant interference. A number of plasma specimens have been measured both by mouse breast bioassay and by radioimmunoassay and the results correlated. As shown in Fig. 2, there has been

References p. 320–321

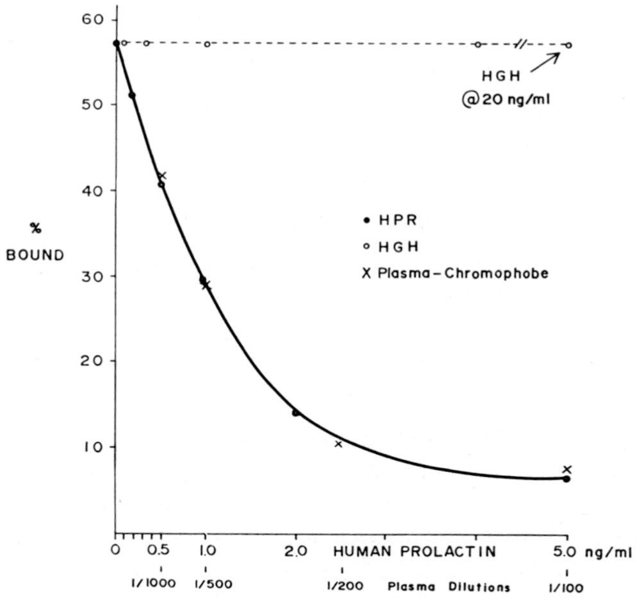

Fig. 1. Standard curve of homologous human prolactin radioimmunoassay employing [^{131}I]HPr (Friesen) and anti-human prolactin antibody. (From Frantz *et al.*, 1972a). HPR, human prolactin, HGH, human growth hormone.

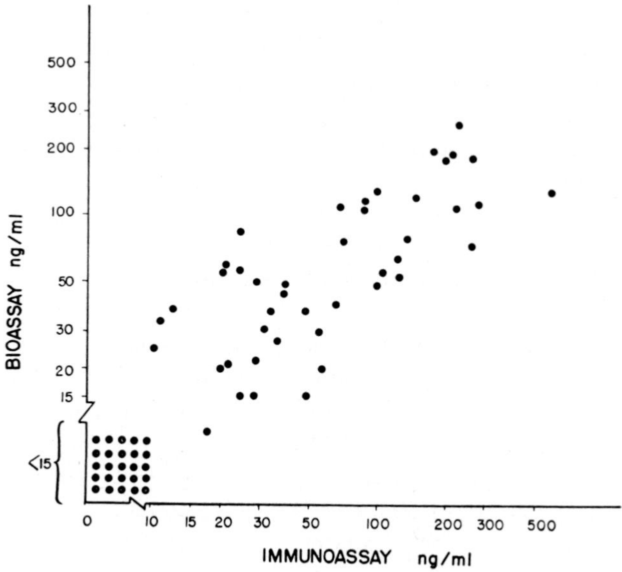

Fig. 2. Scatter diagram showing correlation between results of bioassay and radioimmunoassay for human prolactin in plasma samples. (From Frantz *et al.*, 1972a).

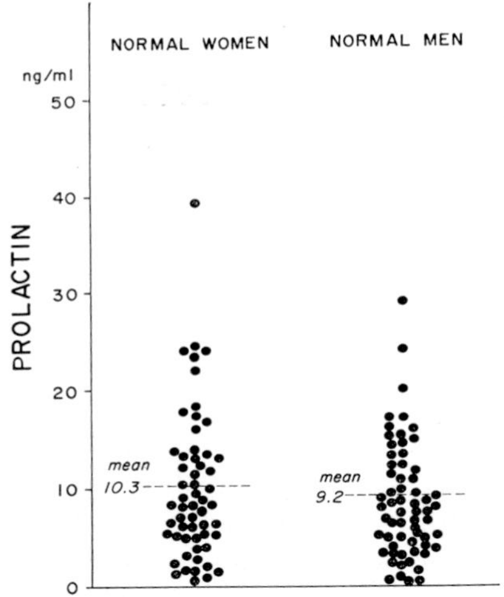

Fig. 3. Plasma prolactin concentrations in normal men and women, as measured by radioimmunoassay. (From Frantz *et al.*, 1972a).

generally good agreement between assays, with a mean ratio of bioassay/radioimmunoassay values of 1.09 in 50 samples with measurable values by both assays. Thus the bioassay supplies evidence that what is being measured in plasma by radioimmunoassay is biologically active prolactin.

For comparative purposes, the results of 120 prolactin determinations in normal men and women are shown in Fig. 3. Samples were drawn at various times of day, and subjects were not necessarily fasting. Although the mean level for women is slightly higher than for men, the difference is not significant in this group because of the large overlap. As will be seen later on, it appears that women are considerably more reactive than men in their responses to certain stimuli for prolactin release.

TABLE I

FACTORS AFFECTING PROLACTIN SECRETION IN HUMANS

Physiological:	
Nursing	(Frantz *et al.*, 1972a; Tyson *et al.*, 1972; Noel *et al.*, 1972b)
Sleep	(Sassin *et al.*, 1972)
Stress	(Frantz *et al.*, 1972a; Noel *et al.*, 1972a; Friesen *et al.*, 1972a)
Pregnancy	(Hwang *et al.*, 1971)
Estrogens	(Frantz *et al.*, 1972a)
Sexual intercourse	(Noel *et al.*, 1972a)
Hypoglycemia	(Frantz *et al.*, 1972a; Friesen *et al.*, 1972a; Noel *et al.*, 1972a)
Pharmacological:	
Neuroleptic drugs	(Kleinberg *et al.*, 1971; Friesen *et al.*, 1972b)
L-DOPA	(Kleinberg *et al.*, 1971; Malarkey *et al.*, 1971; Friesen *et al.*, 1972b; Frantz *et al.*, 1972b)
TRF	(Bowers *et al.*, 1971; Jacobs *et al.*, 1971)

PHYSIOLOGICAL FACTORS AFFECTING PROLACTIN RELEASE

Some of the physiological and pharmacological factors which have been shown to affect prolactin release in humans are listed in Table I, together with references. These factors, some but not all of which had been anticipated from earlier work with animals, are discussed briefly below:

Nursing

The act of suckling, in post-partum women, is one of the most powerful and specific of all stimuli to prolactin release. Plasma samples obtained at frequent intervals before, during and after nursing indicate that prolactin begins to rise within 5 to 10 min after the onset of suckling, continues to rise throughout its duration, and begins to fall almost immediately after the cessation of nursing. It is unrelated to milk let-down and occurs just as readily with the application of a breast pump in the absence of the infant. Growth hormone is unaffected by suckling (Frantz *et al.*, 1972a; Noel *et al.*, 1972b). In non-post-partum women breast stimulation produces a slight prolactin rise in some women and no change in others (see below).

Sleep

A diurnal rhythm of prolactin secretion in humans has recently been documented,

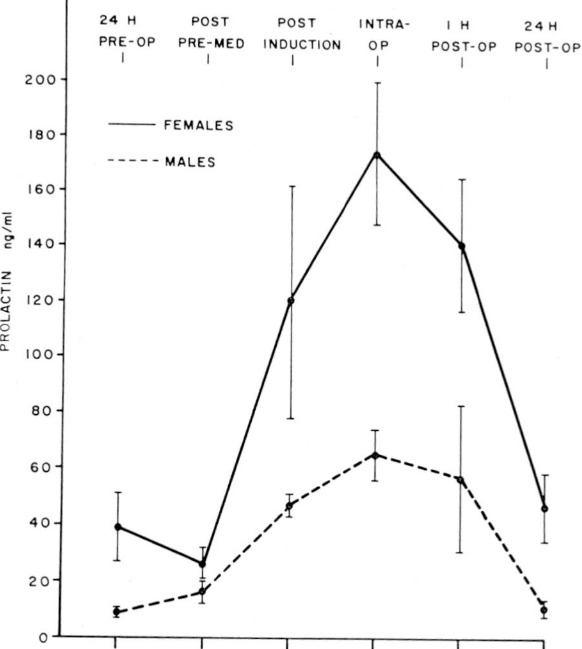

Fig. 4. Plasma prolactin concentrations during surgery with general anesthesia in 19 women and 7 men. Vertical lines indicate standard error of the mean. (From Noel *et al.*, 1972a).

with rising levels in plasma beginning shortly after the onset of sleep and continuing, with considerable variation, throughout much of the night. The pattern differs from that of growth hormone and does not appear to be directly correlated with the electroencephalogram (EEG) (Sassin *et al.*, 1972).

Stress

Prolactin in plasma has been noted to rise in association with several kinds of stressful procedures, the most potent stimulus so far investigated being that of major surgery with general anesthesia (Frantz *et al.*, 1972a; Noel *et al.*, 1972b). As shown in Fig. 4, there is a distinct sex difference in response to surgery. Some of the rise after induction of anesthesia in this figure is attributable to the use of droperidol, a butyrophenone derivative, for induction (see below).

Pregnancy

A progressive rise in prolactin occurs throughout pregnancy in humans. It has been speculated that this phenomenon, which does not occur to any comparable degree in monkeys, may be linked with the rise in estrogen production that takes place in human pregnancy (Hwang *et al.*, 1971).

Estrogens

In preliminary observations, a rise in baseline plasma prolactin of the order of two or three-fold has been observed in males receiving large doses of estrogens (Frantz *et al.*, 1972a). It appears possible that estrogens may sensitize the hypothalamus and/or pituitary to prolactin-releasing stimuli of various kinds in somewhat the same way as has been demonstrated for growth hormone (Frantz and Rabkin, 1965), though definite evidence on this point has not yet appeared.

Sexual intercourse

Prolactin has been reported to be elevated in a minority of normal women following sexual intercourse (Noel *et al.*, 1972a). Further studies are in progress to define more precisely the mechanisms involved.

Hypoglycemia

Severe hypoglycemia induced by insulin, which may be more properly considered a pharmacological than a physiological stimulus, has been shown to stimulate release of prolactin as well as of growth hormone (Frantz *et al.*, 1972a; Noel *et al.*, 1972a). Lesser degrees of hypoglycemia appear to be less effective in releasing prolactin than in releasing growth hormone (Friesen *et al.*, 1972a).

References p. 320–321

PHARMACOLOGICAL FACTORS AND THE ROLE OF CATECHOLAMINES

Neuroleptic drugs: acute administration

For a number of years it has been known that phenothiazine derivatives and other drugs of the neuroleptic class, such as reserpine and butyrophenones, which have the property of depleting or antagonizing cerebral catecholamines, can cause prolactin release in animals (Sulman, 1970). The mechanism of this release has been clearly shown, by *in vitro* studies involving pituitary glands incubated in co-culture with hypothalami from normal and perphenazine-treated rats, to be due to suppression by the drug of prolactin-inhibiting factor (PIF) liberated from the hypothalamus (Danon *et al.*, 1963). Fig. 5 shows plasma prolactin concentrations measured by bioassay in 9 normal volunteers (6 men, 3 women) before and at varying intervals after the intramuscular injection of chlorpromazine, either 12.5 or 25 mg. Prolactin rose from levels which were initially undetectable (less than 15 ng/ml) in all subjects to reach a peak at 1 h, with a slow decline thereafter. Of 4 subjects tested at 24 h, only one had prolactin which was detectable at the threshold of the assay. Patients with

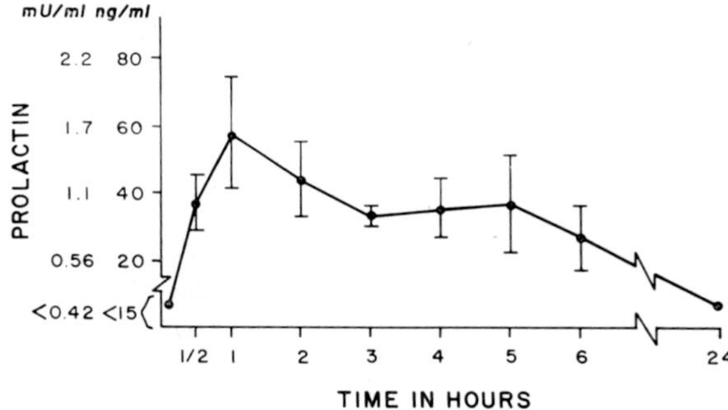

Fig. 5. Plasma prolactin, measured by bioassay, in 9 normal subjects after injection of chlorpromazine intramuscularly at zero time. Prolactin was initially undetectable (less than 15 ng/ml) in all subjects. Vertical bars represent standard error of the mean.

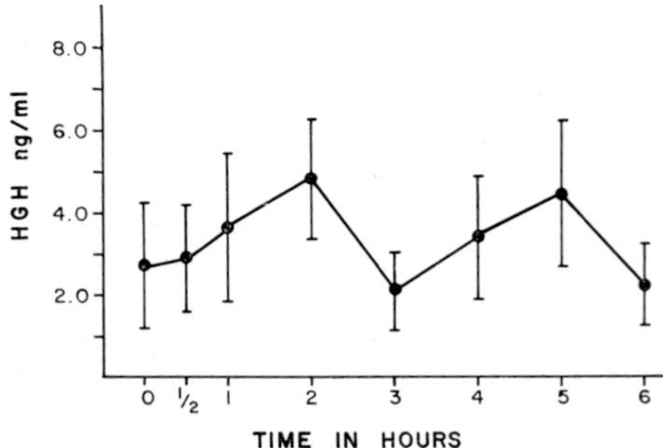

Fig. 6. Plasma growth hormone after chlorpromazine injection, measured in the same subjects as those in Fig. 5.

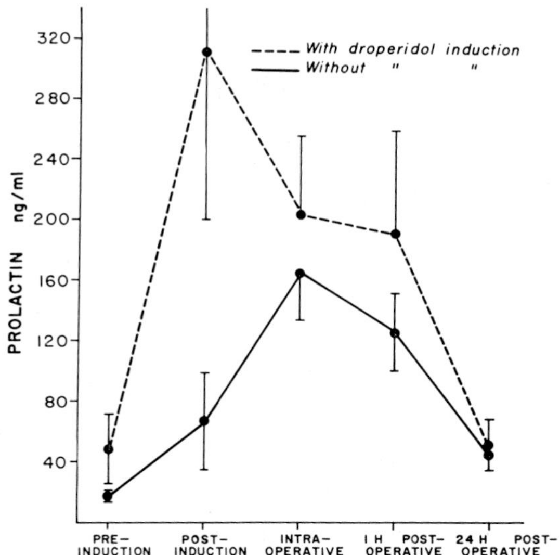

Fig. 7. Plasma prolactin during surgery with general anesthesia in 4 women who received Innovar[R] during induction of anesthesia (dotted line) and 15 women who did not (solid line). (From Noel *et al.*, 1972a).

disease of the hypothalamic-pituitary area have shown no response to chlorpromazine (Kleinberg *et al.*, 1971).

Plasma growth hormone during this same test is shown in Fig. 6. Although a suppressive action of chlorpromazine on growth hormone secretion has been reported (Sherman *et al.*, 1971) and its use advocated in the treatment of acromegaly (Kolodny *et al.*, 1971), no significant effect of chlorpromazine on growth hormone was noted in this study.

The effect of induction of anesthesia with intravenous Innovar, an agent containing droperidol, a butyrophenone derivative, and fentanyl citrate, is shown in Fig. 7. This depicts the responses of the four women included in Fig. 4 who had general anesthesia induced with Innovar *vs.* the 15 who received only pentobarbital. It is evident that much of the post-induction prolactin rise in the group as a whole was due to Innovar, droperidol being presumably the responsible agent. There is at present little experimental evidence to suggest that central nervous system depressants other than those of the neuroleptic class act to release prolactin. We have observed no effect of diazepam (Valium) in 4 volunteers receiving the drug who were studied over a 4-h period (Noel *et al.*, 1972a).

Neuroleptic drugs: chronic administration

We have previously reported elevated prolactin concentrations in patients receiving high doses of phenothiazine derivatives and haloperidol on a chronic basis for psychiatric purposes (Frantz *et al.*, 1972a). To see if chlorpromazine might enhance

References p. 320–321

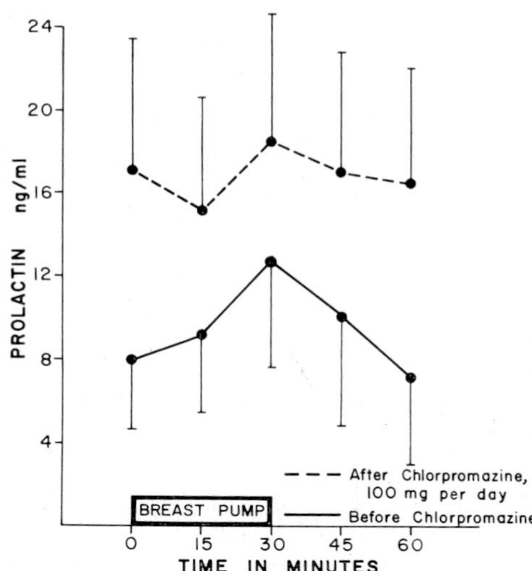

Fig. 8. Radioimmunoassayable plasma prolactin in response to 0.5 h of breast stimulation in 4 normally menstruating women, before and after treatment with chlorpromazine, 25 mg 4 times a day for periods of 2 to 11 days. Vertical bars represent standard error of the mean.

the response of non-post-partum women to breast stimulation, 4 normal women were studied during a standardized one-half hour period of self-stimulation with a breast pump (this same stimulus had produced a major prolactin rise in nursing mothers); the test was then repeated in the same subjects after 2–11 days of oral chlorpromazine treatment, 100 mg/day in divided doses. The results are shown in Fig. 8. Although the mean prolactin level was raised somewhat at all points during the test, the relatively modest response of these subjects to breast stimulation was not enhanced by chlorpromazine.

L-DOPA

Dopamine has been observed to inhibit prolactin secretion in animals, and evidence has been presented indicating a hypothalamic site of action (Kamberi *et al.*, 1971). There is also evidence from *in vitro* studies that dopamine can act directly on the pituitary (Birge *et al.*, 1970; MacLeod *et al.*, 1970; Koch *et al.*, 1970), although to what extent, if any, this site of action is operative in man is uncertain. We have shown that pre-treatment with oral L-DOPA can effectively block the prolactin rise that ordinarily follows chlorpromazine in normal individuals, as indicated in Fig. 9. It has also been shown that L-DOPA can act to depress baseline prolactin concentrations in endocrinologically normal individuals (Malarkey *et al.*, 1971; Friesen *et al.*, 1972b; Frantz *et al.*, 1972b). More surprising to us has been the finding that pre-treatment with L-DOPA, 500 mg 1 h before and 250 mg 0.5 h before the beginning of a thyrotrophin-releasing factor (TRF) test can markedly suppress the acute prolactin response which Bowers *et al.* (1971) and Jacobs *et al.* (1971) have found to intravenous TRF.

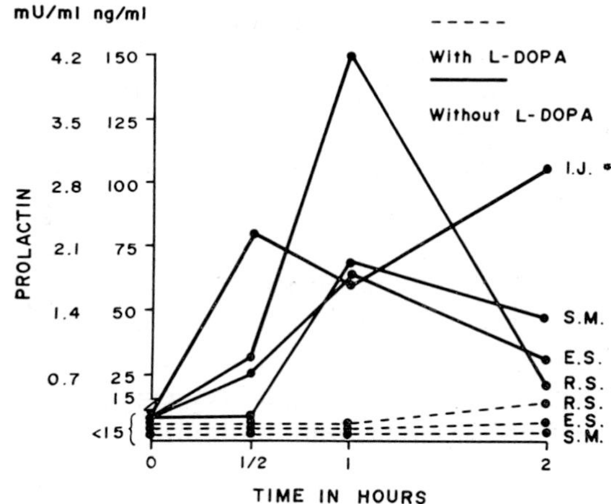

Fig. 9. Plasma prolactin, measured by bioassay, in 4 normal subjects who received 25 mg chlorpromazine (solid lines). The test was repeated in the same individuals several days later after pre-treatment with 500 mg of L-DOPA given orally 0.5 h before the test (dashed lines). Suppression of prolactin response occurred in all subjects, including I.J., whose post L-DOPA response is not shown. (From Frantz *et al.*, 1972a).

Results of TRF testing in men and women with and without L-DOPA pre-treatment are shown in Table II. A high degree of suppression is evident in both sexes (Noel, Suh, and Frantz, unpublished findings). Since TRF has been generally considered to act directly on the pituitary, and has been shown to do so *in vitro* with respect to

TABLE II

PROLACTIN RESPONSE TO TRF WITH AND WITHOUT L-DOPA PRE-TREATMENT

	Prolactin (ng/ml)										
	−60	*−30*	*0*	*+5*	*+10*	*+15*	*+20*	*+30*	*+45*	*+60*	*+120 min*
7 Females											
Without L-DOPA											
Mean:	—	9.39	7.74	27.28	48.33	59.43	67.71	46.57	43.57	31.43	12.81
± SEM:	—	2.31	1.35	9.45	13.39	19.11	23.17	9.14	9.88	7.00	2.52
With L-DOPA											
Mean	7.67	5.97	4.29	6.67	16.44	20.01	20.14	19.37	14.07	10.84	4.59
± SEM	1.78	1.47	1.11	1.82	6.26	8.30	8.24	7.91	5.14	4.33	1.39
7 Males											
Without L-DOPA											
Mean:	—	8.07	8.00	22.48	35.83	44.43	45.14	40.31	34.21	25.57	12.07
± SEM	—	2.28	2.92	7.91	9.93	11.41	13.27	12.05	11.26	7.73	3.80
With L-DOPA											
Mean	3.69	2.06	1.23	2.36	5.04	4.21	5.66	5.97	5.81	4.58	2.60
± SEM	0.95	0.43	0.34	0.35	1.91	1.34	2.74	2.55	2.89	2.39	1.09

References p. 320–321

prolactin stimulation (Tashjian *et al.*, 1971), these results suggest at least three possibilities: (*1*) Dopamine (to which L-DOPA is converted by decarboxylation) may act directly on the pituitary to inhibit prolactin secretion as well as on the hypothalamus. (*2*) Dopamine may act solely on the hypothalamus to liberate PIF, but the PIF inhibition of the pituitary may be strong enough to overcome the TRF stimulation. (*3*) TRF itself may act, in part at least, through the hypothalamus, and its action may be antagonized at this point by dopamine. It should be pointed out that there is no definite evidence as yet for a physiological role of TRF in the regulation of prolactin secretion.

Although it is clear that dopaminergic pathways act as inhibitors of prolactin secretion in humans, the exact loci of their action is still unsettled. Also uncertain is the extent of participation, if any, of noradrenergic pathways in prolactin regulation. Further studies with alpha- and beta-adrenergic blocking agents are being undertaken and may help clarify some of the mechanisms involved.

SUMMARY

The recent development of bioassay and radioimmunoassay techniques has confirmed the existence of a human prolactin and has opened a new field of physiologic studies. Some of the recently identified physiological and pharmacological factors affecting prolactin secretion in man are briefly discussed. The stimulatory effect of neuroleptic drugs, agents which deplete or antagonize cerebral catecholamines, is shown in various situations. Also shown are the suppressive actions of L-DOPA. Possible loci of dopamine-mediated prolactin inhibition are discussed.

REFERENCES

Birge, C. A., Jacobs, L. S., Hammer, C. T. and Daughaday, W. H. (1970) Catecholamine inhibition of prolactin secretion by isolated rat adenohypophyses. *Endocrinology*, **86**, 120–130.

Bowers, C. Y., Friesen, H. G., Hwang, P., Guyda, H. J. and Folkers, K. (1971) Prolactin and thyrotropin release in man by synthetic pyroglutamyl-histidyl-prolinamide. *Biochem. biophys. res. Commun.*, **45**, 1033–1041.

Danon, A., Dikstein, S. and Sulman, F. G. (1963) Stimulation of prolactin secretion by perphenazine in pituitary-hypothalamus organ culture. *Proc. Soc. exp. biol. Med.*, **114**, 366–368.

Frantz, A. G. and Rabkin, M. T. (1965) Effects of estrogen and sex difference on secretion of human growth hormone. *J. clin. Endocr.*, **25**, 1470–1480.

Frantz, A. G. and Kleinberg, D. L. (1970) Prolactin: Evidence that it is separate from growth hormone in human blood. *Science (Wash.)*, **170**, 745–749.

Frantz, A. G., Kleinberg, D. L. and Noel, G. L. (1972a) Studies on prolactin in man. *Recent Progr. Hormone Res.*, **28**, 527–573.

Frantz, A. G., Habif, D. V., Hyman, G. A. and Suh, H. K. (1972b) Remission of metastatic breast cancer after reduction of circulating prolactin in patients treated with L-dopa. *Clin. Res.*, **20**, 864.

Friesen, H., Webster, B. R., Hwang, P., Guyda, H., Munro, R. E. and Read, L. (1972a) Prolactin synthesis and secretion in a patient with the Forbes Albright syndrome. *J. clin. Endocr.*, **34**, 192–199.

Friesen, H., Guyda, H., Hwang, P., Tyson, J. E. and Barbeau, A. (1972b) Functional evaluation of prolactin secretion: A guide to therapy. *J. clin. Invest.*, **51**, 706–709.

Hwang, P., Guyda, H. and Friesen, H. (1971) A radioimmunoassay for human prolactin. *Proc. natl. Acad. Sci. (U.S.A.)*, **68**, 1902–1906.

Hwang, P., Guyda, H. and Friesen, H. (1972) Purification of human prolactin. *J. biol. Chem.*, **247**, 1955–1958.

Jacobs, L. S., Snyder, P. J., Wilber, J. F., Utiger, R. D. and Daughaday, W. H. (1971) Increased serum prolactin after administration of synthetic thyrotropin releasing hormone (TRH) in man. *J. clin. Endocr.*, **33**, 996–998.

Jacobs, L. S., Mariz, I. K. and Daughaday, W. H. (1972) A mixed heterologous radioimmunoassay for human prolactin. *J. clin. Endocr.*, **34**, 484–490.

Kamberi, I. A., Mical, R. S. and Porter, J. C. (1971) Effect of anterior pituitary perfusion and intraventricular injection of catecholamines on prolactin release. *Endocrinology*, **88**, 1012–1020.

Kleinberg, D. L. and Frantz, A. G. (1971) Human prolactin: Measurement in plasma by *in vitro* bioassay. *J. clin. Invest.*, **50**, 1557–1568.

Kleinberg, D. L., Noel, G. L. and Frantz, A. G. (1971) Chlorpromazine stimulation and L-DOPA suppression of plasma prolactin in man. *J. clin. Endocr.*, **33**, 873–876.

Koch, Y., Lu, K. H. and Meites, J. (1970) Biphasic effects of catecholamines on pituitary prolactin release *in vitro*. *Endocrinology*, **87**, 673–675.

Kolodny, H. D., Sherman, L., Singh, A., Kim, S. and Benjamin, F. (1971) Acromegaly treated with chlorpromazine. A case study. *New Engl. J. Med.*, **284**, 819–822.

Lewis, U. J., Singh, R. N. P., Sinha, Y. N. and Van der Laan, W. P. (1971) Electrophoretic evidence for human prolactin. *J. clin. Endocr.*, **33**, 153–156.

Loewenstein, J. E., Mariz, I. K., Peake, G. T. and Daughaday, W. H. (1971) Prolactin bioassay by induction of *N*-acetyllactosamine synthetase in mouse mammary gland explants. *J. clin. Endocr.*, **33**, 217–224.

MacLeod, R. M., Fontham, E. H. and Lehmeyer, J. E. (1970) Prolactin and growth hormone production as influenced by catecholamines and agents that affect brain catecholamines. *Neuroendocrinology*, **6**, 283–294.

Malarkey, W. B., Jacobs, L. S. and Daughaday, W. H. (1971) Levodopa suppression of prolactin in nonpuerperal galactorrhea. *New Engl. J. Med.*, **285**, 1160–1163.

Noel, G. L., Suh, H. K., Stone, G. and Frantz, A. G. (1972a) Human prolactin and growth hormone release during surgery and other conditions of stress. *J. clin. Endocr.*, **35**, 840–851.

Noel, G. L., Suh, H. K. and Frantz, A. G. (1972b) Induction of prolactin release by breast stimulation in humans. In *Fourth Int. Congr. Endocrinol., Washington, D.C., June, 1972*, Excerpta Med., Int. Congr. Series, Amsterdam, (Abstract No. 256)

Sassin, J. F., Frantz, A. G., Weitzman, E. D. and Kapen, S. (1972) Human prolactin: 24-hour pattern with increased release during sleep. *Science*, **177**, 1205–1207.

Sherman, L., Kim, S., Benjamin, F. and Kolodny, H. D. (1971) Effect of chlorpromazine on serum growth-hormone concentration in man. *New Engl. J. Med.*, **284**, 72–74.

Sulman, F. G. (1970) *Hypothalamic Control of Lactation*, Springer, New York.

Tashjian, A. H. Jr., Barowsky, N. J. and Jensen, D. K. (1971) Thyrotropin releasing hormone: Direct evidence for stimulation of prolactin production by pituitary cells in culture. *Biochem. biophys. res. Commun.*, **43**, 516–523.

Tyson, J. E., Hwang, P., Guyda, H. and Friesen, H. G. (1972) Studies of prolactin secretion in human pregnancy. *Amer. J. Obstet. Gynec.*, **113**, 14–20.

DISCUSSION

McCann: This is a fascinating presentation. It is remarkable that there is almost complete parallelism between the responses that you have described in the human and those that have been described in the rat. Regarding nocturnal secretion of prolactin, Neil has recently reported that during pseudopregnancy in the rat there is a nocturnal surge of prolactin and it appears at almost exactly the same time after turning off the lights as the maximum you see during sleep in the human. There is one discrepancy, and that is that during the normal estrous cycle of the rat one gets a proestrous surge of prolactin. The question is, does this occur during the menstrual cycle in man? I also wonder what a more physiological stimulation than a breast pump might do in non-lactating women, because at a recent meeting in Acapulco a dramatic rise of prolactin was reported after suckling in non-lactating women.

FRANTZ: In one woman who responded very strongly with a prolactin response to sexual intercourse, 0.5 h of nipple stimulation failed to stimulate prolactin release. In response to your first question, we have not studied prolactin levels during the menstrual cycle but others have found no changes associated with the menstrual cycle. It is possible that finer sampling times during the cycle would reveal characteristic changes.

DICKEY: I wanted to congratulate Dr. Frantz on this excellent work and to report on some clinical studies in humans with breast cancer. Earlier this year Stone reported on his attempts to suppress metastatic breast cancer with L-DOPA in a series of women all of whom were post-menopausal or post-oophorectomy. He found no response until he pretreated these women with premarin. Then he found a decrease in the size of breast cancer metastases. We also measured prolactin level in women treated with L-DOPA for metastatic breast cancer. In two women who did respond we saw a 50% fall, as much as you've seen with L-DOPA. Furthermore, in one of the women who responded and who was premenopausal we subsequently did an oophorectomy and three days later found that her prolactin levels had fallen again by 50%. This made us believe that perhaps the action of steroid treatment in breast cancer, either by removal of the ovaries, giving high doses of estrogen, or adrenalectomy, may be mediated through prolactin. This is Stone's idea originally, and I would like your comments on it.

FRANTZ: It is very interesting but we have been unable to correlate the incidence of remissions in breast cancer patients with the degree of prolactin suppression. Also, two of our best responses came from males who showed objective as well as subjective remissions and they had not been treated at any time with estrogen.

PODOLSKY: Have you had a chance to measure prolactin levels in patients with Huntington's chorea either in the basal state or after chlorpromazine or L-DOPA administration?

FRANTZ: No we have not. That would be most interesting to do.

Pituitary-Adrenal Activation and Related Responses to Δ^1-Tetrahydrocannabinol

HERBERT BARRY, III, ROBERT K. KUBENA AND JAMES L. PERHACH, JR.

University of Pittsburgh School of Pharmacy, Pittsburgh, Pa. 15261; ICI America, Inc., Wilmington, Del. 19899; and Mead Johnson Research Center, Evansville, Ind. 47721 (U.S.A.)

The compound Δ^1-tetrahydrocannabinol (Δ^1-THC) was synthesized rather recently (Gaoni and Mechoulam, 1964). Subsequent evidence that it is the main psychoactive ingredient of marihuana has been given by Mechoulam (1970b), who has stated his reasons for using the monoterpenoid nomenclature (Δ^1-THC) instead of the widely used formal nomenclature (Δ^9-THC) for the same compound (Mechoulam, 1970a). The availability of this single, pure compound has been a great advantage for determining the pharmacological effects of marihuana, which is a combination of many chemicals, generally of unknown quantities. An oft-repeated truism is that our knowledge about Δ^1-THC is scant and needs to be expanded.

In the last few years a great many papers have been published on various aspects of the actions of Δ^1-THC and marihuana, with the help of a U.S. Government policy of encouraging research by making the compounds freely available to qualified investigators. A highly consistent effect of Δ^1-THC in laboratory rats is pituitary-adrenal activation. Dewey *et al.* (1970) measured this effect by depletion of ascorbic acid. Kubena *et al.* (1971) reported on a series of experiments, measuring effects of Δ^1-THC by increase in plasma corticosterone, which is more closely related to corticotrophin (ACTH) secretion and thereby a more specific and sensitive indication of pituitary-adrenal activation. A statistically reliable elevation of plasma corticosterone was found at 45 min after a dose of Δ^1-THC as low as 2 mg/kg. This effect of Δ^1-THC (8 mg/kg) was acute, lasting less than 8 h, but it was also stable, being found at 45 min after the eighth daily dose of the drug. A central rather than peripheral site of action of the drug was demonstrated by further experiments showing that the increase in plasma corticosterone was completely blocked in hypophysectomized rats or after pretreatment with anesthetic doses of pentobarbital and morphine.

This entire pattern of endocrinological responses to Δ^1-THC is closely similar to the effects of intoxicating doses of ethyl alcohol in rats (Ellis, 1966). Since alcohol is primarily a central depressant or sedative (Wallgren and Barry, 1970), this is consistent with other evidence for central depression as an important component of the actions of Δ^1-THC (Kubena and Barry, 1970). A number of other depressant drugs also cause pituitary-adrenal activation after a single dose (Marks and Bhattacharya,

References p. 329–330

1970), but unlike the reports for alcohol and Δ^1-THC, their effects tend to disappear with repeated drug administrations (Ellis, 1966).

The present paper reports in greater or more graphic detail some of the findings of Kubena *et al.* (1971). In addition to these effects of Δ^1-THC on plasma corticosterone, effects of the compound are reported on plasma glucose and on urinary electrolytes. These effects are related to corresponding effects of alcohol and to the spectrum of physiological and behavioral effects of Δ^1-THC, reported in a large number of recently published articles.

METHOD

The experiments were performed on male albino rats. All were Wistar descendants, received from Hilltop Laboratory Animals, Inc., Scottdale, Pa., at approximately two months of age. They were housed in groups with food and water continuously available for several days prior to the experimental procedures. The animal quarters were maintained at 22–24° and on a circadian cycle of 12 h light (6:00 *a.m.*–6:00 *p.m.*) and the other 12 h dark. The test procedures were performed during the lighted phase in a nearby room maintained at the same temperature.

The Δ^1-THC was synthesized by Mechoulam. Kubena *et al.* (1971) give details of storage, preparation and administration of the compound. The vehicle was propylene glycol in a Tween 80–saline suspension. The advantages of this vehicle over several alternative ones have been reported by Sofia *et al.* (1971) in a study on mice. The Δ^1-THC and all other compounds were injected intraperitoneally.

Plasma corticosterone was assayed fluorometrically with the method used by Perhach and Barry (1970) modified from Guillemin *et al.* (1959). Plasma glucose was determined photometrically by the method described by Dubowski (1962) with Diagnatest (Dow Chemical Co., Midland, Michigan) glucose reagent (9% w/v, *ortho*-toluidine), glucose standard, and photoelectric colorimeter. Urine was collected in metabolic cages with food and water continuously available. Sodium and potassium concentrations were determined with a Perkin-Elmer (Model 303) atomic absorption spectrophotometer.

In all cases blood was collected by decapitating the rat. The blood was heparinized immediately, centrifuged and frozen within 1 h, and the plasma corticosterone or glucose determinations were made within two weeks.

RESULTS

Fig. 1 summarizes data obtained on plasma corticosterone levels at 45 min after injection of Δ^1-THC or its vehicle. Two experiments are shown, with 8–10 rats under each dosage condition for each experiment. In the first experiment, with doses of 4, 8 and 16 mg/kg, the Δ^1-THC reliably elevated plasma corticosterone levels, with no reliable difference among the three doses. However, the plasma corticosterones of the

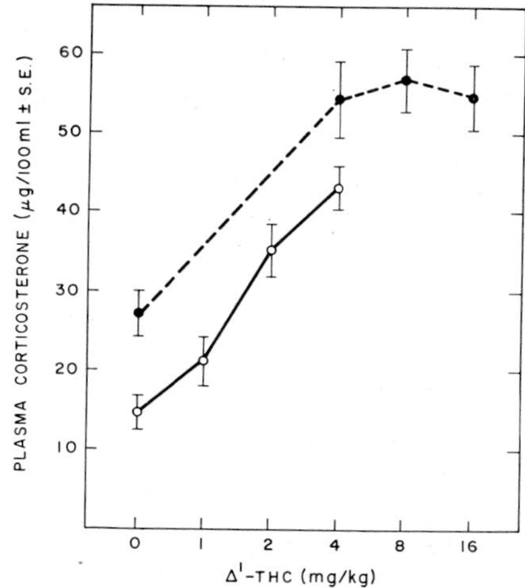

Fig. 1. Plasma corticosterone at 45 min after injection of vehicle or Δ^1-THC, comparing the results of two experiments. In the first experiment (0, 4, 8, 16 mg/kg), the rats were exposed to a more novel and stressful environment prior to decapitation.

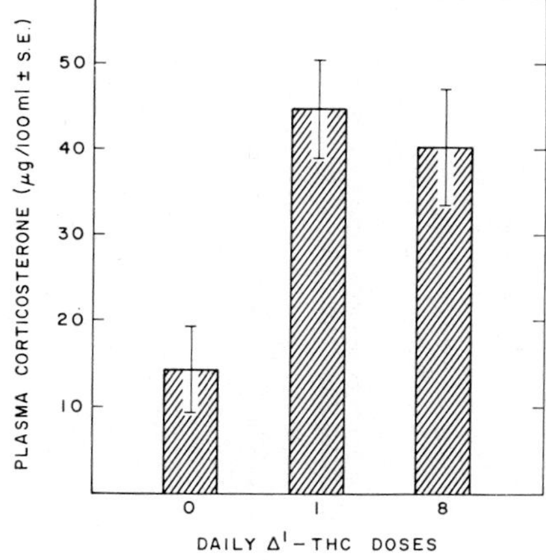

Fig. 2. Plasma corticosterone at 45 min after vehicle or Δ^1-THC injection (8 mg/kg), comparing groups of rats for which the Δ^1-THC was the first or eighth daily dose.

vehicle animals were above the usual normal level. A possible reason for this was an effect of the procedure of transporting all the animals at the same time to the room where they were decapitated at intervals of 1–2 min. Pituitary-adrenal activation might have been induced by the novel environment, including the odor of blood of animals decapitated earlier in the sequence. Therefore, in the second experiment and all the others reported in this paper, the animals were carried individually to the novel environment within 2 min of decapitation. The mean plasma corticosterone for the vehicle animals in the second experiment (Fig. 1) was within the usual normal range and reliably lower than the vehicle mean for the first experiment. Progressively higher

References p. 329–330

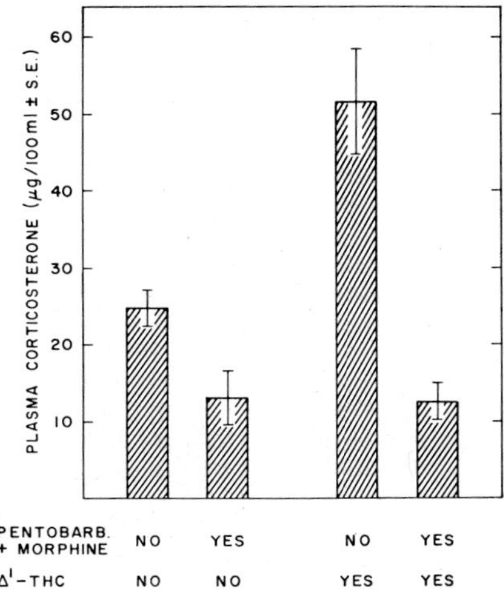

Fig. 3. Effects of pretreatment with pentobarbital (pentobarb.; 50 mg/kg), morphine (20 mg/kg), Δ^1-THC (8 mg/kg), or their vehicles, on plasma corticosterone.

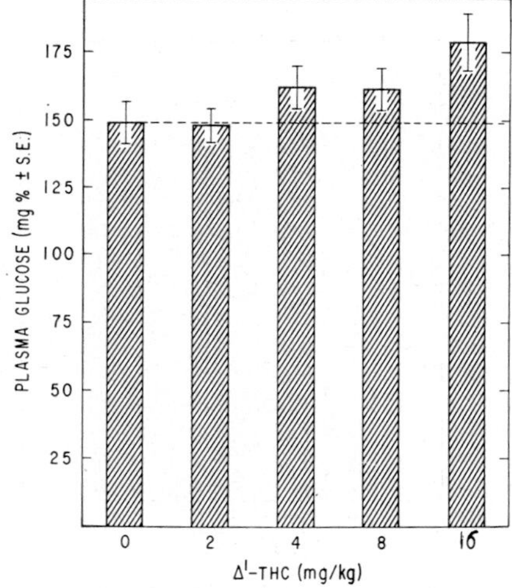

Fig. 4. Plasma glucose at 45 min after injection of Δ^1-THC or its vehicle.

levels were found with increasing doses of Δ^1-THC (1, 2, 4 mg/kg). The average levels for the two higher doses were reliably above the vehicle average. Almost parallel increases from vehicle to 4 mg/kg, in the two experiments, indicate that the effect of Δ^1-THC was independent of the baseline value.

The stability of this effect of Δ^1-THC after repeated doses is portrayed in Fig. 2, showing data for three groups of eight rats each. One group was injected with Δ^1-THC on each of eight successive days. The second group was injected with the vehicle for the first seven days and the drug for the first time on the eighth day. The third group was injected with the vehicle on each of the eight days. The plasma corticosterone, at 45 min after injection on the eighth day, shows a reliable elevation both for the acute Δ^1-THC group (following its first drug dose) and the chronic Δ^1-THC group (eight doses) compared with the vehicle group. A trend toward tolerance or habituation is indicated by the slightly lower corticosterone level for the chronic than the acute drug group, but the difference was short of statistical significance.

An experiment giving evidence for a central site of the Δ^1-THC effect is portrayed in Fig. 3. Data were obtained from 8–10 rats in each of the four groups, all given three injections at 10-min intervals and sacrificed at 45 min after the third injection. The corticosterone of the control group apparently became elevated above the usual normal level after two injections of saline followed by an injection of the vehicle for Δ^1-THC. Pretreatment with an anesthetic dose of pentobarbital sodium (20 mg/kg) followed by morphine sulfate (20 mg/kg) has been shown to block the secretion of corticotrophin-releasing factor from the hypothalamus, thereby preventing centrally acting stimuli from evoking pituitary-adrenal activation (Briggs and Munson, 1955). Fig. 3 shows that this treatment reduced plasma corticosterone reliably below the control level. When the vehicles for pentobarbital and morphine were followed by Δ^1-THC instead of its vehicle, corticosterone was greatly elevated. However, this effect of Δ^1-THC was completely blocked by the pentobarbital-morphine pretreatment. Therefore, the pituitary-adrenal activating effect of Δ^1-THC occurs at a central rather than peripheral site.

Plasma glucose was measured in a total of 50 rats, divided equally among the five dosage conditions shown in Fig. 4. The animals were sacrificed at 45 min after injection of vehicle or drug. Fig. 4 shows that all except the lowest dose of Δ^1-THC increased plasma glucose, although a statistically reliable difference from the vehicle group was found only with the highest dose of Δ^1-THC (16 mg/kg).

Urine was collected during 6 h after injection of Δ^1-THC (8 mg/kg) or its vehicle; 20 rats given each treatment were housed in pairs in metabolism cages. Table I shows a reliable diuretic effect of Δ^1-THC. The concentrations of electrolytes (mequiv./l) indicate sodium retention and elevated potassium excretion.

In a further experiment, urine was collected for only 1.5 h after injection with Δ^1-THC (16 mg/kg). Sufficient urine was obtained from 6 of 8 rats to allow comparison with predrug control. The urinary excretion of sodium after drug was decreased to 60.7 $\pm$ 14.7 mequiv./l compared with the control value of 211.1 $\pm$ 22.3. This difference was statistically highly reliable. Potassium concentration was slightly increased to 15.2 mequiv./l, compared with a preinjection control of 14.2. Therefore, the effects of Δ^1-THC after 1.5 h agree closely with the effects shown in Table I after 6 h.

DISCUSSION

Similarity between Δ^1-THC and alcohol effects on plasma corticosterone was previously noted by Kubena *et al.* (1971). In common with the further effects of Δ^1-THC reported in the present paper, intoxicating doses of alcohol generally give rise to

References p. 329–330

TABLE I

URINE VOLUME AND ELECTROLYTES AT 6 h AFTER INJECTION OF Δ^1-THC (8 mg/kg) OR ITS VEHICLE

	Vehicle	*Δ^1-THC*
Volume (ml; mean ± S.E.M.)	5.3 ± 0.5	12.0 ± 0.6[b]
Sodium (mequiv./l; mean ± S.E.M.)	218.2 ± 12.5	179.6 ± 8.5[a]
Potassium (mequiv./l; mean ± S.E.M.)	13.2 ± 0.1	14.1 ± 0.1[b]

[a] $p < 0.01$ for difference from vehicle.
[b] $p < 0.001$ for difference from vehicle.

hyperglycemia and to increased urinary excretion, with lower sodium and higher potassium concentrations (Wallgren and Barry, 1970). The hyperglycemia and changes in urinary electrolytes are those which would be expected from a centrally mediated stress response, which causes pituitary-adrenal activation and stimulates secretion of both glucocorticoids and mineralocorticoids. Contrary to the usual effect of acute stressors is the diuresis, and this effect of alcohol has been attributed to central inhibition of antidiuretic hormone (Wallgren and Barry, 1970).

The pituitary-adrenal activation in response to stressors is also elicited by a variety of depressant and sedative drugs (Marks and Bhattacharya, 1970; Ellis, 1966). This drug effect is paradoxical because at sufficiently high doses the same drugs block the endocrinological response, as seen in the present paper for two of these drugs, pentobarbital and morphine (Fig. 3). The pituitary-adrenal activation in response to lower doses may reflect a homeostatic, compensatory response to counteract the depressant effect on functions of the central nervous system.

Pituitary-adrenal activation is a non-specific response to various stressors and drugs. Both Δ^1-THC and alcohol are differentiated from most of the depressant drugs by the continuing corticosterone elevation after several daily doses and by the diuretic effect. Therefore, the effects of Δ^1-THC on urine excretion (Table I) emphasize the similarity already noted between Δ^1-THC and alcohol in endocrinological effects.

Both physiological and behavioral measures are needed to obtain a full understanding of drug effects (Barry and Buckley, 1966). The physiological effects of Δ^1-THC indicate resemblances of this compound to central depressants, in particular alcohol. At present, behavioral data seem necessary for identification of a unique profile of effects for Δ^1-THC, differentiating it from all other drugs. Behavioral experiments with Δ^1-THC (Kubena and Barry, 1970) indicate a predominantly depressant effect of the doses used in the present experiment, but stimulant effects of this drug have also been found (Barry and Kubena, 1969). The depressant or sedative effect of alcohol appears to be more generalized and consistent (Wallgren and Barry, 1970). A high degree of specificity in the subjectively perceived effects of Δ^1-THC is indicated by rats trained to make one response when injected with Δ^1-THC (4 mg/kg) and a different response when injected with the vehicle. The Δ^1-THC response is elicited by marihuana, which contains this compound, but not in tests with a variety of stimulants, depressants and hallucinogens (Barry and Kubena, 1972; Kubena and Barry, 1972).

Pituitary-adrenal activation, which characterizes human patients with adrenal hyperfunction or during ACTH or cortisone treatment, may account for their emotional reactions of elation, depression, and sometimes psychosis (Schildkraut *et al.*, 1968). This endocrinological response to Δ^1-THC, demonstrated in rats, is a plausible explanation for observations (Schultes, 1969) of the same emotional reactions in some users of marihuana. Hollister *et al.* (1970) measured plasma cortisol in humans given Δ^1-THC orally in doses up to approx. 1 mg/kg. Cortisol was elevated only as a concomitant of a severe anxiety reaction which occurred in a minority of the individuals. This gives further evidence for involvement of a centrally mediated stress response in the effects of Δ^1-THC in rats, reported in the present paper.

SUMMARY

Assays of plasma corticosterone in male albino rats indicated strong pituitary-adrenal activation at 45 min after intraperitoneal injection of Δ^1-tetrahydrocannabinol (Δ^1-THC), with doses of 2–16 mg/kg. Pretreatment with high doses of pentobarbital and morphine indicated a hypothalamic or other central locus of this action of Δ^1-THC. This steroid activation is an effect of various depressant drugs. The Δ^1-THC also caused plasma hyperglycemia, measured after 45 min, retention of sodium and increased excretion of potassium, measured in the urine during 6 h, suggesting pituitary-adrenal activation, such as is elicited by stressors. Additional findings were diuresis and continuation of the increase in corticosterone after a week of daily doses of Δ^1-THC. This profile of physiological effects is similar to that reported for ethyl alcohol, differentiating these two compounds from other depressant or sedative drugs.

ACKNOWLEDGMENTS

This research was partially supported by U.S. Public Health Service Research Scientist Development Award K2-MH-5921 and Research Grant MH-13595, both from the National Institute of Mental Health, and by Public Health Service Training Grant GM-1217 from the National Institute of General Medical Sciences.

REFERENCES

BARRY, H., III AND BUCKLEY, J. P. (1966) Drug effects on animal performance and the stress syndrome. *J. pharm. Sci.*, **55**, 1159–1183.

BARRY, H., III AND KUBENA, R. K. (1969) Acclimation to laboratory alters response of rats to Δ^1-tetrahydrocannabinol. *Proc. 77th ann. Conv. Amer. Psychol. Assoc.*, **4**, 865–866.

BARRY, H., III AND KUBENA, R. K. (1972) Discriminative stimulus characteristics of alcohol, marihuana and atropine. In *Drug Addiction, Vol 1, Experimental Pharmacology*, J. M. SINGH, L. H. MILLER AND H. LAL (Eds.), Futura, Mt. Kisco, N.Y.

BRIGGS, F. N. AND MUNSON, P. C. (1955) Studies on the mechanism of stimulation of ACTH secretion with the aid of morphine as a blocking agent. *Endocrinology*, **57**, 205–219.

DEWEY, W. L., PENG, T.-C. AND HARRIS, L. S. (1970) The effect of 1-*trans*-Δ^9-tetrahydrocannabinol on the hypothalamo-hypophyseal-adrenal axis of rats. *European J. Pharmacol.*, **12**, 382–384.

DUBOWSKI, K. M. (1962) An *O*-toluidine method for body-fluid glucose determination. *Clin. Chem.*, **8**, 215–235.

ELLIS, F. W. (1966) Effect of ethanol on plasma corticosterone levels. *J. Pharmacol. exp. Ther.*, **153**, 121–127.

GAONI, Y. AND MECHOULAM, R. (1964) Isolation, structure, and partial synthesis of an active constituent of hashish. *J. Amer. chem. Soc.*, **86**, 1646–1647.

GUILLEMIN, R., CLAYTON, G., SMITTY, J. AND LIPSCOMB, H. (1959) Fluorimetric measurement of rat plasma and adrenal corticosterone concentration. *J. lab. clin. Med.*, **53**, 830–832.

HOLLISTER, L. E., MOORE, F., KANTER, S. AND NOBLE, E. (1970) Δ^1-Tetrahydrocannabinol, synhexyl, and marijuana extract administered orally in man: Catecholamine excretion, plasma cortisol levels and platelet serotonin content. *Psychopharmacologia*, **17**, 354–360.

KUBENA, R. K. AND BARRY, H., III (1970) Interactions of Δ^1-tetrahydrocannabinol with barbiturates and methamphetamine. *J. Pharmacol. exp. Ther.*, **173**, 94–100.

KUBENA, R. K. AND BARRY, H., III (1972) Stimulus characteristics of marihuana components. *Nature (Lond.)*, **235**, 397–398.

KUBENA, R. K., PERHACH, J. L., JR. AND BARRY, H., III (1971) Corticosterone elevation mediated centrally by Δ^1-tetrahydrocannabinol. *European J. Pharmacol.*, **14**, 89–92.

MARKS, B. H. AND BHATTACHARYA, A. N. (1970) Psychopharmacological effects and pituitary-adrenal activity. In *Pituitary, Adrenal and the Brain* (Progr. Brain Res., Vol. 32), D. DE WIED AND J. A. W. M. WEIJNEN (Eds.), Elsevier, Amsterdam, pp. 57–70.

MECHOULAM, R. (1970a) Marijuana chemistry. *Science*, **168**, 1159–1166.

MECHOULAM, R. (1970b) Chemical basis of hashish activity. *Science*, **169**, 611–612.

PERHACH, J. L., JR. AND BARRY, H., III (1970) Stress responses of rats to acute body or neck restraint. *Physiol. Behav.*, **5**, 443–448.

SCHILDKRAUT, J. H., DAVIS, J. M. AND KLERMAN, G. L. (1968) Biochemistry of depressions. In *Psychopharmacology: A Review of Progress*, D. H. EFRON (Ed.), U.S. Public Health Service Publ. No. 1836, Washington, D.C., pp. 625–648.

SCHULTES, R. E. (1969) Hallucinogens of plant origin. *Science*, **163**, 245–254.

SOFIA, R. D., KUBENA, R. K. AND BARRY, H., III (1971) Comparison of four vehicles for intraperitoneal administration of Δ^1-tetrahydrocannabinol. *J. Pharm. Pharmacol.*, **23**, 889–891.

WALLGREN, H. AND BARRY, H., III (1970) *Actions of Alcohol. Vol. 1: Biochemical, Physiological and Psychological Aspects. Vol. 2: Chronic and Clinical Aspects*, Elsevier, Amsterdam.

Discussion on p. 336.

Δ^1-Tetrahydrocannabinol and Luteinizing Hormone Secretion

BERNARD H. MARKS

Department of Pharmacology, The Ohio State University, Columbus, O. 43210 (U.S.A.)

Despite the widespread use of marijuana, and some popular anecdotal reports of disturbances in menstrual cycling associated with the use of marijuana, there are no quantitative studies of the effect of this agent upon gonadotrophin secretion. For no apparent reason, it would appear that most experimental pharmacologic studies have been carried out solely on males (LeDain, 1972). However, females of some species have been reported to be more responsive to cannabis effects than males (Braude *et al.*, 1971). For these reasons we decided to examine the effect of an active principle derived from marijuana, Δ^1-tetrahydrocannabinol (THC) upon gonadotrophin secretion in female rats. In this report we will show the effect of Δ^1-THC upon luteinizing hormone (LH) secretion in rats which had been ovariectomized 3–5 weeks previously. Serum LH was measured by double antibody radio-immunoassay, using the antibody and standard LH provided by the Pituitary Hormone Program, NIAMD-NIH (Monroe *et al.*, 1968). Results are expressed in terms of rat LH reference preparation, RP-1, which has a biological potency of 0.03 $\times$ the purified standard, NIH-LH-SI.

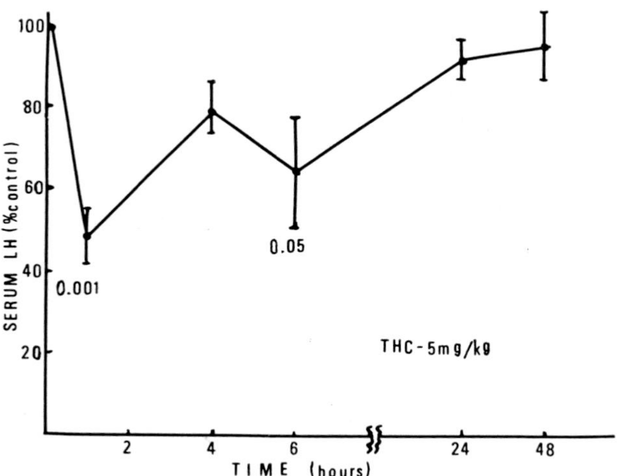

Fig. 1. Time course of changes in serum LH following intravenous administration of Δ^1-THC emulsion. Solvent control used for each group. Groups consist of 4–6 rats ovariectomized for 3–5 weeks. Vertical bars are S.E.M.

References p. 336-337

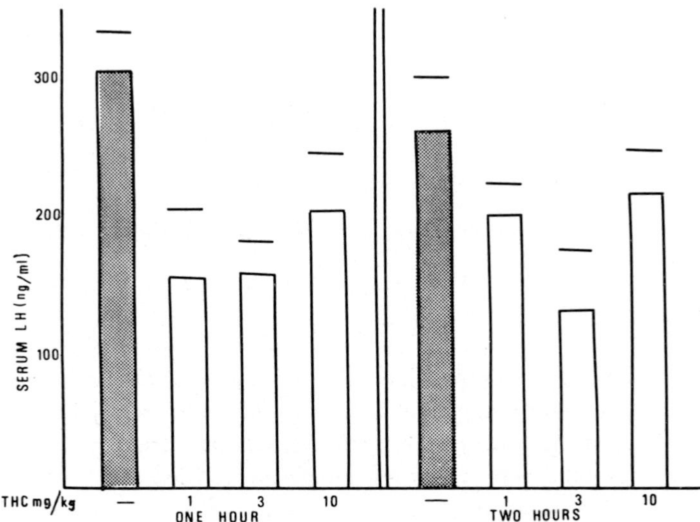

Fig. 2. Dose-dependent changes in serum LH 1 and 2 h after intravenous administration of Δ^1-THC emulsion. LH expressed as ng of reference standard RP-1. Groups consist of 4–6 rats ovariectomized for 3–5 weeks. Shaded bars are solvent controls, horizontal lines above each bar are S.E.M.

Purified Δ^1-THC was administered intravenously after brief ether anesthesia. The Δ^1-THC was emulsified immediately before injection, in a solvent system of 5% Tween 80, 1% ethanol, and 10% glycerol in water (Wall *et al.*, 1970). Solvent injection controls were included in all experiments.

Initial experiments were performed using 5 mg/kg Δ^1-THC, an amount which was known to produce readily evident behavioral changes in rats, consisting of marked

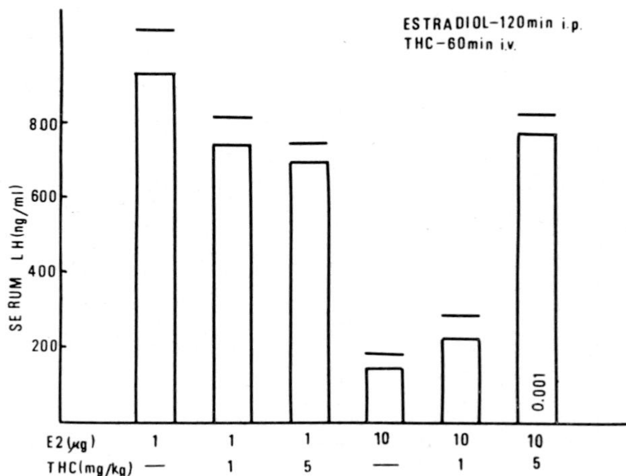

Fig. 3. Changes in serum LH following i.v. administration of Δ^1-THC to estradiol pre-treated rats. Estradiol-treated rats were given either solvent or Δ^1-THC emulsion intravenously 1 h later. Rats were sacrificed 1 h after Δ^1-THC or solvent. Other conditions as in Fig. 2. *P* values as indicated on bars.

reduction of spontaneous motor activity and a cataleptic state in which the muscles appear to be rather tense and rigid. These changes are maximal about 30 min after intravenous injection. Fig. 1 shows that 5 mg/kg of Δ^1-THC inhibits secretion of LH. The inhibition is marked at 1 h, and somewhat less at 4 h and 6 h. By 24 and 48 h after administration of Δ^1-THC, the inhibitory effect had dissipated. Each group in this figure had its own solvent control, and since these data were combined from several groups of ovariectomized rats, and different immunoassay runs, they are presented as the percent of their individual control groups.

In order to get some idea of the dose-dependence of these effects, LH concentration of serum was measured at 1 and at 2 h after doses of Δ^1-THC ranging from 1 to 10 mg/kg. It is evident in Fig. 2 that 1 mg/kg, the lowest dose tested, produced marked reduction of LH in 1 h, but the effect had partially dissipated by 2 h. With 3 mg/kg Δ^1-THC, the effect was maintained and even increased at 2 h. With 10 mg/kg Δ^1-THC, we were clearly dealing with supramaximal doses, acting by additional mechanisms, since the effect of this large dose was less than that of smaller doses. The dose range of Δ^1-THC, over which conventional dose-response relationships exist, has not yet been defined.

What is of considerable interest in relation to the significant inhibition of LH secretion produced by Δ^1-THC is the neurochemical basis for this phenomenon. One way of approaching this kind of question with an agent with possibly varied effects on the brain, is to determine how the inhibitory effects of Δ^1-THC interact with the known physiologically active mechanisms. One such mechanism that would be of interest to study is the complex action of estrogens on gonadotrophin secretion. A preliminary examination of the interaction of Δ^1-THC with estradiol reveals a curious antagonism (Fig. 3). Ovariectomized rats were pretreated with either a large (10 μg) or a small (1 μg) dose of estradiol. Δ^1-THC was given 1 h later and rats

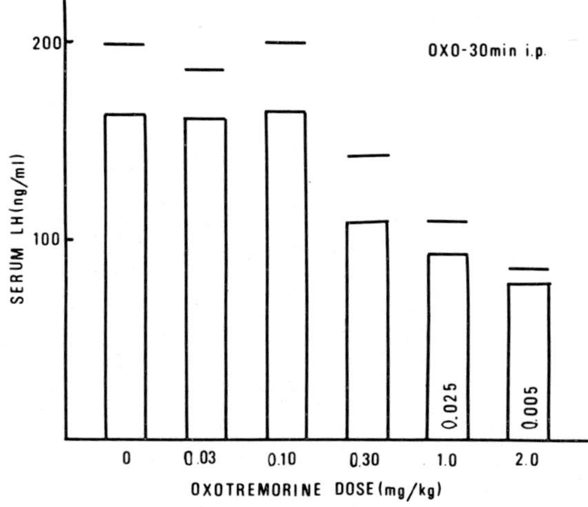

Fig. 4. Dose dependence of oxotremorine (OXO) effect upon serum LH. OXO given i.p. in saline, rats sacrificed 30 min later. Other conditions as in Fig. 2. *P* values indicated on bars.

References p. 336-337

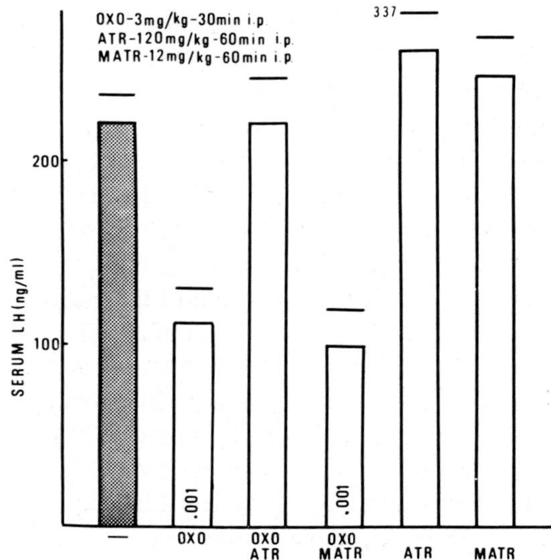

Fig. 5. Reversal of OXO effect on serum LH by atropine. Atropine (ATR) or *N*-methyl atropine (MATR) given i.p.; 30 min later OXO given i.p. Saline injections used as control in each instance in which no drug was given. *P* values on bars refer to control group, shaded bar. Other conditions as in Fig. 2.

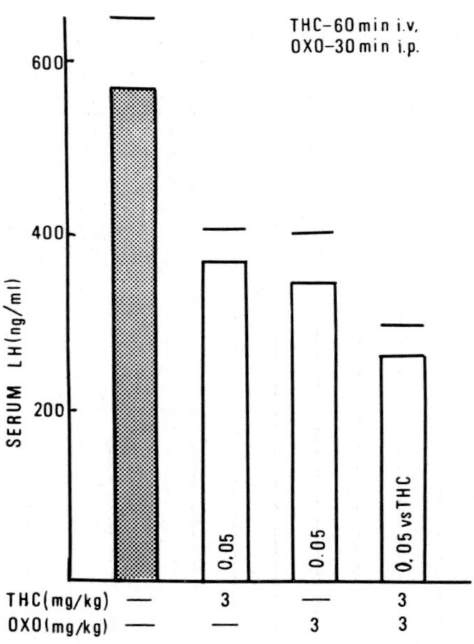

Fig. 6. Effect of Δ^1-THC combined with OXO on serum LH of ovariectomized rats. Each group treated with the appropriate solvent control injections as indicated by the dashes under each bar. *P* values are against solvent control (shaded bar) except for THC plus OXO group which is against THC group. Other conditions as in Fig. 2.

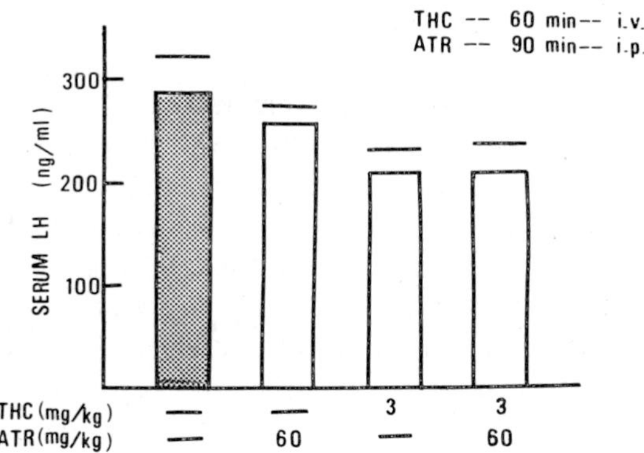

Fig. 7. Effect of ATR on LH response to Δ^1-THC. Each group given solvent control injections indicated by the dashes under each bar. Other conditions as in Fig. 2.

sacrificed 1 h after Δ^1-THC. With a large dose of estradiol, which inhibits LH secretion, Δ^1-THC appears to prevent and reverse the estrogen effect. With a low dose of estradiol, which did not inhibit LH secretion, the Δ^1-THC appears to exert less than its usual depressant effect. The mechanism of this antagonistic action of Δ^1-THC and estrogen is still not at all clear and will require further study.

Another possible mechanism of Δ^1-THC effect that we have had occasion to examine is the interaction with agents that act upon muscarinic receptors. The reasons for selecting this mechanism for study were reports (Phillips *et al.*, 1971) that Δ^1-THC toxicity was associated with peripheral cholinergic symptoms, and that Δ^1-THC increased the toxicity of physostigmine (Rosenblatt *et al.*, 1972). We chose to use the drug oxotremorine in studying central muscarinic effects on LH secretion. Oxotremorine acts upon muscarinic receptors both centrally and peripherally, producing a rhythmic tremor of central origin as well as a peripheral cholinergic syndrome. Data presented here are for 30 min after injection, when the effects of oxotremorine appear to be maximal. It produces dose-dependent inhibition of LH secretion (Fig. 4) in ovariectomized rats. The effect of oxotremorine is blocked by atropine but not by the quaternary nitrogen derivative methylatropine (Fig. 5), which antagonizes all the peripheral muscarinic effects of oxotremorine. This suggests that the action of oxotremorine in inhibiting LH secretion is due in fact to central muscarinic activation.

In view of this central muscarinic mechanism which inhibits LH secretion, it was interesting to find that when both Δ^1-THC and oxotremorine are administered, their effects on LH secretion are less than additive (Fig. 6). In addition, it was noted that the marked tremor associated with oxotremorine administration was considerably attenuated in those rats also given Δ^1-THC. The actions of Δ^1-THC on LH secretion cannot, therefore, be attributed to cholinergic activation. Independence of the actions of Δ^1-THC from cholinergic mechanisms is further shown by lack of interference in the effects of Δ^1-THC by administered atropine (Fig. 7).

These initial experiments demonstrate clearly that Δ^1-THC can reduce LH secretion in ovariectomized rats. The mechanism by which Δ^1-THC produces this effect is quite

References p. 336-337

obscure, as is still the neurochemical basis for the effect of Δ^1-THC on sensory perception and on motor behavior. What is quite clear is that the action of Δ^1-THC is not related to activation of muscarinic receptors. It is possible, on the other hand, that the action of Δ^1-THC may be related to its observed ability to increase the uptake and retention of catecholamines by brain tissues (Fuxe and Jonsson, 1972; Truitt and Anderson, 1972). Thus, if catecholamines released from hypothalamic nerve terminals increase the secretion of LH-releasing factor (LRF) (Schneider and McCann, 1969; Kamberi *et al.*, 1970; Schneider and McCann, 1970; Kamberi *et al.*, 1971), an increase in the rate of catecholamine re-uptake, resulting in a reduced post-synaptic effect of catecholamines, is compatible with the observed inhibition of LH secretion. Such a mechanism should be amenable to experimental study, given existing techniques.

There is increasing evidence that the chronic administration of Δ^1-THC produces central nervous effects somewhat different from those associated with acute treatment (Thompson *et al.*, 1971), and further that the central effects of this agent may be due to hydroxylated metabolites (Lemberger *et al.*, 1970). Thus it may be desirable in the future to compare the chronic effects of Δ^1-THC and its metabolites with those of single doses upon endocrine regulation in order to appreciate the full endocrine consequences of exposure to marijuana.

REFERENCES

BRAUDE, M. C., MANSAERT, R. AND TRUITT, E. B., JR. (1971) Some pharmacologic correlates to marihuana use. *Seminars in Drug Therapy*, **1**, 229–244.

FUXE, K. AND JONSSON, G. (1972) Effect of tetrahydrocannabinol on central monoamine neurons. *Acta pharm. suec.*, **8**, 695.

KAMBERI, I. A., SCHNEIDER, H. P. G. AND MCCANN, S. M. (1970) Action of dopamine to induce release of FSH-releasing factor (FRF) from hypothalamic tissue *in vivo*. *Endocrinology*, **86**, 278–284.

KAMBERI, I. A., MICAL, R. S. AND PORTER, J. C. (1971) Effect of anterior pituitary perfusion and intraventricular injection of catecholamines on FSH release. *Endocrinology*, **88**, 1003–1011.

LEDAIN, G., Chairman (1972) *Cannabis: A Report of the Commission of Inquiry into the Nonmedical Use of Drugs*, Ottawa, p. 35.

LEMBERGER, L., SILBERSTEIN, S. D., AXELROD, J. AND KOPIN, I. J. (1970) Studies on the disposition and metabolism of delta-9-tetrahydrocannabinol in man. *Science*, **170**, 1320–1322.

MONROE, S. E., PARLOW, A. F. AND MIDGLEY, A. R. (1968) Radioimmunoassay for rat luteinizing hormone. *Endocrinology*, **83**, 1004–1012.

PHILLIPS, R. N., TURK, R. F. AND FORNEY, R. B. (1971) Acute toxicity of Δ^9-tetrahydrocannabinol in rats and mice. *Proc. Soc. exp. biol. Med.*, **136**, 260–263.

ROSENBLATT, J. E., JANOWSKY, D. S., DAVIS, J. M. AND EL-YOUSEF, M. K. (1972) The augmentation of physostigmine toxicity in the rat by Δ^9-tetrahydrocannabinol. *Res. Comm. chem. path. Pharmacol.*, **3**, 479–482.

SCHNEIDER, H. P. G. AND MCCANN, S. M. (1969) Possible role of dopamine as transmitter to promote discharge of LH-releasing factor. *Endocrinology*, **85**, 121–132.

SCHNEIDER, H. P. G. AND MCCANN, S. M. (1970) Release of LH-releasing factor (LRF) into the peripheral circulation of hypophysectomized rats by dopamine and its blockade by estradiol. *Endocrinology*, **78**, 249–253.

THOMPSON, G. R., ROSENKRANTZ, H. AND BRAUDE, M. C. (1971) Neurotoxicity of cannabinoids in chronically treated rats and monkeys. *Pharmacologist*, **13**, 296.

TRUITT, E. B., JR. AND ANDERSON, S. H. (1972) Biogenic amine alterations produced in the brain by tetrahydrocannabinol and their metabolites. *Ann. N.Y. Acad. Sci.*, **191**, 68–71.

WALL, M. E., BRINE, D. R., BRINE, G. A., PITT, C. G., FREUDENTHAL, R. I. AND CHRISTENSEN,

H. D. (1970) Isolation, structure, and biological activity of several metabolites of Δ^9-tetrahydrocannabinol. *J. Amer. chem. Soc.*, **92**, 3466–3468.

DISCUSSION

HODGES: I should like to ask Dr. Barry why he thinks the effects of THC are unique. After all, the injection of any drug may elevate plasma corticosterone levels and the degree of elevation is likely to be directly proportional to the intensity of local irritation that the drug produces. Moreover, lots of drugs will elevate blood glucose, many drugs have a diuretic effect, and it is not terribly difficult to think of drugs that would do all three things.

BARRY: I agree with you. I did not describe the unique effects of THC because of the present state of our knowledge these all seem to be behavioral. Observations and experiments on various species of laboratory animals under the influence of THC indicate an unusual combination of depressant and stimulant effects. For example, complete motionless changes suddenly to squeaking and other strong startle responses to mild stimulation. A particular basis for concluding a high degree of specificity in effects of this drug is our behavioral technique of training rats to make a differential response on the basis of whether they are under the THC or non-drug condition, thereby establishing the drug as a discriminative stimulus for a differential response (Barry and Kubena, 1972; Kubena and Barry, 1972). These animals select the non-drug response in tests with a number of other compounds, including mescaline, LSD, DMT, chlorpromazine, chlordiazepoxide, alcohol, amphetamine and cocaine, but the animals do make the THC response in tests with a large enough dose of marijuana which contains that compound.

ALIVISATOS: Has anyone tried antabuse in connection with marijuana?

MARKS: It might be appropriate to do that, but I don't know of anyone who has.

BARRY: It is an interesting idea because THC and alcohol seem to have so many physiological effects in common.

SHASKAN: Few drugs increase the uptake of catecholamines. As a matter of fact, this is the first report that I've heard of THC increasing the reuptake of catecholamines. Was there any difference in the effect of THC on dopamine or noradrenaline re-uptake?

MARKS: I did not say that we have done these studies. These were things that have been reported. Perhaps Dr. Harris, who is more familiar with this area, could amplify that.

HARRIS: I just want to put forth a word of caution about the effects of this particular drug on catecholamines and indoleamines. There are, in the literature many reports on studies of this drug and its relationship with these amines. You can find reports which say that it increases levels, decreases levels, or has no effect, and I think this is a picture that you, endocrinologists, are seeing over and over again as you start working with these neurotransmitter substances. Our own studies at this time would point towards the drug having no specific interaction with neurotransmitter substances in the indole or catecholamine systems.

MARKS: Lou, are you referring to THC effects on brain content of catecholamines? But there have been reports in which synaptasomes, for example, from THC-treated animals seem to show an unusually rapid rate of noradrenaline uptake and you are in a better position to evaluate them than I am.

HARRIS: I look at such reports and I am very cool toward them. I submit to you who are also beginning to work very actively in this field that the technical aspects of the assay of these various amines are not simple. One must carry out extremely careful and sophisticated studies. Just taking pieces or fractions of brain tissue and placing them in the presence of various amines or assaying their amine content can lead to a great deal of confusion. For instance, the day-to-day, or even hour-to-hour variations in catecholamine and indoleamine levels in the brain are greater than most of the effects produced by drugs that have been described at this meeting.

PODOLSKY: In line with the interesting presentations of Dr. Barry and Dr. Marks, I would like to present some preliminary data on the growth hormone levels in chronic marijuana users. The drug, dose and route of administration were selected to approximate the way in which marijuana is commonly used. Dr. Monique Braude kindly arranged for extraction and analysis of the street marijuana used in these studies (Δ^1-THC content of the marijuana was 1.1%). Four healthy psychologically stable chronic marijuana users (21–24) abstained from cannabis and other drugs for seven days before getting the first of two oral glucose tolerance tests (GTT). After the baseline GTT, all subjects returned to heavy marijuana use in the form of deeply inhaled cigarettes. The cigarettes were rolled from the same batch of marijuana and all subjects reported a definite euphoriant effect. After one week the subjects had repeat GTT carried out under identical conditions except that one half of the mariujana cigarette was smoked by each subject immediately prior to glucose ingestion. Plasma glucose levels were higher after marijuana. But there were no definite abnormalities of insulin or growth hormone. There was little difference in growth hormone levels and in the control and post-marijuana GTT's. It is interesting that there was no suppression of fasting growth hormone levels after glucose in the marijuana experiment; however, this is sometimes seen in healthy subjects. The rebound elevation of growth hormone late in the course of the GTT appears to be higher after marijuana. At this time, however, it is quite speculative to relate these apparent changes in growth hormone to the modest deterioration in glucose tolerance in these subjects. The data have been published (Ann. N.Y. Acad. Sci., 191, 54, 1971).

Effects of Narcotic Analgesics on Hypothalamo-Pituitary-Thyroid Function

ROBERT GEORGE

Department of Pharmacology and Brain Research Institute, Center for the Health Sciences, University of California, Los Angeles, Calif. 90024 (U.S.A.)

Most of the early publications regarding the interrelationship of morphine and the thyroid dealt chiefly with the effects of administration of thyroid preparations or thyroidectomy on morphine toxicity. Data from studies in mice, rats, guinea pigs, dogs and rabbits have been conflicting, although in man the consensus is that hypothyroidism may lead to increased sensitivity to morphine (Krueger *et al.*, 1941).

In view of our present knowledge about thyroid physiology and neuroendocrine control mechanisms it is rather surprising that very few studies have been done to determine the effects of narcotic analgesics, agents which are widely used clinically, on thyroid activity.

The first studies in which ^{131}I was used for assessing pituitary-thyroid activity during morphine administration were reported by Sámel (1958). He injected rats subcutaneously for 5 days with morphine (10 mg/kg) and then measured ^{131}I uptake by the thyroid and the level of protein-bound ^{131}I in blood. Both were reduced significantly when compared with uninjected controls, as were the pituitary and thyroid weights. In another experiment Sámel determined the effect of morphine on the rate of release of thyroid hormone by measuring the radioactivity of the neck region of ^{131}I-labeled thyroids. Injection of morphine was found to inhibit significantly the normal release rate.

Redding *et al.* (1966) have reported similar findings in mice following the administration of morphine, codeine, dihydromorphinone, levorphan, dextrorphan or meperidine. The injection of 500 μg daily of each drug for 5 days significantly inhibited thyroidal ^{131}I uptake. On the other hand, when each drug was administered acutely as a single injection of 500 μg per mouse, there was a marked increase in release of ^{131}I from the thyroid and this effect was abolished by hypophysectomy. The inhibitory effect of chronic codeine administration on thyroid activity has been confirmed by Schreiber *et al.* (1968). They found that daily feeding of codeine (approximately 5 mg/kg) for a period of 14 days significantly reduced the uptake of ^{131}I by rat thyroids. However, hypertrophy of the pituitary and thyroid glands produced by methylthiouracil was not altered by chronic codeine administration. Thus, it would seem that

References p. 344–345

codeine can lower the basal rate of thyroid function but does not interfere with hypersecretion of thyrotrophin (TSH) where there is thyroid hormone deficiency.

Histological findings also have indicated that chronic morphine administration inhibits pituitary-thyroid function. Hohlweg *et al.* (1961) observed that injection of morphine twice daily (30 and 60 mg/kg) decreased significantly thyroid weights and pituitary TSH content, and prevented the appearance of thyroidectomy cells in the pituitaries of rats.

Although all of the data described above show that narcotic analgesics can modify thyroid gland activity, none show that their action is mediated *via* the hypothalamic-pituitary-thyroid axes. Thus, in collaboration with Doctors Peter Lomax and Norio Kokka, we have attempted to determine the site(s) and the mechanism(s) by which morphine alters thyroid function.

In all of our studies we have measured thyroid activity by studying the rate of loss of organically bound ^{131}I from the thyroid gland of rats. This is a more reliable method for measuring thyroid activity than the ^{131}I uptake method and provides a continuous measure of thyroid activity (Brown-Grant *et al.*, 1954a). The procedure consisted of injecting each rat with carrier-free radioiodine as [^{131}I] Na (5–20 μCi intraperitoneally for 3 days prior to the experiments. The radioactivity of the thyroid gland was measured then by placing the animal's neck over a flat field, 5-cm diameter scintillation detector. Prior conditioning of the animals ensured fairly constant positioning without struggling and the mean of three 10-sec counts was recorded. Decay curves of thyroid radioactivity, after correction for isotopic decay, against time and the release rate was calculated from the graph.

In an early study (George and Lomax, 1965) we noted that repeated administration of small doses of morphine sulfate (5–10 mg/kg) inhibited thyroid hormone release within 24 h following the first injection. This inhibition persisted throughout the injection period of 66 h and for 24–30 h following the last injection; the release rate then returned to normal (Table I). The injection of chlorpromazine (5 mg/kg) also promptly inhibited thyroid hormone release whereas reserpine, even in near lethal doses, was ineffective. Since morphine and chlorpromazine are known to increase

TABLE I

SUMMARY TABLE OF THE EFFECTS OF SYSTEMIC ADMINISTRATION OF MORPHINE ON THYROID ^{131}I RELEASE RATES IN INTACT, ADRENALECTOMIZED AND HYPOTHALAMIC LESIONED RATS

	Number of animals	*Mean initial release rate ± S.E.M. (% per 24 h)*	*Mean release rate after morphine (%)*	*P*
Intact	10	16.9 ± 0.7	3.0 ± 0.8	<0.01
Adrex[a]	11	19.5 ± 1.7	1.5 ± 0.6	<0.01
Rostral hypothalamic lesions	9	14.8 ± 0.6	3.0 ± 1.1	<0.01
Caudal hypothalamic lesions	9	13.4 ± 0.8	13.0 ± 1.0	>0.5

[a]Adrenalectomized.

adrenal corticosteroid secretion, and since a variety of stresses and corticosteroid administration (Brown-Grant *et al.*, 1954b, c) inhibit thyroid activity, the effects of morphine and chlorpromazine were investigated in adrenalectomized animals.

It was found that adrenalectomy did not interfere with the thyroid-inhibiting effect of both morphine and chlorpromazine; in fact, the effect was slightly enhanced (Table I). In addition, experiments were done to determine whether morphine inhibited thyroid activity by interfering with the action of TSH on the thyroid. It was noted that administration of TSH stimulated release of thyroid hormone in morphinized rats to the same degree as that found in the controls. Thus, on the basis of these findings and those reported by others, it appeared that the inhibitory action of morphine on thyroid activity is mediated at the level of the pituitary gland or the central nervous system (CNS).

In order to further localize this inhibitory site of morphine action, studies were designed to investigate the effects of systemic morphine administration on thyroid release rates in rats with hypothalamic lesions (Lomax and George, 1966). Bilateral electrolytic lesions were made in two groups of rats: one in the region of the anterior hypothalamic/ventromedial nuclei and the other in the medial mammillary nuclei. Repeated injections of morphine (5–10 mg/kg) produced a marked inhibition in thyroid activity in rats with anterior lesions. The inhibition was comparable to that found in intact animals. On the other hand, lesions in the mammillary nuclei completely blocked the thyroid-inhibitory effect of morphine and the release curves were virtually identical with those of untreated controls (Table I). The lesion sites, on histological examination were found to involve, rostrally, the paraventricular and anterior hypothalamic nuclei and, caudally, all or part of the medial mammillary nuclei. Most importantly, the median eminence and the infundibular tract were left intact. From these data it would appear that the thyroid inhibitory effect of morphine is mediated *via* the caudal hypothalamus in the region of the medial mammillary nuclei.

It is well established that the anterior region of the median eminence of the hypothalamus is concerned with the regulation of pituitary TSH secretion. Electrolytic lesions in this area reduce the basal level of thyroid secretion and prevent propylthiouracil-induced goiter formation while electrical stimulation of this region increases thyroid activity (Harris and George, 1969), and recently it has been shown by Martin and Reichlin (1970) that such stimulation increases plasma TSH levels as measured by radioimmunoassay in rats. And finally, the presence of thyrotrophin-releasing factor (TRF) in this region has been clearly documented.

Also, it is apparent that many regions of the CNS which relay to the hypothalamus participate in the regulation of TSH secretion, and the anterior median eminence region probably represents the final pathway through which reflex inhibition or activation of TSH secretion takes place. Supporting evidence for such a concept comes from the following reports: lesions in the region of the habenular nuclei abolish iodine-deficiency goiter and reduce the inhibitory effect of thyroxine on TSH secretion (Szentágothai and Mess, 1958; Bogdanove, 1962); midbrain transection in the dog inhibits thyroidal ^{131}I release (Anderson *et al.*, 1957); electrical stimulation of the hippocampus elicited an increase in release of ^{131}I-labeled thyroid hormone in

References p. 344–345

dogs (Shizume *et al.*, 1962). Inhibition of thyroid hormone release has been noted also following electrical stimulation of the mesencephalic reticular formation in rats (Kovacs *et al.*, 1965) and caudal hypothalamus in rats (Vertes *et al.*, 1965) and rabbits (Harris and Woods, 1958).

Morphine is a compound which has a dual action on the CNS, *i.e.* it may act as a stimulant or a depressant. The dose of morphine used in these studies (5 mg/kg) was found to cause an elevation in body temperature in the rat in contrast to higher doses which produced a marked hypothermia. These temperature changes are due to a direct action of morphine on the thermoregulatory centers in the anterior hypothalamus (Lotti *et al.*, 1965a). Also, injection of morphine into rats pretreated with nalorphine, or into rats made tolerant to morphine, frequently produced a rise in their body temperature (Lotti *et al.*, 1965b; 1966).

If one assumes that tolerance develops to the depressant and not the stimulant effects of morphine (Seevers and Deneau, 1963) and that nalorphine antagonizes, primarily, the depressant effects of morphine (Woods, 1956), then the increase in core temperature in the rats studied by Lotti *et al.* (1965a and b) must be due to a stimulant effect of morphine on the thermoregulatory centers in the hypothalamus. Thus, if we can extrapolate from these studies to the effect of morphine on thyroid activity, it would seem possible that the dose of morphine used (5 mg/kg) could have had an excitatory effect on the hypothalamic neurons resulting in a reduction in thyroid activity by activation of inhibitory areas in the posterior hypothalamus.

To test this hypothesis, studies were undertaken to determine the effects of microinjection of morphine into various regions of the hypothalamus on thyroid function in the rat (Lomax *et al.*, 1970). Guides for injection cannulae were implanted symmetrically on each side of the midline. The guides were positioned so as to allow injection at various sites, within 1 mm of the mid-sagittal plane, extending from the preoptic to the supramammillary nuclei. The position of the injection sites were verified on completion of the experiments by injecting 1 μl of methyl red at the same point as the drug and sectioning the brains on a freezing microtome. For intracerebral injection, morphine sulfate was dissolved in 0.9% NaCl. The concentration was adjusted so as to allow a constant injection volume of 1 μl. Doses of 5 or 10 μg of morphine were injected.

A total of 36 rats received bilateral injections of morphine sulfate into various regions of the hypothalamus. They were injected with 5 μg in each site at 48 and 56 h, then 10 μg at 72 and 80 h after the onset of thyroid counting. Of the animals so treated, 14 exhibited marked inhibition of thyroid ^{131}I release during the period of injections. The injection sites in these 14 rats were found to lie in two principal areas: between the preoptic nuclei and the chiasma or in the region of the posterior and supramammillary nuclei. In the 6 rats with rostral injection sites, morphine completely arrested the release of ^{131}I, but the release returned to normal after the 72nd h, before the final injection of morphine. In contrast to these animals, the release of ^{131}I was abolished throughout the period of morphine administration in the 8 animals injected into the caudal hypothalamic regions. Injection of morphine into other hypothalamic sites failed to alter normal thyroid activity.

The inhibition of thyroid secretion following morphine injection into the rostral hypothalamus was a rather unexpected finding and indicates that the drug does not have a single site of action. These data pointed out that morphine has a more complex action on pituitary-thyroid function than we had visualized from our earlier experiments.

As mentioned previously, morphine has a dual action on the CNS, both stimulation and depression of neurons can occur. Tolerance develops to the depressant but not to the stimulant action of morphine. Therefore, it is interesting to note that, in the case of injections into the rostral hypothalamic sites, there was a reversion to the normal thyroid release rate even during the period of morphine administration. This suggests the development of tolerance to morphine. A similar type of tolerance was seen to the hypothermic effect of morphine by Lotti *et al.* (1966). In contrast to this, tolerance was not detected when morphine was injected into the caudal hypothalamus. It would seem then that there are two target sites for morphine in the hypothalamus: both activation of a caudal site and depression of a rostral site leading to decreased pituitary-thyroid activity. This possibility is further supported by the studies of Lotti *et al.* (1965a) who found that injection of microquantities of morphine into the rostral hypothalamus produced hypothermia, catatonia, respiratory depression and an increase in pain threshold, effects which are commonly noted after a large systemic dose of morphine. Conversely, injection of morphine into the caudal hypothalamus produced hyperthermia and marked excitation, associated with increased motor activity and agressive behavior.

SUMMARY

It appears that narcotic analgesics have a dual action on the secretion of thyrotrophin (TSH) secretion, however, the predominant effect appears to be one which produces inhibition of pituitary-thyroid function. The inhibitory effect of morphine on TSH secretion is mediated *via* the hypothalamic-pituitary axis and probably by an excitation of inhibitory neurons that lie in the caudal hypothalamus.

Although the mechanism(s) by which narcotic analgesics influence hypothalamic-pituitary activity has not been clearly elucidated, two possibilities arise. The first is that analgesics exert their effect on the pituitary through a direct action on the hypothalamic neurosecretory cells that contain releasing factors. The second possibility focusses on the presence of the "neurotransmitters", acetylcholine, dopamine, noradrenaline and serotonin which are found in the hypothalamus. If these transmitters lie in a presynaptic position to neurosecretory cells, it is conceivable that narcotic analgesics can exert their action on the pituitary by interfering with the synthesis and/or release of the neurotransmitters at the presynaptic site, thereby altering the activity of the neurosecretory cells.

Of these two possibilities, the latter seems more likely since there is evidence that narcotic analgesics may alter release and turnover of the neurotransmitters (Smith

References p. 344–345

1972) and that the neurotransmitters have been implicated in the control of pituitary function (George, 1971).

ACKNOWLEDGEMENT

The preparation and part of the work reported in this manuscript were supported by research grants from USPHS, MH-17691, and MH-20787.

REFERENCES

Anderson, E., Bates, R. W., Hawthorne, E., Haymaker, W., Knowlton, K., Rioch, D. McK., Spence, W. R. and Wilson, H. (1957) The effects of midbrain and spinal cord transection on endocrine function with postulation of a midbrain hypothalamico-pituitary activating system. *Recent Progr. Hormone Res.*, **13**, 21–66.

Bogdanove, E. M. (1962) Regulation of TSH secretion. *Fed. Proc.*, **21**, 623–627.

Brown-Grant, K., Von Euler, C., Harris, G. W. and Reichlin, S. (1954a) The measurement and experimental modification of thyroid activity in the rabbit. *J. Physiol. (Lond.)*, **126**, 1–28.

Brown-Grant, K., Harris, G. W. and Reichlin, S. (1954b) The effect of emotional and physical stress on thyroid activity in the rabbit. *J. Physiol. (Lond.)*, **126**, 29–40.

Brown-Grant, K., Harris, G. W. and Reichlin, S. (1954c) The influence of the adrenal cortex on thyroid activity in the rabbit. *J. Physiol. (Lond.)*, **126**, 41–51.

George, R. (1971) Hypothalamus: anterior pituitary gland. In *Narcotic Drugs Biochemical Pharmacology*, D. H. Clouet (Ed.), Plenum, New York, pp. 283–299.

George, R. and Lomax, P. (1965) The effects of morphine, chlorpromazine and reserpine on pituitary-thyroid activity in rats. *J. Pharmacol.*, **150**, 129–134.

Harris, G. W. and George, R. (1969) Neurohumoral control of the adenohypophysis and the regulation of the secretion of TSH, ACTH and growth hormone. In *The Hypothalamus*. W. Haymaker, E. Anderson and W. J. H. Nauta (Eds.), Thomas, Springfield, Ill., pp. 326–388.

Harris, G. W. and Woods, J. W. (1958) The effect of electrical stimulation of the hypothalamus or pituitary gland on thyroid activity. *J. Physiol. (Lond.)*, **143**, 246–274.

Hohlweg, V. W., Knappe, G. and Dörmer, G. (1961) Tierexperimentelle Untersuchungen über den Einfluss von Morphin auf die Gonadotrope und thyrotrope Hypophysenfunktion. *Endokr. Bd.*, **40**, 152–159.

Krueger, H., Eddy, N. B. and Sumwalt, M. (1941) Pharmacology of the opium alkaloids. *U.S. Public Health Service, Public Health Report Suppl. 165*, parts 1 and 2.

Kovacs, S., Vertes, Z., Sandor, A. and Vertes, M. (1965) The effect of mesencephalic lesions and stimulation on pituitary-thyroid function. *Acta physiol. acad. sci. hung.*, **26**, 227–233.

Lomax, P. and George, R. (1966) Thyroid activity following administration of morphine in rats with hypothalamic lesions. *Brain Res.*, **2**, 361–367.

Lomax, P., Kokka, N. and George, R. (1970) Thyroid activity following intracerebral injection of morphine in the rat. *Neuroendocrinology*, **6**, 146–152.

Lotti, V. J., Lomax, P. and George, R. (1965a) Temperature responses in the rat following intracerebral microinjection of morphine. *J. Pharmacol.*, **156**, 135–139.

Lotti, V. J., Lomax, P. and George, R. (1965b) *N*-allylnormorphine antagonism of the hypothermic effect of morphine in the rat following intracerebral and systematic administration. *J. Pharmacol.*, **156**, 420–425.

Lotti, V. J., Lomax, P. and George, R. (1966) Acute tolerance to morphine following systemic and intracerebral injection in the rat. *Int. J. Neuropharmacol.*, **5**, 35–42.

Martin, J. B. and Reichlin, S. (1970) Thyrotropin secretion in rats after hypothalamic electrical stimulation or injection of synthetic TSH-releasing factor. *Science*, **168**, 1366–1388.

Redding, T. W., Bowers, C. Y. and Schally, A. V. (1966) The effects of morphine and other narcotics on thyroid function in mice. *Acta endocrinol.*, **51**, 391–399.

Sámel, M. (1958) Blocking of the thyrotrophic hormone secretion by morphine and chlorpromazine in rats. *Arch. int. Pharmacodyn.*, **117**, 151–157.

SCHREIBER, V., ZBUSEK, V. AND ZBUZKOVA-KMENTOVA, V. (1968) Effect of codeine on thyroid function in the rat. *Physiol. bohemoslov.*, **17**, 253–258.

SEEVERS, M. H. AND DENEAU, G. A. (1963) Physiological aspects of tolerance and physical dependence. In *Physiological Pharmacology*, vol. 1, W. S. ROOT AND F. G. HOFMAN (Eds.), Academic Press, New York, pp. 565–640.

SHIZYME, K., MATUZAKI, F., IINO, S., MATSUDA, K., NAGATAKI, S. AND OKINAKA, S. (1962) Effect of electrical stimulation of the limbic system on pituitary-thyroidal function. *Endocrinology*, **71**, 456–463.

SMITH, C. B. (1972) Neurotransmitters and the narcotic analgesics. In *Chemical and Biological Aspects of Drug Dependence*, S. J. MULÉ AND H. BRILL (Eds.), CRC Press, Cleveland, pp. 495–504.

SZENTÁGOTHAI, J. AND MESS, B. (1958) Central control of thyrotropic activity of the anterior pituitary lobe; functional significance of nucleus medialis habenulze. *Wien. Klin. Wschr.*, **70**, 259–261.

VERTES, M., VERTES, Z. AND KOVACS, S. (1965) Effect of hypothalamic stimulation on pituitary-thyroid function. *Acta physiol.*, **27**, 229–235.

WOODS, L. A. (1956) The pharmacology of nalorphine. *Pharmacol. Rev.*, **8**, 175–198.

DISCUSSION

ALIVISATOS: In view of our previous reports that morphine interferes competitvely with certain serotoninergic receptors, I wonder whether serotonin was tried in counteracting this effect of morphine?

GEORGE: The mechanism by which morphine inhibits thyroid activity is complicated and does not seem to be serotonin-linked. We know that the amines in the hypothalamus are concerned with secretion of the anterior lobe hormones. We also know that morphine influences the levels or the turnover rates of these amines. In studies I didn't include here, we morphinized animals over a 6 week period and then challenged them with TRF. TRF, in the doses used, produced an increase in the release of thyroid hormone of normal animals but was blocked in the morphine-treated animals. On the basis of these preliminary findings we suspect that possibly the blocking effect is somewhere between TRF and the pituitary gland.

KASTIN: Just to extend to humans, your last remark, although methadone certainly isn't morphine, we have tested, in collaboration with Drs. Ruiz and Vargas, TRH administration in 4 patients treated with methadone. Three of them gave perfectly normal responses and one gave no response so we are further looking at that.

KRIVOY: Would you like to speculate on the relevance of these data to the addiction cycle?

GEORGE: I don't think the pituitary hormones are directly involved in addiction although they may still play a secondary role in the addiction cycle. We all know that the addiction problem is a serious and complex one. For example, the controversy regarding the role of serotonin in the development of physical dependence to morphine has not been resolved.

MESS: It appeared that the anterior hypothalamic lesions were ventral and the posterior ones were localized more dorsally. If so, your data would correlate with thermal regulatory data of my experiments with Dr. Donhoffer.

GEORGE: The drug effect was most pronounced when placed in the thermoregulatory area and reduced when the drug was injected into a more dorsal site.

Effects of Acute and Chronic Administration of Narcotic Analgesics on Growth Hormone and Corticotrophin (ACTH) Secretion in Rats

NORIO KOKKA*, JOSEPH F. GARCIA** AND HENRY W. ELLIOTT*

*Department of Medical Pharmacology and Therapeutics, California College of Medicine, University of California, Irvine;**Lawrence Radiation Laboratory, University of California, Berkeley, Calif. (U.S.A.)

The effects of narcotic analgesics on corticotrophin (ACTH)-secretion and on hypothalamo-pituitary systems have been reviewed recently by Sloan (1971) and by George (1971). The latter review cited relatively few references to the effects of acute and chronic administration of morphine on growth hormone (GH) secretion in comparison to the numerous reports of its effect on ACTH release. We recently reported an inverse relationship between GH and ACTH secretion in rats (Kokka *et al.*, 1972). In agreement with the findings of Takahashi *et al.* (1971), common stressful stimuli that produce an elevation of plasma corticosterone were shown to simultaneously cause a significant fall of plasma GH. The only exception to this inverse correlation between plasma concentrations of corticosterone and GH occurred after injection of morphine, which caused significant increases in plasma concentrations of both hormones (Kokka *et al.*, 1972). Although morphine is known to have both depressant and excitant effects on the central nervous system (CNS), the rise of plasma GH was attributed to suppression of an inhibitory mechanism since pentobarbital produces a similar increase of GH.

The present experiments were designed (*a*) to compare the acute effects of various narcotic analgesics on GH and ACTH secretion, and (*b*) to examine endocrine aspects of tolerance in rats treated chronically with morphine or methadone.

METHODS

Only male Sprague-Dawley rats weighing between 200–300 g were used in these experiments. Variations of plasma corticosterone concentration due to "transfer stress" or to circadian changes were minimized by keeping the animals in the laboratory overnight and by performing all experiments between 8:30 to 11:30 *a.m.*

For the acute studies, all drugs were administered intraperitoneally (i.p.). The animals were observed continuously after drug injection and gently moved whenever ventilation could have been impaired by body position or close contact with other rats.

References p. 358

The rats were decapitated with a guillotine at 30, 60, or 120 min after drug injection to avoid stress stimulation of ACTH release which occurs with other methods involving restraint or ether anesthesia and venipuncture. Blood was collected in heparinized beakers, and after removal of 0.1 ml for glucose determination (Washko and Rice, 1961), the remainder was transferred to tubes and centrifuged; plasma was separated for analysis of GH and corticosterone (indirect measure of ACTH). Plasma GH was measured by radioimmunoassay (Garcia and Geschwind, 1968) and corticosterone by fluorescence assay (Guillemin *et al.*, 1959).

For the chronic studies, rats received subcutaneous injections of drugs twice daily at 8:00 to 8:30 *a.m.* and 4:30 to 5:30 *p.m.* Therefore, the time between the last chronic dose and the test dose the following day was approx. 15–16 h. The effects of chronic treatment were determined by measuring corticosterone and GH in plasma 30 min after injection of the test dose of morphine or methadone.

The following drugs were dissolved in 0.9% saline and administered in doses calculated as the free base; morphine sulfate, methadone hydrochloride, codeine phosphate, thebaine hydrochloride, apomorphine hydrochloride, nalorphine hydrochloride and naloxone hydrochloride. Statistical evaluation of the data was performed by Student's "*t*" test; a value of $P < 0.05$ was considered statistically significant.

RESULTS

Effects of narcotic analgesics

Dose-response studies with various narcotic analgesics were done, because it is generally accepted that in rodents morphine-like drugs have a biphasic effect on the CNS characterized by depression with low doses and by stimulation with high doses. The results of these experiments are shown in Table I. The lowest dose of morphine, 5 mg/kg, produced sedation and, with the exception of an increase of GH at 60 min, blood glucose and plasma corticosterone and GH concentrations were the same as the saline controls. Rats injected with 10 mg/kg of morphine exhibited catatonia, respiratory depression and analgesia to toe or tail pinch. The results show that plasma GH of these rats was elevated at all 3 sampling times, whereas corticosterone showed an increase only at 60 min. Doses of 20 mg/kg or more were required for consistent stimulation of ACTH secretion. Table I also shows that the 20 mg/kg dose was as potent as the 40 and 80 mg/kg doses in stimulating ACTH release. On the other hand, these high doses of morphine were less effective than the 10 mg/kg dose in stimulating GH release. 20 mg/kg of morphine produced significant increases of plasma GH as well as corticosterone at 30 and 60 min, and 40 and 80 mg/kg doses of morphine had the shortest duration of stimulant action on GH secretion. The results also show that the graded doses of morphine employed in this study did not produce hyperglycemia in fasted rats. On the contrary, the largest dose, 80 mg/kg, produced a significant hypoglycemia at 60 min as well as the greatest changes of behavior and signs of toxicity.

TABLE I

EFFECTS OF NARCOTIC ANALGESICS ON BLOOD GLUCOSE, PLASMA CORTICOSTERONE AND GH OF FASTED RATS

	Dose mg/kg	min after injection								
		30			60			120		
		Blood glucose mg/100 ml	Cortico-sterone μg/100 ml	GH ng/ml	Blood glucose mg/100 ml	Cortico-sterone μg/100 ml	GH ng/ml	Blood glucose mg/100 ml	Cortico-sterone μg/100 ml	GH ng/ml
Saline	—	(5) 71 ± 2[a]	17 ± 3	9 ± 3	(5) 80 ± 3	8 ± 2	24 ± 4	(6) 75 ± 2	12 ± 3	19 ± 6
Morphine	5	(4) 78 ± 9	8 ± 4	25 ± 10	(4) 72 ± 5	13 ± 5	44 ± 6[c]	(4) 78 ± 2	14 ± 5	15 ± 5
	10	(7) 74 ± 2	29 ± 5	77 ± 14[b]	(7) 73 ± 2	41 ± 7[b]	49 ± 4[b]	(5) 92 ± 12	21 ± 9	49 ± 10[c]
	20	(6) 71 ± 4	51 ± 5[b]	65 ± 20[c]	(6) 76 ± 6	37 ± 4[b]	65 ± 14[c]	(6) 90 ± 11	51 ± 5[b]	32 ± 7
	40	(6) 80 ± 6	60 ± 7[b]	33 ± 6[c]	(7) 82 ± 8	50 ± 4[b]	33 ± 4	(6) 63 ± 14	59 ± 9[b]	30 ± 7
	80	(4) 60 ± 4	53 ± 6[b]	46 ± 2[b]	(5) 37 ± 10	63 ± 7[b]	33 ± 4	(4) 65 ± 14	50 ± 6[b]	20 ± 5
Methadone	5	(4) 87 ± 7	35 ± 10	50 ± 3[b]	(4) 75 ± 5	25 ± 10	37 ± 7	(4) 89 ± 8	21 ± 15	40 ± 14
	10	(4) 76 ± 13	67 ± 8[b]	32 ± 6[c]	(4) 41 ± 15	41 ± 4[b]	21 ± 8	(4) 49 ± 11	34 ± 5[b]	11 ± 5
	20	(4) 24 ± 1[b]	37 ± 4[b]	45 ± 6[b]	(6) 24 ± 4[c]	47 ± 5[b]	39 ± 7	(5) 39 ± 6[c]	39 ± 4[b]	14 ± 2
Codeine	10	(4) 88 ± 4	14 ± 3	51 ± 12[b]	(4) 75 ± 4	16 ± 5	47 ± 11[c]	(4) 82 ± 3	14 ± 5	15 ± 3
	20	(4) 75 ± 4	26 ± 10	87 ± 14[b]	(4) 83 ± 9	35 ± 17	38 ± 4[c]	(4) 77 ± 6	6 ± 1	36 ± 9
	40	(4) 86 ± 9	70 ± 3[b]	13 ± 4	(4) 80 ± 12	42 ± 3[b]	16 ± 6	(4) 79 ± 10	38 ± 2[b]	19 ± 6
Thebaine	5	(5) 84 ± 4	29 ± 5[c]	18 ± 9	(5) 72 ± 3	11 ± 2	52 ± 13[c]	(5) 78 ± 2	8 ± 3	16 ± 7
	10	(5) 96 ± 10	34 ± 5[c]	18 ± 12	(5) 90 ± 8	12 ± 1	27 ± 9	(5) 90 ± 6	7 ± 3	26 ± 8
	15	(6) 80 ± 5	30 ± 5	49 ± 14	(5) 72 ± 1	16 ± 5	14 ± 4	(5) 81 ± 2	6 ± 2	13 ± 4
Apomorphine	5	(5) 85 ± 11	37 ± 4[b]	3 ± 2[c]	(4) 79 ± 5	37 ± 10[c]	4 ± 4[b]			
	10	(4) 88 ± 8	48 ± 2[b]	5 ± 2	(4) 77 ± 7	48 ± 8[b]	9 ± 4[c]	(4) 85 ± 4	15 ± 9	11 ± 7

[a]Mean ± S.E.M. Number of rats in parentheses.
[b]$P < 0.01$.
[c]$P < 0.05$.

References p. 358

Experiments with methadone were done with lower doses of 5, 10 and 20 mg/kg since it is relatively toxic to rats. The highest dose approximated the LD_{25}. As shown in Table I, 5 mg/kg of methadone produced increases of plasma corticosterone and GH which were not statistically significant except for the rise of GH at 30 min. The gross effects of 10 and 20 mg/kg of methadone on behavior as well as the endocrine effects were similar to those produced by 40 and 80 mg/kg of morphine. 10 and 20 mg/kg of methadone caused an initial rise of both plasma corticosterone and GH. The effect on corticosterone persisted for 120 min whereas plasma GH fell to control levels after 30 min. A marked hypoglycemia, similar to that occurring after 80 mg/kg of morphine, was also found in the rats injected with methadone. Since these rats were cyanotic, the hypoglycemia may be attributable to hypoxia which is known to increase glucose uptake by peripheral tissues (Russell *et al.*, 1944; Randle *et al.*, 1958; Morgan *et al.*, 1961).

Codeine, a weaker analgesic than morphine and methadone, in doses of 10 and 20 mg/kg produced a rise of plasma GH but not of corticosterone. A reversal in response was obtained with the highest dose of 40 mg/kg which stimulated ACTH secretion but had little or no effect on GH secretion. In contrast to morphine and methadone, high doses of codeine did not produce simultaneous increases of plasma corticosterone and GH.

The effects of thebaine were also studied because this compound is closely similar in structure to morphine but is reported to have mainly excitant effects and little or no depressant activity. Thebaine was found to be an extremely potent convulsant. The LD_{50} in mice as determined in this laboratory was 2.0 mg/kg when given intravenously. 5, 10 and 15 mg/kg of thebaine, doses that are non-convulsant when administered i.p., had no consistent effect on ACTH and GH secretion in rats. Table I shows that a moderate increase of plasma corticosterone occurred 30 min after 10 mg/kg of the baine, whereas plasma GH but not corticosterone was elevated 30 min after 15 mg/kg. Thus, plasma corticosterone and GH concentrations of rats treated with sub-convulsant doses of thebaine generally did not differ significantly from those of the saline-treated controls. Experiments with higher doses of thebaine were not feasible because of its toxicity. For example, 5 of 6 rats convulsed and died within 15 min when the dose of thebaine was increased to 20 mg/kg.

The effects of apomorphine on GH and ACTH secretion were studied because this drug, in contrast to morphine, produces a stereotyped, excitatory behavior characterized by gnawing, sniffing and increased motor activity, resembling in many respects the effects of amphetamine in rats. The results in Table I show that 5 mg/kg of apomorphine produced inverse changes in ACTH and GH secretion. Plasma corticosterone rose and GH decreased significantly when compared to the saline controls. A dose of 10 mg/kg produced similar changes except that plasma GH was not significantly diminished at 30 min.

Effects of narcotic antagonists

The effects of the narcotic antagonists, nalorphine and naloxone, are shown in Table II.

TABLE II

EFFECTS OF NARCOTIC ANTAGONISTS ON BLOOD GLUCOSE, PLASMA CORTICOSTERONE AND GH OF FASTED RATS

	Dose mg/kg	min after injection								
		30			60			120		
		Blood glucose mg/100 ml	Cortico-sterone μg/100 ml	GH ng/ml	Blood glucose mg/100 ml	Cortico-sterone μg/100 ml	GH ng/ml	Blood glucose mg/100 ml	Cortico-sterone μg/100 ml	GH ng/ml
Saline[b]	—	(5) 71 ± 2[a]	17 ± 3	9 ± 3	(5) 80 ± 3	8 ± 2	24 ± 4	(6) 75 ± 2	12 ± 3	19 ± 6
Nalorphine	11	(4) 80 ± 3	32 ± 6	25 ± 3[c]	(4) 74 ± 6	44 ± 10[a]	16 ± 5	(4) 81 ± 1	4 ± 2	22 ± 7
	22	(4) 86 ± 3	37 ± 8[d]	55 ± 12[c]	(3) 91 ± 3	46 ± 9[c]	60 ± 32	(5) 91 ± 2	27 ± 6	14 ± 4
	44	(4) 70 ± 2	52 ± 6[c]	39 ± 9[c]	(4) 64 ± 2	49 ± 3[c]	42 ± 8	(4) 80 ± 3	14 ± 5	21 ± 6
Naloxone	2	(4) 72 ± 2	17 ± 3	5 ± 2	(4) 72 ± 4	7 ± 3	17 ± 5	(4) 71 ± 3	2 ± 1	22 ± 13
	11	(5) 75 ± 2	20 ± 4	12 ± 6	(15) 74 ± 2	16 ± 4	31 ± 6	(12) 79 ± 2	5 ± 1	35 ± 5
	23	(7) 82 ± 4	30 ± 3[c]	14 ± 3	(7) 81 ± 2	8 ± 3	39 ± 9	(9) 93 ± 6	4 ± 2	22 ± 8
	46	(4) 68 ± 3	19 ± 2	14 ± 1	(4) 68 ± 3	19 ± 2[d]	27 ± 8	(4) 77 ± 4	3 ± 2	20 ± 9

[a]Mean ± S.E.M. Number of rats in parentheses.
[b]From Table I.
[c]$P < 0.01$.
[d]$P < 0.05$.

TABLE III

EFFECTS OF NALOXONE PRETREATMENT ON BLOOD GLUCOSE, PLASMA CORTICOSTERONE AND GH OF RATS

	Dose mg/kg	Naloxone mg/kg − 30 min	min after injection					
			30			60		
			Blood glucose mg/100 ml	Cortico-sterone μg/100 ml	GH ng/ml	Blood glucose mg/100 ml	Cortico-sterone μg/100 ml	GH ng/ml
Morphine	20	(5) 11	78 ± 3[a]	24 ± 6	41 ± 11[a]	(5) 80 ± 1	11 ± 3	60 ± 24
	40	(5) 11	82 ± 4	23 ± 6	48 ± 14[c]	(6) 76 ± 2	10 ± 3	70 ± 17[c]
Thebaine	10	(6) 10	85 ± 4	29 ± 3	9 ± 4	(6) 73 ± 2	12 ± 3	41 ± 10
Apomorphine	5	(5) 10	71 ± 6	50 ± 4[b]	3 ± 0.2[c]	(5) 69 ± 7	43 ± 6[b]	6 ± 3[c]
	10	(5) 10	84 ± 8	49 ± 6[b]	3 ± 0.1[c]	(5) 78 ± 6	39 ± 4[b]	3 ± 0.6[b]

[a]Mean ± S.E.M. Number of rats in parentheses.
[b]$P < 0.01$.
[c]$P < 0.05$.

Nalorphine, which has many of the agonist actions of morphine, in doses equimolar to 10, 20 and 40 mg/kg of morphine produced simultaneous increases of plasma corticosterone and GH at 30 but not at 60 and 120 min. The major difference from morphine was its weaker stimulatory effect and shorter duration of action. In contrast to nalorphine, naloxone, which is reported to have none of the agonist properties of morphine, had no effects on GH and only minor effects on ACTH secretion. A small but statistically significant increase of plasma corticosterone occurred 30 and 60 min after injection of 23 and 46 mg/kg of naloxone, respectively.

Effects of naloxone pretreatment

The effects of nalorphine and naloxone indicate a relationship between agonist activity of narcotic antagonists and their effects on ACTH and GH secretion. Since it is generally accepted that narcotic antagonists block mainly the depressant but not the stimulant actions of morphine, the effects of morphine on GH and ACTH secretion in rats pretreated with naloxone were determined to help decide whether the stimulation of GH and ACTH release by morphine is due to a depressant or an excitatory effect on the CNS.

As shown in Table III, 20- and 40-mg/kg doses of morphine that produced marked increases of plasma corticosterone had no effect in rats previously injected with 11 mg/kg of naloxone. Morphine stimulation of GH release, on the other hand, was not antagonized by naloxone. The increases of plasma GH were statistically significant when compared either to the saline controls (Table I) or to the naloxone-injected rats (Table II). Since naloxone blocks the effects of morphine on ACTH but not on GH secretion, the stimulatory effects of morphine on the mechanisms that regulate the secretion of these two pituitary hormones are apparently attributable to different actions of morphine. Failure to achieve complete blockade with naloxone is possible but considered unlikely since high antagonist:agonist ratios of 1:2 and 1:4 were used and overt behavioral signs of depression or stimulation were never observed.

As shown in Table III, the endocrine effects of thebaine and apomorphine are not modified by naloxone. Blood glucose, plasma corticosterone and GH after injection of thebaine in naloxone-treated rats were not significantly different when compared to the groups injected with saline or naloxone alone. Also, the rise of corticosterone and the fall of GH in plasma produced by apomorphine were not altered by naloxone. Although apomorphine and morphine both activate ACTH release, the results obtained with naloxone suggest these two drugs act by different mechanisms. In addition, the lowering of plasma GH by apomorphine, in contrast to the rise produced by morphine, provides further support for the hypothesis that the endocrine effects in rats are due to different pharmacologic properties of these drugs.

Effects of chronic treatment

The effects of chronic drug administration on GH and ACTH secretion were studied because tolerance is reportedly acquired more readily to the depressant than to the

References p. 358

TABLE IV

EFFECTS OF CHRONIC DRUG TREATMENT ON BLOOD GLUCOSE, PLASMA CORTICOSTERONE AND GH OF RATS

		Days of chronic treatment						
		0[b] *(30 min)*	*1*	*2*	*4*	*6*	*8*	*12*
Morphine (*a*) 20 mg/kg	Blood glucose mg/100 ml	(6) 71 ± 4[a]	(5) 106 ± 5	(5) 101 ± 3	(8) 90 ± 4		(7) 109 ± 6	(4) 118 ± 4
	Cortico-sterone μg/100 ml	51 ± 5	22 ± 9[c]	25 ± 7[c]	10 ± 4[c]		24 ± 5[c]	16 ± 8[c]
	GH ng/ml	65 ± 20	63 ± 5	53 ± 11	44 ± 7		66 ± 16	83 ± 6
(*b*) 40 mg/kg	Blood glucose mg/100 ml	(6) 80 ± 6		(7) 123 ± 5	(7) 115 ± 3	(8) 108 ± 4	(8) 103 ± 3	(8) 107 ± 3
	Cortico-sterone μg/100 ml	60 ± 7		32 ± 5[c]	24 ± 6[c]	26 ± 7[c]	15 ± 4[c]	16 ± 4[c]
	GH ng/ml	33 ± 6		42 ± 3	43 ± 3	58 ± 10	44 ± 4	82 ± 12[c]
Methadone 10 mg/kg	Blood glucose mg/100 ml	(4) 76 ± 13			(4) 111 ± 7		(5) 119 ± 5	(5) 102 ± 5
	Cortico-sterone μg/100 ml	67 ± 9			15 ± 6[c]		16 ± 5[c]	7 ± 3[c]
	GH ng/ml	32 ± 6			71 ± 4[c]		103 ± 21[c]	100 ± 16[c]

[a]Mean ± S.E.M. Number of rats in parentheses.
[b]From Table I.
[c]$P < 0.01$.

stimulant effects of opiates. As shown in Table IV, with twice daily injections of 20 and 40 mg/kg of morphine, tolerance to the stimulant effect on ACTH secretion was present at 1 and 2 days, respectively. The rapid endocrine tolerance was somewhat unexpected because these rats still exhibited marked catatonia and respiratory depression. Secretion of GH, on the other hand, was not diminished and, instead, the data suggest that its release was moderately enhanced as rats acquired tolerance to the stressful effects of morphine. The greater rise of plasma GH occurring with chronic treatment was most evident in rats injected with 40 mg/kg of morphine or 10 mg/kg of methadone. It was noted earlier that these doses of morphine and methadone have comparable behavioral and endocrine effects, and the data in Table IV additionally show an augmentation of GH secretion following chronic administration of these two drugs.

Effects of withdrawal and stress

Experiments were undertaken next to determine whether chronic administration of morphine altered the endocrine response to various stimuli known to alter GH and ACTH secretion. For these studies, rats were injected twice daily with 40 mg/kg of morphine for 12 days, then subjected to the test procedures described in Table V. Naloxone produced a distinct withdrawal response consisting of hypermotility, aggressiveness, diarrhea and "wet-dog shakes". Acute drug-induced withdrawal concomitantly caused a sharp increase of plasma corticosterone and a decrease of plasma GH, the typical endocrine response of rats to stress. Since ACTH and GH secretion are inversely related in rats, the data show that chronic administration of morphine did not alter the normal release of these hormones in response to the stress

TABLE V

EFFECTS OF NALOXONE, ACTH AND STRESS ON BLOOD GLUCOSE, PLASMA CORTICOSTERONE AND GH OF RATS TREATED CHRONICALLY WITH MORPHINE

	Dose mg/kg	*30 min after injection*			
			Blood glucose mg/100 ml	*Cortico-sterone μg/100 ml*	*GH ng/ml*
Morphine[b]	40	(6)	107 ± 3[a]	16 ± 4	82 ± 12
Naloxone	10	(5)	193 ± 9	50 ± 5[c]	3 ± 0.1[c]
ACTH$_{\beta 1-24}$	1 U./kg	(5)	99 ± 3	37 ± 4[c]	8 ± 0.5[c]
Pentylenetetrazol	50	(3)	190 ± 4	48 ± 2[c]	2 ± 0.2[c]
Insulin	5 U./kg	(4)	63 ± 11	38 ± 7[d]	5 ± 2[c]
1 h cold exposure, 1 °		(4)	114 ± 5	45 ± 3[c]	2 ± 0.3[c]

[a]Mean ± S.E.M. Number of rats in parentheses.
[b]From Table IV (Morphine 40 mg/kg on 12th day).
[c]$P < 0.01$.
[d]$P < 0.05$.

References p. 358

of acute abstinence. In addition, the rise of plasma corticosterone following injection of synthetic ACTH shows that chronic injection of morphine did not impair adrenal steroid secretion.

The assumption that the development of tolerance to the morphine dose of 40 mg/kg employed in the present study did not impair the endocrine response to stress is supported by data obtained with pentylenetetrazol, insulin hypoglycemia and cold exposure which are known to elicit reciprocal changes of ACTH and GH secretion in normal rats. The data in Table V show that rats injected twice daily with 40 mg/kg of morphine also exhibit the same endocrine response to these stresses. Under the present experimental conditions, it would seem clear that although chronic administration of morphine both produces tolerance to its stimulant effect on ACTH and appears to enhance its effect on GH secretion, the secretion of these two pituitary hormones in response to various stresses is not impaired in tolerant rats.

DISCUSSION

In contrast to the numerous reports of increased GH secretion in man under conditions known to stimulate ACTH release, recent studies show that the secretion of these two pituitary hormones is inversely related in rats since diverse stressful stimuli that produce a rise of plasma corticosterone simultaneously cause inhibition of GH release. Enhanced GH secretion in rats, on the other hand, has been observed only after "gentling" (Schalch and Reichlin, 1968), electrical stimulation of the ventromedial nucleus of the hypothalamus (Frohman *et al.*, 1968) and administration of CNS depressants (Takahashi *et al.*, 1971). Morphine, which has both depressant and stimulant effects in rats, causes increases of both GH and corticosterone in plasma, thus altering the reciprocal relationship between GH and ACTH secretion (Kokka *et al.*, 1972).

The stimulation of both GH and ACTH secretion after administration of morphine is dose-dependent. The lower doses of 5 and 10 mg/kg of morphine used in this study produced mainly sedation, elevation of plasma GH and minimal stimulation of ACTH secretion, similar to the results obtained with pentobarbital. The higher doses of morphine had a short stimulant effect on GH secretion, and a longer action on ACTH release. The diminished effectiveness of high doses of morphine on GH secretion is probably a manifestation of the toxic, stressful effects of morphine which tend to abolish its own stimulant action on GH secretion.

This view is supported by the findings from the chronic injection experiments with morphine and methadone. High doses that produce a moderate, short-lasting increase of plasma GH in non-tolerant rats were found to have a marked stimulant effect in rats pretreated with these two drugs, suggesting that tolerance to the stress-mediated inhibitory effects on GH secretion developed without loss of its stimulant action. According to the view that tolerance is more readily acquired to the depressant than to the excitant effects of morphine-like drugs, diminution of ACTH secretion would be attributable to the former and the augmentation of GH secretion would be due to the latter property of these drugs. The results obtained with naloxone are consistent with this view. Narcotic antagonists blocked the acute stimulant effect of morphine on ACTH but had no effect on GH secretion, suggesting that the enhanced secretion of these two pituitary hormones is mediated by different pharmacological actions of morphine.

The present study is in agreement with previous reports of a dual action of morphine on ACTH secretion. Stimulation of ACTH release following acute administration and inhibition with chronic injection of morphine have been reported by several investigators (for recent reviews, see George, 1971 and Sloan, 1971). Morphine stimulation of ACTH secretion is probably mediated additively by a direct action on the hypothalamus (Lotti *et al.*, 1969) and by non-specific stress effects such as hypotension, hypoxia, hypothermia and adrenaline secretion (Fortier, 1966; Gold and Ganong, 1967).

Previous work (see George, 1971), showing inhibition of the stimulant effects of morphine on ACTH secretion by chronic drug administration and by nalorphine have been confirmed in this study. Similarly, the rise of plasma corticosterone observed during naloxone-precipitated abstinence is in agreement with that of Paroli and Melchiorri (1961) who found increased urinary excretion of corticosteroids during abstinence due to withdrawal of drug or administration of nalorphine.

Separation of the stimulant effects of morphine on GH from its action on ACTH secretion by chronic drug administration or by pretreatment with naloxone could be interpreted as evidence that separate systems govern the release of these two pituitary hormones. This interpretation would be in contrast to that of Takahashi *et al.* (1971) who recently suggested that GH and ACTH secretion are mediated by a final common pathway, possibly in the hypothalamus.

SUMMARY

The effects of narcotic analgesics on GH and ACTH secretion in rats appear to be dose-related. The lower doses of morphine, methadone and codeine employed in this study mainly caused a rise of plasma GH and had little or no effect on plasma corticosterone. Higher doses of morphine and methadone produced increases of both plasma corticosterone and GH. A greater stimulation of ACTH secretion than of GH secretion occurred with high doses since plasma corticosterone was elevated for 120 min, whereas plasma GH was not significantly different from the controls after 30 to 60 min. Subconvulsant doses of thebaine had little effect on ACTH and GH secretion. Apomorphine, which produces a marked increase of motor activity in rats, caused a significant rise of corticosterone and a fall of GH concentration in plasma. Naloxone did not antagonize the effects of apomorphine.

Dose-response studies with narcotic antagonists showed that nalorphine produced simultaneous increases of plasma corticosterone and GH, while naloxone had no consistent effects on GH or ACTH secretion. Separation of the stimulant effects of morphine on ACTH and GH secretion was achieved with naloxone, which blocked

References p. 358

the rise of plasma corticosterone but not of GH produced by morphine. Daily administration of morphine or methadone resulted in tolerance to the stimulant effects of test-doses of these drugs on ACTH secretion. Tolerance to the stimulant action on GH secretion could not be demonstrated. Acute abstinence produced by naloxone resulted in a marked increase of plasma corticosterone and a diminution of plasma GH. Similar changes of plasma corticosterone and GH were observed in morphine-tolerant rats after pentylenetetrazol, insulin hypoglycemia or cold exposure.

ACKNOWLEDGMENT

This work was supported in part by grants from the University of California, Irvine, California College of Medicine Research and Education Foundation, and the United States Atomic Energy Commission.

REFERENCES

FORTIER, C. (1966) The nervous control of ACTH secretion. In *The Pituitary Gland*, Vol. II, G. W. HARRIS AND B. T. DONOVAN (Eds.), Butterworth, London, pp. 195–234.

FROHMAN, L. A., BERNARDIS, L. L. AND KANT, K. J. (1968) Effect of hypothalamic stimulation on pituitary and plasma GH levels in rats. *Science*, **162**, 580–582.

GARCIA, J. F. AND GESCHWIND, I. I. (1968) Investigation of growth hormone secretion in selected mammalian species. In *Growth Hormone*, A. PECILE AND E. E. MULLER (Eds.), Excerpta Medica, Amsterdam, pp. 267–291.

GEORGE, R. (1971) Hypothalamus: anterior pituitary gland. In *Narcotic Drugs Biochemical Pharmacology*, D. H. CLOUET (Ed.), Plenum, New York, pp. 283–299.

GOLD, E. M. AND GANONG, W. F. (1967) Effects of drugs on neuroendocrine processes. In *Neuroendocrinology*, Vol. II, L. MARTINI AND W. F. GANONG (Eds.), Academic Press, New York, pp. 377–437.

GUILLEMIN, R., CLAYTON, G. W., LIPSCOMB, H. S. AND SMITH, J. D. (1959) Fluorometric measurement of rat plasma and adrenal corticosterone concentration. *J. lab. clin. Med.*, **53**, 830–832.

KOKKA, N., GARCIA, J. F., GEORGE, R. AND ELLIOTT, H. W. (1972) Growth hormone and ACTH secretion: evidence for an inverse relationship in rats. *Endocrinology*, **90**, 735–743.

LOTTI, V. J., KOKKA, N. AND GEORGE, R. (1969) Pituitary-adrenal activation following intrahypothalamic microinjection of morphine. *Neuroendocrinology*, **4**, 326–332.

MORGAN, H. E., HENDERSON, M. J., REGEN, D. M. AND PARK, C. R. (1961) Regulation of glucose uptake in muscle, I. The effects of insulin and anoxia on glucose transport and phosphorylation in the isolated, perfused hearts of normal rats. *J. biol. Chem.*, **236**, 253–261.

PAROLI, E. AND MELCHIORRI, P. (1961) Urinary excretion of hydroxysteroids, 17-ketosteroids and aldosterone in rats during a cycle of treatment with morphine. *Biochem. Pharmacol.*, **6**, 1–17.

RANDLE, P. J. AND SMITH, G. H. (1958) Regulation of glucose uptake by muscle, 1. The effects of insulin, anaerobiosis and cell poisons on the uptake of glucose and release of potassium by isolated rat diaphragm. *Biochem. J.*, **20**, 490–500.

RUSSELL, J. A., LONG, C. N. H. AND ENGEL, F. L. (1944) Biochemical studies on shock. *J. exp. Med.*, **79**, 1–7.

SCHALCH, D. S. AND REICHLIN, S. (1968) Stress and growth hormone release. In *Growth Hormone*, A. PECILE AND E. E. MULLER (Eds.), Excerpta Medica, Amsterdam, pp. 211–225.

SLOAN, J. W. (1971) Corticosteroid hormones. In *Narcotic Drugs Biochemical Pharmacology*, D. H. CLOUET (Ed.), Plenum, New York, pp. 262–282.

TAKAHASHI, K., DAUGHADAY, W. H. AND KIPNIS, D. M. (1971) Regulation of immunoreactive growth hormone secretion in male rats. *Endocrinology*, **88**, 909–917.

WASHKO, M. E. AND RICE, E. W. (1961) Determination of blood glucose by an improved enzymatic procedure. *Clin. Chem.*, **7**, 542–545.

DISCUSSION

DANELLIS: Perhaps it would be more judicious in discussing your results to talk strictly in terms of corticosterone. It would be most surprising to find circulating ACTH levels maintained at elevated levels for 120 min or longer after treatment with some of these drugs. Do you have any information based on direct measurement of ACTH concentrations?

KOKKA: Dr. Garcia and I have been working on an ACTH immunoassay for over 2 years to answer that question. At present, we have an assay that will detect ACTH in plasma at levels of 60 pg/ml. We did not measure ACTH in the present study because resting plasma ACTH values are reported to be well below this concentration. Whether plasma ACTH does or does not remain elevated after morphine administration will have to be determined by further studies in which ACTH is measured directly by radioimmunoassay.

SCAPAGNINI: Your results with apomorphine are very fascinating, since, as you know, it has recently been shown that apomorphine is a rather specific stimulant of dopaminergic receptors. Your findings fit beautifully with what Dr. Collu showed us last night.

KOKKA: I was also very interested in Dr. Collu's work on GH secretion, intraventricular injections, and hypothalamic deafferentation. We have reserpinized rats by giving an initial injection of 5 mg/kg followed by daily injection of 1 mg/kg for 5 days. On the 6th day, the rats were injected with morphine. However, we found no impairment in the GH response to morphine, but we did find a small decrease in the corticosterone response.

KITAY: Dr. Danellis was concerned about your findings at 120 min. I would like to express interest in your earlier values. Did you attempt to measure corticosterone levels at 10, 15 or 20 min? We have used morphine in small doses and we do frequently see in male rats values in plasma corticosterone levels that peak at 15 min or at 20 min but which have fallen close to the resting level at 30 min. However, this is not true in females.

KOKKA: One of the reasons we did not make more measurements at 15 min was because of the results obtained with $ACTH_{1-24}$. We gave $ACTH_{1-24}$ in doses of 0.10 and 0.25 U/kg i.p. and observed a rise in plasma corticosterone which remained elevated for 30 min. Therefore we thought it unlikely that a comparable rise produced by morphine was followed by a return to normal at 30 min.

KITAY: That's true, but 100 mU. of $ACTH_{1-24}$ could be a supramaximal dose so that its effects would last well after 30 min.

KNIGGE: I am trying to find some correlation now between the dose of morphine that you used to produce the increase in both GH and corticosterone and the dose of morphine that Dr. George used to get a depressant effect on TSH. It seems to me that you have high corticosterone with decreased TSH, yet control of both of these hormones seems to be related to the posterior hypothalamic region.

KOKKA: I've discussed this many times with Dr. George. I can't explain it. You saw the results we obtained with a wide range of doses of morphine, where low doses produced significant increases of GH with minimal effects on corticosterone, and higher doses produced a rise of both plasma GH and corticosterone. I can't account for the fact that 5 mg/kg of morphine inhibits TSH secretion and has no effect on corticosterone secretion except to point out that these two hormones are regulated by different systems which may exhibit different sensitivities to morphine.

CARROLL: As a clinician, I want to take exception to Dr. Kokka's statement that stress situations that cause a cortisol response do not induce a GH response because clinically there are a number of standard procedures such as insulin hypoglycemia, lysine vasopressin, and probably pyrogen, not to mention surgery, which predictably induce GH and cortisol responses. I assume you are talking only about rats.

KOKKA: That's right. I apologize for not mentioning the well-known rise of plasma GH produced by many procedures that simultaneously cause a rise of cortisol in primates. However, our studies in cats and rabbits, in addition to those done in rats, show that various stimuli that elicit a rise of GH in man are ineffective in these species.

Effects of Morphine and Related Drugs on the Corticotrophin (ACTH)-Stress Reaction

PAUL L. MUNSON

Department of Pharmacology, School of Medicine, University of North Carolina, Chapel Hill, N. C. 27514 (U.S.A.)

The corticotrophin (ACTH)-stress reaction was first clearly recognized and conceptualized in 1936 by Hans Selye (1936), who gave it the name, "general alarm reaction". This paper has to do mainly with the inhibitory effect of morphine on the reaction but, indeed, morphine can itself provoke the reaction; it was one of the drugs that led Selye to his discovery.

Selye (1936) found that high doses of morphine and certain other drugs and procedures produced a decrease in weight of the thymus and enlargement of the adrenal cortex in rats. Morphine and the other stimuli, denominated "stressors" by Selye, lost their endocrine effects after hypophysectomy or adrenalectomy, leading to the conclusion, still valid, that the stressor acts to increase the secretion of ACTH and in turn the glucocorticoids, which then act on the thymus and other target tissues. The concept was later expanded by Green and Harris (1947) to include the central nervous system, particularly the hypothalamus, and the corticotrophin-releasing factor (CRF) (so named by Saffran *et al.*, 1955) as mediators between the stressor and increased ACTH secretion.

18 years after Selye's initial experiments Briggs and I discovered accidentally that under the proper circumstances, morphine can be a powerful inhibitor of the stress reaction (Briggs and Munson, 1955).

The dose of morphine used by Selye (1936) to stimulate ACTH secretion was quite large, about 300 mg/kg, but it is known from the work of other investigators (George and Way, 1955; Nikodijevic and Maickel, 1967) that a much lower dose, in the range of 2 to 8 mg/kg, is effective in the rat.

This dose is about the same as the dose customarily used as a standard in the rat hot-plate assay for analgesic agents (Harris and Pierson, 1964). The dose needed for inhibition of ACTH secretion is also near this range (Briggs and Munson, 1955; Burdette *et al.*, 1961).

As noted above, the discovery of the inhibitory effect of morphine on ACTH secretion was accidental (Munson and Briggs, 1955). Briggs and I were attempting to extend Gray's and my work (Gray and Munson, 1951) on the time course of the stress reaction to intravenous histamine in rats anesthetized with pentobarbital. We were hampered and annoyed by the fact that a standard dose of pentobarbital failed to

References p. 371–372

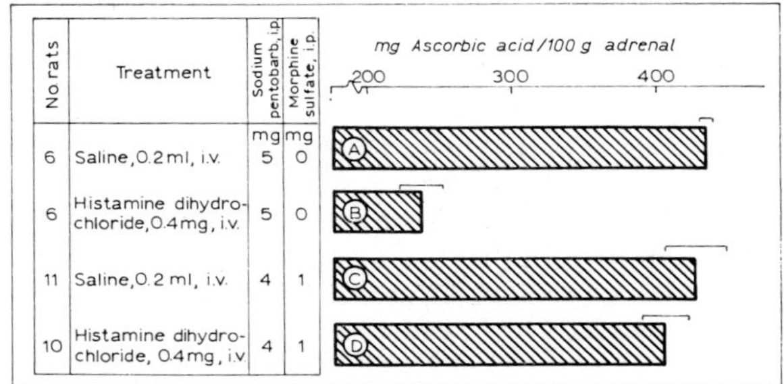

Statistical significance: B *vs.* D, *P* <0.01

Fig. 1. The effect of pretreatment with morphine on the adrenal ascorbic acid response of anesthetized rats to histamine. The doses shown were administered per 100 g body weight. The brackets represent the standard errors (Briggs and Munson, 1955). Pentobarb. = pentobarbital.

anesthetize some rats adequately and was lethal to others. We attempted to improve the anesthesia by giving morphine in addition to the barbiturate, and were amazed to find, as shown in Fig. 1, that an ordinarily stressful dose of histamine had no detectable effect on ACTH secretion whatsoever in these animals, in addition to the fact that morphine itself was no longer acting as a stressor (Briggs and Munson, 1955). In these experiments, conducted 18 years ago, the measure of increased ACTH secretion was the unsophisticated but still reasonably reliable decrease in adrenal ascorbic acid concentration (Sayers *et al.*, 1944). If we were doing these experiments in the 1970's instead of the earlier 1950's we would want to measure CRF directly or if that were not possible, ACTH. Even so, the adrenal ascorbic acid method has some advantages. The unstimulated value is usually between 400 and 450 mg/100 g, and the maximum decrease usually seen is 35 to 50% (Sayers *et al.*, 1948).

Other experiments quickly followed and we soon found that morphine, in the pentobarbital-anesthetized rat, inhibited or blocked the stressful effect on ACTH secretion of all our standard stressing agents and procedures, including, in addition to histamine, vasopressin, adrenaline, laparotomy, sham adrenalectomy, and unilateral adrenalectomy (Figs. 2–5) (Briggs and Munson, 1955). Others have extended this list

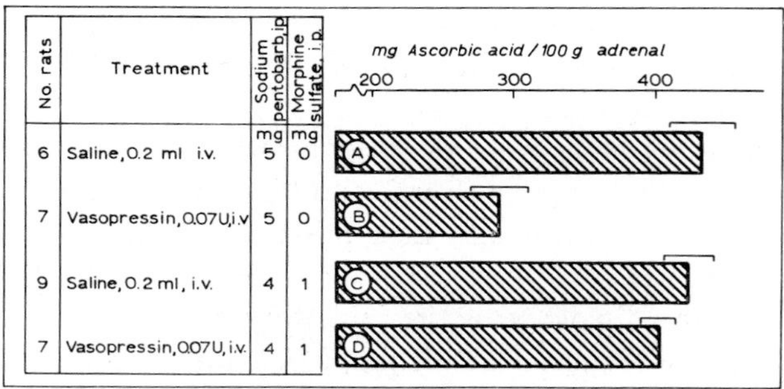

Statistical significance: B *vs.* D, *P*<0.001

Fig. 2. The effect of pretreatment with morphine on the adrenal ascorbic acid response of anesthetized rats to vasopressin. For details, see Fig. 1. (Briggs and Munson, 1955).

No. rats
Treatment
Sodium pentobarb, i.p.
Morphine sulfate, i.p.
mg Ascorbic acid/100g adrenal
200
300
400
mg
mg
9
Saline, 0.2 ml, s.c.
5
0
9
l-Adrenaline hydrochloride, 0.03 mg, s.c.
5
0
8
Saline, 0.2 ml, s.c.
4
2
8
l-Adrenaline hydrochloride, 0.03 mg, s.c.
4
2
A
B
C
D
Statistical significance: B *vs* D, *P*<0.01

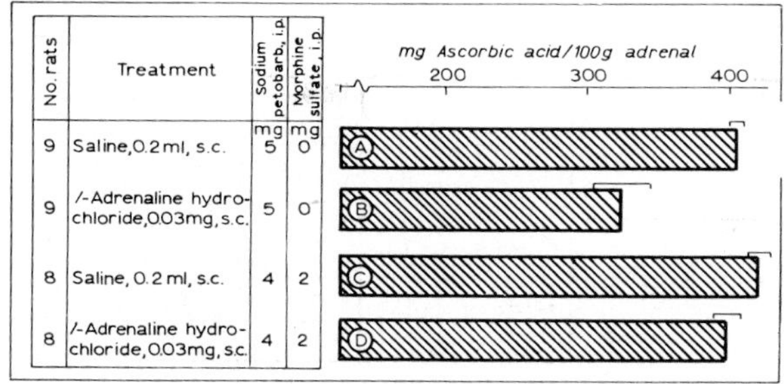

Fig. 3. The effect of pretreatment with morphine on the adrenal ascorbic acid response of anesthetized rats to adrenaline. For details, see Fig. 1 (Briggs and Munson, 1955).

No. rats
Treatment
Sodium pentobarb, i.p.
Morphine sulfate, i.p.
mg Ascorbic acid/100g adrenal
200
300
400
mg
mg
6
Control
5
0
8
Surgery
5
0
10
Control
4
1
13
Surgery
4
1
8
Control
4
2
9
Surgery
4
2
A
B
C
D
E
F
Statistical significance: B *vs* D, *P* <0.05; B *vs*. F, *P*< 0.001

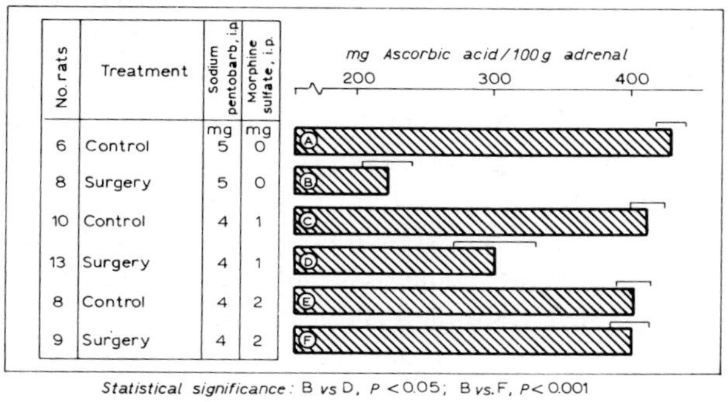

Fig. 4. The effect of pretreatment with morphine on the adrenal ascorbic acid response of anesthetized rats to surgery (laparotomy and bile duct dissection). For details, see Fig. 1 (Briggs and Munson, 1955).

No. rats
Treatment
Sodium pentobarb, i.p.
Morphine sulfate, i.p.
mg Ascorbic acid/100g adrenal
200
300
400
mg
mg
15
Sham unilateral adrenalectomy
5.5
0
13
Unilateral adrenalectomy
5.5
0
14
Sham unilateral adrenalectomy
4
2
11
Unilateral adrenalectomy
4
2
A
B
C
D
Statistical significance: B *vs*. D, *P*< 0.001

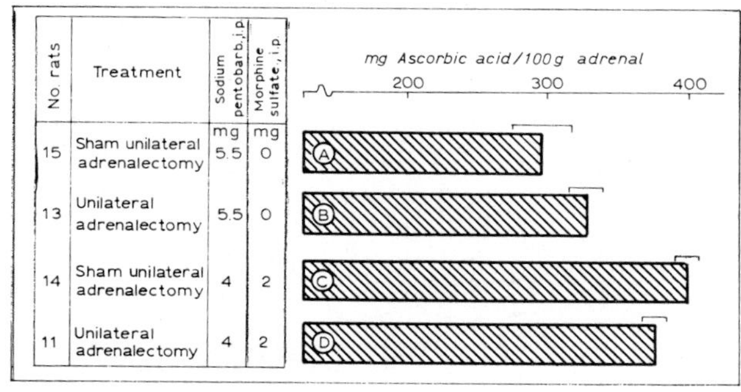

Fig. 5. The effect of pretreatment with morphine on the adrenal ascorbic acid response of anesthetized rats to unilateral adrenalectomy. For details, see Fig. 1 (Briggs and Munson, 1955).

of stressors, whose effects on ACTH release are blocked or inhibited by morphine, and recently, Peng, Six, and I (Peng *et al.*, 1970), showed that the stressful effect of prostaglandin E_1 is strongly inhibited by morphine (Fig. 6), results in agreement with De Wied *et al.*, (1969) that CRF is probably not a prostaglandin.

References p. 371–372

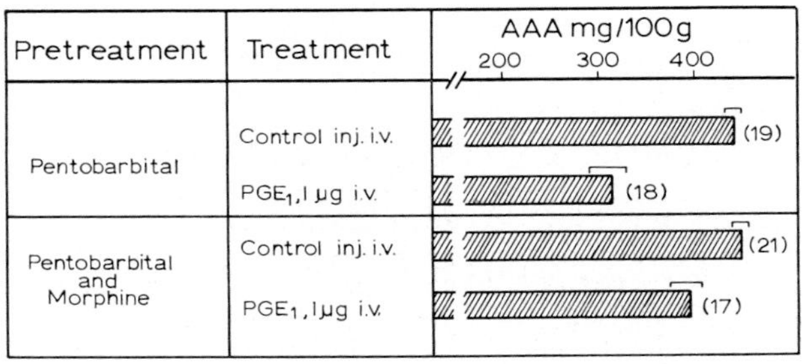

Pretreatment	Treatment	AAA mg/100g (200 300 400)
Pentobarbital	Control inj. i.v.	(19)
	PGE$_1$, 1 μg i.v.	(18)
Pentobarbital and Morphine	Control inj. i.v.	(21)
	PGE$_1$, 1μg i.v.	(17)

Fig. 6. The effect of pretreatment with morphine (10 mg/kg i.p., as the sulfate) on the adrenal ascorbic acid (AAA) response of anesthetized rats (sodium pentobarbital, 40–50 mg/kg i.p.) to prostaglandin E$_1$ (PGE$_1$). Number of rats per group in parentheses. The brackets represent the standard errors (Peng *et al.*, 1970).

We found only one exception to the rule hypothalamic extract containing CRF (Leeman and Voelkel, 1959; Leeman *et al.*, 1962), which was logical according to the hypothesis that the site of action of morphine is not in the anterior pituitary gland but in the hypothalamus or higher center (Munson and Briggs, 1955; George and Way, 1959; Munson, 1962).

Morphine can inhibit ACTH secretion in man as well as in rats. In man, unlike the unanesthetized rat, a dose of morphine sufficient to inhibit ACTH secretion does not stimulate ACTH secretion. Therefore, it is unnecessary to pretreat with a barbiturate. Fig. 7, illustrating one of the experiments conducted by McDonald *et al.* (1959), clearly demonstrates the inhibitory effect of morphine on ACTH secretion in man. Two groups of 7 subjects each were used; one group injected with morphine (16 mg of morphine sulfate) and the other with a placebo were both given 2 units of vasopressin intravenously. Morphine or the control solution was injected 60 min before the vasopressin. Within 30 min after administration of vasopressin there was a sharp rise

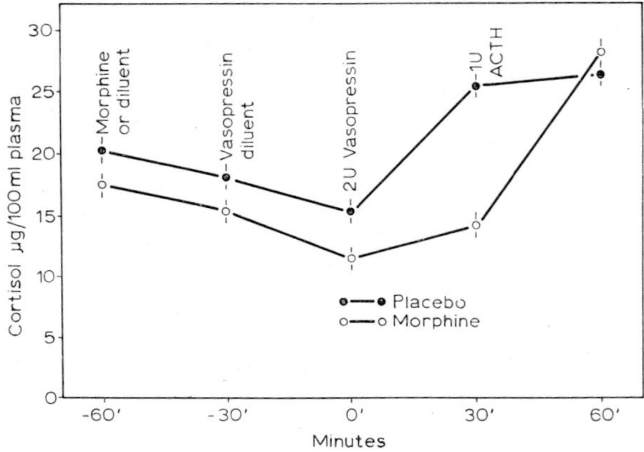

Fig. 7. Effect of morphine on ACTH response to vasopressin in 7 human subjects. The vertical lines through the points represent the standard errors. See text for further details (McDonald *et al.*, 1959).

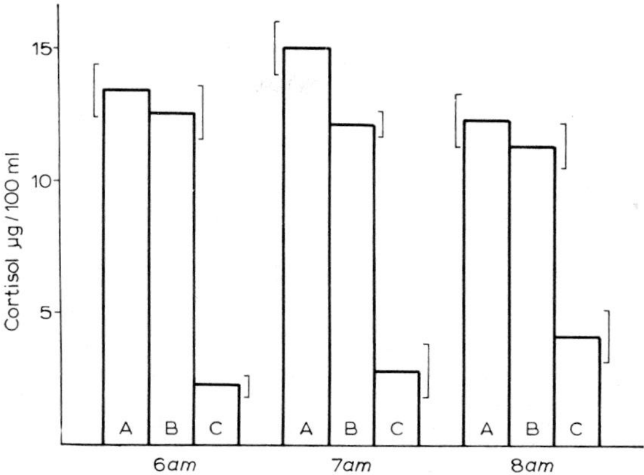

Fig. 8. Effect of morphine on plasma free cortisol in 5 human subjects. A and B were control series. Morphine was given in series C. The brackets represent the standard errors. See text for further details (McDonald *et al.*, 1959).

in plasma cortisol in the subjects given the placebo solution instead of morphine and no significant effect in the group that had been given morphine. The response of the placebo group to ACTH demonstrates that the adrenal glands of this group were responsive to ACTH and indicates that the failure of the morphine group to respond to vasopressin was because, under the influence of morphine, vasopressin did not stimulate release of endogenous ACTH.

Fig. 8, also from McDonald *et al.* (1959), shows that morphine prevented the normal early morning rise in plasma cortisol in 5 human subjects. In control series A, these subjects were given placebos at 10 *p.m.* and 3 *a.m.* In control series B, they were given oral pentobarbital at 10 *p.m.* and a placebo injection at 3 *a.m.* In series C the same subjects were given pentobarbital at 10 *p.m.* and 16 mg of morphine sulfate at 3 *a.m.* The placebo and pentobarbital values were in the normal range and did not differ significantly from each other, whereas the effect of morphine was strikingly to prevent or reduce the early-morning high cortisol values.

Nalorphine can antagonize the action of morphine, both as a stressor and as an inhibitor of the ACTH-stress reaction, and it can do so both in man and the rat (Briggs and Munson, 1955; George and Way, 1955; McDonald *et al.*, 1959; Burdette *et al.*, 1961), just as it does for other pharmacological properties of morphine.

Nalorphine, like morphine, if given in a high enough dose, can act as a stressor in rats. Burdette, Leeman, and I (Burdette *et al.*, 1961) found that doses of 40 mg/kg or higher stimulated ACTH release, but that a dose of 20 mg/kg was inactive in this respect. Therefore, doses of 20 mg/kg or less could be used to test the antagonistic effect of nalorphine on the inhibitory action of morphine on the ACTH-stress reaction. As shown in Fig. 9, from the work of Burdette *et al.* (1961), the fully inhibitory effect of 20 mg/kg of morphine sulfate against the stressful effect of histamine was strongly antagonized by 0.5 mg/kg of nalorphine HCl and fully antagonized by 2 mg/kg. The lower dose of morphine, not fully inhibitory, was antagonized by an even lower dose of nalorphine.

References p. 371–372

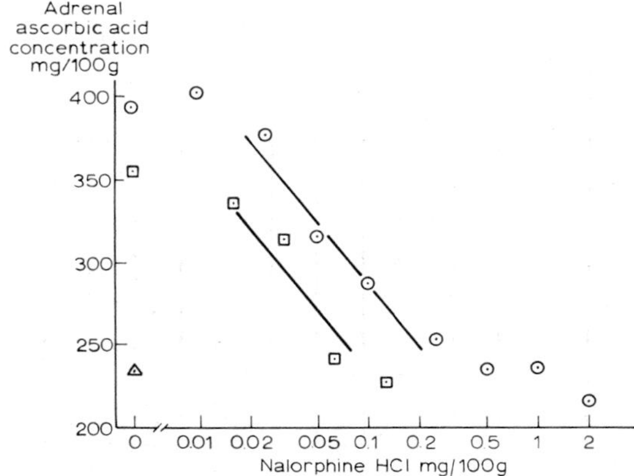

Fig. 9. Log dose response lines for the antagonistic effect of nalorphine against the inhibitory action of morphine on the adrenal ascorbic acid response to histamine.

All rats were injected with an anesthetic dose (40 mg/kg) of sodium pentobarbital 10 min before administration of morphine. The nalorphine was injected immediately after the morphine. Histamine (10 mg/kg) was administered to all rats 10 min after nalorphine (or morphine). All injections were i.p. Each point represents the mean of 5 to 23 rats; total number, 148. ⊙, morphine sulfate, 20 mg/100 g; ⊡, morphine sulfate, 0.5 mg/100 g; △, no morphine. (Burdette *et al.*, 1961)

George and Way (1955) demonstrated that the stimulation of ACTH secretion by morphine in previously untreated nonanesthetized rats could be antagonized by nalorphine. A dose 1/6 that of morphine was effective. These investigators showed, furthermore, that lesions in the median eminence also prevented morphine from stimulating ACTH secretion (George and Way, 1959).

These findings strengthened our view that both the stimulating and inhibitory actions of morphine were exerted in the central nervous system and not in the anterior pituitary gland.

The relation between pentobarbital and morphine in inhibiting ACTH secretion has been termed "synergistic" by Gold and Ganong (1967). We have taken a somewhat different point of view (Munson and Briggs, 1955). Sodium pentobarbital has been a favorite anesthetic agent for the investigation of acute stimulation of ACTH secretion, because, unlike ether, it does not itself provoke ACTH release and because it effectively prevents the pain or alarm that the awake rat would otherwise experience from restraint or intravenous injections. Pain and alarm are themselves sufficient to stimulate ACTH secretion and thus would tend to obscure the effects of the drug or stimulus under study. Thus, the barbiturate by its anesthetic effect facilitates study of the stress reaction by blocking the effects of some stimuli without at the same time interfering with the pituitary response to other stimuli that have more deep-seated consequences. It seemed to us most logical to assign the acute stressful effect of a first dose of morphine on a rat to this same category of pain, fear, loud noise, restraint, and the like that require the wakeful state for their effectiveness.

That the blocking action of morphine in stress is not always dependent on pentobarbital anesthesia is suggested by the results shown in Fig. 10 (Briggs and Munson,

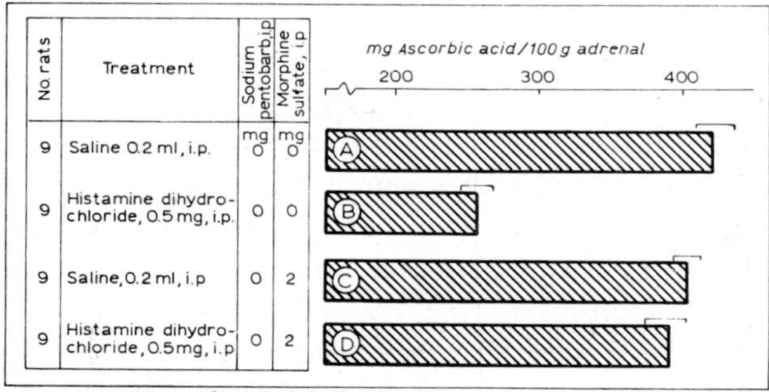

Fig. 10. The effect of pretreatment with morphine on the adrenal ascorbic acid response of non-anesthetized rats to histamine. Groups C and D had been given morphine sulfate (2 mg/100 g) once daily for 4 days immediately before the experiment. For other details, see Fig. 1. (Briggs and Munson, 1955)

1955). In this experiment, rats were accustomed to morphine by a daily injection for 4 days. On the 5th day an injection of morphine was no longer an effective stimulus for ACTH secretion in the unanesthetized rat, and yet it was still an effective inhibitor of the normal histamine effect. Thus, morphine alone, under these circumstances, appeared to be entirely responsible for the observed blocking action and we hypothesized that this was also true in experiments in which morphine was being given for the first time and in which anesthesia was necessary merely to circumvent its alarming effects.

The findings after chronic treatment with morphine led us into similar experiments with reserpine, which, like morphine, is a stressful drug itself in rats the first time it is injected. However, Wells, Briggs, and I (Wells *et al.*, 1956) found that, like morphine, reserpine, after repeated daily injections, was no longer a stressor and, furthermore, other stressful stimuli, such as ether and histamine, no longer produced an increase in ACTH secretion.

Our results with chronic reserpine were confirmed by Kitay *et al.* (1959) and Maickel *et al.* (1961), but they offered a different interpretation. Both of these groups of investigators found that 20 to 24 h after the first injection of reserpine the ACTH content of the treated rats' pituitary glands had decreased substantially (62 to 73%), and they suggested that the failure of rats to respond to stressful stimuli after reserpine was due not to inhibition of the stress reaction at the hypothalamic level but to depletion of pituitary ACTH stores. In further support of the hypothesis it was shown by Kitay *et al.* (1959) that adrenaline, and by Maickel *et al.* (1961) that exposure to cold had effects similar to reserpine both in depleting pituitary ACTH stores and in reducing the effects of subsequent stressful stimuli.

Several objections can be raised against this plausible hypothesis (Munson, 1963). In the first place, the amount of ACTH left in the pituitary gland after reserpine treatment is far in excess of that required to produce the type of adrenal cortical stimulation ordinarily observed in acute stress. Furthermore, van Peenen and Way (1957) showed that 12 to 15 h after a single large injection of reserpine, at a time when considerable pituitary ACTH depletion had already undoubtedly occurred, the ACTH

References p. 371–372

response to aspirin and to histamine appeared to be unimpaired, although the responses to adrenaline and morphine were indeed considerably reduced.

It is also difficult to explain the adrenal enlargement reported by some investigators to occur after continued reserpine administration (reviewed by Munson, 1963) if stress secretion of ACTH is seriously compromised by reduction in pituitary ACTH stores. Certainly, a cause–effect relationship between pituitary ACTH depletion and failure to respond to stress has not been established. Nevertheless, a clear understanding of the mechanism responsible for the change in the character of the stress response after reserpine and similarly acting drugs is still lacking.

Most of the evidence supporting the inhibitory effect of morphine on ACTH secretion in both rat and man is based on experiments in which it is unlikely that there was any decrease in ACTH content from the pituitary gland. In the rat, essentially all the data are from experiments in which the morphine was administered under pentobarbital anesthesia and there was no resulting increase in ACTH secretion. If there was no increase in ACTH secretion, it is reasonable to assume that there was no decrease in pituitary ACTH content. Even so, in these experiments the stressful stimulus was applied within 10 to 20 min after administration of the morphine, which would be an inadequate interval for the loss of much ACTH from the pituitary gland. Finally, we have shown that an increase in intensity of the stressful stimulus surmounted the morphine blockade and resulted in ACTH secretion (Briggs and Munson, 1955), indicating that there was an adequate amount of ACTH present in the pituitary gland for the response.

Even after chronic morphine, there are data, as from Paroli and Melchiorri (1961), indicating that whatever effects there may have been on the pituitary gland, they did not prevent a rise in ACTH secretion after cessation of chronic morphine treatment for 10 to 40 days. Tanabe and Cafruny (1958), as well as Selye (1936) in his original work, reported adrenal enlargement after repeated injections of morphine.

In man, in contrast to the rat, the evidence indicates that an ordinary single dose of morphine does not stimulate ACTH secretion (Eisenman *et al.*, 1961). Therefore, it should have no effect on pituitary ACTH content. Eisenman *et al.* (1958, 1961) also found that chronic administration of morphine in man resulted in a marked fall in plasma and urinary corticoids. However, after several months of addiction to morphine, abrupt withdrawal of the drug resulted, associated with development of the abstinence syndrome, in a tremendous rise in plasma free cortisol as well as in urinary 17-ketosteroids (Fig. 11), indicating adequate pituitary ACTH reserve to respond to a stressful situation as soon as the effect of a long series of morphine injections had ended.

Whatever the interpretation of the depressant effect of reserpine on the ACTH-stress reaction, the evidence that morphine inhibits this reaction independently of depletion of pituitary ACTH stores appears to be overwhelming.

One of the by-products of our investigations on the effect of morphine on the ACTH-stress reaction was the development of a test system to be used in monitoring purification of CRF (Munson, 1962) and it was employed for this purpose to a certain extent by Guillemin, and coworkers (Guillemin *et al.*, 1959; Schally and Guillemin,

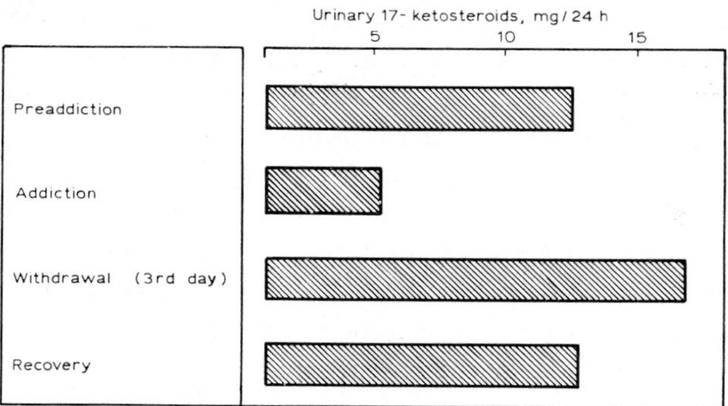

Fig. 11. Effect of morphine addiction and withdrawal on 17-ketosteroid excretion, as an indicator of ACTH secretion, in 9 men. Additional details in text (Data from Eisenman *et al.*, 1958).

1960). The test system that Leeman and I originally proposed (Leeman and Munson, 1958) involved testing each fraction in three different rat preparations, rats anesthetized with pentobarbital alone, rats given both pentobarbital and morphine, and hypophysectomized rats. A negative result in hypophysectomized rats indicated the absence of ACTH contamination in the fraction. If a submaximal dose of extract produced the same effect (adrenal ascorbic acid decrease) in pentobarbital-anesthetized rats with and without morphine it indicated that the entire effect of the extract was not inhibitable by morphine, therefore it was due to CRF (or ACTH), whereas if the effect was greater in the rats not given morphine this indicated that part or possibly all of the effect was due to contamination of the extract with a non-CRF constituent, such as vasopressin or histamine. The complexity of this system might appear to be one of its drawbacks. The need for parallel assays in rats with and without morphine arises because of the surmountable nature of the morphine "blockade". A dose of extract being tested that produces the maximum effect on the morphine-treated rat may represent the effect of a stressful substance at a dose high enough to surmount morphine inhibition. It is necessary first to obtain a dose–response curve in rats not given morphine, then to administer a submaximal dose in rats both with and without morphine. Only then can one be certain that the effect of the extract is not inhibitable by morphine and that it can be assumed to be CRF (if it is not ACTH).

In practice, if the starting extract being purified has been shown to be relatively free of ACTH and stressful substances, it is only necessary to assay the fractions produced during further purification for ACTH-releasing potency in pentobarbital-anesthetized rats without morphine. The morphine-treated rat and the hypophysectomized rat need only be used at less frequent intervals to assure the investigator that ACTH and stressful substances which did not seriously contaminate the starting extract have not become concentrated during later purification to the point that they constitute a problem.

Others have attempted to devise assay methods for CRF using other drugs in conjunction with or in place of morphine in order to overcome major defects of the original morphine assay method, which are principally the surmountability of morphine blockade and the toxicity of the combined treatment with morphine and pentobarbital. In a recent comparison of assay methods for CRF, Chan *et al.* (1969), concluded that an assay in which intracarotid injections are given to rats with median eminence lesions and the response is taken as adrenal steroidogenesis, was superior to our method. In a subsequent publication by De Wied *et al.* (1969), still other assay methods were employed, suggesting that the ideal method, combining convenience, specificity, and precision, has not yet been devised. One conclusion that does appear to have emerged is that it is undesirable to include a glucocorticoid in the pretreatment of the assay rat, because of the inhibitory effect of this class of steroids on the pituitary response to CRF (De Wied *et al.*, 1969).

It has been stated repeatedly that one of the obstacles in the way of purification and isolation of CRF is the lack of a reliable assay method. In concluding this paper, I should like to offer a recommendation for circumventing this problem. It is *not* to recommend the pentobarbital–morphine rat as the basic method of assay. Instead, I suggest the simplest method conceivable, intravenous injection of the fractions obtained into pentobarbital-anesthetized rats coupled with a convenient method for measuring ACTH release. No doubt several active fractions will be identified. Each of these should be further purified and then subjected to a battery of tests, which might include assays for ACTH and vasopressin, tests in morphine-inhibited rats, atropine-inhibited rats, rats with median eminence lesions, in fact, every challenge that can be devised before it is concluded that the natural CRF has finally been isolated.

SUMMARY

The effects of morphine and related drugs on the ACTH-stress reaction are reviewed with emphasis on morphine. Morphine was one of the drugs with a stimulant effect on the pituitary-adrenal axis that led Selye in 1936 to the concept of the "general alarm reaction". Years later, Briggs and Munson discovered that under certain circumstances morphine could be a powerful inhibitor of the stress reaction. This inhibitory effect has been demonstrated in man as well as in rats. Both the stimulant and inhibitory effects of morphine on the stress reaction can be antagonized by nalorphine. The controversy over whether the inhibitory effect of chronic morphine or reserpine treatment on the pituitary-adrenal axis is primarily neural in character or is merely due to depletion of pituitary ACTH is evaluated. The utility of morphine in the bioassay of ACTH-releasing factor is discussed and a practical suggestion for the simplification of this assay problem is presented.

ACKNOWLEDGMENTS

Original work of the author reviewed in this paper was supported in part by research grants from the National Science Foundation (GB-6752) and the Air Force Office of Scientific Research (1339-67).

REFERENCES

BRIGGS, F. N. AND MUNSON, P. L. (1955) Studies on the mechanism of stimulation of ACTH secretion with the aid of morphine as a blocking agent. *Endocrinology*, **57**, 205–219.

BURDETTE, B. A., LEEMAN, S. E. AND MUNSON, P. L. (1961) The reversal by nalorphine of the inhibitory effect of morphine on the secretion of adrenocorticotropic hormone in stress. *J. Pharmacol. exp. Ther.*, **132**, 323–328.

CHAN, L. T., DE WIED, D. AND SAFFRAN, M. (1969) Comparison of assays for corticotrophin-releasing activity. *Endocrinology*, **84**, 967–972.

DE WIED, D., WITTER, A., VERSTEEG, D. H. G. AND MULDER, A. H. (1969) Release of ACTH by substances of central nervous system origin. *Endocrinology*, **85**, 561–569.

EISENMAN, A. J., FRASER, H. F., SLOAN, J. AND ISBELL, H. (1958) Urinary 17-ketosteroid excretion during a cycle of addiction to morphine. *J. Pharmacol. exp. Ther.*, **124**, 305–311.

EISENMAN, A. J., FRASER, H. F. AND BROOKS, J. W. (1961) Urinary excretion and plasma levels of 17-hydroxycorticosteroids during a cycle of addiction to morphine. *J. Pharmacol. exp. Ther.*, **132**, 226–231.

GEORGE, R. AND WAY, E. L. (1955) Studies on the mechanism of pituitary-adrenal activation by morphine. *Brit. J. Pharmacol. Chemother.*, **10**, 260–264.

GEORGE, R. AND WAY, E. L. (1959) The role of the hypothalamus in pituitary-adrenal activation and antidiuresis by morphine. *J. Pharmacol. exp. Ther.*, **125**, 111–115.

GOLD, E. M. AND GANONG, W. F. (1967) Effects of drugs on neuroendocrine processes. In *Neuroendocrinology*, Vol. II, L. MARTINI AND W. F. GANONG (Eds.), Academic Press, New York, pp. 377–437.

GRAY, W. D. AND MUNSON, P. L. (1951) The rapidity of the adrenocorticotropic response of the pituitary to the intravenous administration of histamine. *Endocrinology*, **48**, 471–481.

GREEN, J. D. AND HARRIS, G. W. (1947) The neurovascular link between the neurohypophysis and adenohypophysis. *J. Endocrinol.*, **5**, 136–146.

GUILLEMIN, R., DEAR, W. E., NICHOLS, B. JR. AND LIPSCOMB, H. S. (1959) ACTH releasing activity *in vivo* of a CRF preparation and lysine vasopressin. *Proc. Soc. exp. biol. Med.*, **101**, 107–111.

HARRIS, L. S. AND PIERSON, A. K. (1964) Some narcotic antagonists in the benzomorphan series. *J. Pharmacol. exp. Ther.*, **143**, 141–148.

KITAY, J. I., HOLUB, D. A. AND JAILER, J. W. (1959) "Inhibition" of pituitary ACTH release after administration of reserpine or epinephrine. *Endocrinology*, **65**, 548–554.

LEEMAN, S. E. AND MUNSON, P. L. (1958) An *in vivo* system for detection of the neural hormone responsible for ACTH secretion in stress. *Fed. Proc.*, **17**, 387.

LEEMAN, S. E. AND VOELKEL, E. F. (1959) Preparation and bioassay of a hypothalamic extract that stimulates ACTH secretion *in vivo*. *Fed. Proc.*, **18**, 89.

LEEMAN, S. E., GLENISTER, D. W. AND YATES, F. E. (1962) Characterization of a calf hypothalamic extract with adrenocorticotropin-releasing properties: Demonstration of a central nervous system site for corticosteroid inhibition of adrenocorticotropin release. *Endocrinology*, **70**, 249–262.

MAICKEL, R. P., WESTERMANN, E. O. AND BRODIE, B. B. (1961) Effects of reserpine and cold-exposure on pituitary-adrenocortical function in rats. *J. Pharmacol. exp. Ther.*, **134**, 167–175.

MCDONALD, R. K., EVANS, F. T., WEISE, V. K. AND PATRICK, R. W. (1959) Effect of morphine and nalorphine on plasma hydrocortisone levels in man. *J. Pharmacol. exp. Ther.*, **125**, 241–247.

MUNSON, P. L. (1962) Pharmacological control of the secretion of ACTH. *Proc. 1st int. pharmacol. Meeting, Stockholm, 1961*, **1**, 11–25.

MUNSON, P. L. (1963) Pharmacology of neuroendocrine blocking agents. In *Advances in Neuroendocrinology*, A. V. NALBANDOV (Ed.), University of Illinois Press, Urbana, Ill., pp. 427–444.

MUNSON, P. L. AND BRIGGS, F. N. (1955) The mechanism of stimulation of ACTH secretion. *Recent Progr. Hormone Res.*, **11**, 83–117.

NIKODIJEVIC, O. AND MAICKEL, R. P. (1967) Some effects of morphine on pituitary-adrenocortical function in the rat. *Biochem. Pharmacol.*, **16**, 2137–2142.

PAROLI, E. AND MELCHIORRI, P. (1961) Urinary excretion of hydroxysteroids, 17-ketosteroids and aldosterone in rats during a cycle of treatment with morphine. *Biochem. Pharmacol.*, **6**, 1–17.

PENG, T-C., SIX, K. M. AND MUNSON, P. L. (1970) Effect of prostaglandin E_1 on the hypothalamo-hypophyseal-adrenocortical axis in rats. *Endocrinology*, **86**, 202–206.

SAFFRAN, M., SCHALLY, A. V. AND BENFEY, B. G. (1955) Stimulation of the release of corticotropin from the adenohypophysis by a neurohypophysial factor. *Endocrinology*, **57**, 439–444.

SAYERS, G., SAYERS, M. A., LEWIS, H. L. AND LONG, C. N. H. (1944) Effect of adrenotropic hormone on ascorbic acid and cholesterol content of the adrenal. *Proc. Soc. exp. biol. Med.*, **55**, 238–239.

SAYERS, M. A., SAYERS, G. AND WOODBURY, D. M. (1948) The assay of adrenocorticotrophic hormone by the adrenal ascorbic acid depletion method. *Endocrinology*, **42**, 379–393.

SCHALLY, A. V. AND GUILLEMIN, R. (1960) Corticotropin-releasing factor: Ion-exchange chromatography of pituitary preparations. *Tex. Rep. Biol. Med.*, **18**, 133–146.

SELYE, H. (1936) Thymus and adrenals in the response of the organism to injuries and intoxications. *Brit. J. exp. Pathol.*, **17**, 234–248.

TANABE, T. AND CAFRUNY, E. J. (1958) Adrenal hypertrophy in rats treated chronically with morphine. *J. Pharmacol. exp. Ther.*, **122**, 148–153.

VAN PEENEN, P. F. D. AND WAY, E. L. (1957) Effect of certain central nervous system depressants on pituitary-adrenal activating agents. *J. Pharmacol. exp. Ther.*, **120**, 261–267.

WELLS, H., BRIGGS, F. N. AND MUNSON, P. L. (1956) The inhibitory effect of reserpine on ACTH secretion in response to stressful stimuli. *Endocrinology*, **59**, 571–579.

DISCUSSION

HEDGE: I am somewhat surprised that we have reached the final day of this symposium on endocrine pharmacology before any mention was made of a very interesting class of compounds, namely the prostaglandins (PGs). Dr. Munson has shown us pharmacological studies indicating that PGs of the E series stimulate ACTH by acting above the anterior pituitary, and he has referred to the similar studies of De Wied *et al.* Perhaps it is now appropriate for me to mention some of our related work. We have taken a different approach to this problem and in doing so we have confirmed and extended the findings presented. We have shown that microinjections of PGE_1 into the hypothalamus are quite effective in causing ACTH secretion, at doses that are without effect when injected into the anterior pituitary or a tail vein. In addition, we have found that PGs of the F series share this property with those of the E series; a finding that is in apparent discordance with the data of others. The explanation for this seems to reside in differing rates of inactivation. When administered intravenously the F PGs (in contrast to those of the E series) are apparently inactivated to a large extent before reaching the hypothalamus. However, when administered directly into the hypothalamus, this problem is not present and the effectiveness of the F series can be seen.

GEORGE (JACK): I would like to tell you of a study which relates Dr. Munson's classic findings to clinical medicine. As you may know, morphine is being increasingly used as the sole anesthetic agent in major surgery. This is particularly the case with open-heart surgery because morphine is less of a cardiac depressant than the usual anesthetic agents. The doses used range from about 1–4 mg per kg. In a patient of 70 kg this involves giving anywhere from 70 to 280 mg morphine rapidly intravenously and this results in anesthesia for the entire procedure. To my knowledge there has been no reported study of the effects of these doses of morphine on cortisol or growth hormone in man. One mg/kg morphine gave a curve identical to the control, 2 mg/kg caused some suppression, but not statistically significant and 4 mg/kg produced significant suppression ($p < 0.01$). We got exactly parallel results with growth hormone. You might ask what's happening to these patients with the 4 mg/kg morphine. Actually nothing bad seems to be happening to them. Their blood pressures don't fall, and their pulse rates don't particularly rise. This had led us to hypothesize that the cortisol response usually seen in response to surgical stress is not necessary to maintain life.

MUNSON: That's a very interesting study. I am still uncertain as to what beneficial effect the increase in ACTH secretion and glucocorticoid secretion does have in stress.

HODGES: I should like to ask Dr. Munson and Dr. Jack George whether their remarks were meant to imply that a normal hypothalamo-pituitary-adrenocortical response involving a marked rise in plasma cortisol is not essential for the patient's well being during surgery.

MUNSON: In surgery or other stress, the patient needs adrenal cortical steroids, but I know of no evidence that the patient needs a higher level of steroids than normal.

DE WIED: As you know, morphine is a potent histamine releaser. Unpublished studies done in 1956 in Dr. Mirsky's laboratory showed that repeated administration of histamine gradually prevents the release of ACTH in response to histamine injection but not to other stresses. It is therefore possible that histamine does not release ACTH in rats treated chronically with morphine because of this effect of morphine on the release of histamine.

Human Pharmacology of Drugs of Abuse with Emphasis on Neuroendocrine Effects

LEO E. HOLLISTER

Medical Investigator, Veterans Administration Hospital and Associate Professor of Medicine, Stanford University School of Medicine, Palo Alto, Calif., 94304 (U.S.A.)

The present discussion will consider as drugs of abuse opiates, sedatives, stimulants, hallucinogens and marihuana. Alcohol might properly be included, but traditionally has not been considered as a drug of abuse.

OPIATES

Morphine was first isolated from opium early in the 19th century; a little less than a century ago a diacetyl derivative, heroin, was produced by exposure of morphine to acetic anhydride. Most opiates, with the exception of codeine, are much more potent when taken parenterally. The usual custom in the USA is to take opiates intravenously, as contrasted to smoking or sniffing in other parts of the world. The impact of a bolus of intravenously administered heroin is considerable, both in terms of the clinical effects and the concentrations of drug attained. As many experimental studies employ subcutaneous or intraperitoneal routes of administration, these may not properly reflect the effects from intravenous dosage. Monoacetylmorphine, as well as morphine itself, are active metabolites of heroin, the former passing readily into the brain and possibly accounting for the increased potency. For practical purposes, the effects of heroin are similar to, if not identical with, those of morphine.

Tolerance to opiates is well known, and many pharmacological theories abound as to its mechanisms. The nature of the withdrawal syndrome from opiates is well known, many of the symptoms resembling those of increased cholinergic activity. The need for ever increasing amounts of drug to maintain the expected euphoriant effects, as well as the discomfort of withdrawal, have the expected consequence of strongly reinforcing the addiction once it is started.

For ethical reasons clinical pharmacological studies of heroin have mainly been confined to postaddicts. Such subjects usually show quite well the typical symptoms and signs expected from the drug: an initial "buzz" or "rush" centered in the abdomen and then spreading to the throat and the rest of the body; a sleepy, euphoric state ("nodding"); deepened voice; and constricted pupils (Zaks *et al.*, 1969). Normal subjects often find the effects somewhat dysphoric; the visceral sensations often are

References p. 379–280

considered akin to physical illness; the sleepiness and mental impairment outweigh any sense of euphoria. Such subjects usually show considerable signs of mental impairment under the drug (Smith *et al.*, 1962). Addicts may develop a certain amount of behavioral tolerance with less evident impairment of function.

Medical complications of addiction to opiates are numerous, including acute pulmonary edema (often associated with overdoses and severe respiratory depression), acute or chronic hepatitis, and bacterial endocarditis, among others. Curiously, clinical reports of endocrinological or metabolic complications have been exceedingly rare, despite the diverse actions of morphine on the release of corticotrophin (ACTH), pituitary gonadotrophins, thyrotrophin (TSH) and vasopressin. The decrease in gonadotrophin release seen in addicts and manifested by decreased urinary excretion of 17-ketosteroids (17-KS) is only partial; response to exogenous chorionic gonadotrophins is increased (Eisenman *et al.*, 1958). Diminished gonadal activity may be related to some of the loss of sexual desire universally experienced by addicts, but part may also be attributable to the orgastic sensation evoked by each "fix" and the subsequent sedation. Gynecological problems, such as abnormal menses, infertility and spontaneous abortion are frequent in addicted women. Diminished or absent menstrual periods may be regarded as evidence of diminished release of pituitary gonadotrophins (Stoffer, 1968). Gynecomastia in male heroin addicts is more likely attributable to chronic liver disease than to a neuroendocrine effect of the drug (Camiel *et al.*, 1967).

Although morphine diminishes adrenal cortical secretion, addicts are normally responsive to exogenous ACTH (Eisenman *et al.*, 1961). Stress may overcome the suppressed release of ACTH, as patients who react to the drug with vomiting or unpleasant neuropsychiatric experiences have increased adrenal function. Heroin addicts, not on methadone, had normal plasma concentrations of 17-hydroxysteroids (17-OHCS), which were normally responsive to insulin stimulation (Cushman *et al.*, 1970). The same situation prevailed in patients being treated with methadone maintenance. Normal resting 17-KS also rose normally after stimulation with metapyrone or exogenous ACTH. Thus, there is no convincing evidence that a clinically important state of relative adrenal insufficiency exists, despite the evidence suggesting that morphine depresses ACTH release. Animal studies have indicated inhibition of thyroid function by interference with the normal release of TSH from the adenohypophysis, but no instances of clinical hypothyroidism of myxedema have been encountered. The well-known effect of morphine in releasing vasopressin may only be transient, as judged by animal studies (Mills and Wang, 1964). In fact, one might consider strongly the possibility that tolerance may develop to many neuroendocrine effects of morphine, just as they do to other pharmacological actions of the drug. Hyperglycemia is occasionally reported but is generally clinically insignificant in man. One instance of diabetic ketoacidosis which occurred during heroin abstinence was very likely fortuitous (Desser and Arvan, 1969).

With maintenance of normal hygiene and nutrition, as well as the availability of pure drug and sterile methods for administering it, a morphine addict can live a normally healthy life. The most famous figure in American surgery was a long-time morphine addict whose addiction was inapparent to all but a few of his closest confidantes.

STIMULANTS

Amphetamines, such as methamphetamine and dextroamphetamine, as well as amphetamine surrogates, such as phenmetrazine or methylphenidate, are sympathomimetic stimulants widely abused. The pharmacological actions of each of these drugs are essentially similar, including euphoria, increased mental alertness, decreased physical fatigue, suppression of appetite, and a variety of physical signs indicating stimulation of the sympathetic nervous system (Martin *et al.*, 1971). Clinical uses of the drug, now being repudiated, are all clearly derived from these well established pharmacological effects.

Abuse of amphetamines follows three patterns. In one, the drug may be used only sporadically. Doses are small, taken by mouth, may not be repeated and only are used for specific situations. A second pattern employs oral doses chronically, with doses tending to become larger although still measured in tens of mg per day. Some of this use evolves from poorly supervised treatment of chronic depression or obesity. This pattern may involve the use of other drugs, principally alcohol and barbiturates. During the last decade, a new pattern of use has developed which represents a radical departure from previous patterns. The drug is used on a "spree" basis, is taken by intravenous injection and repetitively, and doses are measured in hundreds or thousands of mg per day. This type of amphetamine abuse is part of a drug culture in which many drugs are tried, including heroin.

The effects obtained from intravenous injection of massive doses are qualitatively different from those obtained from smaller oral doses (Kramer *et al.*, 1967). Just as with heroin, an initial "rush" is experienced which is described as a visceral numbness and tingling something akin to a diffuse orgasm. The subject then becomes highly loquacious, physically active and claims great powers of mind and body. The physical activity may be manifested by peculiar stereotyped grimacing movements, something akin to those produced in animals with large doses. Injections are taken at periodic intervals, to reinforce the pleasurable aspects of the rush. Such a sequence might be repeated over several days during which overexcitement, sleeplessness, and poor nutrition are the rule. Discontinuation is frequently associated with some symptoms of withdrawal: restlessness, aching, and mental depression. These withdrawal symptoms may be treated by the user with either barbiturates or, all too frequently, with heroin.

The major effect of repeated use of amphetamines is diminution in food intake, an effect generally believed to be located in the lateral hypothalamus. The subsequent weight loss is generally attributed to the diminished food intake, although the mobilization of free fatty acids from stimulants may also contribute. Even relatively small oral doses, such as two 10-mg tablets taken 3 h apart, can produce an increase in plasma free fatty acid levels without any appreciable change in plasma glucose levels (Hollister and Gillespie, 1970). The general belief is that the stimulants release

References p. 379–380

noradrenaline which acts through adenosine 3′,5′-cyclic monophosphate to activate lipases to split fatty acids from triglycerides in fatty tissue. Thus, this change in fat metabolism is mediated by a peripheral, rather than a central neuroendocrine mechanism.

A recent report of a rapid increase in plasma immunoassayable insulin in rats and mice, independent of hypo- or hyperglycemia, could be an instance of a species-specific phenomenon (McMahon *et al.*, 1971). Hypoglycemia was consistently found in mice but not in rats. As yet, there is no evidence of clinically detectable hypoglycemia associated with stimulant abuse, although one might speculate that some of the clinical manifestations of the "rush" might be attributed to a brief period of hypoglycemia.

HALLUCINOGENS

Lysergic acid diethylamide (LSD) and mescaline are the two major hallucinogens in use. Psilocybin, dimethyltryptamine, and various hallucinogenic amphetamine analogs are simply variants, producing mainly similar effects.

Most use of hallucinogens is sporadic, an isolated "trip". Continued daily use is unlikely as tolerance quickly develops on such a schedule. With customary doses, the clinical syndrome appears within minutes and lasts for several hours, usually reaching a peak at about 3 to 4 h. The somatic symptoms, perceptual changes and psychic alterations are well known. Comparisons indicate that the clinical syndromes, as well as most of the other effects of the drugs, are essentially identical between LSD, mescaline and psilocybin (Hollister, 1968). The doses vary over quite a wide range, however.

The endocrinological effects of these drugs in man are not very clear. Data from a few chronic schizophrenics revealed no change in urinary excretion of adrenaline or noradrenaline following small doses of LSD. The same doses increased excretion of catecholamines in manic-depressive patients, and increased adrenaline excretion while decreasing noradrenaline excretion in involutional patients, both of whom showed more clinical reactions (Elmadjian *et al.*, 1958). LSD, 2 μg/kg orally, produced a small rise in adrenaline excretion during the first 2 h after administration, but over an 8-h period, the excretion rates of adrenaline, noradrenaline, total metanephrines and vanylmandelic acid (VMA) did not differ from a control period. Mescaline (6 mg/kg) had a somewhat different effect in recovered schizophrenics, both adrenaline and VMA excretion being decreased transiently during a 4-h period. Excretion of 17-OHCS and 17-KS by subjects taking 1.5 to 2 μg/kg of LSD was not much changed, although a significant increase in excretion of 17-ketogenic steroids was noted during the first 8 h after the drug (Hollister, 1969). No effects were noted on serum protein-bound iodine levels within the first 4 h after the drug.

An antidiuretic effect following oral doses of 1.5 to 2 μg/kg of LSD was produced in 10 of 14 subjects (Hollister et al., 1970a). As compared with a control day during which a water load was administered, LSD decreased urine formation, decreased free water clearance, and increased urine osmolarity. These changes occurred promptly and lasted 4 h or more. Similar changes in urine formation were noted after doses of 5 to 6 mg/kg of mescaline, effects being more constant and profound. Attempts to relate the degree of antidiuresis with another measure of physiologic stress, the rise in plasma free fatty acids, or clinical indicators of stress as reported by subjects, were unsuccessful. Compared to the antidiuretic action of usual doses of morphine, hallucinogens appear to be much more potent. Except for a delayed excretion of urine, the effect has no clinical significance.

Hallucinogens produce a marked mobilization of plasma free fatty acids, almost approaching adrenaline itself in this action (Hollister and Moore, 1965). The rise can not be correlated with urinary excretion of catecholamines or their metabolites, which raises the question of whether these drugs may act directly rather than by release of catecholamines, or whether they may release the pituitary lipid-mobilizing material. The skinny look of many hippies could conceivably be due to their extensive use of fat as a source of energy.

SEDATIVES

The most popular sedatives for abuse are short-acting barbiturates, especially secobarbital sodium. Other so-called non-barbiturate sedatives are also subject to abuse, such as methaqualone, glutethimide and meprobamate. Drugs with a slower onset and longer duration of action, such as chlordiazepoxide and diazepam, tend to be abused far less frequently, as is also the case with phenobarbital.

The pattern of sedative abuse has not greatly changed in the past thirty years. Mostly drugs are taken orally with daily doses tending to stay in the range of 1000 mg of secobarbital sodium. The dose may be divided during the day so as to maintain a steady state of intoxication somewhat akin to that of alcohol. Prolonged use in such a way sets the stage for a withdrawal reaction which is quite similar to that from alcohol.

Many of the neuroendocrine effects observed from barbiturates in animals are similar to those described for morphine: decreased release of ACTH and decreased plasma concentrations of adrenal hormones; decreased release of pituitary gonadotrophins; and increased release of vasopressin. The latter could conceivably play a role in the acute oliguria noted in overdoses of barbiturates but its importance is much less than that of diminished glomerular filtration associated with hypotension.

MARIHUANA

Marihuana is one of the oldest of all socially used drugs, its use being recorded several millennia ago. It may also be the most frequently used drug; current estimates vary between 200 and 300 million users throughout the world. Of the three principal constituents in marihuana—cannabidiol, tetrahydrocannabinol (THC), and cannabinol—only THC has been proved to be active. A number of THC isomers and homologs have been synthesized, and appear to be active.

References p. 379–380

Clinically, the drug has a biphasic effect with initial symptoms of "stimulation" and euphoria followed later by sleepiness and dreamlike states. These effects are highly dose-dependent, ranging from a brief and mild "high" with minimal sleepiness from smoking weak marihuana preparations to a prolonged intoxication with many features similar to psychotomimetic drugs when high doses are taken orally (Hollister, 1971). Analogies have been made on the bases of various clinical and pharmacological studies to other drugs, such as hallucinogens, amphetamines, alcohol, atropine, morphine, and tricyclic antidepressants, but so far as the entire profile of pharmacological actions is concerned, marihuana is unique.

For many years, marihuana was alleged to cause hypoglycemia, without any evidence that it really did. A number of recent studies have indicated clearly that it has no appreciable effect on fasting plasma glucose concentrations (Hollister *et al.*, 1968; Weil *et al.*, 1968). On the contrary, one report indicated a deterioration in oral glucose tolerance following a brief and mild use (0.5 to 1 marihuana cigarette daily for seven days) of the drug. No impairment of insulin release or elevation of growth hormone levels was found (Podolsky *et al.*, 1971). A report of a single case of severe diabetic ketoacidosis following oral ingestion of marihuana seems more likely to be fortuitous than a consequence of the use of the drug (Hughes *et al.*, 1970).

THC and synhexyl in substantial oral doses had no appreciable effect of plasma free fatty acid concentrations, unlike the situation with the hallucinogens (Hollister *et al.*, 1968). To some extent, this is a reflection of the degree of excitation or sympathetic stimulation evoked by the drug and is consistent with the mixed stimulant-sedative properties of marihuana.

Despite evidence of increased ACTH secretion in rats (Dewey *et al.*, 1970) and increased plasma corticosterone in rats (Barry *et al.*, 1970), neither THC or synhexyl had any effect on plasma cortisol in man in the absence of secondary fear or anxiety (Hollister *et al.*, 1970b). THC elicited an increased excretion of adrenaline in the first 2 h after its use in man, which was first attributed to some anticipatory stress from the experiment or the rapid onset of unfamiliar symptoms. Subsequently, we have seen reactions in subjects which suggest that some of the early increase in pulse rate and elevations of blood pressure may be due to this mechanism, although it is virtually impossible to be sure that these responses are not of emotional origin. Nonetheless, such an effect in man would be consistent with the finding of a rapid (within 10 min) and marked (25 to 36%) reduction of adrenal adrenaline in mice given 10 mg/kg doses of THC (Welch *et al.*, 1971).

Although some lines of evidence in animals suggest depression of thyroid uptake of radioactive iodine (Miras, 1965) or an inhibition of pituitary-thyroid function with diminished release of TSH (Lomax, 1970), in man the clinical consequences of such changes have not yet been observed.

CONCLUSIONS

Although drugs of abuse have been shown in animal studies to have many actions on neuroendocrine systems, few of these have any relevance in man to clinical effects or to complications. These differences might be due to species, to the magnitude of doses used, to routes of administration, to duration of dosage, or to various mechanisms of tolerance. The leap from animal to man is as precarious here as it is elsewhere in pharmacology.

SUMMARY

The neuroendocrine functions of various drugs of abuse are difficult to relate to their clinical manifestations or complications. Decreased sexual desire and performance, menstrual irregularities, and increased fetal loss among heroin addicts may be attributed in part to decreased gonadotrophin release. The weight loss, almost to the point of emaciation, seen in amphetamine users may be related both to a direct central effect on appetite as well as to peripheral mobilization of free fatty acids. Hallucinogens tend to be used only sporadically, so long-term neuroendocrine effects are not evident. Barbiturates share many of the neuroendocrine effects of opiates, but these do not seem to play a prominent role in the clinical syndromes of chronic use. An early release of adrenaline after marihuana or THC may account for the initial stimulated phase of the clinical syndrome. At best, the number of systematic studies of neuroendocrine effects of these drugs in man are limited. Therefore, only limited conclusions can be drawn now.

ACKNOWLEDGEMENTS

Work of the author cited in this paper was supported in part by PHS grant MH-03030.

REFERENCES

BARRY, H., PERHACH, J. L. AND KUBENA, R. K. (1970) Δ^1-tetrahydrocannabinol activation of pituitary-adrenal function. *Pharmacologist*, **12**, 258.

CAMIEL, M. R., ALEXANDER, L. L. AND BENNINGHOFF, D. L. (1967) Drug addiction and gynecomastia. *New York J. Med.*, **67**, 2494–2495.

CUSHMAN, P. JR., BORDIER, B. AND HILTON, J. G. (1970) Hypothalamic-pituitary-adrenal axis in methadone-treated heroin addicts. *J. clin. Endocrinol.*, **30**, 24–29.

DESSER, K. B. AND ARVAN, S. (1969) Diabetic ketoacidosis during acute heroin abstinence. *Lancet*, **2**, 689–690.

DEWEY, W. L., PENG, T. C. AND HARRIS, L. S. (1970) The effect of 1-*trans*-Δ^9-tetrahydrocannabinol on the hypothalamo-hypophyseal-adrenal axis of rats. *Europ. J. Pharmacol.*, **12**, 382–384.

EISENMAN, A. J., FRASER, H. F., SLOAN, J. AND ISBELL, H. (1958) Urinary 17-ketosteroid excretion during a cycle of addiction to morphine. *J. Pharmacol. exp. Ther.*, **124**, 305–311.

EISENMAN, A. J., FRASER, H. F. AND BROOKS, J. W. (1961) Urinary excretion and plasma levels of 17-hydroxycorticosteroids during a cycle of addiction to morphine. *J. Pharmacol. exp. Ther.*, **132**, 226–231.

ELMADJIAN, F., HOPE, J. M. AND LAMSON, E. T. (1958) Excretion of epinephrine and norepinephrine under stress. *Recent Progr. Hormone Res.*, **14**, 513–553.

HOLLISTER, L. E. (1968) *Chemical Psychoses. LSD and Related Drugs*, Thomas, Springfield, Ill.

HOLLISTER, L. E. (1969) Steroids and moods: Correlations in schizophrenics and subjects treated with lysergic acid diethylamide (LSD), mescaline, tetrahydrocannabinol, and synhexyl. *J. clin. Pharmacol.*, **9**, 24–29.

HOLLISTER, L. E. (1971) Marihuana in man: three years later. *Science*, **172**, 21–29.

HOLLISTER, L. E. AND MOORE, F. (1965) Increased plasma free fatty acids following psychotomimetic drugs. *J. psychiat. Res.*, **3**, 199–204.

HOLLISTER, L. E. AND GILLESPIE, H. K. (1970) A new stimulant, prolintane hydrochloride, compared with dextroamphetamine in fatigued volunteers. *J. clin. Pharmacol.*, **10**, 103–109.

HOLLISTER, L. E., RICHARDS, R. K. AND GILLESPIE, H. K. (1968) Comparison of tetrahydrocannabinol and synhexyl in man. *Clin. pharmacol. Ther.*, **9**, 783–791.

HOLLISTER, L. E., KANTER, S. L. AND DRONKERT, A. (1970a) Antidiuresis in man following lysergic acid diethylamide and mescaline. *Behav. Neuropsychiat.*, **2**, 50–54.

HOLLISTER, L. E., MOORE, F., KANTER, S. L. AND NOBLE, E. (1970b) Δ^1-tetrahydrocannabinol, synhexyl and marihuana extract administered orally in man: Catecholamine excretion, plasma cortisol levels and platelet serotonin concentration. *Psychopharmacologia (Berl.)*, **17**, 354–360.

HUGHES, J. E., STEAHLY, L. P. AND NIER, N. M. (1970) Marihuana and the diabetic coma. *J. Amer. med. Ass.*, **214**, 1113–1114.

KRAMER, J. C., FISHMAN, V. S. AND LITTLEFIELD, D. C. (1967) Amphetamine abuse. *J. Amer. med. Ass.*, **201**, 305–309.

LOMAX, P. (1970) The effect of marihuana on pituitary-thyroid activity in the rat. *Agents and Actions*, **1**, 252–257.

MARTIN, W. R., SLOAN, J. W., SAPIRA, J. D. AND JASINSKI, D. R. (1971) Physiologic, subjective, and behavioral effects of amphetamine, methamphetamine, ephedrine, phenmetrazine and methylphenidate in man. *Clin. pharmacol. Ther.*, **12**, 245.

MCMAHON, E. M., ANDERSEN, D. K., FELDMAN, J. M. AND SCHANBERG, S. M. (1971) Methamphetamine-induced insulin release. *Science*, **174**, 66–68.

MILLS, E. AND WANG, S. C. (1964) Liberation of antidiuretic hormones. Pharmacologic blockade of ascending pathways. *Amer. J. Psychiat.*, **207**, 1405–1410.

MIRAS, C. J. (1965) Some aspects of cannabis action. In *Hashish. Its Chemistry and Pharmacology* (Ciba Foundation Study Group No. 21), G. E. W. WOLSTENHOLME (Ed.), Little Brown, Boston, pp. 37–47.

PODOLSKY, S., PATTAVINA, C. G. AND AMARAL, M. A. (1971) Effect of marihuana on the glucose-tolerance test. *Ann. N. Y. Acad. Sci.*, **191**, 54–60.

SMITH, G. M., SEMKE, C. W. AND BEECHER, H. K. (1962) Objective evidence of mental effects of heroin, morphine and placebo in normal subjects. *J. pharmacol. exp. Ther.*, **136**, 53–58.

STOFFER, S. S. (1968) A gynecologic study of drug addicts. *Amer. J. Obstet. Gynecol.*, **101**, 779–783.

WEIL, A. T., ZINBERG, N. E. AND NELSEN, J. M. (1968) Clinical and psychological effects of marihuana in man. *Science*, **162**, 1234–1242.

WELCH, B. L., WELCH, A. S., MESSIHA, F. S. AND BERGER, H. J. (1971) Rapid depletion of adrenal epinephrine and elevation of telencephalic serotonin by (-)-trans-Δ^9-tetrahydrocannabinol in mice. *Res. Commun. chem. pathol. Pharmacol.*, **2**, 382–391.

ZAKS, A. M., BRUNER, A., FINK, M. AND FREEDMAN, A. M. (1969) Intravenous diacetylmorphine (heroin) in studies of opiate dependence. *Dis. nerv. Syst.*, **30**, 89–92.

DISCUSSION

TABAKOFF: Did you use any alpha or beta blockers in trying to suppress free fatty acid response to LSD?

HOLLISTER: No, I haven't. I have really little doubt that it would block the free fatty acid rise. What would be of greater interest from a psychopharmacological point of view is whether it would attenuate the mental effects of LSD. We have plans to test propranolol with THC as a blocking agent.

BARRY: What was the previous history of marihuana use in your subjects?

HOLLISTER: We aren't allowed to use "virgins", even if we could find them. On the other hand, we don't like to use "pot-heads". What we generally take is what we would describe as "casual users".

People who may smoke a reefer on a weekend or something of that sort. Thus, we try to get people who aren't so well habituated that they'll provide unreliable results due to pharmacodynamic or metabolic tolerance or simply psychic habituation. Getting back to the rats; so many of these experiments with THC are done with intraperitoneal injections. This is a poor way to give the drug. There is evidence that really very little of it is absorbed and it creates a chemical peritonitis. This raises the question of whether some effects seen in animals with this route of administration may not simply be due to an inapparent stressful effect of sticking this stuff into the peritoneal cavity.

PEARSON: In your studies relative to the antidiuretic action of LSD you didn't show when the water-loaded LSD users got rid of the water. Does it last as long as the hallucinogenic effect or when does it return to normal levels?

HOLLISTER: Unfortunately, I can't answer that. We designed these experiments to do them over the course of the normal working day and without hospitalizing people. I suppose that it would have been more logical to follow a couple of them over a 24 h period. However, we never heard of anyone who didn't get rid of the water load eventually.

PEARSON: At these doses of LSD how long do the subjects report the presence of the hallucinogenic effects?

HOLLISTER: Usually by about 8 h, which was the end of the experiment, but while the antidiuretic effect was still persisting. Subjects were fairly clear, although mild degrees of impairment lasted throughout the remaining part of the evening. In fact, we got into the regular habit of giving people a sedative at bedtime and many of them continued to be stimulated. I thought that adding a night of insomnia to what they had been through during the day was to add insult to insult.

KRIVOY: How do the changes in urinary adrenaline levels follow the hallucinations?

HOLLISTER: We haven't been able to correlate urinary catecholamine levels with anything. We tried to correlate them with the free fatty acids, we tried to correlate them with clinical manifestations, and we tried to correlate changes in water clearance with clinical stress as reported by the patients, changes in plasma free fatty acids and changes in urinary catecholamines. We just couldn't make any reasonable correlations between these.

Antagonism Between Morphine and the Polypeptides ACTH, $ACTH_{1-24}$, and β-MSH in the Nervous System

E. ZIMMERMANN* AND W. KRIVOY

National Institute of Mental Health, Addiction Research Center, Lexington, Ky. (U.S.A.)

The literature contains a number of observations indicating an interaction between morphine and the polypeptides corticotrophin (ACTH) and beta-melanocyte stimulating hormone (β-MSH). However, few studies have been conducted to test the hypothesis that ACTH or β-MSH might play a causal role in any part of the addiction cycle to morphine. This possibility was raised by Cohen *et al.* (1965) who observed that actinomycin D inhibits the development of tolerance to morphine. These authors suggested that the development of tolerance to morphine is associated with the production of new RNA, and consequently, a peptide or protein which is capable of antagonizing the actions of morphine on the nervous system. Since Krivoy and Guillemin (1961, 1962) had observed that β-MSH stimulates neural activity, Cohen *et al.* (1965), as well as Krivoy and Zimmermann (1973), postulated that β-MSH might be one of the peptides involved in the development of tolerance to morphine.

The purpose of this communication is to review the literature relative to the antagonism which exists between the neural actions of morphine and those of the peptides ACTH, $ACTH_{1-24}$, and β-MSH, and to examine the possible role of ACTH–MSH-like peptides in the development of tolerance to morphine.

I. Intact animals

Early evidence of antagonism of morphine by ACTH was reported by Winter and Flataker (1951) who demonstrated that pretreatment of adult male rats with four hourly intraperitoneal injections of ACTH (2 mg/rat) partially reduced the analgesic effect of morphine sulfate (4 or 8 mg/kg) administered subcutaneously immediately following the fourth injection of ACTH. ACTH itself exerted no analgesic action, *i.e.* it did not alter the reaction time to thermal stimulation of the tail. A fifth injection of ACTH (2 mg/rat), given 45 min after the administration of morphine, was followed by an apparent increased responsivity to stimulation, so that the reaction time was actually reduced relative to that of the ACTH-injected controls. During the period of

* Present address: Department of Anatomy, University of California School of Medicine, Los Angeles, Calif. (U.S.A.).

References p. 391–392

the "rebound" reaction (Winter and Flataker, 1951) the ACTH–morphine-treated animals exhibited signs of arousal and increased activity.

The findings of Winter and Flataker (1951) were confirmed and extended by Paroli (1967) who found that the intramuscular administration of ACTH (1 U./kg) 45–60 min prior to intraperitoneal injection of 20 mg/kg morphine markedly reduced the analgesic effect of morphine. He also pretreated mice with ACTH in varying doses (5.0–600.0 mU./kg) and found that the effect was dose related. Although Paroli (1967) failed to observe the morphine-antagonistic effect in adrenalectomized rats, he also failed to observe antagonism of morphine by hydrocortisone (100 μg/kg) in adrenalectomized rats. Moreover, in intact animals, the antimorphine effect of ACTH did not parallel the levels of circulating 11-hydroxycorticosteroids. From these results, he concluded that the antagonistic action of ACTH on the analgesic action of morphine depends upon the presence of the adrenal gland, but is not determined by the plasma level of corticosteroids.

Ferrari *et al.* (1963) and Gessa *et al.* (1967) described a peculiar stereotyped behavioral syndrome which follows the intraventricular or intracerebral administration of ACTH-like peptides, including $ACTH_{1-24}$ and β-MSH. This syndrome, the stretching crisis, is characterized by frequent and repeated stretching and yawning movements, accompanied by electroencephalographic and behavioral signs of arousal. The stretching crises occur at frequent intervals starting 30–120 min following the intracisternal administration of microquantities of these peptides and persist for several hours thereafter. A single intravenous injection of 1 or 5 mg/kg of morphine caused complete cessation of these stretching crises for 30 and 60 min, respectively, in dogs treated with 1 U./kg ACTH intracisternally 3 h earlier (Ferrari *et al.*, 1963). Several other centrally active drugs including chlorpromazine, atropine, and diethazine, were also effective in antagonizing this effect of ACTH. The authors attributed their findings to antagonism of the excitatory action of ACTH by inhibitory effects of these agents on the brain stem reticular formation.

II. Spinal animals

The tail flick response to heat studied by Winter and Flataker (1951) and by Paroli (1967) involves a reflex which is integrated at the spinal level, but which may be influenced by supraspinal activity. To determine whether or not the antagonism of morphine by ACTH occurred at a spinal level, Winter and Flataker (1951) transected the spinal cord of rats. They observed that morphine still inhibited the tail flick, and that ACTH antagonized this action of morphine. However, they also noted that, unlike intact animals, morphine-treated spinal rats failed to exhibit reduced reaction times following the administration of ACTH. These observations were taken to indicate that while the "rebound" phenomenon observed in intact animals may be due to supraspinal actions, the antagonism of morphine depression of spinal reflex activity may be explained by a direct action of ACTH on the spinal cord.

Recent experiments in our laboratory (Krivoy *et al.*, in preparation) were designed to determine if β-MSH or $ACTH_{1-24}$, administered prior to morphine, alters the inhibitory action of morphine on the segmental reflex of the cat spinal cord. Using conventional electrophysiological techniques, this series of experiments was performed on decerebrate spinal cats. Details of this preparation and its use in similar studies is described elsewhere (Krivoy, *et al.*, 1973). Briefly, adult cats of either sex were anesthetized with ether, decerebrated by electrocoagulation, and the spinal cord was exposed from L_1 to S_2. The spinal cord was transected at L_1. Dorsal and ventral roots of spinal segments L_7 or S_1 were used for stimulation and recording, respectively, of the segmental reflex. Succinylcholine was given by intravenous drip, and the cat artificially respired. Blood pressure was measured continuously, but in the absence of an anticoagulant. The segmental reflex was evoked every 400 msec throughout the experiment using a stimulus which produced a submaximal reflex response. Following a control period lasting 30 min, the peptide being tested was injected intravenously. 1 min later, the first of three doses of morphine sulfate (0.5 mg/kg) was given intravenously. The second (2.5 mg/kg) and third (12.5 mg/kg) doses of morphine were administered intravenously at 30-min intervals thereafter. In some experiments the

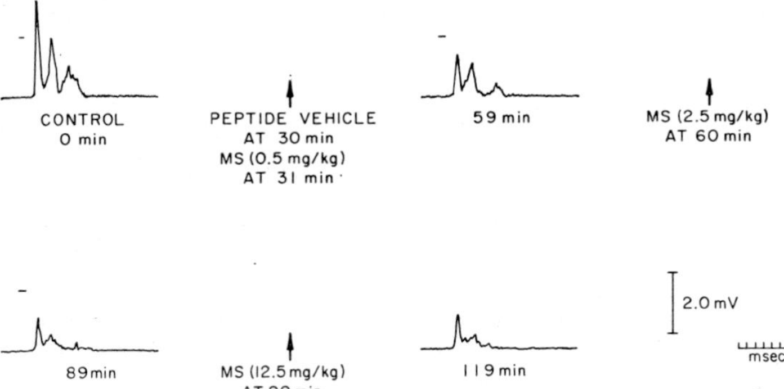

Fig. 1. Actions of morphine (MS) on amplitudes of mono- and polysynaptic potentials reflexly evoked in a lumbar ventral root of a decerebrate-spinal cat. In this figure and in Figs. 2–4, the relative time intervals are used to indicate when a given trace was recorded and when a given drug was administered.

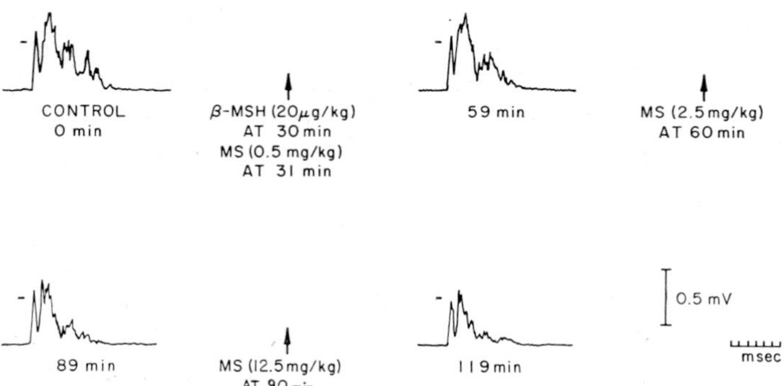

Fig. 2. Antagonism by β-MSH of MS-induced depression of amplitudes of mono- and polysynaptic potentials reflexly evoked in a lumbar ventral root of a decerebrate-spinal cat.

References p. 391–392

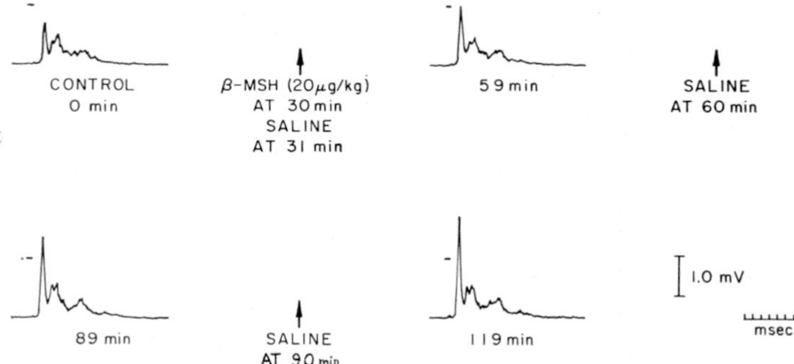

Fig. 3. Actions of β-MSH on amplitudes of mono- and polysynaptic potentials reflexly evoked in a lumbar ventral root of a decerebrate-spinal cat.

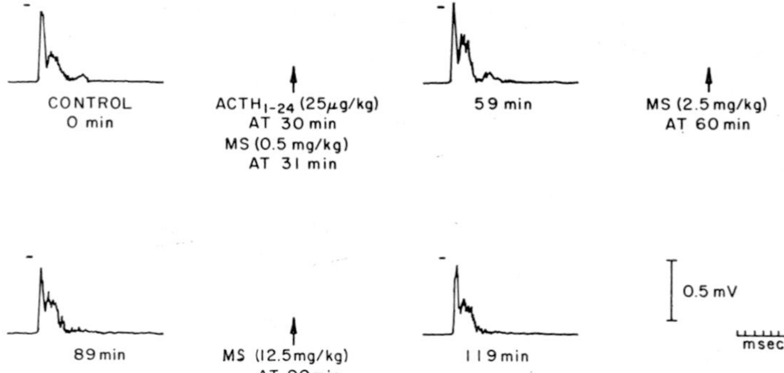

Fig. 4. Antagonism by $ACTH_{1-24}$ of MS-induced depression of mono- and polysynaptic potentials reflexly evoked in a lumbar ventral root of a decerebrate-spinal cat.

peptide vehicle was used in place of the peptide. In other experiments, saline was used in place of morphine.

From the experiments outlined in the preceding paragraph, it was observed that morphine injection is followed by a dose-related diminution of the amplitudes of evoked mono- and polysynaptic reflex activity (Fig. 1). In this, and all subsequent figures, the first upward deflection after the shock-artefact is monosynaptic, whereas subsequent potentials are considered to be polysynaptic. When cats were injected with β-MSH (20 μg/kg) before morphine, the depressant action of morphine on mono- and polysynaptic reflexes was not significant (Fig. 2). Consistent with results obtained earlier (Krivoy and Guillemin, 1961), the administration of the same dose of β-MSH, followed by saline, caused selective enhancement of the amplitude of the monosynaptic reflex discharge (Fig. 3). Administration of 25 μg/kg $ACTH_{1-24}$, a dose equimolar to that of β-MSH used above, also antagonized the depressant action of morphine on evoked mono- and polysynaptic reflexes (Fig. 4); however, in contrast to the effects of β-MSH, $ACTH_{1-24}$, followed by saline, failed to alter the magnitude of the evoked reflex response.

During the studies related in the preceding paragraph, morphine administration was followed by a dose-related decrease of systolic and diastolic blood pressures to approximately 75 and 65%, respectively, of control values. Despite their antagonism of the spinal depressant actions of morphine, neither β-MSH nor $ACTH_{1-24}$ significantly altered the cardiovascular response to morphine. This dissociation of morphine's actions by administration of β-MSH or $ACTH_{1-24}$ suggests that these peptides may selectively antagonize the neural depressant effects of morphine. Plasma corticosteroid levels were determined before, and at intervals following the administration of peptide and/or morphine. These levels were found to be highly elevated during the control periods and did not vary significantly from this during the course of these experiments. This probably reflects the fact that prior to obtaining blood samples each cat was exposed to ether vapor, extensive surgery, and coagulation of its midbrain. As a result, pituitary-adrenal activation was likely maximal prior to and during the entire period of observation. From these observations, it appeared unlikely that the morphine-antagonistic actions of β-MSH or of $ACTH_{1-24}$ were mediated by a change in circulating levels of corticosteroids.

III. Experiments in vitro

In order to circumvent some of the problems involved in interpreting results obtained in intact and spinal animals, the actions of morphine and $ACTH_{1-24}$, have been

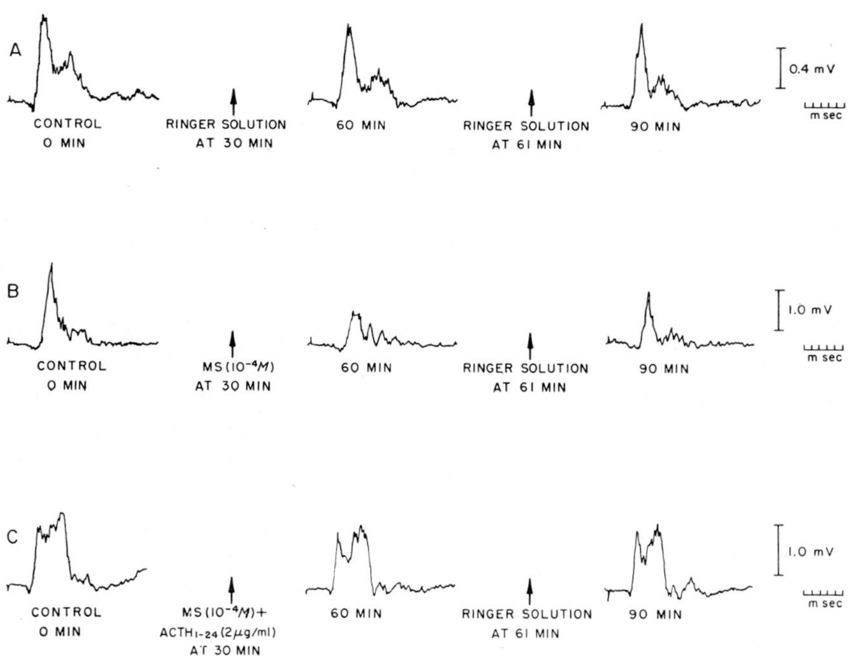

Fig. 5. Antagonism by $ACTH_{1-24}$ of MS-induced depression of monosynaptic potentials evoked in a lumbar ventral root of the frog isolated spinal cord. The relative time intervals are used to indicate when a given trace was recorded or when the superfusion solution was changed. A, B, and C indicate separate experiments.

References p. 391–392

studied alone, and in combination, using the isolated frog spinal cord (Zimmermann and Krivoy, in preparation). These experiments were based on those of Brookhart *et al.* (1959) who described a monosynaptic pathway which could be studied by recording the electrical activity evoked in the ventral spinal root after stimulation of the lateral aspect of the cord several segments cephalad to the lumbar segment under investigation. Using this preparation, frog spinal cords were superfused with Ringer's solution, or Ringer's solution containing morphine, $ACTH_{1-24}$, or morphine plus $ACTH_{1-24}$. Superfusion with Ringer's solution alone did not significantly alter the amplitude of the evoked monosynaptic potential. Exposure for 30 min to morphine ($10^{-4}M$) dissolved in the superfusate reduced the amplitude of the potential to 68.1 $\pm$ 5.7% of the mean predrug control amplitude, and this reduction (observed in 5 cords) was significantly different from the mean amplitude of 5 cords exposed to Ringer's solution alone (100.9 $\pm$ 8.1). When $ACTH_{1-24}$ (2 μg/ml) was superfused along with morphine ($10^{-4}M$), the mean amplitude of the evoked response in 5 cords did not change significantly (101.4 $\pm$ 8.8). Superfusion of $ACTH_{1-24}$ (2 μg/ml) alone in Ringer's solution did not alter the response. Fig. 5 illustrates representative potentials recorded before, during, and after superfusion of Ringer's solution alone (A), with morphine ($10^{-4}M$) (B), or with morphine ($10^{-4}M$) plus $ACTH_{1-24}$ (2 μg/ml) (C). These findings are consistent with reported effects of morphine on spinal cord reflexes in the frog (Angelucci, 1955) but further indicate that the antagonism between morphine and $ACTH_{1-24}$ is a consequence of their direct actions on spinal cord.

DISCUSSION

The observations reviewed above are consistent with the hypothesis of Cohen *et al.* (1965) in that they illustrate antagonism of the actions of morphine on neural structures by naturally occurring β-MSH and ACTH, as well as by $ACTH_{1-24}$. Although the precise site of this antagonism is not clear, the evidence available indicates that it can occur at several levels within the neuraxis. Thus, while the findings of Ferrari *et al.* (1963) and Gessa *et al.* (1967) indicate a cerebral site of action, our studies (Section II), and those of Winter and Flataker (1951) have demonstrated that the antagonism can occur within the spinal cord. Although the antagonism between these polypeptides and morphine has been described at a number of sites within the neuraxis, there does appear to be a degree of specificity. We say this because of the failure both of $ACTH_{1-24}$ and of β-MSH to antagonize the actions of morphine on the blood pressure of the decerebrate low-spinal Lloyd preparation, despite the fact that naloxone does antagonize these actions of morphine (Krivoy *et al.*, in press).

The mechanism, or mechanisms, by which these peptides act on the nervous system or antagonize morphine is not clear. There are structural similarities (*e.g.*, $ACTH_{4-10}$) between β-MSH, ACTH and $ACTH_{1-24}$ which have been used to explain certain aspects of their pharmacology which are similar and imply a common mechanism of action on the nervous system. These include the ability of these peptides to produce stretching crises (Ferrari *et al.*, 1963, Gessa *et al.*, 1967), sexual excitement (Bertolini *et al.*, 1969), synchronization of the electroencephalogram (Sandman *et al.*, 1971, Torda and Wolf, 1952), and their ability to enhance acquisition and inhibit extinction of conditioned avoidance behavior (De Wied, 1966, 1969). However, until the precise mechanism of one of these peptides is determined and compared to the others, it is not possible to state that a single mechanism explains their actions on the nervous system, their ability to antagonize morphine, or the ability of morphine to antagonize these peptides. Alternatively, it might be reasonable to espouse the concept of a single mechanism if each of the peptides had the same array of specific antagonists or agonists. Unfortunately, it is not known if such an array exists. Therefore, although the suggestion is a tempting one, we do not yet have sufficient information to determine whether or not the neurotrophic actions of MSH–ACTH-like peptides depend upon a common mechanism of action.

The fact that β-MSH augments transmission of monosynaptic reflex activity (Krivoy and Guillemin, 1961) suggests that it may be a non-specific antagonist of morphine. This possibility is supported by the observation that β-MSH also antagonizes chlorpromazine-induced depression of spinal reflexes (Krivoy and Guillemin, 1962). On the other hand, as pointed out in Section II above, whereas β-MSH does not facilitate polysynaptic reflex activity, it does appear to antagonize morphine-induced depression of polysynaptic activity. This would suggest that at least part of the morphine-antagonistic actions of β-MSH can be dissociated from its stimulant properties.

Winter and Flataker (1951) found that cortisone antagonized the analgesic action of morphine. This finding was used to suggest that the morphine-antagonistic actions of ACTH were due to its ability to stimulate secretion of adrenocortical hormones. However, Paroli (1967) found that although ACTH did not antagonize morphine in the adrenalectomized rat, neither did corticosteroids. From this observation it was concluded that the antagonistic action of ACTH depended upon the presence of the adrenals, but not upon the corticotrophic action of ACTH. In experiments from these laboratories (Section II above), the circulating levels of corticosteroids did not appear to change in concert with the actions of morphine on spinal reflexes, or with the antagonism of this action either by β-MSH or by $ACTH_{1-24}$, suggesting the lack of a causal relationship between the actions of these agents on the reflexes studied and the levels of corticosteroids. Finally, adrenocortical involvement would not explain the action of β-MSH on the cat spinal cord since β-MSH is only a very weak corticotrophic agent (Guillemin *et al.*, 1957), or the capacity of $ACTH_{1-24}$ to antagonize the action of morphine on the isolated frog spinal cord (Section III above). Taken together, it seems unlikely that the antagonism of the spinal depressant or analgesic actions of morphine depends upon adrenocortical activation. However, one cannot exclude the possibility that elevated levels of circulating corticosteroids are a prerequisite for the morphine-antagonistic action of ACTH, since corticosteroids are known to augment other activities of this peptide (Braun and Hechter, 1970).

Cohen *et al.* (1965) reasoned that because morphine administration subjects neural cells to new information and results in a decreased response to subsequent injections of the drug, the development of tolerance may be considered a form of learning. This concept is consistent with the evidence that learning involves the synthesis of RNA and that the inhibition of RNA and protein synthesis blocks the development of tolerance to morphine (Cohen *et al.*, 1965, Cox *et al.*, 1968, 1970). In this regard, it is interesting that the administration of ACTH augments protein synthesis in brain and spinal cord (Semiginovsky and Jakoubek, 1971), and that ACTH and related polypeptides, including $ACTH_{1-24}$ and MSH, augment acquisition and/or decrease extinction of conditioned avoidance responses in rats (De Wied, 1966, 1969). From these observations, it becomes tempting to speculate that β-MSH and $ACTH_{1-24}$ antagonize the actions of morphine on the nervous system by facilitating the development of tolerance.

One mechanism postulated for the antagonism of morphine by β-MSH (Krivoy and Zimmermann, 1973) is based upon two observations. The first is that morphine reduces the supernormal period residual after detonation of the nerve cell (Krivoy and Huggins, 1961). The second is that when the synapse in not being maximally activated, β-MSH enhances the supernormal period residual after synaptic activation (Krivoy *et al.*, 1963). The former observation has been used to explain some of the depressant actions of morphine on spinal cord (Krivoy and Zimmermann, 1973) since, if morphine reduces the supernormal period following synaptic detonation, the next succeeding nerve impulse would find the synaptic zone less excitable than normal and produce detonation of fewer cells than it normally would. On the other hand, since β-MSH has an action opposite to that of morphine, it would antagonize morphine and lead to more normal synaptic transmission.

In view of the antagonism of morphine by the two naturally occurring polypeptides ACTH and β-MSH, it is appropriate to consider if these two peptides might be involved in the development of tolerance to and physical dependence upon morphine. One of the major concepts underlying theories to explain these two aspects of the pharmacology of morphine assumes that homeostatic mechanisms are brought into play and counteract the actions of the drug. When morphine is withheld from the tolerant and physically dependent subject, tissue levels of morphine are reduced by metabolism or excretion of the drug, but the augmented level of homeostatic adjustment not only persists, but persists unopposed thus giving rise to the abstinence syndrome. One of the homeostatic mechanisms involved in the development of tolerance has been suggested to be the increased production of a peptide which counteracts the actions of morphine (Cohen *et al.*, 1965). We propose that two of the peptides involved in this process could be ACTH and β-MSH. We submit this for the following reasons. The evidence reviewed in Sections I and II illustrate that these two naturally occurring polypeptides antagonize at least some of the actions of morphine. It has been shown that morphine administration, at least initially, causes increased secretion of ACTH (Paroli and Malchiorri, 1961a) and of MSH (Kastin *et al.*, 1969) from the pituitary. Unfortunately, evidence relative to the secretion of MSH after repeated injections of morphine is lacking, and the evidence for sustained increased secretion of ACTH is conflicting. Thus, several investigators have reported adrenal enlargment (Sung *et al.*, 1953, Tanabe and Cafruny, 1958). Paroli and Melchiorri (1961a) observed increased urinary levels of hydroxysteroids in rats during the first

5–10 days of treatment with morphine. Whereas these findings suggest prolonged increased secretion of ACTH, Paroli and Melchiorri (1961a) found that the continued administration of morphine resulted in decreased levels of urinary steroids, and Eisenman *et al.* (1961, 1969) observed reduced levels of 17-hydroxycorticosteroids in plasma and urine of man during addiction to morphine, suggesting diminished release of ACTH. These latter two observations might be a result of the fact that repeated administration of morphine can cause direct inhibition of corticosteroid synthesis by the adrenal (Paroli and Melchiorri, 1961b). This reduced production of corticosteroids following chronic treatment with morphine might be expected to promote the secretion of ACTH by reducing corticosteroid feedback inhibition (Liddle *et al.*, 1961). Therefore, to evaluate the role of ACTH or MSH in the addiction cycle it becomes important to measure blood levels of these peptides using direct techniques, but this has not yet been done.

SUMMARY

The information reviewed illustrates that the peptides, ACTH, $ACTH_{1-24}$, and β-MSH, can antagonize the depressant action of morphine on the central nervous system. The mechanism underlying this antagonism is not known, although the antagonism has been demonstrated to occur at the spinal cord level. Based upon evidence that morphine decreases, whereas β-MSH increases the period of supernormality following detonation of the nerve cell, the possibility is discussed that these agents exert opposing actions on synaptic transmission, and thereby modulate the central excitatory state in opposite directions. Although much more evidence is needed to critically evaluate this hypothesis, it might help explain, in part at least, the development of tolerance to morphine.

REFERENCES

Angelucci, L. (1955) Experiments with perfused frog's spinal cord. *Brit. J. Pharmacol.*, **11**, 161–170.

Bertolini, A., Vergoni, W., Gessa, G. L. and Ferrari, W. (1969) Induction of sexual excitement by the action of adrenocorticotrophic hormone in brain. *Nature (Lond.)*, **221**, 667–669.

Braun, T. and Hechter, O. (1970) Glucocorticoid regulation of ACTH sensitivity of adenyl cyclase in rat fat cell membranes. *Proc. natl. Acad. Sci.*, **66**, 995–1001.

Brookhart, J. M., Machne, X. and Fadiga, E. (1959) Patterns of motor neuron discharge in the frog. *Arch. Ital. Biol.*, **97**, 53–67.

Cohen, M., Keats, A., Krivoy, W. and Ungar, G. (1965) Effect of actinomycin D on morphine tolerance. *Proc. Soc. exp. biol. Med.*, **119**, 381–384.

Cox, B., Ginsburg, M. and Osman, O. H. (1968) Acute tolerance to narcotic analgesic drugs in rats. *Brit. J. Pharmacol.*, **33**, 245–256.

Cox, B. and Osman, O. H. (1970) Inhibition of the development of tolerance to morphine in rats by drugs which inhibit ribonucleic acid or protein synthesis. *Brit. J. Pharmacol.*, **38**, 157–170.

De Wied, D. (1966) Inhibitory effect of ACTH and related peptides on extinction of conditioned avoidance behavior in rats. *Proc. Soc. exp. biol. Med.*, **122**, 28–31.

De Wied, D. (1969) Effects of peptide hormones on behavior. In *Frontiers in Neuroendocrinology*, Martini, L. and Ganong, W. F. (Eds.), Academic Press, New York, pp. 97–140.

Eisenman, A. J., Fraser, H. F. and Brooks, J. W. (1961) Urinary excretion and plasma levels of

17-hydroxycorticosteroids during a cycle of addiction to morphine. *J. Pharmacol. exp. Ther.*, **132**, 226–231.

EISENMAN, A. J., SLOAN, J. W., MARTIN, W. R., JASINSKI, D. R. AND BROOKS, J. W. (1969) Catecholamine and 17-hydroxycorticosteroid excretion during a cycle of morphine dependence in man. *J. Psychiat.*, **7**, 19–28.

FERRARI, W., GESSA, G. AND VARGIU, L. (1963) Behavioral effects induced by intracisternally administered ACTH and MSH. *Ann. N.Y. Acad. Sci.*, **104**, 330–343.

GESSA, G. L., PISANO, M., VARGIU, L., CRABAI, F. AND FERRARI, W. (1967) Stretching and yawning movements after intracerebral injection of ACTH. *Rev. Canad. Biol.*, **26**, 229–236.

GUILLEMIN, R., HEARN, W., CHEEK, W. AND HOUSEHOLDER, D. (1957) Control of corticotropin release: further studies with *in vitro* methods. *Endocrinology*, **60**, 448–506.

KASTIN, A. J., SCHALLY, A. V., VIOSCA, S. AND MILLER, M. C. (1969) MSH activity in plasma and pituitaries of rats after various treatments. *Endocrinology*, **84**, 20–27.

KRIVOY, W. AND GUILLEMIN, R. (1961) On a possible role of B-melanocyte stimulating hormone (β-MSH) in the spinal cord of the cat. *Endocrinology*, **69**, 170–175.

KRIVOY, W. AND HUGGINS, R. (1961) The action of morphine, methadone, meperidine, and nalorphine on dorsal root potentials of cat spinal cord. *J. Pharmacol. exp. Ther.*, **134**, 210–213.

KRIVOY, W. AND GUILLEMIN, R. (1962) Antagonism of chlorpromazine by Beta-melanocyte stimulating hormone (β-MSH). *Experientia*, **18**, 20–21.

KRIVOY, W., LANE, M. AND KROEGER, D. C. (1963) The action of certain polypeptides on synaptic transmission. *Ann. N.Y. Acad. Sci.*, **104**, 312–329.

KRIVOY, W. A. AND ZIMMERMANN, E. (1973) A possible role of polypeptides in synaptic transmission. In *James E. P. Toman Memorial Volume on Neurobiology and Behavior*, H. SABELLI, R. GREENBURG, A. ABRAMS AND S. ALIVISATOS (Eds.), Raven, New York.

KRIVOY, W., KROEGER, D. AND ZIMMERMANN, E. (1973) Actions of morphine on the segmental reflex of the decerebrate spinal cat. *Brit. J. Pharmacol.*, in press.

LIDDLE, G. W., ISLAND, D. AND MEADOR, C. (1961) Normal and abnormal regulation of corticotrophin secretion in man. *Recent Progr. Hormone Res.*, **18**, 125–166.

PAROLI, E. (1967) Indagini sull'effeto antimorfinico dell'ACTH, I. Relazioni con il corticosurrene ed i livelli ematici degli 11-OH steroidi. *Arch. Ital. Sci. Farmacol.*, **13**, 234–237.

PAROLI, E. AND MALCHIORRI, P. (1961a) Urinary excretion of hydroxysteroids, 17-ketosteroids, and aldosterone in rats during a cycle of treatment with morphine. *Biochem. Pharmacol.*, **6**, 1–17.

PAROLI, E. AND MELCHIORRI, P. (1961b) Inhibitory effect of morphine on metabolism of adrenal and testicular steroids. *Biochem. Pharmacol.*, **6**, 18–20.

SANDMAN, C. A., DENMAN, P. M., MILLER, L. H., KNOTT, J. R., SCHALLY, A. V. AND KASTIN, A. J. (1971) Electroencephalographic measures of melanocyte-stimulating hormone activity. *J. comp. Physiol. Psych.*, **76**, 103–109.

SEMIGINOVSKY, B. AND JAKOUBEK, B. (1971) Effect of ACTH on the incorporation of ^{14}C-leucine in the brain and spinal cord of inbred mice. *Brain Res.*, **35**, 319–323.

SUNG, C. Y., WAY, E. L. AND SCOTT, K. G. (1953) Studies on the relationship of metabolic fate and hormonal effects of d,l-methadone to the development of drug tolerance. *J. Pharmacol. exp. Ther.*, **107**, 12–23.

TANABE, T. AND CAFRUNY, E. J. (1958) Adrenal hypertrophy in rats treated chronically with morphine. *J. Pharmacol. exp. Ther.*, **122**, 148–153.

TORDA, C. AND WOLF, H. G. (1952) Effects of various concentrations of adrenocorticotrophic hormone on electrical activity of brain and on sensitivity to convulsion-inducing agents. *Amer. J. Physiol.*, **168**, 406–413.

WINTER, C. A. AND FLATAKER, L. (1951) The effect of corticosterone, desoxycorticosterone, and adrenocorticotrophic hormone upon the responses of animals to analgesic drugs. *J. Pharmacol. exp. Ther.*, **103**, 93–105.

DISCUSSION

PEARSON: The morphine doses in the frog were quite high. Did you examine the effect of antagonists or inactive narcotic isomers in the frog preparation?

ZIMMERMANN: I agree that the dose 10^{-4} M is high. It is similar to the concentration found by Angelucci (Brit. J. Pharmacol., 11, 161, 1955) to depress spinal reflex activity in frog cord. We used an equimolar dose of naloxone and found that it antagonized the depressant action of morphine.

STRAND: I would like to comment on Dr. Zimmermann's very interesting results in the central nervous system and to suggest that ACTH and β-MSH may have similar effects on the peripheral nervous system or the neuromuscular junction. We have been working with the sciatic nerve gastrocnemius muscle *in situ* and found that the amplitudes of both nerve and muscle action potentials are increased and the effect of fatigue is decreased by ACTH and even more effectively by β-MSH using about the same dosage that you have been using.

ZIMMERMANN: Thank you Dr. Strand, those are very interesting findings. They may help explain the beneficial effects of ACTH in the treatment of myasthenia gravis.

MILLER: We have studied effects of β-MSH on electrocortical activity of the rat. Interestingly, we found that methadone produces a pattern of activity in the rat EEG which is similar to that of β-MSH, namely, high-voltage slow activity with some spiking. This seems to follow the development of tolerance to methadone in that animals when they were first placed on methadone, in their drinking water, exhibit this particular pattern a very high percentage of the time which diminishes over a 3-day period and seems to follow the course of the development of tolerance. I think that this is very interesting that we have a similar kind of electrographic effect at the higher levels in the nervous system.

ZIMMERMANN: In 1952, Dr. Torda demonstrated a EEG pattern similar to this following injection of ACTH in rats. Thus, again we see a parallel between the effects of ACTH and β-MSH on the nervous system.

KASTIN: Congratulations on a very fine piece of work. I have two brief questions. First, did you try α-MSH? Secondly, do you know anything about the vasopressin content of your β-MSH preparation?

ZIMMERMANN: In answer to your first question, we have not tried α-MSH. Regarding the vasopressin content of the β-MSH used I would like to ask Dr. Krivoy if he wouldn't mind commenting on that.

KRIVOY: When we intially got the sample I was told that it was quite free of anything else and I have no evidence to the contrary. The β-MSH we used was obtained from Joe Fisher of Armour Pharmaceuticals. When Joe Fisher extracted the β-MSH with which he provided us, he divided the peak into three parts. We used the center of the peak hoping to avoid just these problems of contamination. Subsequent samples he sent out were of the total peak of β-MSH.

KASTIN: I would be extremely surprised if your preparation did not contain vasopressin. I know of no natural preparation, even after being repurified, that doesn't have it. However, that does not detract from your studies since similar effects were obtained with the synthetic ACTH.

KRIVOY: If you would bioassay our material for vasopressin, I should be delighted to send an ampule of it.

DE WIED: In addition to what is being said about the vasopressin contamination of the purified β-MSH it should be noted that Dr. Zimmermann measured blood pressure in the cat following administration of β-MSH and observed no effect. I wish to complement Dr. Zimmermann on his fine experiments.

LANDE: Can you say anything about the effects of vasoactive or myoactive peptides in your assay system? Secondly, does administration of these peptides in intact addicted animals cause withdrawal symptoms?

ZIMMERMANN: The bioassay system is too new and we have not had time to determine the number of peptides that it will detect. The system probably requires some modification before it will be useful for that purpose. In the cat spinal cord preparation we do know that in the presence of chlorpromazine, bradykinin is active and in the presence of LSD, substance P is active. In terms of withdrawal, there is some suggestion of this in a paper by Fraser and Isbell (Ann. Int. Med., 38, 234, 1953) indicating that the severity of the symptoms during acute abstinence increases during ACTH administration. This is, I think the only statement in the literature. The question you have raised should be looked at but I don't know anyone who has done so.

KRIVOY: I would like to close this session with a very brief note that Dr. Porter in his initial comments indicated the extent of the interests of neuroendocrinology. This morning, I think demonstrates the potential interaction between drugs of abuse and the neuroendocrine system and further points out that in some instances there could be important causal relationships between drug abuse and the endocrine systems. This underscores, even more, the greater need for research devoted to clarifying these relationships.

Adrenocortical Mediation of the Effects of Early Life Experiences

ROBERT ADER AND LEE J. GROTA

Department of Psychiatry, University of Rochester School of Medicine and Dentistry Rochester, N.Y. 14642 (U.S.A.)

Progress in any field cannot necessarily be gauged in terms of the quantity of new data collected. Sometimes it is necessary to stop for a moment to see where we have been in order to see where we are going. The classic procedure of generating and testing hypotheses based on personal bias, conviction, and, even, data is not to be denied. Conviction, in the absence of data, is an unending and immensely valuable source of ideas, hypotheses, and theories. However, conviction in the face of contradicting data is not simply wrong, it may be compelling enough to lead away from more productive lines of research and, thereby, retard real progress. It will be our purpose, then, to reevaluate some of the data regarding the effects of early life experiences—specifically, the hypothesis that the behavioral and neuroendocrine effects of environmental stimulation experienced during infancy are mediated by early changes in the pituitary-adrenal system.

Handling infant rats will influence adult behaviors and adrenocortical reactivity. The most explicit statement of the hypothesis that the effects of early life experiences such as handling are mediated by the pituitary-adrenal axis is given in a recent paper by Denenberg and Zarrow (1971). Based on the proposition that emotional reactivity is reduced as a function of the amount of stimulus input experienced during infancy and the further assumption of a relationship between "emotionality" and adrenocortical activity, it is hypothesized that the neonatal rat responds to the stimulation of being handled by releasing corticosterone from the adrenal cortex. This steroid, acting upon the immature brain, serves to modify neural organization in such a way as to reduce emotional and adrenocortical reactivity in response to subsequent environmental stimulation. This is essentially the hypothesis developed by Levine (Levine, 1962, 1970; Levine and Mullins, 1966). In terms of subsequent adrenocortical function, early stimulation enables the individual to respond "more appropriately" to the demands of its environment, *i.e.*, the stimulated animal will be more reactive in response to intense stimulation but less reactive to relatively innocuous stimuli. In short, the handled animal is considered to be more adaptive in its physiological response to "stressful" stimuli than its unstimulated counterpart.

We will not comment on the adaptive significance of changes in adrenocortical reactivity. Any such statement can only reflect a value judgment since the adaptive

References p. 404–405

value of an increased or decreased adrenal reactivity or an increase or decrease in "emotionality", for that matter, has not been established—nor is it likely to be established without rephrasing the problem, *i.e.*, changes in behavioral or physiological reactivity are more or less adaptive with respect to what? This issue has been discussed elsewhere (Ader, 1970a).

"Handling" refers to the procedure by which infant rats are removed from the mother and nest and either held in the experimenter's hand or placed into individual containers for varying periods of time—usually daily, and usually for a period of 3 min. In reviewing the literature, Denenberg and Zarrow (1971) have chosen to exclude all techniques for stimulating infant animals except "handling". We will not limit our remarks accordingly. First of all, the hypothesis, implicitly at least, purports to account for the effects of stimulation during infancy without being restrictive with respect to the techniques used to provide stimulation. Secondly, if one were permitted to argue that the data from subjecting infant animals to electric shock, for example, were not immediately relevant, one could logically object to studies in which the handling procedures were not exactly the same as those described by these authors, and, finally, to any handling procedures not conducted in one particular laboratory. However correct, any theory with no generalizability would, of course, be meaningless.

It is commonly observed that animals stimulated during early life are less "emotional" than unmanipulated controls when observed in a reaction-to-handling test or in the commonly used open field. The evidence suggests that this is, in fact, an "early" experience effect. Rats handled after they have been weaned (21 days) do not show the same reduction in emotional reactivity relative to unmanipulated controls as do animals handled during the preweaning period. It is also commonly observed that handling or electric shock stimulation experienced during the first 3 weeks of life reduces subsequent adrenocortical reactivity in the rat (Ader, 1968, 1970b; Ader and Grota, 1969; Denenberg and Haltmeyer, 1967; Haltmeyer *et al.*, 1967; Hess *et al.*, 1969; Levine *et al.*, 1967b). There are, however, data which cast serious doubt on the assumptions (*a*) that there is a relationship between "emotionality" and adrenal function in the rat, (*b*) that the adrenocortical reactivity of differentially manipulated animals is a function of the intensity of stimulation used to elicit an adrenocortical response, (*c*) that the reduction in adrenocortical reactivity is a function of "early" as opposed to "prior" experience, and (*d*) that the effects of such early experiences are mediated *via* the adrenocortical system.

THE RELATIONSHIP BETWEEN EMOTIONAL AND ADRENOCORTICAL REACTIVITY

The assumption of a relationship between emotional and adrenocortical reactivity (Denenberg and Haltmeyer, 1967) is based on the study by Levine *et al.* (1967b) in which rats handled during the first 20 days of life were found to be less emotional than unmanipulated controls and also displayed a lesser adrenocortical response to testing in an open field. Based on such data, Denenberg and Haltmeyer (1967) used adrenocortical reactivity as a direct measure of emotional reactivity. The data obtained by Levine *et al.* (1967b) certainly suggest that such a relationship may exist, but these data do not establish the relationship. The implicit correlation was not sufficiently pervasive to hold under repeated testing in the open field (though this could relate to the relative rate of habituation), the corticosterone levels determined immediately after repeated testing tended to show smaller and smaller differences between the handled and non-handled animals whereas the absolute differences in open-field behavior tended to increase on subsequent trials, and no within-group correlations were reported. These considerations would seem to warrant some caution in promoting a documented relationship. Denenberg and Zarrow (1971) failed to note that their proposed relationship was not observed in other studies involving differentially manipulated animals (*e.g.*, Ader, 1968; Ader and Plaut, 1968; Hess *et al.*, 1969). In the study by Hess *et al.* (1969), for example, animals handled during the preweaning period showed a reduced adrenocortical reactivity relative to controls in response to open-field testing, but there were *no* differences in open-field behavior between the handled and non-handled groups. Conversely, consistent behavioral differences between rats that have been handled or shocked during early life have been reported (Ader, 1965, 1968; Goldman, 1969; Henderson, 1968; Levine, 1957, 1958; Levine *et al.*, 1956; Salama and Hunt, 1964) yet both handled and shocked animals show an attenuated adrenocortical response to external stimulation relative to unmanipulated controls (Ader, 1968; Ader and Grota, 1969). Moreover, in one of these studies (Ader, 1968) a recombination of animals on the basis of emotional reactivity, independent of differences in experiential history, failed to disclose any differences in adrenocortical reactivity. Although not directly relevant to the kind of "early" experiences being discussed here, it is of interest that Meyer and Bowman (1972) observed no differences in adrenocortical reactivity between monkeys with different experiential histories known to result in dramatic differences in the affective repertoire of these animals.

Finally, there are studies (Ader, 1969; Ader *et al.*, 1967; Moyer, 1958; Pare and Cullen, 1965; Paul and Havlena, 1962) in which the hypothesis of a relationship between emotionality and adrenocortical function has been approached directly. In the study by Ader *et al.* (1967) emotional reactivity was measured in an open-field and in a reaction-to-handling procedure; adrenocortical function was assessed by determinations of adrenal weight, adrenal corticosterone, and plasma corticosterone. Because of the known rhythm in adrenocortical function and its effects on reactivity (Ader and Friedman, 1968), measures of behavior and adrenal function were sampled at both the crest and trough in the 24-h adrenocortical cycle. Furthermore, two different strains of rats and one strain of mouse were tested. Under no combination of circumstances was there any evidence to suggest a relationship between adrenal activity and emotional reactivity. The conclusion drawn from these data was that if one conceives of "emotionality" as a characteristic of behavior which is related to the activity of the adrenal cortex, then the reaction-to-handling and open-field tests do not measure "emotionality". Alternatively, one may retain the concept of "emotionality" as that which is measured by tests such as the open-field, in which case it becomes necessary to question the assumption that such a behavioral characteristic is

References p. 404–405

related to adrenocortical function. It should be kept in mind that we are not here concerned with the qualitative or quantitative evaluation of specific affective states which would be exceedingly difficult to document in the rat—and for which there might well be steroid concomitants; we are concerned only with the commonly held operational definition of behaviors noted in specific test situations. It is these behaviors which fail to reveal any relationship to adrenal activity in experientially naive rats and mice. In view of these data, it is difficult to accept Denenberg's contention (Denenberg and Haltmeyer, 1967; Denenberg and Zarrow, 1971) that they have documented a relationship between emotional reactivity and adrenal function. On the contrary, it would appear that the reduction of emotional and adrenocortical reactivity effected by extra stimulation administered to animals during infancy are independent effects of the early life experience.

INTENSITY OF STIMULATION AND ADRENOCORTICAL REACTIVITY

In all of the experiments conducted thus far it has been consistently found that handling or electric shock stimulation administered during the preweaning period will influence the rat's subsequent adrenocortical response to environmental events. In response to relatively innocuous stimulation it has been consistently observed that the adrenocortical reactivity of the previously manipulated animals is less than that of non-manipulated controls. The results have not been nearly so consistent when the plasma corticosterone response to more intense stimulation was measured. Levine (1962) found that handled animals had a greater plasma corticosterone response than control animals as early as 15 sec and as late as 15 min following electric shock stimulation. On the basis of these data, it was proposed that handled animals are less reactive physiologically to relatively mild forms of stimulation but would show a greater initial reactivity and a more rapid recovery in response to relatively intense stimulation. This hypothesis which characterizes the handled animal as being more adaptive than the non-handled animal has been accepted by Denenberg and Zarrow (1971). But are there data to support this hypothesis?

Denenberg and Haltmeyer (1967) handled animals for varying periods of time or throughout the preweaning period. At weaning some of the animals were placed into a novel environment for 10 min following which they were killed. The results revealed a linear decrease in plasma corticosterone levels as a function of the number of days of handling. Other animals were placed into the same novel environment for 10 min where they received a 30-sec electric shock (0.8 mA). These animals did not show any change in adrenocortical reactivity as a function of the amount of previous handling experienced. Also, in contrast to the data reported by Levine (1962), there was no difference between the plasma corticosterone response of any of the handled groups relative to the non-handled controls in response to electric shock. The authors assumed that the intensity of the electric shock acted to mask the effects of the earlier experiences. As part of a more elaborate study, Levine and Mullins (1966) also observed a population of handled and non-handled animals stimulated by electric shock at weaning. Again, in contrast to earlier data (Levine, 1962), previously handled animals showed the lower plasma corticosterone response to 0.1 mA of electric shock.

Using adult animals, Haltmeyer *et al.* (1967) did find some support for the greater initial reactivity of handled relative to control animals. Having found (in weanlings) no difference between the adrenocortical reactivity of previously handled and non-handled animals in response to 0.8 mA of shock, the animals in this study were subjected to 0.2, 0.5, or 0.8 mA of shock for periods ranging from 2 to 60 min. Independent of shock intensity or duration, the level of corticosterone sampled immediately after shock was greater for the handled than the control animals. 15 min after electric shock stimulation there was no apparent difference between these groups. The magnitude of stimulation did not exert any influence on the reactivity of the differentially manipulated animals and, again, it was suggested that all these shock levels were too intense to allow for any differentiation.

The possibility that differences in adrenocortical reactivity between differentially manipulated animals might be related to the magnitude of stimulation to which such animals were exposed was also directly tested by Ader and Grota (1969). Unmanipulated control animals and rats that were subjected to handling or electric shock stimulation during the preweaning period were subsequently stimulated by being placed into a novel environment. Magnitude of stimulation was manipulated by varying the duration of this experience—5 sec or 3 min. Plasma corticosterone levels were sampled 5, 15, or 30 min following this stimulation. There were no differences between the handled and shocked animals. As a group, however, the manipulated animals showed a lesser adrenocortical response to the novel environment than controls irrespective of the duration of exposure. In still another study (Ader, 1970b), magnitude of stimulation was manipulated by varying the number of electric shocks received during a constant period of time. Plasma corticosterone was sampled from handled and non-handled animals given no additional stimulation or 5, 15, 30, or 60 min after a 60-sec exposure to a novel environment in which different groups were subjected to 0, 1, 4, or 12 2-sec electric shocks. Steroid levels rose significantly in response to the novel environment and in females there was an additional elevation in corticosterone levels in response to 4 and 12 shocks, indicating that the levels of stimulation used did not result in maximal steroid elevations. Again, the adrenocortical reactivity of handled animals was less than that of controls, irrespective of the magnitude of stimulation to which the animals were exposed.

Considering all the available data, then, an unresolved discrepancy remains. Levine (1962) observed that handled animals are more reactive than controls in response to electric shock stimulation. However, subsequent studies designed to repeat and extend these observations have failed to provide any compelling confirmation of these results or any support for the hypothesis that the differences in adrenocortical reactivity between animals with different experiential histories is a function of the intensity of stimulation used to elicit an adrenocortical response.

References p. 404–405

"EARLY" *versus* "PRIOR" EXPERIENCE

There is still another relevant feature of the studies conducted by Ader (1970b) and Ader and Grota (1969). These are the only studies dealing with adrenocortical reactivity in differentially manipulated animals in which the manipulations were imposed after as well as before weaning; these are the only studies in which the effects of "early" experience, *per se*, have been investigated with respect to adrenocortical reactivity. Denenberg and Zarrow (1971) suggest that the manner in which adrenocortical steroids released in response to stimulation of the neonate modify brain development and organization to influence subsequent emotional reactivity is analogous to the manner in which the administration of sex hormones during critical periods of infancy acts to modify subsequent sexual behavior. According to Denenberg and Zarrow, "When one looks at the data on infantile stimulation and compares them with the neonatal sex hormone data, certain interesting parallels are seen. First of all, the effects of infantile stimulation are limited to the period of infancy, and the sex hormones also have their impact during very early infancy". As far as adrenocortical reactivity is concerned, however, none of the studies cited by Denenberg and Zarrow (1971) were discussed in this context and no evidence was presented bearing on the validity of this hypothesis. These authors evidently assume that, because many of the behavioral effects of stimulating infant animals are, in fact, "early" experience effects, the same would be the case for adrenocortical reactivity—or, that it is unnecessary to examine this basic assumption. Although not discussed by Denenberg and Zarrow (1971), relevant data do exist. The studies we conducted on the effects of early life experiences on adrenocortical reactivity to different magnitudes of stimulation (Ader, 1970b; Ader and Grota, 1969) included groups of animals manipulated throughout the 21-day preweaning period or during the 21 days immediately after weaning. In both of these studies there were no differences between the animals manipulated before and after weaning. Handling *and* electric shock stimulation experienced during the immediate postweaning period were as effective as stimulation prior to weaning in reducing adrenocortical reactivity to subsequent environmental stimulation. There was, then, no evidence that the extra stimulation to which animals are subjected must occur "early" in life in order to be effective—or maximally effective—in modifying subsequent adrenocortical reactivity.

Hess *et al.* (1969) subjected rats to handling during the first 5 or first 20 days of life. There were no differences between these groups; both reduced subsequent adrenocortical reactivity. Since stimulation during the first 5 days of life was as effective as stimulation during the first 20 days, it was concluded that if there is a critical period for this phenomenon it occurs during the first 5 days of life. The issue, however, is not whether stimulation during the first 5 days of life is *as* effective as stimulation during the first 20 days, but whether stimulation at any particular stage of development is critical in determining the subsequent response or magnitude of that response. Moreover, Denenberg and Haltmeyer (1967) observed animals handled during the first, second, or third 5 days of life and found no evidence that stimulation during the first 5 days was critical in modifying subsequent adrenocortical reactivity.

Let us review briefly the results and implication of this re-examination of the data thus far. The stimulation of animals during infancy influences subsequent emotional and adrenocortical reactivity, and it is assumed that there is a relationship between emotional and adrenocortical reactivity. In fact, no such relationship has been established. The data with respect to a correlation between these behavioral and physiological characteristics in differentially manipulated animals are inconsistent and attempts to document such a relationship in experimentally naive animals have failed. However, the more conservative suggestion that the reduction in emotional and adrenocortical reactivity are independent effects of the previous stimulation to which these animals were exposed does not depreciate the phenomena observed. Stimulation during infancy does reduce subsequent emotional reactivity and does influence adrenocortical function. For the most part, these are highly reliable findings which have yet to be explained.

Although there is some indication that animals stimulated during infancy can show an increased adrenocortical reactivity relative to controls—presumably because of the use of relatively intense stimulation—there has been no unequivocal replication of such results. It has been repeatedly demonstrated, though, that there is a reduction in adrenocortical reactivity in previously stimulated relative to unmanipulated control animals which is independent of the magnitude of stimulation to which such animals were subsequently exposed. The discrepancy among these data, then, remains unresolved. This issue is relevant only to the extent that one conceives of stimulation in infancy as increasing the adaptive capacity of the individual by virtue of its ability to show a greater variation or modulation in its adrenal response to environmental events. Quite apart from the data cited above, there have been several reviews of the literature on susceptibility to a variety of somatic diseases as a function of early life experiences (Ader, 1966, 1967, 1970a; Friedman *et al.*, 1969). On the basis of these data, it is apparent that the effects of early stimulation as measured by the individual's response to potentially pathogenic stimulation are neither uniformly beneficial or detrimental. Handling, for example, increases resistance to experimentally induced gastric erosions and retards the growth rate of a transplanted tumor, but handling decreases subsequent resistance to a transplanted leukemia and to electroconvulsive shock while having no effect on susceptibility to alloxan diabetes, encephalomyocarditis virus, or the spontaneous development of leukemia in AKR mice. In short, the direction in which animals manipulated during early life may differ from unmanipulated controls depends upon the subsequent stimulation to which they may be exposed.

Finally, there is the issue of whether the reduction in adrenocortical reactivity that results from stimulating animals during infancy is an "early" experience phenomenon in the first place. Despite assumptions to the contrary, the available data indicate that stimulation prior to weaning is no more effective than stimulation after weaning. But the issue is not closed. Plasma levels of corticosterone represent the summation of adrenocortical secretion and rate of metabolism. Therefore, the possibility remains that the reduced adrenocortical reactivity observed in animals manipulated before and after weaning reflect different physiological processes, *i.e.*, animals manipulated

References p. 404–405

before and after weaning show a reduction in plasma corticosterone levels, but for different reasons—and this represents a testable hypothesis.

ADRENOCORTICAL MEDIATION OF THE EFFECTS OF "EARLY" EXPERIENCE

The above arguments are based on a re-examination of the data cited by Denenberg and Zarrow (1971) as well as existing data omitted from their review. These arguments raise serious questions regarding the underlying assumptions, some of the predictions, and the generalizability of the hypothesis that the effects of early experience on emotional and adrenocortical reactivity are mediated *via* early changes in the pituitary-adrenal system. These arguments, however, do not constitute a direct test of the hypothesis.

Consistent with the hypothesis advanced by Denenberg and Zarrow (1971) and Levine (1962, 1970) are the observations that the infant rat is capable of responding to intense or prolonged stimulation with an elevation in plasma levels of corticosterone (Haltmeyer *et al.*, 1966; Zarrow *et al.*, 1966). One experiment (Denenberg *et al.*, 1967) indicated that the 2-day-old rat could show elevated steroid levels in response to the relatively innocuous stimulus of handling (which, incidentally, includes the additional stimulation provided by the mother when pups are returned to the nest). Considering the variability between the populations tested in the Denenberg *et al.* (1967) study, these single results should be accepted with caution—especially since their observations on the adrenal response of infant rats to even more severe forms of stimulation, (Haltmeyer *et al.*, 1966; Zarrow *et al.*, 1966), are not consistent with data reported by Levine and Mullins (1966), Levine *et al.* (1967a), or Gray (1971). Assuming that these data are reliable and that the discrepancies between studies are due to procedural differences, it is still true that, as Denenberg and Zarrow (1971) point out, such results do not constitute a direct test of the hypothesis. There are, however, recent data from a more critical kind of experiment.

If the reduction in adrenocortical reactivity in stimulated animals is the result of changes effected by the release of steroids by the neonate in response to the early stimulation, blocking the release of these steroids should eliminate the subsequent difference in adrenocortical reactivity between stimulated and non-stimulated animals. Two such experiments have been conducted (Grota, 1972; Grota and Ader, 1972). Lactating rats were provided with drinking water containing dexamethasone, a synthetic glucocorticoid which blocks the release of corticotrophin (ACTH) in response to environmental stimulation. The doses used (63, 125, or 250 μg/8 oz. drinking bottle) were sufficient to block the release of corticosterone in the mother alone or in the mother and the pups in response to removing the pups from the nest and subjecting them to electric shock stimulation. Dexamethasone treatment was discontinued when the pups were 17 days old. In the study by Grota (1972) animals were killed at weaning either before or 15 min after being subjected to 3 min of electric shock. In the study by Grota and Ader (1972) adult animals were sampled following avoidance conditioning. In both weanling and adult rats plasma corticosterone levels of animals subjected to electric shock stimulation during early life were less than those of unmanipulated control animals whether or not the adrenocortical response to electric shock stimulation had been blocked during infancy. These results, then, provide no support for the hypothesis that an adrenocortical response on the part of either the mother or the young is responsible for the effects of stimulation during infancy on subsequent adrenocortical reactivity.

None of the above remarks should be interpreted as a rejection of the effects of "early experience". On the contrary, it is our conviction—and there are even some data to support it—that we have not yet even fully appreciated the potential significance of early life experiences for the development and subsequent adaptation of the individual. There is little argument that one or another of the kinds of stimulation to which animals have been exposed during early life influence the development of basic neuroendocrine processes as well as subsequent behavior and even the organism's response to potentially pathogenic stimulation. We submit, however, that there is probably no *single* "early experience" effect. Further, the search for a single physiological pathway by which the variety of stimuli experienced by infant animals exert their effects and which, in turn, influences adaptation in some uniform or unidirectional manner is misdirected and naive. Certainly, on the basis of the data reviewed above there is little support for the proposition that pituitary-adrenal changes mediate the effects of early experience, in general, or altered emotional and adrenocortical reactivity, in particular. The pituitary-adrenal axis represents only one of the systems that could be modified by early life experiences, but there are undoubtedly many ways in which the individual is changed as a result of experiences which occur during infancy. The adaptive significance of these changes can only be evaluated in terms of the relevance of one or another of such changes to the demands of the subsequent environment. It is the interaction between the responses unconditionally elicited by the demands of the environment and the chronic changes in psychophysiological function resulting, in part, from early life experiences that will ultimately define the adaptive capacity of the individual.

SUMMARY

It has been hypothesized that the stimulation of infant rats results in a release of corticosterone which acts to modify brain organization in such a way as to reduce subsequent emotional and adrenocortical reactivity. The present paper consists of a re-examination of the data relevant to the assumptions underlying this proposition. The following conclusions are drawn from this critical evaluation of the available data:

(*1*) There is no evidence to support the assumption of a relationship between emotional and adrenocortical reactivity; these would appear to be independent effects of the previous experiences of the animals.

(*2*) There has been no compelling verification of the observation that stimulation during infancy increases subsequent adrenocortical reactivity in response to relatively intense stimulation. On the contrary, the data indicate that the consistently reported

References p. 404–405

reduction in adrenocortical reactivity in stimulated relative to unstimulated animals is independent of the magnitude of stimulation to which such animals are subsequently exposed.

(*3*) There has been no demonstration that the reduction in adrenocortical reactivity effected by stimulation during infancy is an "early" experience effect; stimulation before weaning is no more effective in reducing subsequent adrenocortical reactivity than stimulating after weaning. It has yet to be determined, however, whether the attenuation in adrenocortical reactivity could reflect different physiological processes in the animals that experienced extra stimulation before or after weaning.

(*4*) If the release of corticosterone in response to stimulation experienced during infancy is blocked by chronic treatment of the mother with drinking water containing dexamethasone, such animals still show the reduced adrenocortical reactivity characteristic of stimulated animals.

ACKNOWLEDGMENTS

Preparation of this manuscript and research conducted by the authors were supported by U.S.P.H.S. grant MH-16741 and a Research Scientist Award (MH-6318) to the senior author (R.A.) from the National Institute of Mental Health.

REFERENCES

Ader, R. (1965) Effects of early experience and differential housing on behavior and susceptibility to gastric erosions in the rat. *J. comp. Physiol. Psychol.*, **60**, 233–238.

Ader, R. (1966) Early experience and adaptation to stress. *Res. Publ. Ass. nerv. ment. Dis.*, **43**, 292–306.

Ader, R. (1967) The influence of psychological factors on disease susceptibility in animals. In *Husbandry of Laboratory Animals*, M. L. Conalty (Ed.), Academic Press, London, pp. 219–236.

Ader, R. (1968) Effects of early experience on emotional and physiological reactivity in the rat. *J. comp. Physiol. Psychol.*, **66**, 264–268.

Ader, R. (1969) Adrenocortical function and the measurement of "emotionality". *Ann. N.Y. Acad. Sci.*, **159**, 791–805.

Ader, R. (1970a) The effects of early life experiences on developmental processes and susceptibility to disease in animals. In *Minnesota Symposium on Child Psychology*, J. P. Hill (Ed.), Univ. of Minnesota Press, Minneapolis, Minn., pp. 3–35.

Ader, R. (1970b) The effect of early experience on the adrenocortical response to different magnitudes of stimulation. *Physiol. Behav.*, **5**, 837–839.

Ader, R. and Friedman, S. B. (1968) Plasma corticosterone response to environmental stimulation: Effects of duration of stimulation and the 24-hour adrenocortical rhythm. *Neuroendocrinology*, **3**, 378–386.

Ader, R. and Grota, L. J. (1969) The effects of early experience on adrenocortical reactivity. *Physiol. Behav.*, **4**, 303–305.

Ader, R. and Plaut, S. M. (1968) Effects of prenatal maternal handling and differential housing on offspring emotionality, plasma corticosterone levels, and susceptibility to gastric erosions. *Psychsom. Med.*, **30**, 277–286.

Ader, R., Friedman, S. B. and Grota, L. J. (1967) "Emotionality" and adrenal cortical function: Effects of strain, test, and the 24-hour corticosterone rhythm. *Animal Behav.*, **15**, 37–44.

Denenberg, V. H. and Haltmeyer, G. C. (1967) Test of the monotonicity hypothesis concerning infantile stimulation and emotional reactivity. *J. comp. Physiol. Psychol.*, **63**, 394–396.

DENENBERG, V. H. AND ZARROW, M. X. (1971) Effects of handling in infancy upon adult behavior and adrenocortical activity: Suggestions for a neuroendocrine mechanism. In *Early Childhood: The Development of Self-regulatory Mechanims*, D. H. WALCHER AND D. L. PETERS (Eds.), Academic Press, New York, pp. 39–64.

DENENBERG, V. H., BRUMAGHIM, J. T., HALTMEYER, G. C. AND ZARROW, M. X. (1967) Increased adrenocortical activity in the neonatal rat following handling. *Endocrinology*, **81**, 1047–1052.

FRIEDMAN, S. B., GLASGOW, L. A. AND ADER, R. (1969) Psychosocial factors modifying host resistance to experimental infections. *Ann. N.Y. Acad. Sci.*, **164**, 381–392.

GOLDMAN, P. S. (1969) The relationship between amount of stimulation in infancy and subsequent emotionality. *Ann. N.Y. Acad. Sci.*, 1959, 640–650.

GRAY, P. (1971) Pituitary-adrenocortical response to stress in the neonatal rat. *Endocrinology*, **89**, 1126–1128.

GROTA, L. J. (1972) Dexamethasone treatment and the effects of early experience on adrenocortical reactivity. Presented at the meetings of the Eastern Psychological Association, Boston, Mass.

GROTA, L. J. AND ADER, R. (1972) Effects of early experience with electric shock and dexamethasone on avoidance conditioning at adulthood. *Psychon. Sci.*, **28**, 10–12.

HALTMEYER, G. C., DENENBERG, V. H., THATCHER, J. AND ZARROW, M. X. (1966) Response of the adrenal cortex of the neonatal rat after subjection to stress. *Nature*, **212**, 1371–1373.

HALTMEYER, G. C., DENENBERG, V. H. AND ZARROW, M. X. (1967) Modification of the plasma corticosterone response as a function of infantile stimulation and electric shock parameters. *Physiol. Behav.*, **2**, 61–63.

HENDERSON, N. D. (1968) Physiological and behavioral effects of different sequences of preweaning shock in rats. *Psychosom. Med.*, **30**, 62–71.

HESS, J. L., DENENBERG, V. H., ZARROW, M. X. AND PFEIFER, W. D. (1969) Modification of the corticosterone response curve as a function of handling in infancy. *Physiol. Behav.*, **4**, 109–111.

LEVINE, S. (1957) Infantile experience and consummatory behavior in adulthood. *J. comp. Physiol. Psychol.*, **50**, 609–612.

LEVINE, S. (1958) Noxious stimulation in infant and adult rats and consummatory behavior. *J. comp. Physiol. Psychol.*, **51**, 230–233.

LEVINE, S. (1962) Plasma-free corticosteroid response to electric shock in rats stimulated in infancy. *Science*, **135**, 795–796.

LEVINE, S. (1970) The pituitary-adrenal system and the developing brain. In *Pituitary, Adrenal and the Brain* (Progress in Brain Research, Vol. 32), D. DE WIED AND J. A. W. M. WEIJNEN (Eds.), Elsevier, Amsterdam, pp. 79–85.

LEVINE, S. AND MULLINS, R. J. JR. (1966) Hormonal influence on brain organization in infant rats. *Science*, **152**, 1585–1592.

LEVINE, S., CHEVALIER, J. A. AND KORCHIN, S. J. (1956) The effects of early shock and handling on later avoidance learning. *J. Personal.*, **24**, 475–493.

LEVINE, S., GLICK, D. AND NAKANE, P. K. (1967a) Adrenal and plasma corticosterone and vitamin A in rat adrenal glands during postnatal development. *Endocrinology*, **80**, 910–914.

LEVINE, S., HALTMEYER, G. C., KARAS, G. G. AND DENENBERG, V. H. (1967b) Physiological and behavioral effects of infantile stimulation. *Physiol. Behav.*, **2**, 55–59.

MEYER, J. S. AND BOWMAN, R. E. (1972) Rearing experience, stress and adrenocortico-steroids in the Rhesus monkey. *Physiol. Behav.*, **8**, 339–343.

MOYER, K. E. (1958) Effects of adrenalectomy on the startle response in the rat. *J. Genet. Psychol.*, **92**, 11–16.

PARE, W. P. AND CULLEN, J. W. JR. (1965) Emotional behavior and adrenal function in the rat. *Psychol. Rep.*, **16**, 283–286.

PAUL, C. AND HAVLENA, J. (1962) Maze learning and open-field behavior of adrenalectomized rats. *J. psychosom. Res.*, **6**, 153–156.

SALAMA, A. A. AND HUNT, J. MCV. (1964) "Fixation" in the rat as a function of infantile shocking, handling, and gentling. *J. Genet. Psychol.*, **105**, 131–162.

ZARROW, M. X., HALTMEYER, G. C., DENENBERG, V. H. AND THATCHER, J. (1966) Response of the infantile rat to stress. *Endocrinology*, **79**, 631–634.

DISCUSSION

McEwen: I wonder if you would comment on two points: First, in Dr. Grota's dexamethasone treatment experiments, how do you eliminate the possibility that dexamethasone is itself mimicking the glucocorticoid secretion which it is suppressing? Second, in view of the relatively small stress response which occurs in the rat in the first two weeks of life, is the elevation of glucocorticoids sufficient to be the signal or causal factor for the "stress" effects on behavior and pituitary-adrenal reactivity?

Ader: In answer to your first question, yes, we are "flooding the system" so to speak, with the glucocorticoid, dexamethasone. However, the distinction is that the elevation in steroid level is dissociated from any external stimulation that we are providing. Moreover, it is available in control animals as well, we have dexamethasone-treated animals that are not stimulated as well as dexamethasone-treated animals that are stimulated. As far as the magnitude of the stress response is concerned, I think that you are absolutely correct. The only studies that show a magnitude of response that would seem sufficient to be implicated in these effects involve stimulation which is far more intense than has been used to get these behavioral effects. The small effects seen when relatively "mild" stimulation is used are not impressive in terms of their replicability or in terms of the very high variability obtained. On the other hand, I could say that even though the response is a small one, it doesn't bother me considering that you are getting such a response to stimulation everyday. Now, unless there is some critical period (for which there is no evidence) this cumulative effect could have some influence.

Gorski: What is your opinion of the view that the effects of early experience are in fact mediated by the response of the mother to her handled pups?

Ader: This is a hypothesis for which there are data in the sense that there are changes in the adrenocortical response to manipulating the young, and these could influence a response to the young. However, the amount of empirical data is really very slim. Denenberg and Zarrow (1971) raise this possibility, but also point out that one can obtain these effects even after eliminating the mother as a variable. Our measures of subtle differences in maternal behavior are not that precise. As it happens, though, we are currently monitoring maternal behavior 24 h per day in litters of manipulated and non-manipulated pups. Another problem with the hypothesis is that different kinds of experiences produce different effects. Therefore, to be entirely consistent you are now going to have to hypothesize that the mother is capable of responding differently to the pups depending upon the kind of stimulation that the pups experienced. That's a differentiation which theoretically could exist but I do not find it very compelling.

Smelik: I wonder if you would mention work with animals that have been reared in complete isolation. Such animals behave completely different in adult life and it seems that there is a critical period for learning social behavior from parents and litter-mates.

Ader: The question you asked could prompt an hour's discussion, but the point of it, I think, is the issue of "critical periods". I do not think that there is a *single* "critical period" that is "critical" in the sense that all subsequent behavior is determined by events occurring during that period. I think it makes more sense to ask, critical for what? In addition, there are species differences and you can't rear a rat in isolation from birth on. Monkeys reared in isolation do display altered social and affective responses. Still, a "critical period" in the course of development for one species would have no necessary bearing on a "critical period" in another species.

Kellar: Do pups stimulated during infancy weigh more when they reach sexual maturity?

Ader: We frequently find that the growth rate of animals manipulated early in life is faster than that of controls and often we find no differences. In any case, this does not appear to have any effect on the consistent behavioral differences between these same groups of animals.

Pituitary-Adrenal Influences on Avoidance and Approach Behavior of the Rat

BELA BOHUS

Rudolf Magnus Institute for Pharmacology, Medical Faculty, University of Utrecht, Vondellaan 6, Utrecht (The Netherlands)

It is well established that the pituitary-adrenal system plays an essential role in the organism's adaptive reactions towards environmental stimuli. Beside physical somatic factors, neurogenic or emotional stimuli such as anxiety or fear invariably induce the discharge of corticotrophin (ACTH) from the adenohypophysis and the subsequent increase in the production of adrenal corticosteroids. Although several aspects of so-called stress-induced pituitary-adrenal activation have been explored in relation to the "peripheral" mechanisms of adaptation, relatively little attention has been paid to studying the brain as a possible target organ for these hormones. In the course of clinical assessment of adrenocortical steroids and ACTH as therapeutic agents, it was frequently noticed that a number of psychological changes, including mood alterations and disturbance, occurred. Excitability changes in seizure threshold, as observed clinically, were also observed in animals after administration of ACTH or corticosteroid.

The experimental studies on the role of pituitary-adrenal hormones in behavioral adaptation took their origin from very different starting points. For example, my studies were primarily stimulated by the recognition of the involvement of discrete brain regions in the "feedback" effect of steroids on the release of pituitary ACTH (Bohus *et al.*, 1968a). De Wied's interest originated from observations in posterior lobectomized rats showing impaired ACTH release to emotional but not to somatic stimuli (De Wied, 1969). Certain relationships between the performance of avoidance behavior and pituitary-adrenal responsiveness also stimulated several groups to study the behavioral influence of these hormones (Lissák and Endröczi, 1964; Levine, 1968; Weiss *et al.*, 1970). Recently a number of observations on this subject indicate that the behavioral effects of these hormones are now well established.

The aim of this paper is to summarize our knowledge on the behavioral effects of pituitary and adrenal hormones with special attention to the mode, the site and the specificity of their actions on central nervous mechanisms.

Several aspects of the influence of pituitary-adrenal hormones on avoidance behavior of rodents were studied by us and by other groups. Acquisition of active avoidance response is markedly impaired by hypophysectomy (Applezweig and Baudry, 1955; Applezweig and Moeller, 1959; De Wied, 1964). Administration of

References p. 418–419

ACTH-like peptides reverses the learning deficit of the operated rats. Response performance of hypophysectomized rats can also be restored by supplementary treatment with thyroxine, cortisone and testosterone (De Wied, 1964) or by growth hormone (De Wied, 1969). Accordingly, metabolic factors are important in the impaired learning capacity of hypophysectomized rats. However, normalizing the acquisition rate by pituitary peptides is independent of a metabolic effect and not mediated by the adrenal cortex as was demonstrated by using peptides structurally related to ACTH but devoid of corticotrophic and anabolic activities (De Wied, 1969). The influence of ACTH-like peptides depends on the actual presence of the peptide. Daily administration of $ACTH_{4-10}$ improves the acquisition of a shuttle-box avoidance response in hypophysectomized rats. Cessation of the treatment results in a gradual impairment of avoidance performance (Bohus *et al.*, 1973). While the removal of the pituitary markedly influences avoidance acquisition, adrenalectomy has no substantial effect on it, *i.e.* acquisition of active avoidance can take place in the absence of corticosteroids. Slight improvement of shuttle-box avoidance performance as observed by Beatty *et al.* (1970) and Weiss *et al.* (1970) is presumably due to the increase in release of pituitary ACTH in adrenalectomized rats. Slight temporary facilitation of active avoidance acquisition was observed in intact rats after administration of ACTH. This influence, which appeared also to be present in the absence of the adrenals, depended on a certain development of conditioned behavior (Bohus and Endröczi, 1965; Bohus *et al.*, 1968b).

Extinction of active avoidance behavior appeared to be substantially affected by alteration of pituitary-adrenal function. Administration of ACTH results in a delay of extinction. This effect also appeared to be extra-adrenal; the peptide is effective in adrenalectomized rats as well (Miller and Ogawa, 1962; Bohus *et al.*, 1968b). Corticosteroids on the other hand seemed to affect the extinction rate of active avoidance response in an opposite way: enhancement of extinction was observed not only with corticosterone, which is the physiological glucocorticoid of the rat, but with cortisone and dexamethasone as well (De Wied, 1967; Bohus and Lissák, 1968). It was also shown that this effect of steroids is not closely related to the glucocorticoid activity, since other steroids such as pregnenolone and progesterone but not testosterone and estradiol were equipotently active (Van Wimersma Greidanus, 1970).

These first results on the effect of pituitary-adrenal hormones stimulated at least two major directions in further research. The extra-adrenal nature of ACTH on the function of the central nervous systems raised the question as to whether the full peptide molecule is essential for the behavioral effects. A series of experiments in De Wied's laboratory clearly demonstrated that even the heptapeptide $ACTH_{4-10}$ has full behavioral activity in avoidance responding (De Wied, 1966, 1969; De Wied *et al.*, 1968). More details and recent developments on this line of research are described by Greven and De Wied in this volume (p. 429–442).

The other line of research has attempted to explore the site of action of pituitary-adrenal hormones in the brain. The first suggestion of the involvement of the thalamic parafascicular region in the mediation of peptide effects on avoidance extinction was given by experiments in rats bearing mid-posterior thalamic lesions. Melanocyte-stimulating hormone (α-MSH, acetyl-$ACTH_{1-13}$) in amounts which in intact rats increase resistance to extinction, failed to delay the rapid extinction of a shuttle-box avoidance response in rats with bilateral lesions in the parafascicular area (Bohus and De Wied, 1967). Subsequent experiments with intracerebral implantation of $ACTH_{4-10}$ extended this observation: the extinction of a pole-jumping avoidance response is delayed in rats when the peptide is implanted in the parafascicular area of the thalamus (Van Wimersma Greidanus and De Wied, 1971).

Intracerebral implantation of various steroids revealed the importance of this thalamic area as one site of action of corticosteroids on avoidance extinction. Corticosteroids implanted in the parafascicular nuclei of the thalamus or in the rostral mesencephalic reticular formation enhance the extinction of active avoidance response (Bohus, 1968; Van Wimersma Greidanus and De Wied, 1969; Bohus, 1970a). It has also been demonstrated that the opposite behavioral effect of ACTH and steroids involves their action on the thalamic area. The stronger the suppression of avoidance performance by intrathalamic steroid implants, the larger the amount of ACTH necessary to prevent the steroid action (Bohus, 1970b).

In the meantime it was shown that corticosteroids may also act through forebrain mechanisms. Cortisone implanted in the anterior hypothalamus, septum, amygdala or dorsal hippocampus of the rat enhances the extinction of an active avoidance response (Bohus, 1970a). These observations were in favor of previous suggestions based upon both behavioral and electrophysiological experiments (Lissák and Endröczi, 1964; Bohus and Endröczi, 1965; Endröczi, 1969) in which corticosteroids enhanced forebrain-inhibitory processes, thus leading to enhanced internal inhibition. The suppressive influence on the ascending reticular function and the enhancement of forebrain inhibition by steroids presupposed a dual character of their behavioral action (Bohus, 1971). Facilitation of active avoidance extinction may be interpreted as a synergistic influence of steroids on both systems. One might then expect that the effect of steroids on passive avoidance behavior based upon the inhibition of a motivated response may have even an antagonistic-like action on the two systems unless the enhancement of forebrain inhibition by hormones has a suppressive effect on fear motivation rather than on the performance.

Corticosteroids such as cortisone or dexamethasone suppress passive avoidance responses in both aversive *vs.* aversive and thirst *vs.* fear conflict situations. Suppression of passive avoidance depended on the shock-intensity and the dose of cortisone administered before learning in an aversive *vs.* aversive situation (Bohus *et al.*, 1970a). Corticosterone, the main glucocorticoid of the rat adrenal cortex, and glucocorticoids such as cortisol were also effective if the passive avoidance behavior of rats was investigated in a thirst *vs.* fear conflict situation. The experimental paradigm has been described in detail elsewhere (Bohus, 1971). Suppression of passive avoidance immediately after the shock trial and 24 h later was seen when high doses of corticosterone, cortisol or 6-dehydro-16-methylene-cortisol were given before the learning trial. The lower doses of steroids were ineffective except for corticosterone 24 h after the learning trial. Deoxycorticosterone was not effective even at a high dose level (Fig. 1). The ACTH suppressive potency of these steroids was also determined by

References p. 418–419

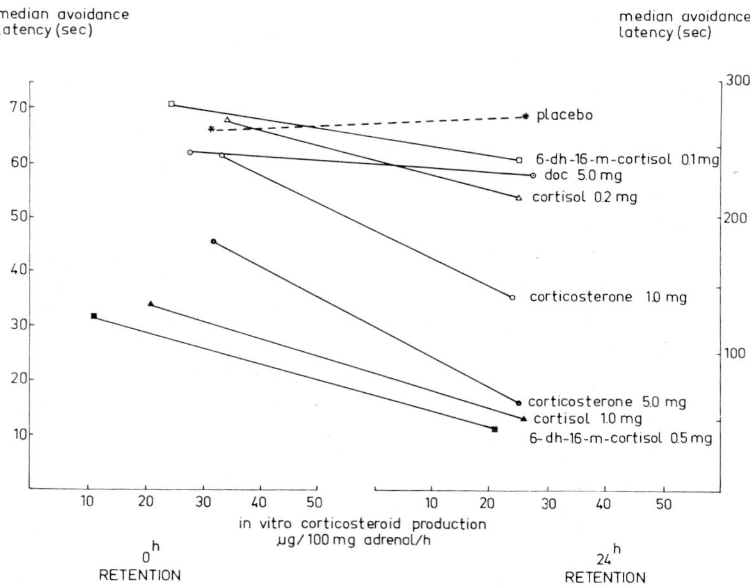

Fig. 1. The influence of naturally occurring and synthetic adrenal steroids on the retention of a passive avoidance response in a thirst *vs.* fear conflict situation and on the activation of pituitary-adrenal system accompanying the behavioral situation. Steroids were given s.c. 2 h before the single shock trial. *In vitro* corticosteroid production of the adrenals served as an index of pituitary ACTH-release. Each point represents 8–10 observations. doc, deoxycorticosterone; 6-dh-16-m-cortisol, 6-dehydro-16-methylene-cortisol.

measuring the corticosteroid production of the adrenals *in vitro* 15 min after the immediate and 24-h trials. ACTH release was suppressed by high doses of cortisol and 6-dehydro-16-methylene-cortisol. The behavioral effect of this latter steroid was positively correlated with the endocrine influence: the stronger the suppression of ACTH release induced by the behavioral stress, the more effective was the suppression of behavior.

As far as the locus of action of these steroids is concerned, corticosterone implants both in the forebrain and the medial thalamus were effective in suppressing passive avoidance in the 24-h retention test, whereas forebrain implants were effective in suppressing immediate passive avoidance as well. Cortisol suppressed passive avoidance both in immediate and 24-h retention tests whenever the implants were located in the forebrain or the medial thalamus. 6-Dehydro-16-methylene-cortisol and deoxycorticosteroid implants in general were ineffective (Fig. 2). The former steroid is known as a potent blocker of ACTH release which presumably acts at lower hypothalamic sites and at the pituitary level (Berthold *et al.*, 1970). Therefore, it seems that suppression of passive avoidance by systemic administration of this steroid is due to suppression of ACTH release. Indeed, ACTHβ_{1-24} administered before the single learning trial enhanced passive avoidance retention if the shock intensity is mild. Hypophysectomy, on the other hand, suppresses the avoidance behavior. These

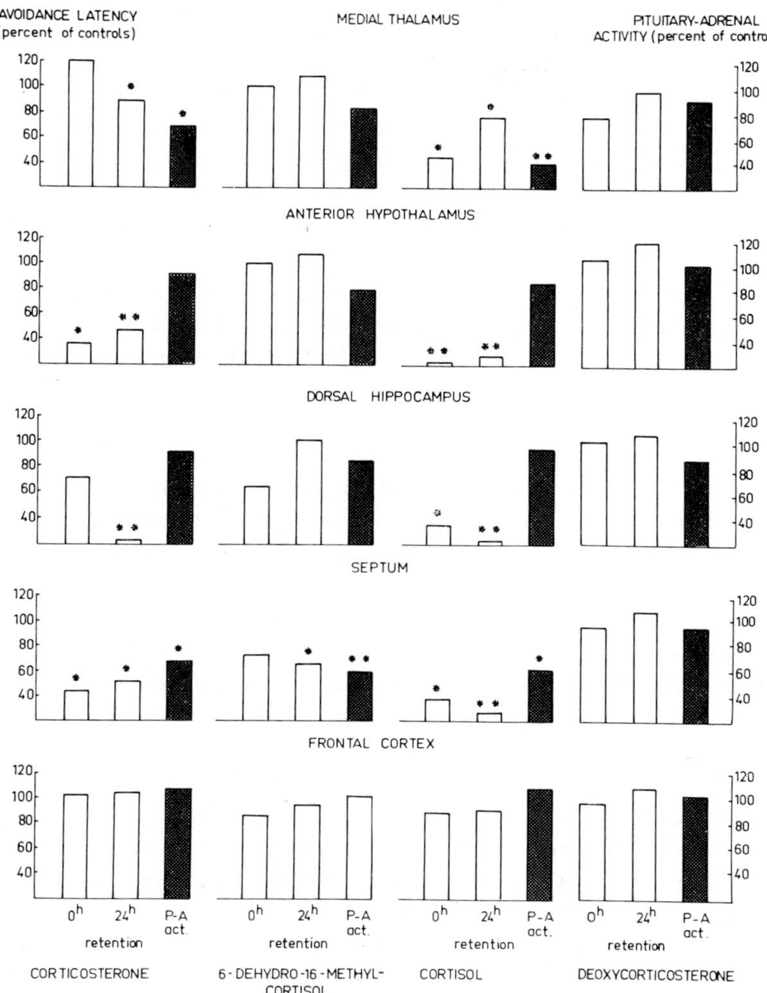

Fig. 2. The effect of intracerebral implantation of various crystalline steroids on the retention of a passive avoidance response in a thirst *vs.* fear conflict situation and on pituitary-adrenal activity as measured by the *in vitro* corticosteroid production of the adrenals determined 15 min after the retention test at 24 h. The steroids were implanted one day before the single avoidance learning trial. The stars on top of the columns represent the level of significance (U-test). 8–10 observations per placement and per steroid. *, $p > 0.05$, **, $p > 0.01$.

effects also depend on the shock intensity (Lissák and Bohus, 1972). Observations of Levine and Jones (1965), Weiss *et al.* (1970) and Guth *et al.* (1971a) are in agreement with these findings.

If one summarizes the behavioral studies in active and passive avoidance situations, the most parsimonious explanation for the effect of ACTH, ACTH-like peptides and corticosteroids seems to be an influence on the fear level which motivates avoidance behavior. The magnitude of the effects appeared to be a function of the drive intensity and the dose of hormones applied. The higher the drive intensity, the less the

References p. 418–419

modification of the behavior. Although the insensitivity of behavioral measures in certain situations cannot be totally excluded, it seems reasonable to postulate that the central nervous system is less sensitive to hormonal effects when the aversive stimuli evoke high drive-intensity levels. A clear dichotomy appears between the behavioral and endocrine feedback effects of most of the steroids. Thus, the primary behavioral influence of steroids is not mediated through the suppression of ACTH release. As far as the mode of action of pituitary-adrenal hormones is concerned, enhancement of internal inhibitory processes by corticosteroids leading to the suppression of fear has been suggested (Bohus and Lissák, 1968). Based upon intracerebral implantation and electrophysiological experiments, this hypothesis was reinforced (Bohus, 1970a), but, in addition, the observation that the steroids affect avoidance behavior through ascending reticular structures at the mesencephalic and thalamic level as well (Bohus, 1968, 1970a; Van Wimersma Greidanus and De Wied, 1969) suggests a "dual character" of steroid action on the brain. However, as shown earlier, the behavioral consequences of this "dual character" were not apparent in passive avoidance situations. Facilitation of forebrain activity results in enhanced passive avoidance. Corticosteroid implants in the forebrain, however, suppressed passive avoidance. Therefore, it is more likely that the influence of corticosteroids on forebrain mechanisms always bears a suppressive property on aversively motivated behavior. Factors such as increased thirst drive in a conflict situation or impairment of pain perception in passive avoidance experiments may play a certain role in the effect of steroids on behavior. Meanwhile, the fact that the steroids affect immediate passive avoidance behavior suggests that attenuation of motivational influence may be the mode of action of these hormones.

In order to decide whether a motivational hypothesis is valid, two further directions of research were introduced: (*1*) the study of autonomic responses evoked by the emotional stimuli and (*2*) the behavioral analysis of pituitary-adrenal system hormones in situations motivated by factors other than aversion.

There exists increasing evidence from psychophysiological literature for the occurrence of marked autonomic response changes in relation to the emotional status of an animal. One of the most significant systems responding to environmental and internal stimuli is the cardiovascular system. Psychological stresses such as fear or anxiety elicit marked alterations in heart rate, blood pressure, blood flow, *etc.* These responses may be of both behaviorally and metabolically relevant changes accompanying the psychological and somatic events during behavioral adaptation (Obrist *et al.*, 1970). Several observations suggest that both classical and instrumental conditioning may occur in the autonomic nervous system (Razran, 1961; Miller, 1969) and that both of these influences may affect the emotional state of the animals. Since it was not clear how ACTH-like peptides and corticosteroids affect these processes, the following experiments were carried out.

Experiments in a classically conditioned fear situation showed that both ACTH and corticosteroids influence the heart rate of rats used as a psychophysiological measure (Bohus *et al.*, 1970b, 1971). When $ACTH_{4-10}$ and corticosterone were given during the extinction of classically conditioned fear, significant alterations of brady-

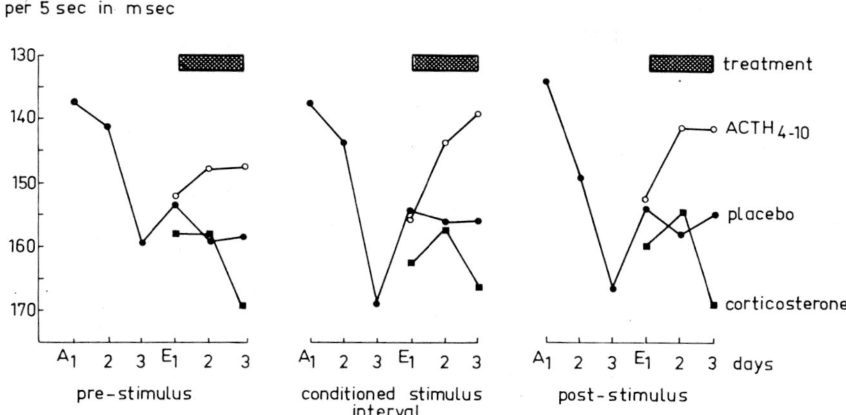

Fig. 3. The effect of $ACTH_{4-10}$ and corticosterone treatment given during the extinction period on the heart rate of rats in a classically conditioned fear situation. Each point represents the mean of 3 non-reinforced trials during acquisition (A) or 12 extinction (E) trials. Heart rate was analysed for 5–5–5 sec, before (pre-stimulus interval), during (conditioned-stimulus interval) and after (post-stimulus interval) the presentation of the conditioned stimulus in each trial.

cardiac heart rate response, as developed during acquisition, occurred. As a consequence of $ACTH_{4-10}$ treatment an increase in heart rate developed, whereas corticosterone resulted in a decrement of cardiac rate during fear extinction. However, these treatment effects were not restricted to the conditioned cardiac response. Similar patterns of heart rate changes appeared in the pre- and post-stimulus intervals (Fig. 3). That is to say, pituitary-adrenal hormones influenced the autonomic consequence of generalized emotional responses of rats which typically developed after this type of classical conditioning. The development of an off-line computer measurement of interbeat interval time allowed a more precise insight into the hormonal effects on conditional cardiac responses. The conditioned heart rate response appeared in a gradually developing bradycardia during the presentation of the conditioned stimulus. The effect of the first 12 extinction trials in control rats is a less pronounced conditioned response. However, both corticosterone and $ACTH_{4-10}$-treated rats showed the response during these trials. The conditioned response was not present after the next 12 extinction trials in control and corticosterone-treated rats, whereas the bradycardiac conditioned response was still marked in rats with $ACTH_{4-10}$ treatment. Continuation of extinction tended to increase the heart rate in response to the conditioned stimulus. This shift in conditioned response was the most pronounced in $ACTH_{4-10}$-treated rats (Fig. 4).

These experiments again strongly suggest the opposite effects of ACTH-like peptides and corticosteroids on a response other than behavioral to aversive conditioning. Further, the hormones seemed to affect both the general emotional status and the conditioned response. The rapid disappearance of bradycardiac heart rate changes in ACTH-treated rats seems to indicate that the generalized autonomic response to classical conditioning has been rapidly extinguished, but, at the same time,

References p. 418–419

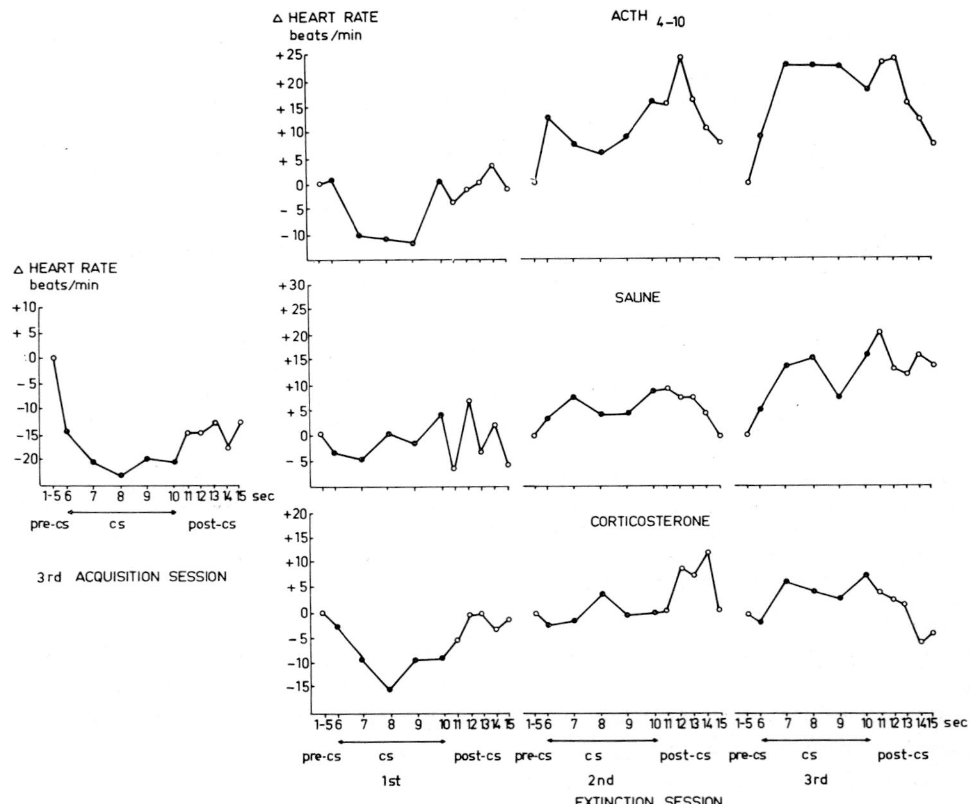

Fig. 4. The effect of $ACTH_{4-10}$ and corticosterone treatment on a conditioned cardiac response during the extinction of classically conditioned fear. Heart rate was calculated from the mean cardiac frequencies of each second of the presentation of the conditioned stimulus minus the mean heart rate for 5 sec before the trial. The differences between the post-stimulus and pre-stimulus heart rate are also given. cs, conditioned stimulus.

the conditioned cardiovascular consequence of fear conditioning is well preserved in peptide-treated rats. The opposite seems to hold for corticosterone-treated rats. If one assumes that emotionality changes, or increase in the level of general arousal, are accompanied by heart rate increase, these preliminary observations are in favor of an effect of hormones on arousal of certain structures in the central nervous system enhancing or attenuating the motivational effect of environmental stimuli.

If one speaks about effects on arousal or motivation, the question immediately arises whether such influences are only related to aversive motives or whether one should expect hormonal influences on approach motives as well. Data are accumulating that pituitary-adrenocortical hormones may affect the acquisition and extinction of appetite and drinking responses (Bohus, 1971; Gray, 1971; Gray *et al.*, 1971; Guth *et al.*, 1971b; Sandman *et al.*, 1969). However, negative observations by Weijnen and Slangen (1970) have also been published. In order to observe any influence of pituitary-adrenal hormones on approach behavior, the importance of stringent

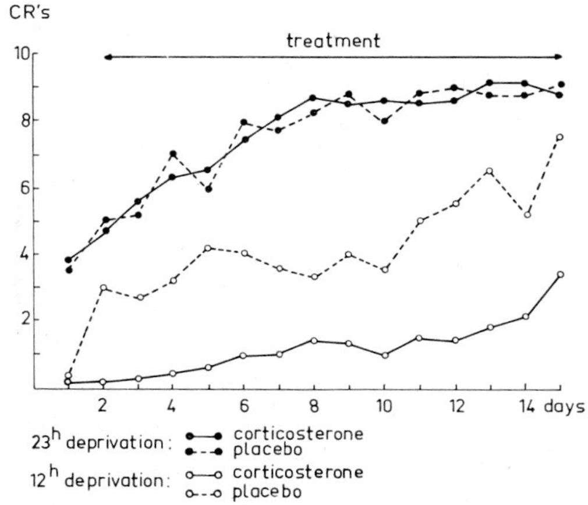

Fig. 5. The effect of corticosterone treatment (1.0 mg/100 g body weight) on the acquisition of a space-discriminative conditioned drinking response as a function of the deprivation time. Each point represents the mean of 8 observations. CR, conditioned response.

controls for extraneous noise and level of motivation (Guth *et al.*, 1971b) and of conflict components in the experimental situation (Bohus, 1971) has been suggested. The following experiments are in favor of these suggestions.

The influence of corticosterone treatment on acquisition of a space-discriminative conditional drinking response is a function of the deprivation level, and consequently of the drive intensity. The acquisition rate was not affected by the treatment if the rats were kept on a 23-h deprivation schedule. However, a marked retardation of the acquisition of the conditioned response was observed in corticosterone-treated rats kept on a 12-h water deprivation (Fig. 5).

Further experiments demonstrated that corticosterone markedly affected the conditioned response performance in a signal-discriminative drinking situation towards both the reinforced and non-reinforced stimulus, if the steroid was administered during reversal training. Corticosterone-treated rats exhibited an enhanced reversal: the response rate was accelerated to the new reinforced stimulus, while the non-reinforced responses were rapidly extinguished (Fig. 6). Similar effects of cortisone have been described previously (Bohus, 1971).

The significance of a conflict component in the behavioral effects of pituitary-adrenal system hormones as shown by this observation is supported by experiments involving "frustrative non-reward". ACTH administration can block the effect of frustrative non-reward during partial reinforcement acquisition or extinction of appetite responses (Gray *et al.*, 1971; Gray, 1971).

The present experiments and the observations of Sandman *et al.* (1969), Gray (1971), Gray *et al.* (1971) and Guth *et al.* (1971b) indicate that ACTH, ACTH-like peptides and corticosteroids have opposite effects on approach behavior as well. Furthermore, the reversal learning data suggest that the attenuation of the response by corticosteroids is not a general property of these hormones. One should not forget

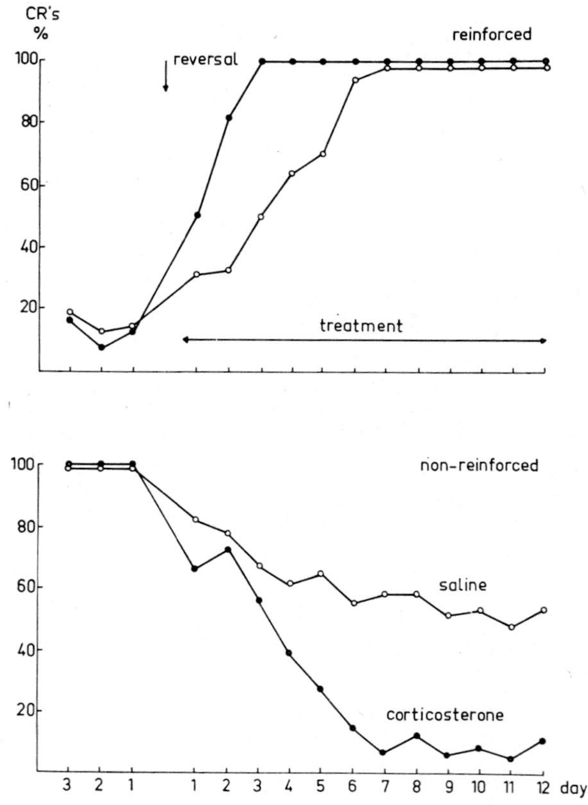

Fig. 6. The effect of corticosterone treatment on the reversal of a signal-discriminative conditioned drinking response. 8–8 observations per point. CR, conditioned response.

that the conditioning procedure employed in these experiments is complex. The original discriminative learning involves the acquisition of the ability to respond towards the reinforced stimulus and to eliminate the motivational property of this stimulus if another signal is also present and not followed by reinforcement. During the reversal training the animal must learn against the background of a well-conditioned inhibitory mechanism and, at the same time, must eliminate the previously reinforced conditioned response. Therefore, it seems that corticosteroids are not only able to eliminate the non-reinforced response by suppressing the motivational value of the conditional stimulus, but are also capable of suppressing the inhibitory value of the previously non-reinforced signal, thus resulting in an enhanced reversal acquisition. On the basis of this experiment with steroid and other studies with ACTH in approach conditioning one would expect an opposite effect of ACTH or ACTH-like peptides on reversal learning.

GENERAL CONCLUSIONS

Although a large number of observations has been collected by us and by others concerning the behavioral effects of pituitary-adrenal hormones, it is still not easy to draw a conclusion on the mode of action of these hormones. It is clear that both pituitary ACTH or ACTH-like peptides and corticosteroids profoundly influence adaptive behavior whether it is motivated by aversive or by approach motives. Furthermore, it is also well established that the peptides and steroids affect adaptive responses of either behavioral or autonomic nature in an opposite manner. The mode of action of pituitary-adrenal hormones may be described in terms of an increase or attenuation of the motivational property of diffuse and specific conditioned environmental cues. Such an influence may be due to a general influence of the excitability of the brain. However, studies that attempted to locate the action of both the peptide and steroid effect in the brain suggest that their influence is restricted to those systems that are involved in the integration of incoming extero- and interoceptive stimuli and/or in motivational processes. Dependence of their effects on drive intensity seems in favor of a motivational hypothesis rather than a non-specific generalized arousal.

Attenuation of the motivational property of external and internal stimuli by ACTH and corticosteroids as a rather specific influence in relation to the pituitary-adrenal responsiveness to specific behavioral stressor stimuli is still obscure. However, a certain specificity, at least concerning the mode of action of ACTH or ACTH-like peptides, is suggested by observations showing facilitation of avoidance learning in intact rats if a certain number of avoidance responses has appeared (Bohus *et al.*, 1968b). This observation suggests that enhancement of the association of environmental signals with the motivational factors may also be responsible for some of the behavioral effects of pituitary-adrenal hormones. Increased ability to detect sensory signals of auditory, gustatory and olfactory modalities by patients after removal of all adrenocortical hormone activity, and decreased sensory detection in patients with excessive glucocorticoid secretion as observed by Henkin (1970), seem to support this assumption. However, if pituitary-adrenal hormones affect associative processes, this influence appears to be limited to the presence of peptides or steroids, since the behavioral changes observed are not seen after the cessation of treatment. For this reason, it is unlikely that permanent associative processes related to learning and memory are affected by pituitary-adrenal hormones. In conclusion, it is suggested that these hormones attenuate or facilitate the motivational property of both conditioned and unconditioned stimuli.

SUMMARY

Pituitary-adrenal system hormones markedly influence adaptive responses of behavioral and autonomic nature. The behavioral effects are present whether a response is motivated by aversive or approach motives. The peptides and steroids have opposite

References p. 418–419

effects on adaptive responses. The mode of action of pituitary-adrenal system hormones may be described in terms of an increase or attenuation of the motivational properties of environmental and internal bodily stimuli. The sites of action of hormones are located in the brain stem and the forebrain.

ACKNOWLEDGEMENTS

The author is greatly indebted to Organon Comp., Oss, The Netherlands, for supplying the steroids, ACTH and ACTH analogs. The generous donation of 6-dehydro-16-methylene-cortisol by Merck Comp., Darmstadt, Germany, is also acknowledged.

REFERENCES

APPLEZWEIG, M. H. AND BAUDRY, F. D. (1955) The pituitary adrenocortical system in avoidance learning. *Psychol. Rev.*, **1**, 417–420.

APPLEZWEIG, M. H. AND MOELLER, G. (1959) Anxiety, the pituitary-adrenocortical system and avoidance learning. *Acta psychol.*, **15**, 602–603.

BEATTY, P. A., BEATTY, W. W., BOWMAN, R. E. AND GILCHRIST, J. O. (1970) The effects of ACTH, adrenalectomy and dexamethasone on the acquisition of an avoidance response in rats. *Physiol. Behav.*, **5**, 939–944.

BERTHOLD, K., ARIMURA, A. AND SCHALLY, A. V. (1970) *In vivo* studies on the mechanism of action of 6-dehydro-16-methylene-hydrocortisone (STC 407) on the hypothalamo-pituitary-adrenal axis in rats. *Neuroendocrinology*, **6**, 301–310.

BOHUS, B. (1968) Pituitary ACTH release and avoidance behavior of rats with cortisol implants in mesencephalic reticular formation and median eminence. *Neuroendocrinology*, **3**, 355–365.

BOHUS, B. (1970a) Central nervous structures and the effect of ACTH and corticosteroids on avoidance behavior: A study with intracerebral implantation of corticosteroids in the rat. In *Pituitary, Adrenal and the Brain* (Progress in Brain Research, Vol. 32), D. DE WIED AND J. A. W. M. WEIJNEN (Eds.), Elsevier, Amsterdam, pp. 171–184.

BOHUS, B. (1970b) The medial thalamus and the opposite effect of corticosteroids and adrenocorticotrophic hormone on avoidance extinction in the rat. *Acta physiol. acad. sci. hung.*, **38**, 217–223.

BOHUS, B. (1971) Adrenocortical hormones and central nervous function: the site and mode of their behavioral action in the rat. *Proc. Second Int. Congr. Hormonal Steroids. Excerpta med. int. Congr. Series*, No. 219, 752–758.

BOHUS, B. AND ENDRÖCZI, E. (1965) The influence of pituitary-adrenocortical function on the avoiding conditioned reflex activity in rats. *Acta physiol. acad. sci. hung.*, **26**, 183–189.

BOHUS, B. AND DE WIED, D. (1967) Failure of α-MSH to delay extinction of conditioned avoidance behavior in rats with lesions in the parafascicular nuclei of the thalamus. *Physiol. Behav.*, **2**, 221–223.

BOHUS, B. AND LISSÁK, K. (1968) Adrenocortical hormones and avoidance behavior in rats. *Int. J. Neuropharmacol.*, **7**, 301–306.

BOHUS, B., NYAKAS, C. AND LISSÁK, K. (1968a) Involvement of suprahypothalamic structures in the hormonal feedback action of corticosteroids. *Acta physiol. acad. sci. hung.*, **34**, 1–8.

BOHUS, B., NYAKAS, C. AND ENDRÖCZI, E. (1968b) Effects of adrenocorticotropic hormone on avoidance behavior of intact and adrenalectomized rats. *Int. J. Neuropharmacol.*, **7**, 307–314.

BOHUS, B., GRUBITS, J., KOVÁCS, G. AND LISSÁK, K. (1970a) Effect of corticosteroids on passive avoidance behavior of rats. *Acta physiol. acad. sci. hung.*, **38**, 381–391.

BOHUS, B., GRUBITS, J. AND LISSÁK, K. (1970b) Influence of cortisone on heart rate during fear extinction in the rat. *Acta physiol. acad. sci. hung.*, **37**, 265–272.

BOHUS, B., DE WIED, D. AND LISSÁK, K. (1971) Heart rate changes during fear extinction in rats treated with pituitary peptides or corticosteroids. *Proc. 25th Int. Congr. Int. Union Physiol. Sci.*, Vol. IX, p. 72.

Bohus, B., Gispen, W. H. and De Wied, D. (1973) Effect of lysine vasopressin and ACTH 4-10 on conditioned avoidance behavior of hypophysectomized rats. *Neuroendocrinology*, **11**, 137–143.
De Wied, D. (1964) Influence of anterior pituitary on avoidance learning and escape behavior. *Amer. J. Physiol.*, **207**, 255–259.
De Wied, D. (1966) Inhibitory effect of ACTH and related peptides on extinction of conditioned avoidance behavior in rats. *Proc. Soc. exp. Biol. (N.Y.)*, **122**, 28–32.
De Wied, D. (1967) Opposite effects of ACTH and glucocorticosteroids on extinction of conditioned avoidance behavior. *Excerpta med. int. Congr. Series*, No. 132, 945–951.
De Wied, D. (1969) Effects of peptide hormones on behavior. In *Frontiers in Neuroendocrinology*, W. F. Ganong and L. Martini (Eds.), Oxford University Press, New York, pp. 97–140.
De Wied, D., Bohus, B. and Greven, H. M. (1968) Influence of pituitary and adrenocortical hormones on conditioned avoidance behavior in rats. In *Endocrinology and Human Behavior*, R. P. Michael (Ed.), Oxford University Press, New York, pp. 188–199.
Endröczi, E. (1969) Brain stem and hypothalamic substrate of motivated behavior. In *Results in Neurophysiology, Neuroendocrinology, Neuropharmacology and Behavior* (Recent Developments of Neurobiology in Hungary, Vol. II), K. Lissák (Ed.), Hung. Acad. Sci., Budapest, pp. 27–49.
Gray, J. A. (1971) Effect of ACTH on extinction of rewarded behavior is blocked by previous administration of ACTH. *Nature*, **229**, 52–54.
Gray, J. A., Mayes, A. R. and Wilson, M. (1971) A barbiturate-like effect of adrenocorticotrophic hormone on the partial reinforcement acquisition and extinction effects. *Neuropharmacology*, **10**, 223–230.
Guth, S., Seward, J. P. and Levine, S. (1971a) Differential manipulation of passive avoidance by exogenous ACTH. *Hormones Behav.*, **2**, 127–138.
Guth, S., Levine, S. and Seward, J. P. (1971b) Appetitive acquisition and extinction effects with exogenous ACTH. *Physiol. Behav.*, **7**, 195–200.
Henkin, R. I. (1970) The effects of corticosteroids and ACTH on sensory systems. In *Pituitary, Adrenal and the Brain* (Progress in Brain Research, Vol. 32), D. de Wied and J. A. W. M. Weijnen (Eds.), Elsevier, Amsterdam, pp. 270–294.
Levine, S. (1968) Hormones and conditioning. In *Nebraska Symposium on Motivation*, W. J. Arnold (Ed.), Univ. of Nebraska Press, Lincoln, Neb., pp. 85–101.
Levine, S. and Jones, L. E. (1965) Adrenocorticotropic hormone (ACTH) and passive avoidance learning. *J. comp. physiol. Psychol.*, **59**, 357–360.
Lissák, K. and Endröczi, E. (1964) Neuroendocrine interrelationships and behavioural processes. In *Major Problems in Neuroendocrinology*, E. Bajusz and G. Jasmin (Eds.), Karger, Basel, pp. 1–16.
Lissák, K. and Bohus, B. (1972) Pituitary hormones and the avoidance behavior of the rat. *Int. J. Psychobiol.*, **2**, 103–115.
Miller, N. E. (1969) Learning of visceral and glandular responses. *Science*, **163**, 434–445.
Miller, R. E. and Ogawa, N. (1962) The effect of adrenocorticotrophic hormone (ACTH) on avoidance conditioning in the adrenalectomized rat. *J. comp. physiol. Psychol.*, **55**, 211–213.
Obrist, P. A., Webb, R. A., Sutterer, J. R. and Howard, J. L. (1970) The cardio-somatic relationship: some reformulations. *Psychophysiology*, **6**, 569–587.
Razran, G. (1961) The observable unconscious and the inferable conscious in current Soviet psychophysiology. *Psychol. Rev.*, **68**, 81–147.
Sandman, C. A., Kastin, A. J. and Schally, A. V. (1969) Melanocyte-stimulating hormone and learned appetitive behavior. *Experientia (Basel)*, **25**, 1001–1002.
Van Wimersma Greidanus, Tj. B. (1970) Effects of steroid on extinction of an avoidance response in rats. A structure-activity relationship study. In *Pituitary, Adrenal and the Brain* (Progress in Brain Research, Vol. 32), D. de Wied and J. A. W. M. Weijnen (Eds.), Elsevier, Amsterdam, pp. 185–191.
Van Wimersma Greidanus, Tj. B. and De Wied, D. (1969) Effects of intracerebral implantation of corticosteroids on extinction of an avoidance response in rats. *Physiol.. Behav.*, **4**, 365–370.
Van Wimersma Greidanus, Tj. B. and De Wied, D. (1971) Effects of systemic and intracerebral administration of two opposite acting ACTH-related peptides on extinction of conditioned avoidance behavior. *Neuroendocrinology*, **7**, 291–301.
Weiss, J. M., McEwen, B. S., Silva, M. T. and Kalkut, M. (1970) Pituitary-adrenal alterations and fear responding. *Amer. J. Physiol.*, **218**, 864–868.
Weijnen, J. A. W. M. and Slangen, J. L. (1970) Effects of ACTH-analogues on extinction of conditioned behavior. In *Pituitary, Adrenal and the Brain* (Progress in Brain Research, Vol. 32), D. de Wied and J. A. W. M. Weijnen (Eds.), Elsevier, Amsterdam, pp. 221–233.

DISCUSSION

KITAY: You showed first that cortisone administration accelerated and that ACTH prolonged extinction of conditioned avoidance behavior. Then you showed that ACTH was equally effective in intact and adrenalectomized animals. It seems to me that if the administration of cortisone or of ACTH were to have some physiologic significance, the 14-day adrenalectomized animal would be a super animal with respect to prolonged extinction of behavior and that exogenous ACTH would not have any particular marked effect because endogenous ACTH would have been working in the absence of endogenous corticosterone. Could you explain this?

BOHUS: The experiments you are referring to were performed on rats adrenalectomized just before the first extinction session. Therefore, increase of endogenous ACTH release in the absence of corticosteroids cannot be the primary mechanism for the delayed extinction of the conditioned avoidance response in adrenalectomized, ACTH-treated rats. On the other hand, if adrenalectomy was performed 14 days before the behavioral experiments—in which case the endogenous ACTH release was already increased at the beginning of extinction period—the delay of extinction appeared similar to that of the ACTH-treated rats. This observation favours a physiological role of endogenous ACTH in the extinction behavior.

MCEWEN: I wonder if you would comment on the relative effectiveness of various glucocorticoids on behavior.

BOHUS: The experiments using passive avoidance situations and comparing the behavioral and ACTH-suppressive potencies of various corticosteroids suggest a "preferential" effect of corticosterone on the behavior of the rat.

KRIVOY: I should like to complement Dr. Bohus on his very fine presentation. Additionally, I should like to point out that in the spinal cord we have not found an action of β-MSH or $ACTH_{1-24}$ in maximally stimulated spinal cords but only in submaximally stimulated, or pharmacologically depressed cords. This seems to parallel Dr. Bohus' observations very nicely.

Unique Pituitary Peptides with Behavioral-affecting Activity

SAUL LANDE, DAVID DE WIED AND ALBERT WITTER

Yale University School of Medicine, Department of Dermatology, New Haven, Conn. (U.S.A.), and Rudolf Magnus Institute for Pharmacology, Medical Faculty, University of Utrecht, Vondellaan 6, Utrecht (The Netherlands)

The profound deficit in acquisition and retention of conditioned avoidance responses (CARs) imposed on rats by hypophysectomy can be substantially reversed by subcutaneous administration of corticotrophin (ACTH) and certain subunits thereof, as well as by the melanotrophins and pitressin (De Wied, 1969). Facilitation of CAR acquisition in these deficient animals is independent of adrenal mediation (De Wied, 1969). The potent behavioral effects of synthetic corticotrophin subunits in conjunction

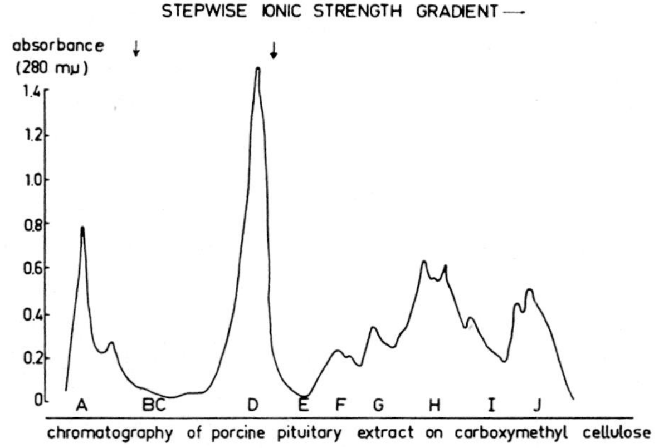

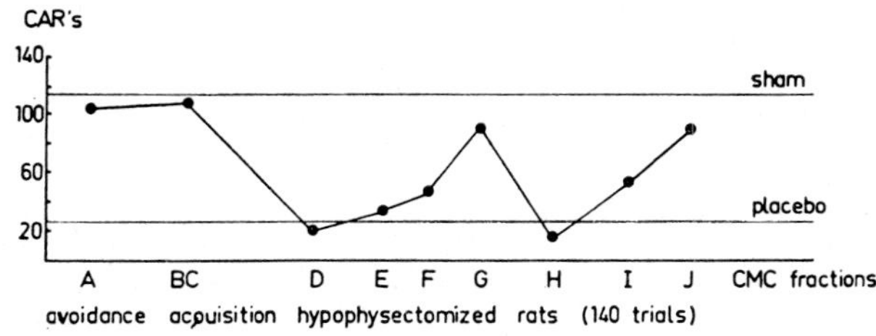

Fig. 1. Effect of peptide subfractions obtained by carboxymethyl-cellulose chromatography on acquisition of a conditioned avoidance response in hypophysectomized rats. The ordinate in the lower curve indicates total conditioned avoidance responses (CAR) out of a possible 140 (De Wied *et al.*, 1970).

References p. 427

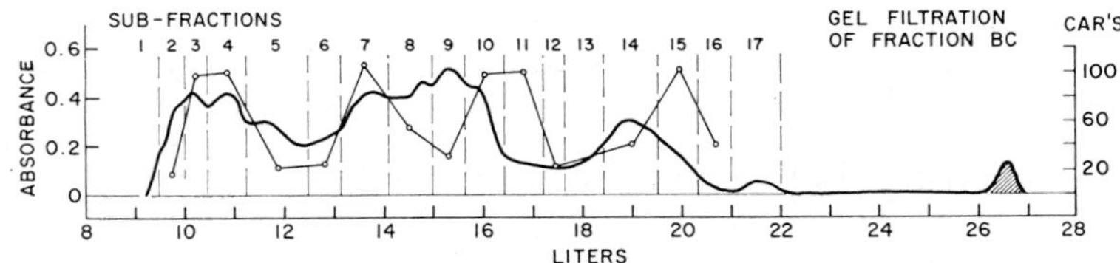

Fig. 2. Effect of peptide subfractions obtained by Sephadex G-25 gel filtration of fraction BC, on acquisition of a conditioned avoidance response in hypophysectomized rats (De Wied *et al.*, 1970). The lighter line indicates distribution of CAR-facilitating activity.

with an apparent lack of peripheral action suggested the possible existence of naturally occurring pituitary peptides with similar biological activity. The availability of a porcine pituitary extract in a large quantity afforded the opportunity to undertake a search for such compounds.

Initial screening studies for activity were performed on hypophysectomized rats. Effects on shuttle-box–CAR acquisition were measured following administration of peptide fractions obtained by ion exchange chromatography on carboxymethyl cellulose (Fig. 1) (Lande *et al.*, 1965). Behavioral results of subcutaneous doses of peptide fractions—20 μg in a stabilizing vehicle every 48 h for the duration of the experiment—are also shown in Fig. 1 (De Wied *et al.*, 1970). Fraction BC was studied further because of its relatively high potency and the expectation that BC would contain a less complex mixture of peptides than unretarded fraction A.

Components of fraction BC, resolved by gel filtration on Sephadex G-25, (Upton *et al.*, 1966), were assayed as described above. Results are shown in Fig. 2 (De Wied *et al.*, 1970). Four peaks of biological activity were revealed, corresponding to materials of molecular size 40, 20, 13 and 8 amino acid residues $\pm 10\%$ respectively. This was determined with use of a Sephadex column calibrated for molecular weight *vs.* elution volume.

The component smallest in size, BC-15, was resolved further by ion exchange chromatography on DEAE-Sephadex as shown in Fig. 3 (Lande *et al.*, 1971). The

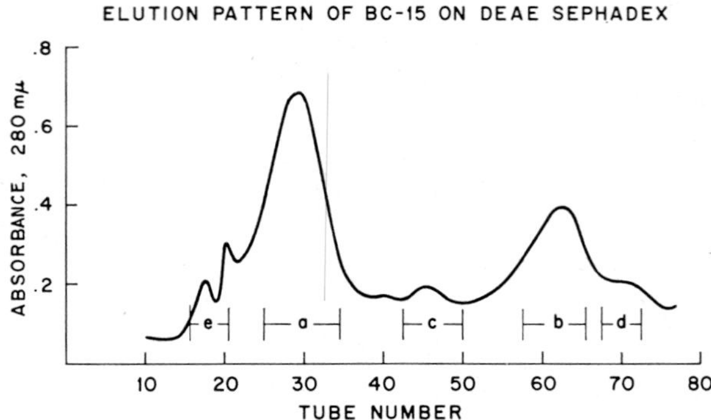

Fig. 3. Chromatography of peptide fraction BC-15 on DEAE-Sephadex, with 0.04 *M* ammonium bicarbonate, pH 8.7 (Lande *et al.*, 1971).

STRUCTURE OF BC 15a

Cys - Tyr - Phe - Gln - Asn - Cys - Pro - Lys

LYSINE VASOPRESSIN

Cys - Tyr - Phe - Gln - Asn - Cys - Pro - Lys - Gly - NH_2

Fig. 4. Structure of lysine[8] vasopressin and desglycinamide-lysine[8] vasopressin.

major component, BC-15a, highly active by the criteria listed above, was not electrophoretically homogeneous. However, the level of purity was sufficient to warrant structure determination by a subtractive Edman degradation technique (Koningsberg, 1967). The product was identified as desglycinamide-lysine[8] vasopressin (Lande *et al.*, 1971) (Fig. 4). Verification of both structure and activity of the natural product was obtained by preparation of identical biologically active material by total synthesis as well as by tryptic hydrolysis of authentic lysine[8] vasopressin. Pure lysine vasopressin appears somewhat more potent than the desglycinamide product (De Wied *et al.*, 1972). Of particular interest, however, is that behavioral activity appears independent of pressor action; the desglycinamide product is highly potent in the CAR assay while exhibiting only about 0.5% of the pressor activity of lysine[8]-vasopressin. Other biologic properties of the desglycinamide molecule have also been studied (De Wied *et al.*, 1972; Wang, 1972).

In guiding the isolation of active components in BC-3, 7 and 10, Fig. 2, a pole-jumping assay was employed, in which inhibition of extinction in conditioned intact rats was measured (Van Wimersma Greidanus and De Wied, 1971). Application of this technique for assay of desglycinamide-lysine[8] vasopressin is shown in Table I. Assay of subfractions of BC-3—*i.e.*, -a and -b, obtained by paper electrophoresis—is shown in the same table. The active component, BC-3b, comprises about 40 amino

TABLE I

EFFECT OF SINGLE INJECTION ON RATE OF EXTINCTION

Effect of a single subcutaneous injection of peptide on extinction of a pole-jumping conditioned avoidance response in rats (Mean ± S.E.M.)

Treatment	*Acquisition (30 trials)*	*Extinction sessions (10 trials each) h after injection*			
		24	*48*	*120*	*268*
DG-LVP[a] 0.1 μg	17 ± 1	8 ± 0	2 ± 0.6	0	0 (4)
0.3 μg	15 ± 0.4	8 ± 0.3	5 ± 0.3	6 ± 0.5	5 ± 0.0(4)
0.9 μg	15 ± 0.7	9 ± 0.5	10 ± 0.3	10 ± 0.3	9 ± 0.5(4)
			24 + 48 h[b]		
Placebo	18 ± 0.7		12 ± 3.5(5)		
BC 3a 5 μg	16 ± 1		11 ± 2.2(5)		
BC 3b 5 μg	17 ± 0.7		17 ± 1.0(5)		

[a]Desglycinamide-lysine[8] vasopressin.
[b]Total number of positive responses of two extinction sessions at 24 and 48 h of 10 trials each.

References p. 427

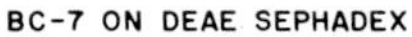

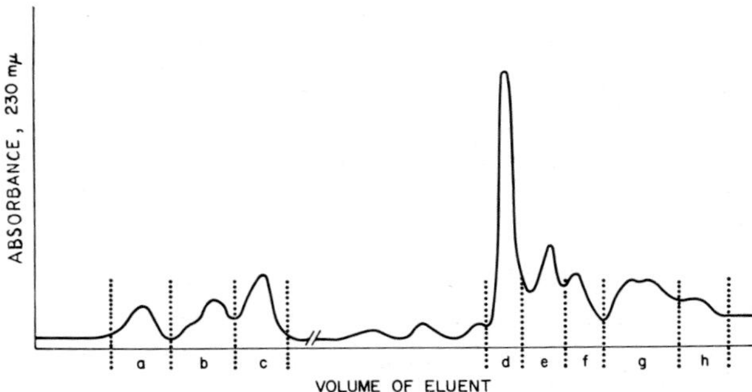

Fig. 5. Chromatography of peptide fraction BC-7 on DEAE-Sephadex, with 0.04 *M* ammonium bicarbonate, pH 8.7.

ELECTROPHORESIS OF BC-7a+b

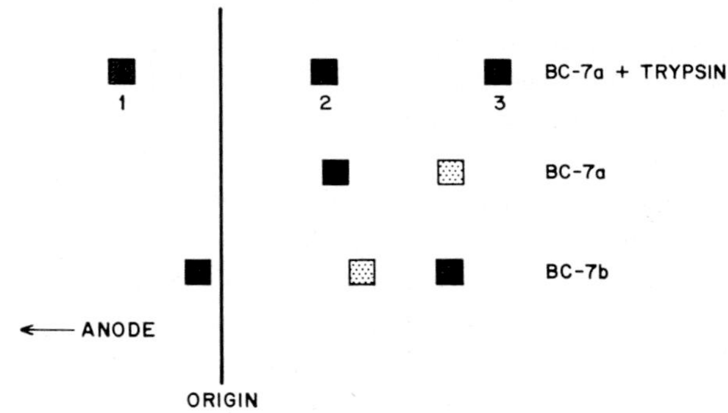

Fig. 6. Diagrammatic representation of BC-7a, -b and a tryptic digest of BC-7a, after high-voltage paper electrophoresis at pH 6.5 and staining with ninhydrin.

acid residues, including 4 half-cystines. Although the molecule contains a number of basic and aromatic residues, it is resistant to hydrolysis by both trypsin and chymotrypsin. Structure determination of this large molecule has, therefore, been deferred.

Components in BC-7 (Fig. 2) were resolved by ion exchange chromatography on DEAE-Sephadex employing conditions previously described (Lande *et al.*, 1971). Results are shown in Fig. 5. In the pole-jumping assay described above, only fractions BC-7a and -b were active at both 5 and 1 μg dose levels. Electrophoresis indicated near homogeneity for BC-7a but the presence of two major components in the b-fraction (Fig. 6). Amino acid analysis of the a-fraction (Table II) revealed the absence of histidine, arginine and half-cystine. The peptide therefore appears unrelated to other behavior-affecting peptides studied previously. Fig. 6 shows the results of trypsin digestion of BC-7a. Three major components were obtained by electrophoresis, in accord with the presence of 2 lysine residues in the parent molecule (Table II). The sum of amino acid compositions of tryptic fragments of BC-7a, shown in the same table, is in close accord with that of the parent molecule. Resistance of BC-7a to

TABLE II

AMINO ACID COMPOSITION OF PEPTIDE BC-7a AND FRAGMENTS PRODUCED BY TRYPTIC DIGESTION OF BC-7a

Amino acid	*Residues per mole*			
	BC-7a	*BC-7a*	+	*Trypsin*
		1	*2*	*3*
Lysine	1.6	1.0	0.2	0.8
Histidine[a]				
Arginine	0.3		0.3	0.2
Aspartic acid	0.7		0.7	0.3
Threonine	2.5	1.0	0.4	1.5
Serine	2.5	1.1	0.8	1.0
Glutamic acid	2.1	1.2	0.7	1.0
Proline	2.0	0.2	1.1	1.0
Glycine	2.0	2.1	0.9	0.4
Alanine	0.8	0.2	1.1	0.3
Half-cystine				
Valine	1.1		0.3	1.0
Methionine	0.8	0.7	0.2	
Isoleucine				
Leucine	2.6		0.8	1.8
Tyrosine	0.8	0.6		
Phenylalanine	2.0	1.0	0.5	1.0
Tryptophan[b]				

[a]Blank means less than 0.1 residues.
[b]Destroyed by acid hydrolysis.

chymotryptic digestion was noted, in spite of the presence of aromatic residues in the peptide (Table II). In addition, BC-7a gave no reaction with Edman- or Dansyl-reagents, indicating a blocked amino terminus in the molecule. Since tryptic peptide BC-7a 1 also appears amino-terminal blocked, and tryptic peptide BC-7a2 contains no lysine, the sequence of peptides in the parent molecule must be BC-7a 1, 3, 2. Further structural determination of the molecule is in progress.

Although the active material in BC-10 and -11 (Fig. 2) is not yet sufficiently pure for chemical characterization, we have demonstrated the presence of at least 4 stable peptides in pituitary extracts that are quite potent in facilitating acquisition or inhibiting extinction of CARs in rats. While the smallest component was identified as desglycinamide-lysine[8] vasopressin, the other peptides do not appear related in structure to the known pituitary hormones. All were isolated from only one of the major subfractions in the starting material, employing a conditioned avoidance assay. Undoubtedly the spectrum of active pituitary peptides will be expanded considerably when other fractions are studied or different modes of assay are employed. The effect of pituitary peptides on levels of behavior unrelated to fear- or pain-motivated responses might be particularly interesting to examine.

A number of questions arise with regard to the studies reported above: whether the

References p. 427

described peptides exist naturally in the pituitary gland or are artifacts; whether such compounds perform physiologic roles or act pharmacologically; what are their sites and modes of action. Presently, these questions can be answered only inferentially.

The starting material employed in these studies—a gift from Armour Pharmaceutical Co.—is a side product of commercial-scale isolation of porcine corticotrophin. The extract consists of peptides falling in a narrow range of physicochemical properties and is therefore not representative of whole pituitary tissue. That certain of the peptides described above were generated during collection and initial extraction procedures is possible, indeed probable. However, a number of pituitary hormones very susceptible to enzymatic degradation have been isolated from the same extract, suggesting that extensive enzymatic degradation did not occur. On the other hand, the rather unusual resistance to hydrolytic enzymes exhibited by a number of the compounds described above might account for their accumulation in pituitary tissue and for their activity when administered subcutaneously. Chromatographic procedures employed in further purification steps were too gentle to induce any significant degree of chemical breakdown.

An indirect demonstration of the physiological role of peptides in affecting behavior may not be beyond current technical capabilities, after the full spectrum of behavioral-affecting peptides has been revealed. One approach would be an immunochemical comparison of peptide distributions in the serum of animals bred for differences in behavior (Bovet *et al.*, 1969). In such a study Levine and Levin (1970) concluded that mice exhibiting a deficit in passive avoidance response acquisition had significantly lower levels of circulating ACTH than did animals capable of rapid acquisition. A second approach might be immunologic comparison of circulating levels of peptides in animals and man spontaneously exhibiting modes of behavior different from an established norm.

Presently little can be said of the site(s) or mode(s) of action of the peptides described above. The role of the pituitary in affecting behavior *via* endocrine organ mediation has been clearly demonstrated (see for example the monograph edited by De Wied and Weijnen, 1970). On the other hand, certain synthetic subunits of ACTH and also the naturally occurring compounds described in this paper appear to exert no peripheral endocrine action. Accordingly, the possibility of direct participation of peptides in central nervous system function is indicated.

SUMMARY

Four unique porcine pituitary peptides have been isolated and partially characterized, which upon subcutaneous administration potently facilitate acquisition of conditioned avoidance responses in hypophysectomized rats and inhibit extinction of avoidance responses in intact rats. Molecular size of the peptides is about 40, 20, 13 and 8 residues, respectively. With the exception of the smallest component, desglycinamide-lysine[8] vasopressin, none appears related in amino acid composition to any pituitary hormone. At dose levels inducing pronounced behavioral effects no peripheral endocrine responses to administration of these peptides have been observed.

ACKNOWLEDGEMENT

This research was supported in part by the National Institute of Health, Grant No. USPH 5 CA-04679, and The American Cancer Society, Grant No. BC-3E.

REFERENCES

BOVET, D., BOVET-NITTI, F. AND OLIVERIO, A. (1969) Genetic aspects of learning and memory in mice. *Science*, **163**, 139–149.

DE WIED, D. (1969) Effects of peptide hormones on behavior. In *Frontiers in Neuroendocrinology, 1969*, W. F. GANONG AND L. MARTINI (Eds.), Oxford University Press, New York, pp. 97–140.

DE WIED, D. AND WEIJNEN, J. A. W. M. (Eds.), 1970. *Pituitary, Adrenal and the Brain* (Progress in Brain Research, Vol. 32), Elsevier, Amsterdam.

DE WIED, D., WITTER, A. AND LANDE, S. (1970) Anterior pituitary peptides and avoidance acquisition of hypophysectomized rats. In *Pituitary, Adrenal and the Brain* (Progress in Brain Research, Vol. 32), D. DE WIED AND J. A. W. M. WEIJNEN (Eds.), Elsevier, Amsterdam, pp. 213–218.

DE WIED, D., WITTER, A., LANDE, S. AND GREVEN, H. M. (1972) Dissociation of the behavioral and endocrine effects of lysine vasopressin by tryptic digestion. *Brit. J. Pharmacol.*, **45**, 118–122.

KONIGSBERG, W. (1967) Subtractive Edman degradation. In *Methods in Enzymology*, Vol. 11, C. H. W. HIRS (Ed.), Academic Press, New York, pp. 461–468.

LANDE, S., LERNER, A. B. AND UPTON, G. V. (1965) Pituitary peptides: isolation of new peptides related to β-melanocyte stimulating hormone. *J. Biol. Chem.*, **240**, 4259–4263.

LANDE, S., WITTER, A. AND DE WIED, D. (1971) An octapeptide that stimulates conditioned avoidance acquisition in hypophysectomized rats. *J. Biol. Chem.*, **246**, 2058–2062.

LEVINE, S. AND LEVIN, R. (1970) Pituitary-adrenal influences on passive avoidance in two inbred strains of mice. *Hormones Behav.*, **1**, 105–110.

UPTON, G. V., LERNER, A. B. AND LANDE, S. (1966) Pituitary peptides: resolution by gel filtration. *J. Biol. Chem.*, **241**, 5585–5589.

VAN WIMERSMA GREIDANUS, TJ. B. AND DE WIED, D. (1971) Effects of systemic and intracerebral administration of two opposite acting ACTH-related peptides on extinction of conditioned avoidance behavior. *Neuroendocrinology*, **7**, 291–301.

WANG, S. S. (1972) Synthesis of desglycinamide lysine vasopressin and its behavioral activity in rats. *Biochem. biophys. Res. Commun.*, **48**, 1511–1515.

DISCUSSION

SACHS: Have you compared any of your peptides with neurophysin degradation products? If care is not taken in the extraction of neural lobes, then considerable degradation of the neurophysin may occur. Saffran some time ago isolated and identified a 40-amino acid peptide from porcine neural lobes. Does it in any way have the properties of any of your peptides?

LANDE: I have considered the possibility that the large peptide which has 2 pairs of disulfide bonds might be a breakdown product of neurophysin, but have not yet compared it to that described by Saffran. It may be possible to find a sequence in neurophysin that is related in amino acid composition. This gets to be a very complicated procedure, however, since these compounds may be much more potent when released endogenously near their site of action than when administered systemically.

MINTZ: What relationship do you think exists between pituitary peptides and learning?

LANDE: In so far as acquisition of avoidance response is a model for learning, and retention of the conditioned avoidance response is a model for memory, the substances described today may reflect molecules that facilitate mechanisms of learning and memory.

The Influence of Peptides Derived from Corticotrophin (ACTH) on Performance. Structure Activity Studies

H. M. GREVEN AND D. DE WIED

Research Laboratories, Organon, Oss, and Rudolf Magnus Institute for Pharmacology Medical Faculty, University of Utrecht, Vondellaan 6, Utrecht (The Netherlands)

INTRODUCTION

Corticotrophin (ACTH) affects performance

To cope with changing or stressful external conditions, mammals have an integrated complex of adaptive reactions termed "General Adaptation Syndrome" (GAS). This term was originally coined by Selye (1950), who gave the following description: "The GAS does not merely represent a transitory 'emergency' adjustment to changes in the environment, but is an adaptive reaction, which comprises the 'learning' of defence against future exposure to stress, and helps to maintain a state of adaptation once this is acquired".

Thus acquisition and extinction of conditioned avoidance behaviour may be considered as aspects of this syndrome. The role of the pituitary-adrenal axis in the GAS was recognized from its inception (Selye, 1950). An effect of ACTH on conditioned avoidance behaviour was demonstrated for the first time by Mirsky *et al.* (1953) and later firmly established in numerous experiments. (Review: De Wied, 1969.)

At first it was not fully realized that ACTH and corticosteroids have different effects on behaviour. However, when synthetic fragments of ACTH became available, which were virtually devoid of intrinsic adrenocorticotrophic activity but which influenced behaviour in a manner similar to that of ACTH, it became clear that the effect of such peptides on conditioned avoidance behaviour was due to their action on the brain and not through their action on the adrenal cortex. This view was further substantiated by the following findings.

(*1*) Intracerebral implantation studies of ACTH-related peptides indicated that the parafascicular nuclei and the rostral parts of the mesencephalon are involved in the behavioural effects of ACTH analogues (van Wimersma Greidanus and De Wied, 1971).

(*2*) Lesions in these regions of the thalamus abolish the behavioural effect of an ACTH analogue (Bohus and De Wied, 1967).

References p. 440–441

(*3*) The effect of ACTH on extinction of conditioned avoidance behaviour is not mediated by the adrenal gland because ACTH has a similar action in adrenalectomized rats (Miller and Ogawa, 1962).

(*4*) Though some investigators suggested a role for the thyroid in acquisition and retention of avoidance behaviour, De Wied and Pirie (1968, see also for references) showed that the inhibitory effect of ACTH analogues on extinction is not mediated by the thyroid gland.

(*5*) Peptides related to ACTH normalize the reduced incorporation of labelled leucine into certain proteins in the brain stem of hypophysectomized rats (Schotman, 1971), and also stimulate leucine incorporation into brain proteins of intact rats (Reading and Dewar, 1971).

From these results we may deduce that the behavioural effect of ACTH and related peptides is a consequence of their action on specific areas of the central nervous system.

The improved performance of hypophysectomized rats treated with ACTH or fragments of ACTH is not due solely to improved motor and/or sensory capacities nor to an increase in the level of general activity (De Wied, 1969; Gispen *et al.*, 1970). Accordingly, ACTH and related peptides appear to improve performance by mechanisms which involve both physical and mental processes. This conclusion is corroborated by the effect of ACTH (Endröczi, 1970), melanocyte-stimulating hormones (MSH) (Kastin *et al.*, 1971) and $ACTH_{4-10}$ (Fink, personal communication) on the electroencephalogram (EEG) in man.

In the study reported here two approaches have been followed. First we sought the smallest peptide sequence of ACTH that possesses essentially the same behavioural effects as ACTH itself. Second we tried to increase the behavioural potency of the sequence $ACTH_{4-9}$ by introducing certain structural modifications. Attention will be focused on the dissociation between behavioural activity and MSH-like potency.

METHODS

Introduction

In the evaluation of the behavioural properties of our synthetic peptides both acquisition and extinction of conditioned avoidance behaviour were studied. In the acquisition trials only hypophysectomized rats were used. Since these are difficult to maintain over a long period of time, this method was applied to certain key compounds only.

Extinction was studied in two different situations: the shuttle-box and the pole-jump apparatus. These methods do not give the same type of information, however (Taber, 1971). The shuttle-box response is indicative of "anti-anxiety activity" since the animal must return repeatedly to an area wherein it was previously shocked, whereas the pole-jump task is more an index of agility and coordination. In practice essentially the same results were obtained when we tested our ACTH-like peptides by both techniques. Since a pole-jumping experiment (in its most recent version) takes only 4–5 days to perfect, whereas a shuttle-box experiment requires several weeks, the former method was used for routine-screening of new synthetic analogues.

Finally, the response latencies in a one-trial passive avoidance paradigm were studied (Ader *et al.*, 1972). Though this technique is the least laborious of all methods discussed, it also proved to be the least discriminative. It was therefore used only in studies in which the peptide chain was shortened. The results obtained from structurally modified analogues, however, appeared to be less informative.

Acquisition studies in a shuttle-box

The experiments reported here were carried out on male white rats weighing between 160 and 180 g, from which the whole pituitary was removed *via* the transauricular route under ether anaesthesia. One week after surgery animals were conditioned in a shuttle-box. The conditioned stimulus (CS) was a buzzer presented for 5 sec before the unconditioned stimulus (US) of shock. Ten conditional trials were given each day for 10 or 14 days using a fixed inter-trial interval procedure (De Wied, 1964). As an index of avoidance learning the quotient of the total number of scored responses divided by the total number of trials was used. All peptides were administered subcutaneously in the form of zinc phosphate complexes (De Wied, 1966) on alternate days during the period of avoidance training. The dose given was 20 μg per rat per 2 days.

Extinction studies

(a) Shuttle-box experiments

Intact male white rats weighing 140–180 g were used. Conditioning was performed in a shuttle-box as described above. Conditioning was continued until the rat had achieved a criterion of 80% or more avoidances during 3 consecutive days. The day after this criterion was reached extinction trials were run with the same schedule and procedure as in conditioning, except that the US was never presented and the CS was terminated after 5 sec if the animal had not crossed the barrier. Extinction was studied for 10 or 14 days (De Wied, 1965). The index of extinction of conditioned avoidance behaviour was the quotient of the total number of scored responses divided by the total number of trials during the extinction sessions. The peptides were administered subcutaneously in the form of zinc phosphate complexes on alternate days during the extinction period.

(b) Pole-jumping experiments

Male white rats were conditioned to jump onto a pole. The CS was a light presented for 5 sec. A rat that did not jump onto the pole, but remained on the grid floor of the cage, received an electric shock which served as the US.

Ten conditioning trials were given each day for 3 days with a fixed intertrial interval. Rats showing positive responses in 10 or more of these 30 conditioning trials were

References p. 440–441

used for extinction trials. Extinction was studied over the next 3 consecutive days using the same procedure as that employed in the acquisition trials, except that the US was not presented. Treatment consisted of a single subcutaneous injection of the peptide in the form of a zinc phosphate complex on the third day of the acquisition period immediately after training (De Wied, 1966). The quotient of the total number of responses scored during extinction divided by the total number of trials again served as an index of extinction of conditioned avoidance behaviour. As an indication of relative potency the ratio of doses that induced a half-maximal effect was used.

In a recent modification of the pole-jumping test, the extinction period was reduced to one day (Van Wimersma Greidanus and De Wied, 1969). On the 4th day, immediately after a first extinction session of 10 trials, all rats which made 8 or more avoidances were injected subcutaneously either with the peptide dissolved in saline or with the vehicle. 2 and 4 h later a second and a third extinction session was run.

To measure facilitation of extinction, rats were made more resistant to extinction by extending the acquisition period by one day. Facilitation of extinction was then studied on the 5th day of the experiment in an extinction session 4 h after injection of the peptide or placebo, this treatment being given immediately after the first extinction session.

One-trial passive avoidance learning

On the first day of the test a male white rat (weighing 130–150 g) was placed inside a square chamber with black walls and a grid floor for 2 min to enable adaptation to occur. This was followed by a single trial in which the rat was placed at the end of an elevated and illuminated runway and then allowed to enter the box. The time required for the rat to enter the box was taken as an index of the latency. The next day, 3 such trials were given. After the third trial, animals upon entering the box received a single electric shock (1 sec, 0.25 mA) through the grid floor. Retention was tested on two successive days (Ader *et al.*, 1972). The quotient of the median latency score of a number of experiments divided by the maximal latency (300 sec) served as an index of passive avoidance learning. In these experiments the peptides were dissolved in saline and injected subcutaneously 1 h before the first retention session.

THE SHORTEST PEPTIDE-AFFECTING BEHAVIOUR

De Wied has shown (1964, 1966, 1967, 1969; De Wied and Bohus, 1966; Bohus and De Wied, 1966) that ACTH not only restores the impaired acquisition capacity of hypophysectomized rats but also delays extinction of an avoidance response in intact rats. Subsequent studies showed that both α- and β-MSH affected acquisition and extinction in the same way as ACTH. Since ACTH, α-MSH and β-MSH share the sequence 4–10 as a common core, this was considered as an indication that the minimal requirements essential for such an activity were located within the heptapeptide $ACTH_{4-10}$. This assumption received support from the finding that $ACTH_{1-10}$

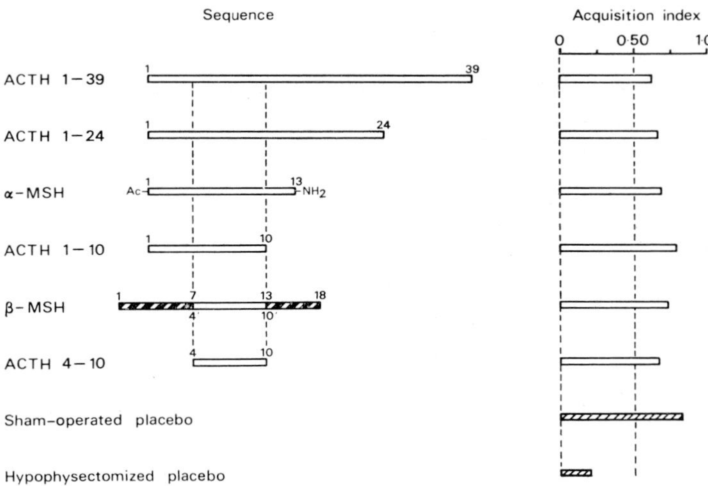

Fig. 1. Avoidance acquisition (hypophysectomized rats). Effect of ACTH, ACTH analogues and placebo, administered subcutaneously in the form of zinc phosphate complexes on alternate days, on avoidance acquisition in the shuttle-box experiment on male hypophysectomized rats. The index of avoidance acquisition of sham-operated controls is also shown. ACTH and β-MSH were of porcine origin. The dose was 1.5 I.U. for ACTH and 20 μg for the analogues.

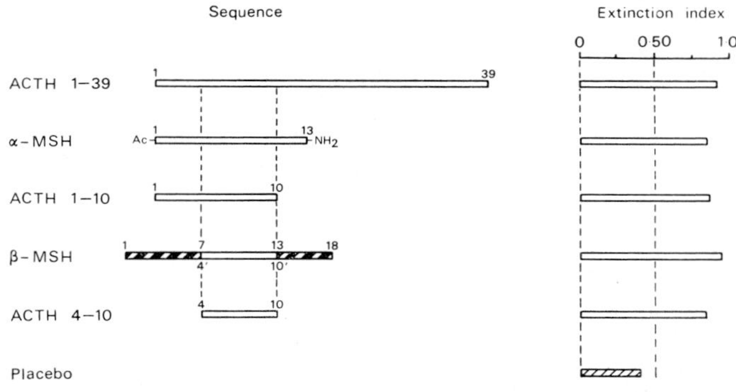

Fig. 2. Extinction of shuttle-box avoidance response. Effect of ACTH, ACTH analogues and placebo, administered subcutaneously in the form of zinc phosphate complexes on alternate days during the extinction period, on extinction of the avoidance response in the shuttle-box experiment on male intact rats. ACTH and β-MSH were of porcine origin. The dose was 1.5 I.U. for ACTH, 6 μg for α and β-MSH, 10 μg for $ACTH_{1-10}$ and 20 μg for $ACTH_{4-10}$.

was as active as ACTH whereas $ACTH_{11-24}$ was inactive. The same conclusion was reached whether the effect was studied on acquisition in hypophysectomized rats or on extinction in intact animals in the shuttle-box or in the pole-jumping test. More recent studies on passive avoidance behaviour support this view. These results are summarized in Figs. 1, 2, 3 and 4.

The relation between chain length and biological activity was then examined in a more systematic way by tracing the effect of progressive shortening of the peptide chain 1–10 at the amino end (Greven and De Wied, 1967). The results (Fig. 5)

References p. 440–441

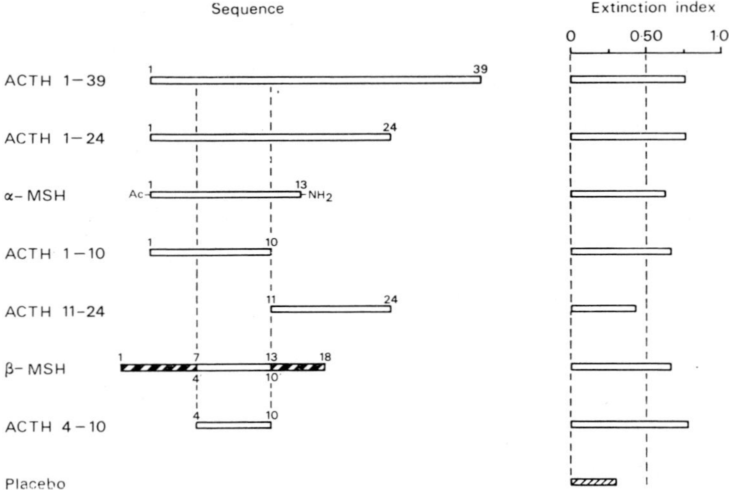

Fig. 3. Extinction of pole-jumping response. Effect of ACTH, ACTH analogues and placebo, administered subcutaneously in the form of zinc phosphate complexes, on extinction of a pole-jumping avoidance response in rats. ACTH and β-MSH were of porcine origin. The dose was 3 I.U. for ACTH, 6 μg for α- and β-MSH, 10 μg for $ACTH_{1-24}$, $ACTH_{1-10}$ and $ACTH_{11-24}$ and 20 μg for $ACTH_{4-10}$.

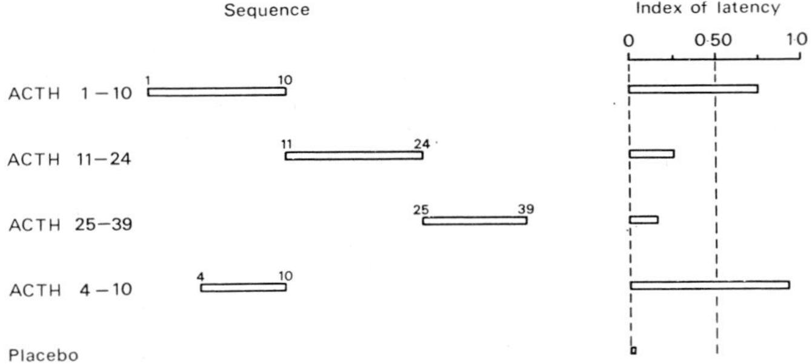

Fig. 4. Passive avoidance test. Effect of ACTH fragments on the response latency in a one-trial passive avoidance test. The peptides were dissolved in saline and injected subcutaneously 1 h before the first retention session in a dose of 30 μg.

confirmed that in this series of peptides with decreasing chain length the sequence 4–10 appears to be the shortest peptide with a behavioural potency comparable to that of the parent molecule.

The outcome of an analogous investigation in which the sequence 4–10 was shortened step by step now starting from the carboxyl terminus was more surprising. The results for both the active and the passive avoidance tests indicated that in this series of peptides the tetrapeptide H-Met-Glu-His-Phe-OH, *i.e.* $ACTH_{4-7}$, can be considered as the shortest peptide that still bears the essential elements required for the behavioural effects.

Although one might imagine that the glycine residue could be removed without loss of activity, it was unexpected that the tryptophan and arginine residues could also

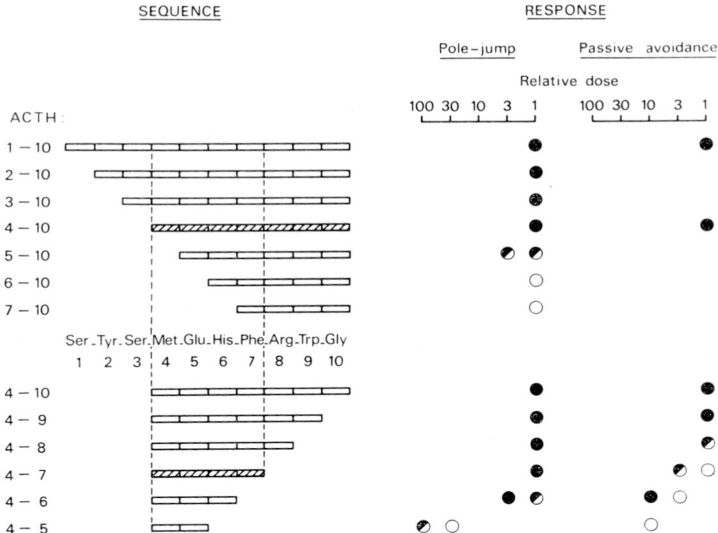

Fig. 5. Effect of progressively shortened ACTH fragments on extinction of a pole-jumping avoidance response and on the response latency of a passive avoidance test. ●, full response; ◐, half-maximal response; ○, response not significantly different from control.

be omitted. This is indicative of a dissociation between the requirements for behavioural activity and MSH potency, since Hofmann (Hofmann *et al.*, 1960) has found that tryptophan is essential for MSH activity, the sequence $ACTH_{1-8}$ without a tryptophan residue in position 9 being inactive. Consequently our results also differ from indications that the minimal requirements for residual MSH activity reside in the sequence 6–9 (Otsuka and Inouye, 1964).

The finding that only such a small part of the ACTH molecule is necessary for behavioural activity is reminiscent of similar observations concerning the "tetragastrin" peptide which exerts essentially the same biological activity as the complete gastrin molecule (Tracy and Gregory, 1964). It may also account for the discovery that in the fractionation of mother liquors of the extractive commercial ACTH production many subfractions appear to be active (Lande *et al.*, 1971). One may speculate that ACTH and MSH are prohormones, from which the active peptide is released by specifically localized peptidases. This has been proposed by Walter for oxytocin acting as a precursor of hormones, which release (Celis *et al.*, 1971a), or inhibit the release (Celis *et al.*, 1971b) of MSH.

STRUCTURALLY MODIFIED ANALOGUES OF ACTH

One of the first analogues of ACTH that we synthesized and that was tested by Bohus and De Wied (1966) was the *N*-terminal decapeptide in which the phenylalanine residue in position seven was replaced by its D-isomer. When assayed for its effect on

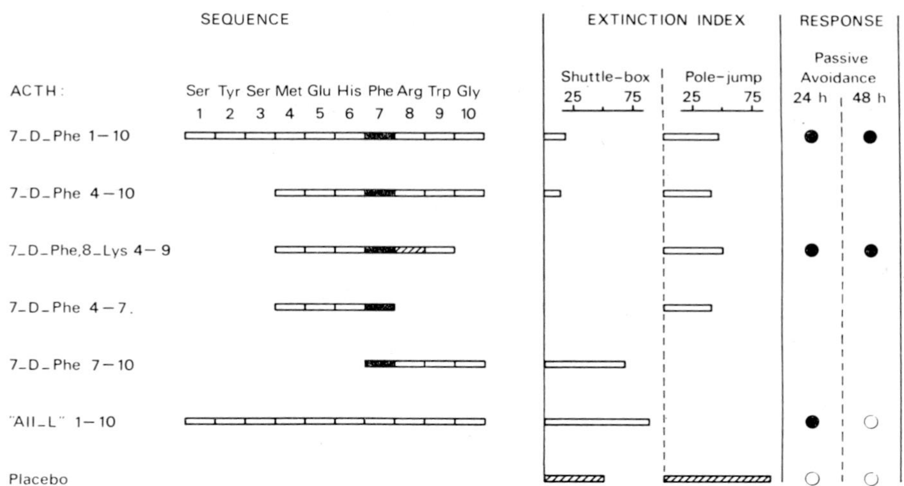

Fig. 6. Effect of various ACTH-related peptides, characterized by a D-phenylalanine residue in position 7, on extinction of an avoidance response in the shuttle-box or in the pole-jumping experiment and on the response latency in a passive avoidance test. In the shuttle-box experiments the peptides were injected subcutaneously in the form of zinc phosphate complexes in a dose of 10 μg for the two 1–10 peptides and 20 μg for the 4–10 and 7–10 analogues. In the pole-jumping test the dose was 100 μg dissolved in saline. In the passive avoidance test the dose was 30 μg dissolved in saline. ●, full response; ○, response not significantly different from control.

extinction of the avoidance response in the shuttle-box, it appeared to induce a facilitation instead of a delay of extinction, as long as the peptide was applied. When treatment was stopped the rate of extinction returned to the level of that of placebo-treated animals. Even in hypophysectomized rats an acceleration of extinction was observed. Thus, the facilitative effect of the D-Phe peptide on extinction of conditioned avoidance response cannot be explained by assuming that there is a direct antagonism between the analogue and such structurally related peptides of pituitary origin as ACTH and MSH. This conclusion may be compared with the recent finding (Ide *et al.*, 1972) that a 7-D-Phe-$ACTH_{1-18}$ analogue appears to be a strong competitive inhibitor for ACTH-stimulated adenyl cyclase activity.

The compound was also investigated for its effect on latency in a passive avoidance situation. $ACTH_{1-10}$ increased the latency for the rat to enter the box when it was administered before the first retention trial. This effect has disappeared 24 h later. Contrary to expectation, the D-Phe peptide was found to increase latency, thus excluding the possibility for the expected facilitation of extinction. This effect even persisted to the following day. One might describe the behavioural effect of the D-Phe peptide in both situations by a common characteristic feature, that is it inhibits an active response. This again supports the view that the peptide has an intrinsic new activity on extinction. The prolonged action of the D-Phe peptide in the passive avoidance test is puzzling but may be caused by an increased resistance to enzymatic degradation, though data from the shuttle-box experiment do not indicate such a mechanism. The 7-D-Phe heptapeptide 4–10 (De Wied and Greven, 1968) and the modified hexapeptide

7-D-Phe,8-Lys-ACTH$_{4-9}$ were found to be as active as the decapeptide analogue, (Fig. 6).

It is noteworthy that the sequence 7-D-Phe-ACTH$_{4-7}$ facilitates extinction of the pole-jump avoidance response in the same way as the corresponding 7-D-Phe hepta- and deca-peptides, whereas the sequence 7-D-Phe-ACTH$_{7-10}$ appears to have lost this property and instead induces a delay of extinction as do "all-L" peptides (De Wied, 1969). The first finding fits in with our observations in the "all-L" series that essential elements for behavioural effect reside in the sequence 4–7; the second finding may be explained by a potentiating effect of the *N*-terminal D-phenylalanine residue on the otherwise inactive tetrapeptide.

Next, the question was studied as to whether the reversal of action on active avoidance behaviour occurred only for analogues with the phenylalanine residue in the D-configuration, or whether this could also be obtained when other residues were inverted to their D-antipodes. Therefore, each of the amino acid residues in the hexapeptide 8-Lys-ACTH$_{4-9}$ was replaced successively by the corresponding D-isomer. The results are shown in Fig. 7.

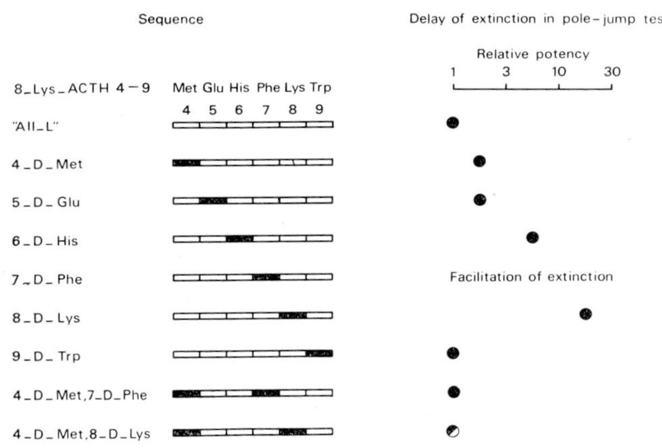

Fig. 7. Effect of ACTH analogues, in which amino acid residues are replaced by corresponding D-isomers, on extinction of a pole-jumping avoidance response. The peptides, dissolved in saline, are injected subcutaneously. ●, full response; ◐, half maximal response.

It appears that the reversed action of the 7-D-Phe analogues is an exception. All the other replacements invariably delayed extinction of avoidance response as has been found with "all-L" peptides derived from ACTH. They even potentiated the inhibitory effect of the original "all-L" 8-Lys-ACTH$_{4-9}$. This potentiation was strongest for the analogue with the lysine residue at position 8 in the D-configuration.

These results again indicate a dissociation between the requirements for behavioural and for MSH-like activity, since Japanese investigators (Koida *et al.*, 1966; Yajima *et al.*, 1966) have found that in the sequence ACTH$_{6-10}$ MSH activity is increased when the aromatic residues phenylalanine or tryptophan are replaced by their D-isomers, whereas this activity is lost when the ionizable residues, *i.e.* the basic histidyl or arginyl residues, are converted to their D-isomer.

References p. 440–441

The possibility was then studied whether a combination of two D-amino acid residues in one peptide sequence would result in a mutual potentiation of the behavioural effect. For two of these analogues this was not so. Thus, combination of the *N*-terminal methionine residue in the D-configuration with a D-lysine resulted in a loss of potentiation for the D-Met,D-Lys-analogue whereas a similar combination with a D-phenylalanine led to a reversal of action for the D-Met,D-Phe analogue, *i.e.* inhibition of extinction (Fig. 7).

Some analogues were then synthesized in which amino acid residues were exchanged for structurally related or simplified groups (Fig. 8). The substitution of lysine for arginine in position 8 has already been mentioned. Although this modification is accompanied by loss of steroidogenic and MSH activity in 8-Lys-$ACTH_{1-17}NH_2$, and of MSH potency in 8-Lys-$ACTH_{6-10}$ (Chung and Li, 1967), the behavioural activity remained unaltered in the peptide 8-Lys-$ACTH_{1-10}$ (Greven and De Wied, 1967) and in 8-Lys-$ACTH_{4-9}$.

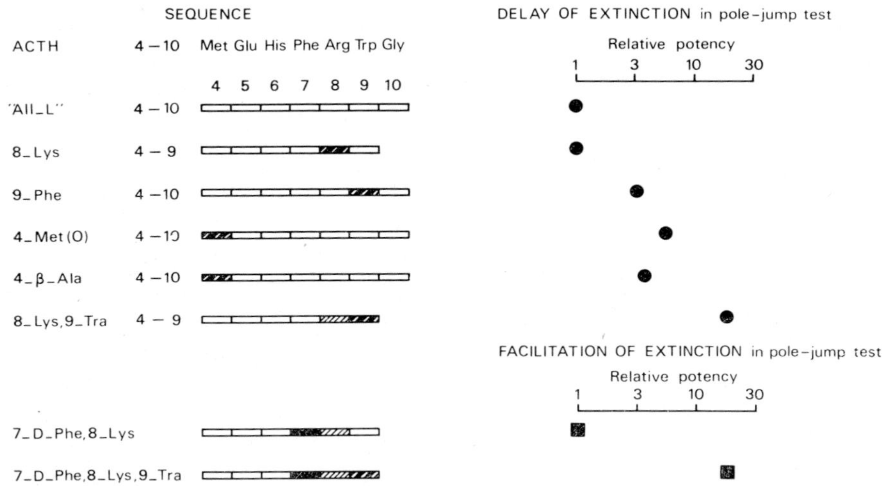

Fig. 8. Effect of ACTH analogues, in which amino acid residues are replaced by structurally related groups, on the rate of extinction of a pole-jumping avoidance response. The peptides, dissolved in saline, are injected subcutaneously.

Subsequently, phenylalanine was substituted for tryptophan in position 9. In the ACTH series such a modification is again accompanied by a marked decrease of adrenocorticotrophic activity in 5-Gln,9-Phe-$ACTH_{1-20}$ NH_2 (Hofmann *et al.*, 1970). On the contrary a three-fold potentiation was found when 9-Phe-$ACTH_{4-10}$ was tested for behavioural activity.

Though oxidation of the methionine residue to the sulfoxide level causes a serious decrease in corticotrophic activity of ACTH A_1 (Dedman *et al.*, 1955) and of melanocyte-stimulating activity of α-MSH (Lo *et al.*, 1961), the same modification in $ACTH_{4-10}$ gives rise to a three-fold increase of behavioural potency. An explanation for this unexpected potentiation may be found in a recently isolated aminopeptidase from brain ribosomes (Kerwar *et al.*, 1971) which has been found to have a higher reactivity towards *N*-terminal methionine than to any other amino acid residue. The specificity of this enzyme for methionyl peptides may account for the cleavage of methionine from the *N*-terminal position of nascent proteins, and may leave the methionine-sulfoxide peptide intact. Similar substitutions with a view to rendering the analogue more resistant to enzymatic degradation were then investigated. When β-alanine instead of methionine-sulfoxide was chosen for the *N*-terminus, potentiation was less. Replacement of tryptophan by tryptamine, however, increased both the facilitation of extinction for the 7-D-Phe analogue and the inhibition of extinction for the "all-L" analogue (Fig. 8).

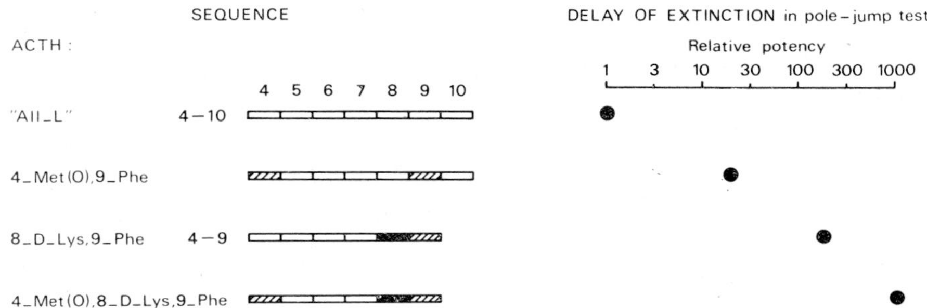

Fig. 9. Effect of ACTH analogues with a combination of modifications on the rate of extinction of a pole-jumping avoidance response. The peptides, dissolved in saline, are injected subcutaneously.

Again a combination of substitutions was investigated to determine whether this would lead to a mutual potentiation of activity, and on this occasion the result was affirmative (Fig. 9). By introducing three different modifications, namely an oxidized residue, a residue in the D-configuration and phenylalanine instead of tryptophan, the behavioural potency of the analogue H-Met(O)-Glu-His-Phe-D-Lys-Phe-OH was increased a thousand-fold, with respect to the inhibitory effect of the parent peptide $ACTH_{4-10}$ on extinction of conditioned avoidance response.

CONCLUSION

From the results of both approaches, that is, the structure of the smallest ACTH fragment with essentially unimpaired behavioural activity and the analogues with a marked increased behavioural activity, it appears that there is a marked difference between the requirements for behavioural activity and those for adrenocorticotrophic or MSH activity.

Finally, we suggest a mechanism of action for the behavioural activity of these to ACTH-related peptides, which is, that they act on membranes of specific target cells in the central nervous system in a way similar to that in which they act on isolated adrenal cells, though with a different substrate specificity (Seelig and Sayers, 1972), *i.e.* by inducing conformational changes which stimulate cyclic AMP production. This in turn may result in a stimulation of the turnover of the target cell and an increased

References p. 440–441

incorporation of labelled leucine which may eventually lead to the establishment of new synaptic junctions.

SUMMARY

The influence of peptides derived from ACTH on acquisition and extinction of conditioned avoidance behaviour in rats was studied. The tetrapeptide $ACTH_{4-7}$ was found to be the shortest peptide which still bears the essential elements required for the behavioural effects. As compared with the inhibitory effect of the parent peptide $ACTH_{4-10}$ on extinction of conditioned avoidance response, the behavioural potency of the analogue H-Met(O)-Glu-His-Phe-D-Lys-Phe-OH was found to be increased a thousand-fold.

REFERENCES

Ader, R., Weijnen, J. A. W. M. and Moleman, P. (1972) Retention of a passive avoidance response as a function of the intensity and duration of electric shock. *Psychon. Sci.*, **26**, 125–128.

Bohus, B. and De Wied, D. (1966) Inhibitory and facilitatory effect of two related peptides on extinction of avoidance behavior. *Science*, **153**, 318–320.

Bohus, B. and De Wied, D. (1967) Failure of α-MSH to delay extinction of conditioned avoidance behavior in rats with lesions in the parafascicular nuclei of the thalamus. *Physiol. Behav.*, **2**, 221–223.

Celis, M. E., Taleisnik, S. and Walter, R. (1971a) Release of pituitary melanocyte stimulating hormone by the oxytocin fragment, H-Cys-Tyr-Ile-Gln-Asn-OH. *Biochem. biophys. res. Commun.*, **45**, 564–569.

Celis, M. E., Taleisnik, S. and Walter, R. (1971b) Regulation of formation and proposed structure of the factor inhibiting the release of melanocyte-stimulating hormone. *Proc. natl. Acad. Sci. (U.S.A.)*, **68**, 1428–1433.

Chung, D. and Li, C. H. (1967) Adrenocorticotropins, XXXVII. The synthesis of 8-lysine-ACTH 1-17 NH_2 and its biological properties. *J. Amer. chem. Soc.*, **89**, 4208–4213.

Dedman, M. L., Farmer, T. H. and Morris, C. J. O. R. (1955) Oxidation-reduction properties of adrenocorticotrophic hormone. *Biochem. J.*, **59**, xii.

De Wied, D. (1964) Influence of anterior pituitary on avoidance learning and escape behavior. *Amer. J. Physiol.*, **207**, 255–259.

De Wied, D. (1965) The influence of the posterior and intermediate lobe of the pituitary and pituitary peptides on the maintenance of a conditioned avoidance response in rats. *Int. J. Neuropharmacol.*, **4**, 157–167.

De Wied, D. (1966) Inhibitory effect of ACTH and related peptides on extinction of conditioned avoidance behavior in rats. *Proc. Soc. exp. Biol. Med. (N.Y.)*, **122**, 28–32.

De Wied, D. (1967) Opposite effects of ACTH and glucocorticosteroids on extinction of conditioned avoidance behavior. In *Proc. Second Int. Congr. on Hormonal Steroids, Milan 1966* (Int. Congr. Series Vol. 132), Excerpta Medica, Amsterdam, pp. 945–951.

De Wied, D. (1969) Effects of peptide hormones on behavior. In *Frontiers in Neuroendocrinology*, W. F. Ganong and L. Martini (Eds.), Oxford University Press, New York, pp. 97–140.

De Wied, D. and Bohus, B. (1966) Long term and short term effects on retention of a conditioned avoidance response in rats by treatment with long acting Pitressin and α-MSH. *Nature (Lond.)*, **212**, 1484–1486.

De Wied, D. and Greven, H. M. (1968) Opposite effect of structural analogues of ACTH on extinction of an avoidance response in rats by replacement of an L-amino acid by a D-isomer. In *Proc. of the Int. Union of Physiological Sciences*, Vol. VII, XXIVth Int. Congr. of Physiological Sciences, Washington D.C., p. 110, abstract No. 329.

De Wied, D. and Pirie, G. (1968) The inhibitory effect of ACTH 1–10 on extinction of a conditioned avoidance response: its independence of thyroid function. *Physiol. Behav.*, **3**, 355–358.

ENDRÖCZI, E., LISSÁK, K., FEKETE, T. AND DE WIED, D. (1970) Effects of ACTH on EEG habituation in human subjects. In *Pituitary, Adrenal and the Brain* (Progress in Brain Research, Vol. 32), D. DE WIED AND J. A. W. M. WEIJNEN (Eds.), Elsevier, Amsterdam, pp. 254–261.

GISPEN, W. H., VAN WIMERSMA GREIDANUS, TJ. B. AND DE WIED, D. (1970) Effects of hypophysectomy and ACTH 1–10 on responsiveness to electric shock in rats. *Physiol. Behav.*, **5**, 143–146.

GREVEN, H. M. AND DE WIED, D. (1967) The active sequence in the ACTH molecule responsible for inhibition of the extinction of conditioned avoidance behaviour in rats. *Europ. J. Pharmacol.*, **2**, 14–16.

HOFMANN, K., THOMPSON, T. A., WOOLNER, M. E., SPÜHLER, G., YAJIMA, H., CIPERA, J. D. AND SCHWARTZ, E. T. (1960) Studies on polypeptides, XV. Observations on the relation between structure and melanocyte-expanding activity of synthetic peptides. *J. Amer. chem. Soc.*, **82**, 3721–3726.

HOFMANN, K., ANDREATTA, R., BOHN, H. AND MORODER, L. (1970) Studies on polypeptides, XLV. Structure-function studies in the β-corticotropin series. *J. med. Chem.*, **13**, 339–345.

IDE, M., TANAKA, A., NAKAMURA, M. AND OKABAYASHI, T. (1972) Stimulation by ACTH analogs of rat adrenal adenyl cyclase activity: Correlation with steroidogenic activity. *Arch. Biochem. Biophys.*, **149**, 189–196.

KASTIN, A. J., MILLER, L. H., GONZALEZ-BARCENA, D., HAWLEY, W. D., DYSTER-AAS, K., SCHALLY, A. V., VELASCO DE PARRA, M. L. AND VELASCO, M. (1971) Psycho-physiologic correlates of MSH activity in man. *Physiol. Behav.*, **7**, 893–896.

KERWAR, S. S., WEISSBACH, H. AND GLENNER, G. G. (1971) An aminopeptidase activity associated with brain ribosomes. *Arch. Biochem. Biophys.*, **143**, 336–337.

KOIDA, M., HANO, K. AND ISO, T. (1966) Evaluation of *in vitro* melanocyte-darkening activities of L-Histidyl-L-Phenylalanyl-L-Arginyl-L-Tryptophyl-Glycine and its nine stereoisomers in *Rana nigromaculata*. *Jap. J. Pharmacol.*, **16**, 243–249.

LANDE, S., WITTER, A. AND DE WIED, D. (1971) Pituitary peptides. An octapeptide that stimulates conditioned avoidance acquisition in hypophysectomized rats. *J. biol. Chem.*, **246**, 2058–2062.

LO, T-B., DIXON, J. S. AND LI, C. H. (1961) Isolation of methionine sulfoxide analogue of α-melanocyte-stimulating hormone from bovine pituitary glands. *Biochim. biophys. acta*, **53**, 584–586.

MILLER, R. E. AND OGAWA, N. (1962) The effect of adrenocorticotropic hormone (ACTH) on avoidance conditioning in the adrenalectomized rat. *J. comp. physiol. Psychol.*, **55**, 211–213.

MIRSKY, I. A., MILLER, R. AND STEIN, M. (1953) Relation of adrenocortical activity and adaptive behavior. *Psychosom. Med.*, **15**, 574–584.

OTSUKA, H. AND INOUYE, K. (1964) Synthesis of peptides related to the *N*-terminal structure of corticotropin, III. The synthesis of L-histidyl-L-phenylalanyl-L-arginyl-L-tryptophan, the smallest peptide exhibiting the melanocyte-stimulating and the lipolytic activities. *Bull. chem. Soc. Jap.*, **37**, 1465–1471.

READING, H. W. AND DEWAR, A. J. (1971) Effects of ACTH 4–10 on cerebral RNA and protein metabolism in the rat. In *Third Int. Meeting of the Int. Soc. for Neurochemistry, Budapest 1971* (Abstract), Akadémiai Kiadó, Budapest, p. 199.

SCHOTMAN, P. (1971) Macromolecular metabolism in the brainstem of the hypophysectomized rat in relation to the conditioned avoidance behaviour. *Thesis, University of Utrecht.*

SEELIG, S. AND SAYERS, G. (1972) ACTH 1–10 and ACTH 4–10 stimulate cyclic AMP production by isolated adrenal cells. *Fed. Proc.* **31**, 252.

SELYE, H. (1950) *The Physiology and Pathology of Exposure to Stress*, Acta, Montreal, p. 6.

TABER, R. I. (1971) Agents affecting learning and retention of conditioned behavior. In *An Introduction to Psychopharmacology*, R. H. RECH AND K. E. MOORE (Eds.), North-Holland, Amsterdam, p. 227.

TRACY, H. J. AND GREGORY, R. A. (1964) Physiological properties of a series of synthetic peptides structurally related to Gastrin I. *Nature (Lond.)*, **204**, 935–938.

VAN WIMERSMA GREIDANUS, TJ. B. AND DE WIED, D. (1969) Effects of intracerebral implantation of corticosteroids on extinction of an avoidance response in rats. *Physiol. Behav.*, **4**, 365–370.

VAN WIMERSMA GREIDANUS, TJ. B. AND DE WIED, D. (1971) Effects of systemic and intracerebral administration of two opposite acting ACTH-related peptides on extinction of conditioned avoidance behavior. *Neuroendocrinology*, **7**, 291–301.

YAJIMA, H., KUBO, K., KINOMURA, Y. AND LANDE, S. (1966) Studies on peptides, XI. The effect on melanotropic activity of altering the arginyl residue in L-histidyl-L-phenylalanyl-L-arginyl-L-tryptophylglycine. *Biochim. biophys. acta*, **127**, 545–549.

DISCUSSION

CIARANELLO: Dr. de Wied, I wonder about the effects of double D-amino acid substitutions. It is possible that the tertiary conformation of such a short peptide might not be affected by substitution of a single D-isomer, but might be affected after a second substitution.

DE WIED: We have done some studies with double substitution of D-amino acids and the interesting thing is that we have found that the facilitation effect of position 7 may disappear when a second D-isomer in the peptide is introduced.

KRIVOY: I should like to compliment Professor De Wied on this typically brilliant presentation. Society has been enriched by a Dutch School of Art, a Dutch School of Physiology, and I am certain we now see before us an equally enriching Dutch School of Pharmacology. The question I wanted to ask is, if you substitute in 4–7 you get a peptide which has less activity? Then if you give the substituted peptide, along with 4–7 what do you see? Do you see an antagonism, potentiation, or addition?

DE WIED: Bill, we haven't done this. I am puzzled about the fact that such a small *sequence* of amino acids can produce an effect. I am reminded of one of the slides Dr. Burgus showed in the first session, in which he showed that after removal of all amino acids but two some FSH releasing activity remains. Maybe this is comparable to what a pharmacologist sees when he deals with acetylcholine in which case choline itself is active as a transmitter but 1000 times less active than the whole molecule. I don't know how to explain this but the experiment that you suggest may be useful.

KRIVOY: I really think it might shed some light on the next step in our understanding how these peptides modify learning. In other words, if we had an antagonist to the ACTH-like peptides which enhance performance, this would be a very useful tool.

SACHS: Do you think it is possible that the peptides which you have been studying are in fact emulating some other unknown peptides which derive from a peptidergic neurone or some other structure instead of the anterior pituitary gland?

DE WIED: The anterior pituitary gland is loaded with peptides and it may be the primary source of the behavioral peptides. We have the feeling that it may be possible that small sequences of pituitary peptides enter the circulation and thereby reach the CNS. It is also possible that pituitary peptides are modified by enzymes in certain structures in the CNS and that these structures may respond to very small sequences of these peptides. This is one of the hypotheses just put forward in our paper.

MCEWEN: Is there any evidence for the endogenous degradation of ACTH to these active fragments?

DE WIED: Not that I know of. ACTH is certainly not broken down to those sequences which we use. However, some natural products of endogenous degradation of ACTH may be active in our tests.

Pituitary-Adrenal System, Learning and Performance: Some Neurochemical Aspects

W. H. GISPEN AND P. SCHOTMAN

Rudolf Magnus Institute for Pharmacology and Laboratory for Physiological Chemistry, University of Utrecht, Medical Faculty, Utrecht (The Netherlands)

INTRODUCTION

The role hormones play in the regulation of cell metabolism is well documented. Numerous results suggest that hormones are in a similar way important to brain cell metabolism. Since cell metabolism underlies cell functioning, it seems logical to expect that chemical events in the brain also underly behavioral processes. Furthermore, assuming that hormones do interact with brain cell metabolism, it is then of interest to study the interrelationship of the three factors mentioned: hormones, brain metabolism and behavior. The present paper is an attempt to describe the results of our own work on this interrelationship, within the framework of current views.

HYPOPHYSECTOMY AND AVOIDANCE LEARNING

Removal of the pituitary or adenohypophysis interferes with avoidance learning in shuttle-box conditioning (Applezweig and Baudry, 1955; Applezweig and Moeller, 1959; De Wied, 1964, 1969). It has been suggested that this result is due to the poor physical condition of hypophysectomized rats and/or to an overall deterioration of behavior. Hypophysectomy does of course produce dramatic changes throughout the body in systems which are normally under the influence of the pituitary (Tepperman, 1962). However, there is evidence that argues against the suggestion that a poor physical condition is the basic cause of the impaired avoidance performance. First, recent experiments showed that hypophysectomized (hypox) rats' behavior does not deteriorate in a novel environment. By observing the behavior of hypox and sham-operated rats in a wire-mesh cage with glass front for 5 min, it was found that hypox rats were more actively engaged in exploratory behavior and climbed and jumped more on the wire-mesh sides than did sham-operated rats (Gispen *et al.*, in press). The rats appeared to be capable of making all bodily movements normally involved in performing the avoidance response in shuttle-box conditioning. That such is true also follows from the observation that hypox rats were all able to escape but

References p. 453–458

not to avoid the foot-shock as the unconditioned stimulus (UCS) in shuttle-box conditioning.

Another study showed that the ability to detect or to respond to the electric foot-shock was certainly not impaired in hypox rats. Hypox rats responded to lower shock intensities of inescapable foot-shock (duration of 1 sec) than did controls (Gispen *et al.*, 1970a). Moreover, treatment of hypox rats with peptides derived from corticotrophin (ACTH), (*e.g.* $ACTH_{4-10}$, $ACTH_{1-10}$) throughout the training period restored their performance to nearly normal levels. Further, under similar conditions, the isomer $ACTH_{4-10}$ (7-D-Phe) had no, or even an inhibiting, effect on the avoidance learning of hypox rats (De Wied, 1969). Since $ACTH_{4-10}$ does not show any endocrine or systemic effect, this important finding suggests that a specific rather than a non-specific mechanism underlies the poor avoidance learning of hypox rats (De Wied, 1969; De Wied *et al.*, 1972). That is, while $ACTH_{4-10}$ had no detectable endocrine or systemic effects, it was sufficient to restore avoidance performance. Thus, although a total hormonal replacement therapy also improved the avoidance performance of hypox rats (De Wied, 1964), it appears that the mechanism of $ACTH_{4-10}$ avoidance improvement is more specific and is not accomplished *via* widespread effects on bodily functions. Further, neither adrenalectomy nor substitution of adrenal steroids in hypox rats affected avoidance conditioning (Applezweig and Moeller, 1959; Bohus and Endröczi, 1965; De Wied *et al.*, 1968, 1972).

Considerable evidence supports the hypothesis that this specific mechanism of ACTH analogs is related to an action of the peptides on central nervous structures. For example, electrophysiological and neuroendocrine research has shown that ACTH, and in some instances its *N*-terminal sequences, are able directly to influence various aspects of nerve cell functioning, including neuronal firing (Sawyer *et al.*, 1968; Krivoy, 1970; Steiner, 1970; Van Delft and Kitay, 1972), electroencephalogram synchronization (Endröczi *et al.*, 1970), ACTH release (Motta *et al.*, 1965) and macromolecular metabolism (see below). The work of Van Wimersma Greidanus and De Wied (1971) strongly supports the concept that ACTH-like peptides regulate avoidance behavior *via* a neurotrophic mechanism of action. They found that in intact rats both subcutaneous and intracerebral administration of the peptide retards extinction of avoidance learning. Recently, a naturally occurring peptide (an analog of vasopressin) was isolated from hog pituitaries and found to possess potent effects on shuttle-box learning in hypox rats (De Wied *et al.*, 1970; Lande *et al.*, 1971). It has been postulated, therefore, that removal of the pituitary would deplete the animal of neurotrophic peptides which in normal circumstances might play an integrating role in the adaptation of the animal to its environment.

HYPOPHYSECTOMY AND MACROMOLECULAR METABOLISM

Periphery

As mentioned before, removal of the pituitary leads to dramatic disorders in a variety of tissues and organs. Such findings are consistent with the concept that protein metabolism in the mammalian cell is under hormonal control (growth hormone, thyroxine). After hypophysectomy the overall impression of the events in the peripheral cell is that the lack of hormones leads to a marked limitation of the cytoplasmic machinery involved in protein synthesis (Cardell, 1967, 1970). In hypox animals both the suggested decrease in RNA synthesis (Korner, 1964, 1965; Gupta and Talwar, 1968) as well as an increase in RNA breakdown as a result of high RNAse activity (Brewer *et al.*, 1969) could account for the reduced polysome content of the cell (Korner, 1964; Staehelin, 1965; Wurfbain-Moolenburgh, 1968). Moreover, there is evidence that hypophysectomy would lead to a defect at the ribosomal level disrupting regular binding capacity to mRNA or to aminocyl-tRNA (Staehelin, 1965; Garren *et al.*, 1967; Korner, 1968, 1969; Liew and Korner, 1969; Barden and Korner, 1969). However, at least in the binding capacity of ribosomes to mRNA, contradictory evidence has been found (Foster and Sells, 1969). Nevertheless, the altered RNA metabolism is likely to modify protein synthesis and, indeed, a marked reduction of incorporation of amino acids into peptide chains was found in hypox rats, concomitant with a reduction in total protein content (Korner, 1968, 1969; Tata and Williams-Ashman, 1967; Herrlich and Lang, 1967; Cheek and Graystone, 1969; Clemens and Korner, 1970).

It appeared that growth hormone treatment alone was sufficient to counteract this deteriorated metabolism of macromolecules in peripheral organs and tissues of the hypox rat (Tata, 1968; O'Malley, 1968; Brewer *et al.*, 1969; Clemens and Korner, 1970; McDonald and Korner, 1971). In contrast with the detailed studies on the effect of hypophysectomy on macromolecules in the periphery, scattered data are present on its effect on brain macromolecules.

Brain

From neuroendocrine studies it is clear how complex the interaction between hormones and the brain can be (Yates *et al.*, 1971). Because of this complexity, neurochemical correlates of hypophysectomy have often appeared to be inconsistent. Critical points to be considered are the age at which the surgery has been performed, the brain region studied, the time between surgery and biochemical analysis, and, very importantly, an appropriate test of the effectiveness of the surgery. For instance, it has been reported that oxygen consumption of brain cortex does not change as a result of hypophysectomy, while anaerobic glycolysis increases by more than 100% (Reiss, 1961). On the other hand, other investigators find a significant increase of oxygen uptake in certain parts of the hypothalamus after hypophysectomy (Libertun *et al.*, 1969; Moguilevsky *et al.*, 1970). Furthermore, De Vellis and Inglish (1968) have reported that glycerophosphate dehydrogenase (EC. 1.1.1.8) was reduced especially in brain stem tissue, and predicted a lower level of anaerobic glycolysis. The reported decrease in RNA, DNA and protein content of the brain of juvenile rats (Cheek and Graystone, 1969) suggests that there is a similar atrophy in brain and liver in young hypox rats. Indeed, some anatomical changes have been reported to take place

References p. 453–458

(Diamond, 1968), but it has also been suggested that the young hypox rat dies, because after hypophysectomy the skull (which has ceased to grow) cannot provide the still growing brain with enough space (Geel and Timiras, 1970). The above-cited evidence illustrates the confusion mentioned before. Regarding the metabolism of macromolecules, indications are present that in the brain both RNA (De Vellis and Inglish, 1968; Cheek and Graystone, 1969) and protein metabolism (Dunn and Korner, 1966; Takahashi *et al.*, 1970) are influenced by hypophysectomy. Previous and current work of our group deals with macromolecular aspects of the effect of hypophysectomy on the brain.

In all our work the experimentals are male rats analyzed three weeks after hypophysectomy. In agreement with preliminary observations, it was found that total cell RNA in the brain was reduced as a result of hypophysectomy. Gross topographical localization of the effect indicated that the decrease was confined to brain stem areas. A more detailed analysis gave more insight into the regional effect of hypophysectomy. Total cell RNA was measured and expressed as mg RNA per mg DNA. The highest RNA/DNA ratio was found in the cortex cerebri (*ca.* 2.15) and hippocampus (2.21), whereas the cerebellum (0.42) and bulbus olfactorius (0.95) showed the lowest values. Hypophysectomy reduced the RNA/DNA ratio by *ca.* 20% in the thalamus, hypothalamus, mesencephalon and medulla oblongata. There was also a small but significant reduction in the rostral part of the cortex cerebri (Gispen *et al.*, 1972).

On the basis of these findings it was decided to use the brain stem to study the change in macromolecular metabolism in greater detail. First, an attempt was made to trace the decrease in total RNA down to the subcellular level. After fractionation of brain stem homogenates into nuclei, crude mitochondria, microsomes and post-microsomal supernatant (Gispen *et al.*, 1970b), the only fraction that showed a significant decrease in RNA content as a result of hypophysectomy was that of the microsomes (−20%) (Versteeg *et al.*, 1972). Moreover, isolating polysomes from the post mitochondrial supernatant showed that hypophysectomy caused an absolute decrease in the amount of polyribosomal aggregates containing 3 or more ribosomes (Gispen *et al.*, 1970; Gispen and Schotman, 1970; Schotman *et al.*, in prep.). Additionally, it was found that hypophysectomy reduced the incorporation of uridine into rapidly labeled messenger-like RNA and into ribosomal RNA (Gispen *et al.*, 1970b; Schotman *et al.*, in prep.; Schotman, 1971) isolated from brain stem tissue. Whether or not such a decrease reflected a decrease in RNA synthesis remains to be shown, since an increased breakdown could also account for most of the observed phenomena. Despite this uncertainty, it seems clear that in the brain stem of hypophysectomized rats there is a modification of RNA metabolism leading to a reduced capacity of the RNA machinery to synthesize proteins. However, overall protein content in the brain stem seems unaltered by removal of the pituitary (De Vellis and Inglish, 1968; Schotman, 1971). The only change observed was a decrease of protein in the polysomal pellet obtained from the brain stem homogenate which is in good agreement with the above data obtained from RNA distribution.

By studying the incorporation of [^{3}H]leucine into proteins over a short period of time (5 min), it was found that hypophysectomy led to a decrease of incorporated radioactivity of *ca.* 20–27%. The decrease was found both in the nuclear and in the cytoplasmic cell fractions. However, we have good reason to believe that the proteins labeled within 5 min after intracranial application of the precursor, are from cytoplasm only. [Treatment of the nuclear fraction with detergent, leaving the nuclei intact, removed all of the label from this fraction (Schotman, 1971).] Analysis of the polysomal fraction showed that preparations obtained from hypox rats contained less label than similar preparations from control rats (Schotman *et al.*, in prep.; Schotman, 1971). It seems reasonable to assume that this reduction reflects a reduced assemblage of amino acids into polypeptide chains. The overall picture therefore is that hypophysectomy changes RNA metabolism in brain stem areas, which indeed has consequences for protein turnover. Using similar techniques, Witter also found, after a pulse length of 60 min, a reduction of incorporation of a mixture of ^{14}C-labeled amino acids in brain stem peptides and proteins (Versteeg *et al.*, 1972). The large effect of hypophysectomy on protein synthesis on the one hand and the absence of an effect on protein content on the other, suggests that the inhibition of protein synthesis pertains to a relatively small fraction of proteins with a high turnover.

AVOIDANCE LEARNING AND MACROMOLECULAR METABOLISM IN THE BRAIN

Various lines of evidence have suggested that chemical events in the brain are involved in the storage of information. A number of reviews, models and hypotheses can be found in the literature which maintain this view, although the available data are limited and often controversial. Among the various possible experimental approaches to the problem, the method in which the fate of a chemical process in the brain is analyzed during or after acquisition of a new behavior pattern, is one of the most important.

Among the first studies which stressed the role of RNA during acquisition of a new behavior, were those by Hydén and coworkers. They found that rats, after learning to climb a wire to obtain food, showed both an increase in cell RNA and a change in base composition of nuclear RNA in the Deiter's nucleus (Hydén and Egyhazi, 1962, 1963). Transfer of handedness resulted in the increased production of DNA-like RNA in certain motoneurons of the "learning" cortical hemisphere (Hydén and Egyhazi, 1964). Although the original interpretations no longer seem fully valid, Hydén's group deserves credit for having been the first to point towards changes in brain RNA related to acquisition of new behavioral patterns.

The work of Glassman and Wilson (Zemp *et al.*, 1966, 1967; Adair *et al.*, 1968a, b; Coleman *et al.*, 1971) seems to be of major importance. They showed that avoidance training of mice and rats resulted in an increased incorporation of radioactive uridine into brain nuclear RNA and polysomes. In these studies, autoradiographic localization pointed towards the diencephalon as a major area of increased incorporation (Zemp *et al.*, 1967; Kahan *et al.*, 1970). A number of experimental variables were studied to determine the conditions responsible for the observed phenomena. Neither yoked training, random foot-shock treatment nor prior trained performing increased the

References p. 453–458

uridine incorporation into brain RNA above the level of that in quiet mice. From this evidence, the investigators concluded that "the process of learning a conditioned avoidance seems to be relevant to the chemical change observed in these studies" (Glassman, 1969). Some laboratories have initiated programs in this type of research in recent years. In a way, the work of Dellweg *et al.* (1968) can be viewed as a partial confirmation of Hydén's data. They reported that rats undergoing wire-balancing training contained more brain polysomes than did controls.

Recently, Uphouse reported results similar to those found by the group of Glassman and Wilson. Using a single-label method, she found that uridine was incorporated to a greater extent into brain RNA in trained mice than in yoked or quiet mice. Moreover, an increase in hippocampal polysome content was also detected as a result of jump-box training (Uphouse, 1971; Uphouse *et al.*, 1972). Others have described an increased incorporation of [^{3}H]cytidine into RNA concomitant with a higher content of nuclear RNA, in rat hippocampal nuclei, as a result of reversal training in a Y-maze spatial discrimination task (Bowman and Strobel, 1969). Also, the incorporation of [^{3}H]UMP into nuclei of hippocampal and cortical neurons was increased as a result of discrimination training, using foot-shock as the reinforcer (Pohle and Matthies, 1971). It is reported that both 50 trials in one 25-min session, and six daily sessions of 30 trials in shuttle-box conditioning, led to an increase in total cell RNA in the hippocampus of female rats. Random treatment with conditioned and unconditioned stimuli did not change the hippocampal RNA content (Nasello and Izquierdo, 1969).

Another, rather preliminary, paper reported a failure to find a change in labeling of hippocampal RNA resulting from the acquisition of a new behavior (Carreres, 1970). Using not histochemical, but rather advanced biochemical, techniques in the search for a correlation between RNA and behavior, it was reported that during shock-avoidance conditioning the synthesis of a unique RNA species took place based upon DNA–RNA hybridization experiments (Machlus and Gaito, 1969). Recently, some doubts have been raised as to the relevance of the reported change (Von Hungen, 1971). Also, in goldfish, acquisition of new behavior patterns seemed to run parallel with qualitative and quantitative changes in RNA metabolism in the brain (Sashoua, 1968, 1970, 1971). Using light as stimulus, Rose *et al.* (1970) found that imprinting behavior in the young chick triggered an increased RNA synthesis in midbrain and roof (at different times after injection of [^{3}H]uracil), not attributable to non-specific factors (Horn *et al.*, 1971). The above-cited literature stresses the belief that changes in macromolecule metabolism can run parallel with the storage of newly acquired information. However, it certainly does not give any explanation of the biological meaning or of the exact mechanism of action by which learning affects brain metabolism or *vice versa*.

Nevertheless, on the basis of the evidence that brain RNA is affected by hypophysectomy and by avoidance learning as well, an effort was made to study brain RNA during shuttle-box training of hypox rats subjected to peptide treatment. Hypox rats were treated with $ACTH_{1-10}$ or β-melanocyte-stimulating hormone (MSH) or with desglycinamide-lysine vasopressin (De Wied *et al.*, 1970; Lande *et al.*, 1971), a peptide isolated from hog pituitaries. On day 7 after surgery, the injection treatment started and lasted throughout the training period which consisted of 10 daily sessions beginning on day 8 after the surgery. After the last training session, the rats were killed and the polysomes of their brain stems were isolated and subsequently analyzed on sucrose gradients (Gispen and Schotman, 1970; Gispen *et al.*, 1970c, 1971). Peptide-treated rats, which mastered the task, contained more brain stem polysomes than those rats treated with placebo suspension and which were therefore unable to acquire the conditioned avoidance response. The ratio of polysomes over monosomes was approximately 1.5–1.6 in the rats that acquired the response, whereas the placebo group showed a ratio of 1.2. In the peptide-treated group, the mean total amount of conditioned avoidance responses out of 100 possible was around 70, and this value was 23 for placebo-treated rats (Gispen *et al.*, 1971). Further study showed that peptide treatment *per se* (at least for $ACTH_{1-10}$) did not affect brain stem polysome profiles in hypox rats. It is of interest to note that treatment of hypox rats with peptide fractions, isolated from hog pituitary, which did not improve avoidance learning in these rats (De Wied *et al.*, 1970), did not result in the increase of polysomes at the end of the training period (Gispen, unpublished). From a number of studies it is clear that environmental stimulation (see Glassman, 1969) and stress (Jakoubek *et al.*, 1970) are able to trigger changes in brain metabolism which directly or indirectly could account for changes in RNA and protein metabolism. Since hypox rats which remained in their home cages throughout the experiment showed brain polysome profiles similar to placebo-treated rats subjected to avoidance training, it seemed clear that the stimulation of the conditioning procedure as such did not trigger the event (*cf.* yoked training of Zemp *et al.*, 1966).

Others have also paid attention to the pituitary-adrenal system and neurochemical events involved in information storage. Flexner and coworkers found that memory of maze learning in mice is blocked for long periods of time by the intracerebral injection of puromycin one or more days after the training period (Flexner *et al.*, 1967). Bilateral adrenalectomy before training protects memory against this action of puromycin (Flexner and Flexner, 1970). This finding led the authors to believe that high circulation levels of ACTH in their adrenalectomized mice would account for the observed "protection". Although it was reported that ACTH administration to intact mice indeed gave protection against memory blockade caused by puromycin (Flexner and Flexner, 1971), it now seems that this result was most likely due to an impurity in the ACTH preparation used, since highly purified ACTH did not give the effect. However, desglycinamide-lysine vasopressin (the natural pituitary peptide, also used by us) did interfere rather strongly with the suppression of memory by puromycin (Lande *et al.*, 1972).

Glassman and coworkers found no differences between sham-operated and adrenalectomized mice in jump-box conditioning, nor did they see differences between sham-operated and hypox rats in short-term avoidance learning in a runway with elevated platform (Adair *et al.*, 1968b; Coleman *et al.*, 1971). Both experiments were conducted 7 days after the surgery, and under both conditions the increased incorporation of uridine into RNA was found. Assuming that the surgery had been performed correctly

References p. 453–458

(no evidence in this respect was provided), these data are of great interest in combination with our work. Hypophysectomy impaired long-term avoidance learning, and peptide treatment restored the ability of the animals to acquire the task and this in turn gave rise to the increase of polysomes. In the short-term situation and 7 days after the surgery, hypophysectomy did not interfere with avoidance learning, and accordingly these untreated rats showed the increase in uridine incorporation into RNA.

The primary conclusion appears to be that hypophysectomy does not interfere with all kinds of avoidance learning, but rather specifically with long-term active avoidance. However, preliminary studies showed that hypophysectomy did interfere with short-term avoidance in rats in jump-box conditioning, tested three weeks after the surgery. The effect was more variable and less marked than in long-term shuttle-box conditioning (Gispen, 1970). From a neurochemical point of view it seems reasonable to assume that the impaired metabolism of macromolecules, in parts of the brain involved in avoidance learning, is not able to provide the cell with, or to maintain, a certain end-product important for the consolidation of information acquired over a longer period of time. In subsequent research we attempted more fully to elucidate the role of the peptides in this respect.

The changes in polysomes suggest that protein synthesis is also affected by acquisition processes. Indeed, in recent years it was found that transfer of handedness was related to an increase in synthesis of a brain-specific acid-soluble protein S-100 in certain hippocampal pyramidal cells (Hydén and Lange, 1969, 1970a, b). Moreover, an increased synthesis of glycoproteins is reported to occur both in pigeons (Bochoch, 1968) and in rats (Dunn *et al.*, in press) as a result of training experience. Also, the incorporation of [^{3}H]leucine into proteins as studied by autoradiographic techniques, is altered in relation to an acquisition of avoidance behavior (Beach *et al.*, 1969). Machlus found that the acquisition of a one-way avoidance resulted in an increased phosphorylation of nuclear acidic proteins in rat brain (Machlus, 1971; Machlus *et al.*, 1973a and b). Current experiments of the same group also indicate that phosphorylation of synaptosomal proteins in mice is increased as a result of acquisition in jump-box training (Dunn *et al.*, in press; Glassman *et al.*, 1972, in press). In so far as polysome profiles can be used as an indication of cell protein synthesis (Henshaw *et al.*, 1971), it is clear that our data fit the concept that acquisition of new behavior is accompanied by changes in brain RNA and proteins.

ACTH ANALOGS AND BRAIN MACROMOLECULAR METABOLISM

That ACTH-like peptides have a role in avoidance learning and performance has been shown before and is the subject of a paper by Greven and De Wied (this volume). In a recent review, Krivoy (1970) stressed as a fundamental hypothesis that certain polypeptides play a role in the nervous system as modulators of nervous activity. ACTH and related peptides are capable of altering transmission in the spinal cord under a variety of conditions (Krivoy, 1970), and, as was pointed out above, a variety of other processes in central nervous system structures seem to be directly influenced by these peptides. From a biochemical point of view, little, if anything, is known about the effect on central nervous system structures. On the other hand, the mechanism by which ACTH stimulates steroidogenesis in the adrenal cortex and exerts its lipolytic effect on the fat cell is relatively well documented.

The interaction of ACTH with the target cell receptor probably consists of a binding of the hormone to the cell membrane (Hofmann *et al.*, 1970) resulting in an activation of adenylcyclase (Garren *et al.*, 1971; Bär and Hechter, 1969; Sutherland *et al.*, 1965; Rodbell, 1967). This in turn leads to an increase in intracellular cyclic AMP levels and subsequently to an activation of a protein kinase (Jost and Rickenberg, 1971; Garren *et al.*, 1971). With respect to the adrenal cell, it has been proposed that the protein kinase would catalyze the transfer of phosphate from ATP to ribosomes. Therefore, it was postulated that ACTH regulates adrenal protein synthesis at the translational level (Garren *et al.*, 1971).

Until now little effort has been made to determine whether or not ACTH acts on the brain cell in a way similar to that on the peripheral target cell. Because ACTH seems to act on rather specific sites in the brain (Steiner, 1970; Motta *et al.*, 1965; Van Delft and Kitay, 1972), it might be difficult to find effects of ACTH on cyclic AMP formation similar to that in the periphery. Work is in progress to elucidate the ACTH-brain receptor mechanism, although with respect to adenylcyclase the observations of Burkhard and Gey (1968) and of Forn and Krishna (1971) do not look promising. Other investigators have found that ACTH treatment of intact mice does affect protein and RNA synthesis in the central nervous system (Jakoubek *et al.*, 1970, 1971a, b), and an extremely high dose of ACTH, injected 60 or 90 min before killing of the animals, resulted in an inhibition of uridine incorporation into RNA of spinal motoneurons and glial cell nuclei (Jakoubek *et al.*, 1971b). Under similar conditions, enhancement of leucine incorporation into proteins was reported (Jakoubek *et al.*, 1971a). However, protein synthesis in whole brain slices seems to be decreased as a result of ACTH treatment (Jakoubek *et al.*, 1970). Since adequate controls were not presented, it is uncertain whether the changes described should be ascribed to ACTH itself, to the increased circulation of corticosteroids resulting from ACTH treatment, or to a combination of both.

In view of the behavioral effects of ACTH analogs, it seemed worthwhile to investigate whether or not these analogs do indeed alter brain stem macromolecular metabolism in hypox rats, despite the observed absence of an effect on the polysome population. Therefore, we treated hypox rats with peptide or placebo (zinc-phosphate) suspension, a procedure similar to that used in the training experiments reported above. A week after the surgery, the rats were injected for 10 days every other day with either peptide suspension (10 μg peptide/ 0.5 ml s.c.) or placebo suspension. The day after the last injection, radioactive labeled uridine or leucine was injected into the rats' brain stems, and the incorporation rate of the precursors into RNA and protein respectively were studied. It appeared that $ACTH_{1-10}$ (7-L-Phe) treatment did not affect the incorporation of labeled uridine into nuclear or cytoplasmic RNA after 70 min of incorporation. However, the same peptide stimulated the incorporation of

[^{3}H]leucine into the acid-insoluble fraction (+ 28%) of both nuclei and cytoplasm after 5 min of incorporation. This fraction represents the same protein fraction whose turnover was affected by hypophysectomy (see above). Under similar conditions it was found that $ACTH_{1-10}$ (7-D-Phe) causes an inhibition of leucine incorporation (−28%) and that $ACTH_{11-24}$ has no effect (Schotman, 1971; Schotman *et al.*, 1972). Work is in progress to characterize the proteins involved and to see whether the observed increased incorporation indeed affects synthesis or is related to uptake and pool phenomena (Reith *et al.*, in press).

These results are therefore of interest because the biochemical effects of these peptides run parallel with their behavioral effects. $ACTH_{1-10}$ (7-D-Phe) has, in both circumstances, an opposite effect to that of the L-form (see also De Wied, 1969). $ACTH_{11-24}$ has an effect neither on avoidance learning nor on brain stem leucine incorporation in hypox rats.

The data with the L-isomer of $ACTH_{1-10}$ are in good agreement with those of Reading and Dewar, who reported a stimulation of glycine and leucine incorporation into brain proteins by treatment of intact rats with $ACTH_{4-10}$ (7-L-Phe). However, under their conditions—incorporation period of 48 h and intact rats—no effect of $ACTH_{4-10}$ (7-D-Phe) was found in this respect (Reading and Dewar, 1971). It is tempting to speculate that the observed neurochemical alterations are indeed related to the action of these peptides on avoidance learning of hypox rats in shuttle-box conditioning.

CONCLUSION AND SUMMARY

Hypophysectomy impaired both avoidance learning and brain-stem macromolecular metabolism in the rat. To study the relationship between the two phenomena, two types of experiment were carried out. First, hypox rats were treated with ACTH-like peptides and trained in a shuttle-box for 10 days. As a result of the peptide treatment, the hypox rats acquired the avoidance task, and showed an increased amount of polysomes in their brain stems. Second, hypox rats were treated with behaviorally active ACTH analogs, one that enhanced avoidance learning of hypox rats ($ACTH_{1-10}$-7-L-Phe), one that had no effect in this respect ($ACTH_{11-24}$) and one whose action was rather opposite to that of $ACTH_{1-10}$ (7-L-Phe), namely $ACTH_{4-10}$ (7-D-Phe).

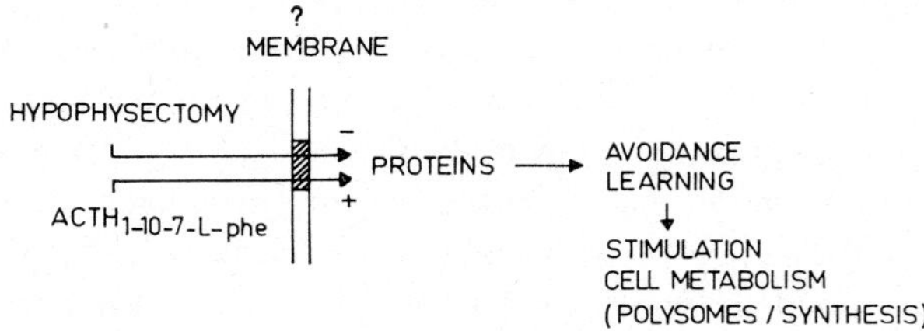

Fig. 1. Hypothetical model of the action of hypophysectomy and $ACTH_{1-10}$ on rat brain and behavior.

Treatment of hypox rats with these peptides enhanced ($ACTH_{1-10}$-7-L-Phe), impaired ($ACTH_{1-10}$-7-L-Phe), or did not affect ($ACTH_{11-24}$) the incorporation of [^{3}H]-leucine into brain stem cytoplasmic proteins. The observation that hypophysectomy *per se* also affected this incorporation of leucine is further evidence that brain stem macromolecular metabolism and avoidance learning of rats are closely related to one another (assuming that the incorporation rate of leucine into proteins under the present conditions reflects synthesis of proteins). In Fig. 1, a tentative scheme is given, representing the current interpretation of our data.

Removal of the pituitary would deplete the rate of pituitary peptides and their breakdown products. These peptides would play a crucial role in certain avoidance learning of the animal. Their mechanism of action would be an interaction with the cell membranes of certain brain centers (adenylcyclase?) leading to an enhanced production of certain proteins which appear to be absent from the hypox rat. As a result of the lack of these pituitary peptides the hypox rat is unable to store the information necessary to master the task in long-term shuttle-box conditioning. Substitution of ACTH-like peptides enhances the production of the proteins involved and therefore leads to a normal acquisition behavior. This in turn would run parallel with a hyperactivity of the circuits involved in the acquisition process and this would account for the observed increase in brain stem polysomes. Therefore, acquisition would trigger an alteration in macromolecular metabolism; and it is likely that subsequent consolidation of the newly acquired information is dependent on this specific alteration. However, it should be kept in mind that the model is only speculative at present. More work is in progress to assess the validity of the hypothesis.

ACKNOWLEDGEMENTS

W. H. G. is greatly indebted to the Division of Chemical Neurobiology, Department of Biochemistry, University of North Carolina, Medical School, Chapel Hill, N.C., for their hospitality and their helpful discussions during the preparation of the manuscript. The authors wish to thank Drs. Landfield and Wilson (Chapel Hill) and Drs. De Wied and Witter (Utrecht) for reading the manuscript.

REFERENCES

Adair, L. B., Wilson, J. E., Zemp, J. W. and Glassman, E. (1968a) Brain function and macromolecules, III. Uridine incorporation into polysomes of mouse brain during short-term avoidance learning. *Proc. natl. Acad. Sci. (U.S.)*, **61**, 606–613.

Adair, L. B., Wilson, J. B. and Glassman, E. (1968b) Brain function and macromolecules, IV. Uridine incorporation during different behavioral experiments. *Proc. natl. Acad. Sci. (U.S.)*, **61**, 917–922.

Applezweig, M. H. and Baudry, F. D. (1955) The pituitary-adrenocortical system in avoidance learning, *Psychol. Rep.*, **1**, 417–420.

Applezweig, M. H. and Moeller, G. (1959) The pituitary-adrenocortical system and anxiety in avoidance learning. *Acta psychol.*, **15**, 602–603.

Bär, H. P. and Hechter, O. (1969) Adenyl cyclase and hormone action, I. Effects of adrenocorticotropic hormone, glucagon and epinephrine on the plasma membrane of rat fat cells. *Proc. natl. Acad. Sci. (U.S.)*, **63**, 351–355.

BARDEN, N. AND KORNER, A. (1969) A defect in the 40s ribosomal subunit after hypophysectomy of the rat. *Biochem. J.*, **114**, 30P.

BEACH, G., EMMENS, M., KIMBLE, D. P. AND LICKEY, M. (1969) Autoradiographic demonstration of biochemical changes in the limbic system during avoidance training. *Proc. natl. Acad. Sci. (U.S.)*, **62**, 692–696.

BOCHOCH, S. (1968) *The Biochemistry of Memory*. Oxford University Press, London.

BOHUS, B. AND ENDRÖCZI, E. (1965) The influence of pituitary-adrenocortical function on the avoiding conditioned reflex activity in rats. *Acta physiol. acad. sci. hung.*, **26**, 183–189.

BOWMAN, R. E. AND STROBEL, D. A. (1969) Brain RNA metabolism in the rat during learning. *J. comp. physiol. Psychol.*, **67**, 448–456.

BREWER, E. N., FOSTER, L. B., SELLS, B. H. (1969) A possible role for ribonuclease in the regulation of protein synthesis in normal and hypophysectomized rats. *J. biol. Chem.*, **244**, 1389–1392.

BURKHARD, W. P. AND GEY, K. F. (1968) Adenyl cyclase in rat brain. *Helv. physiol. pharmacol. acta*, **26**, 197–198.

CARDELL JR., R. R. (1967) Subcellular alterations in rat liver following hypophysectomy. *Biochim. biophys. acta*, **148**, 539–552.

CARDELL JR., R. R. (1970) Effects of hypophysectomy and chronic administration of somatotropin on the fine structure of rat liver cells. *J. Cell Biol.*, **47**, 30a.

CARRERES, Q. J. (1970) RNA, hippocampus and learning. An autoradiographic study. *Acta anat. (Basel)*, **75**, 27–36.

CHEEK, D. B. AND GRAYSTONE, J. (1969) Action of insulin, growth hormone and epinephrine on cell growth in liver, muscle and brain of the hypophysectomized rat. *Pediat. Res.*, **3**, 77–88.

CLEMENS, M. J. AND KORNER, A. (1970) Amino acid requirement for the growth hormone stimulation of incorporation of precursors into protein and nucleic acids of liver slices. *Biochem. J.*, **119**, 629–634.

COLEMAN, M. S., PFINGST, B., WILSON, J. B. AND GLASSMAN, E. (1971) Brain function and macromolecules, VIII. Uridine incorporation into brain polysomes of hypophysectomized rats and ovariectomized mice during avoidance conditioning. *Brain Res.*, **26**, 349–360.

DELLWEG, H., GERNER, R. AND WACKER, A. (1968) Quantitative and qualitative changes in ribonucleic acids of rat brain dependent on age and training experiences. *J. Neurochem.*, **15**, 1109–1119.

DE VELLIS, J. AND INGLISH, D. (1968) Hormonal control of glycerolphosphate dehydrogenase in rat brain. *J. Neurochem.*, **15**, 1061–1070.

DE WIED, D. (1964) Influence of anterior pituitary on avoidance learning and escape behavior. *Amer. J. Physiol.*, **207**, 255–259.

DE WIED, D. (1969) Effects of peptide hormones on behavior. In *Frontiers in Neuroendocrinology*, W. F. GANONG AND L. MARTINI (Eds.), Oxford University Press, New York, pp. 97–140.

DE WIED, D., BOHUS, B. AND GREVEN, H. M. (1968) Influence of pituitary and adrenocortical hormones on conditioned avoidance behaviour in rats. In *Endocrinology and Human Behaviour* (Proc. Conf. Inst. of Psychiat., London, May 9–11, 1967), R. P. MICHAEL (Ed.), Oxford University Press, London, pp. 188–199.

DE WIED, D., WITTER, A. AND LANDE, S. (1970) Anterior pituitary peptides and avoidance acquisition of hypophysectomized rats. In *Pituitary, Adrenal and the Brain* (Progress in Brain Research, Vol. 32), D. DE WIED AND J. A. W. M. WEIJNEN (Eds.), Elsevier, Amsterdam, pp. 213–220.

DE WIED, D., VAN DELFT, A. M. L., GISPEN, W. H., WEIJNEN, J. A. W. M. AND VAN WIMERSMA GREIDANUS, TJ. B. (1972) The role of pituitary-adrenal system hormones in active-avoidance conditioning. In *Hormones and Behavior*, S. LEVINE (Ed.), Academic Press, New York, 135–171.

DIAMOND, M. C. (1968) The effects of early hypophysectomy and hormone therapy on brain development. *Brain Res.*, **7**, 407–418.

DUNN, A. J. AND KORNER, A. (1966) Hypophysectomy and amino acid incorporation in a rat brain-cell-free system. *Biochem. J.*, **100**, 76P.

DUNN, A., BROGAN, L., ENTINGH, D., ENTINGH, T., GISPEN, W. H., MACHLUS, B., PERUMAL, R. AND REES, H. D. (1973) Biochemical correlates of brief behavioral experiences. In *The Neurosciences, The Third Study Program*, F. O. SCHMITT (Ed.), M.I.T. Press, Boston, in press.

ENDRÖCZI, E., LISSÁK, K., FEKETE, T. AND DE WIED, D. (1970) Effects of ACTH and EEG habituation in human subjects. In *Pituitary, Adrenal and the Brain* (Progress in Brain Research, Vol. 32), D. DE WIED AND J. A. W. M. WEIJNEN (Eds.), Elsevier, Amsterdam, pp. 254–262.

FLEXNER, J. B. AND FLEXNER, L. B. (1967) Restoration of expression of memory lost after treatment with puromycine. *Proc. natl. Acad. Sci. (U.S.)*, **57**, 1651–1654.

FLEXNER, J. B. AND FLEXNER, L. B. (1970) Adrenalectomy and the suppression of memory by puromycin. *Proc. natl. Acad. Sci. (U.S.)*, **66**, 48–52.

FLEXNER, J. B. AND FLEXNER, L. B. (1971) Pituitary peptides and the suppression of memory by puromycin. *Proc. natl. Acad. Sci. (U.S.)*, **68**, 2519–2521.

FLEXNER, L. B., FLEXNER, J. B. AND ROBERTS, R. B. (1967) Memory in mice analyzed with antibiotics. *Science*, **155**, 1377–1383.

FORN, J. AND KRISHNA, G. (1971) Effect of norepinephrine, histamine and other drugs on cyclic 3′ 5′-AMP formation in brain slices of various animal species. *Pharmacology*, **5**, 193–204.

FOSTER, L. B. AND SELLS, B. H. (1969) Functional capacity of intact and hybrid ribosomes from livers of normal and hypophysectomized rats. *Arch. Biochem. Biophys.*, **132**, 561–564.

GARREN, D., RICHARDSON JR., A. P. AND CROCCO, R. M. (1967) The role of ribosomes in the regulation of protein synthesis in hypophysectomized and thyroidectomized rats. *J. biol. Chem.*, **242**, 650–656.

GARREN, L. D., GILL, G. N., MASUI, H. AND WALTON, G. M. (1971) On the mechanism of action of ACTH. *Recent Progr. Hormone Res.*, **27**, 433–478.

GEEL, S. E. AND TIMIRAS, P. S. (1970) The role of hormones in cerebral protein metabolism. In *Protein Metabolism of the Nervous System*, A. LAJTHA (Ed.), Plenum, New York, pp. 335–353.

GISPEN, W. H. (1970) On the relation between the deficient conditioned avoidance behaviour of hypophysectomized rats and the RNA metabolism in the brain stem. *Thesis, University of Utrecht.*

GISPEN, W. H. AND SCHOTMAN, P. (1970) Effect of hypophysectomy and conditioned avoidance behavior on macromolecule metabolism in the brain stem of the rat. In *Pituitary, Adrenal and the Brain* (Progress in Brain Research, Vol. 32), D. DE WIED AND J. A. W. M. WEIJNEN (Eds.), Elsevier, Amsterdam, pp. 236–244.

GISPEN, W. H., VAN WIMERSMA GREIDANUS, TJ. B. AND DE WIED, D. (1970a) Effects of hypophysectomy and ACTH 1–10 on responsiveness to electric shock in rats. *Physiol. Behav.*, **5**, 143–146.

GISPEN, W. H., DE WIED, D., SCHOTMAN, P. AND JANSZ, H. S. (1970b) Effects of hypophysectomy on RNA metabolism in rat brain stem. *J. Neurochem.*, **17**, 751–761.

GISPEN, W. H., DE WIED. D., SCHOTMAN, P. AND JANSZ, H. S. (1970c) On the relationship between the deficient performance of hypophysectomized rats in shuttle-box conditioning and the RNA metabolism in their brain stem. (Abstr.) 2nd Annual Meeting European Brain and Behaviour Society, Oxford, September 7th–10th, 1970. *Brain Res.*, **24**, 551.

GISPEN, W. H., DE WIED, D., SCHOTMAN, P. AND JANSZ, H. S. (1971) Brain stem polysomes and avoidance performance of hypophysectomized rats subjected to peptide treatment. *Brain Res.*, **31**, 341–351.

GISPEN, W. H., SCHOTMAN, P. AND DE KLOET, E. R. (1972) Brain RNA and hypophysectomy; A topographical study. *Neuroendocrinology*, **9**, 285–296.

GISPEN, W. H., VAN DER POEL, A. M. AND VAN WIMERSMA GREIDANUS, TJ. B. (1973) Pituitary-adrenal influences on behavior; ethological aspects and responsiveness to electric footshock. *Physiol. Behav.*, in press.

GLASSMAN, E. (1969) The biochemistry of learning; an evaluation of the role of RNA and protein. *Ann. Rev. Biochem.*, **38**, 605–646.

GLASSMAN, E., GISPEN, W. H., PERUMAL, R., MACHLUS, B. AND WILSON, J. (1972) The effect of short experiences on the incorporation of phosphate into synaptosomal and non-histone acid-extractable nuclear proteins from rat and mouse. (Abstr.) *5th International Congress on Pharmacology*, San Francisco, July 23rd–28th, p. 265.

GLASSMAN, E., GISPEN, W. H., PERUMAL, R., MACHLUS, B. AND WILSON, J. (1973) The effect of short experiences on the incorporation of radioactive phosphate into synaptosomal and non-histone acid-extractable nuclear proteins from rat and mouse brain. In *Proceedings of the Symposium on "Pharmacological Agents on Memory and Learning"* (5th Int. Congr. Pharmacol., San Francisco, July 27th, 1972) in press.

GUPTA, S. L. AND TALWAR, G. P. (1968) Effect of growth hormone on ribonucleic acid metabolism. The template activity of the chromatin and molecular species of ribonucleic acid synthesized after treatment with the hormone. *Biochem. J.*, **110**, 401–406.

HENSHAW, E. C., HIRSCH, C. A., MORTON, B. E. AND HIATT, H. (1971) Control of protein synthesis in mammalian tissues. *J. biol. Chem.*, **246**, 436–446.

HERRLICH, P. AND LANG, N. (1967) Influence of growth hormone on template RNA and ribosomes from rat liver. *Z. physiol. Chem.*, **348**, 1377–1380.

HOFMANN, K., WINGERDEN, W. AND FINN, F. M. (1970) Correlation of adrenocorticotropic activity of ACTH analogs with degree of binding to an adrenal cortical particulate preparation. *Proc. natl. Acad. Sci. (U.S.)*, **67**, 829–836.

Horn, G., Horn, A. L. D., Bateson, P. P. G. and Rose, S. P. R. (1971) Effects of imprinting on uracil incorporation into brain RNA in the "split-brain" chick. *Nature (Lond.)*, **229**, 131–132.

Hydén, H. and Egyhazi, E. (1962) Changes in the base composition of nuclear ribonucleic acid of neurons during a short period of enhanced production. *Proc. natl. Acad. Sci. (U.S.)*, **48**, 1366.

Hydén, H. and Egyhazi, E. (1963) Glial RNA changes during a learning experiment in rats. *Proc. natl. Acad. Sci. (U.S.)*, **49**, 618–624.

Hydén, H. and Egyhazi, E. (1964) Changes in RNA content and base composition in cortical neurons of rats in a learning experiment involving transfer of handiness. *Proc. natl. Acad. Sci. (U.S.)*, **52**, 1030–1035.

Hydén, H. and Lange, P. W. (1969) Protein synthesis during learning. *Science*, **164**, 200–201.

Hydén, H. and Lange, P. W. (1970a) Brain-cell protein synthesis specially related to learning. *Proc. natl. Acad. Sci. (U.S.)*, **65**, 898–904.

Hydén, H. and Lange, P. W. (1970b) Protein synthesis in limbic structures during change in behavior. *Brain Res.*, **22**, 423–425.

Jakoubek, B., Semiginovsky, B., Kraus, M. and Erdössova, R. (1970) The alteration of protein metabolism of the brain cortex induced by anticipation, stress and ACTH. *Life Sci.*, **9**, 1169–1179.

Jakoubek, B., Semiginovsky, B. and Dedicova, A. (1971a) The effect of ACTH on the synthesis of proteins in spinal motoneurons as studied by autoradiography. *Brain Res.*, **25**, 133–141.

Jakoubek, B., Pavlik, A., Hajek, I. and Burorescova, M. (1971b) The effect of ACTH on the incorporation of [^{3}H]uridine into RNA of spinal motoneurons. (Abstr.) *3rd Meeting International Society for Neurochemistry, Budapest, July 5th–9th*, J. Domonkos, A. Fonyó, I. Huszák and J. Szentágothai (Eds.), Akadémiai Kaidó, Budapest, p. 198.

Jost, J. P. and Rickenberg, H. V. (1971) Cyclic AMP. *Ann. Rev. Biochem.*, **40**, 741–774.

Kahan, B. E., Krigman, M. R., Wilson, J. E. and Glassman, E. (1970) Brain function and macromolecules, VI. Autoradiographic analysis of the effect of a brief training experience on the incorporation of uridine into mouse brain. *Proc. natl. Acad. Sci (U.S.)*, **65**, 300–308.

Korner, A. (1964) Regulation of the rate of synthesis of messenger ribonucleic acid by growth hormone. *Biochem. J.*, **92**, 449–456.

Korner, A. (1965) Growth hormone control of biosynthesis of protein and ribonucleic acid. In *Recent Progress in Hormone Research*, Vol. 21, G. Pincus (Ed.), Academic Press, New York, pp. 205–240.

Korner, A. (1968) Anabolic action of growth hormone. *Ann. N.Y. Acad. Sci.*, **148**, 408–418.

Korner, A. (1969) The hormonal control of protein synthesis. *Biochem. J.*, **115**, 30P.

Krivoy, W. A. (1970) Effects of ACTH and related polypeptides on spinal cord. In *Pituitary, Adrenal and the Brain* (Progress in Brain Research, Vol. 32), D. de Wied and J. A. W. M. Weijnen (Eds.), Elsevier, Amsterdam, pp. 108–119.

Lande, S., Witter, A. and De Wied, D. (1971) Pituitary peptides. Octapeptide that stimulates conditioned avoidance acquisition in hypophysectomized rats. *J. biol. Chem.*, **246**, 2056–2060.

Lande, S., Flexner, J. B. and Flexner, L. B. (1972) Effect of corticotropin and desglycinamide-lysine vasopressin on suppression of memory by puromycin. *Proc. natl. Acad. Sci. (U.S.)*, **69**, 558–560.

Libertun, C., Moguilevsky, J. A., Schiaffini, O. and Foglia, V. (1969) Effect of hypophysectomy on the oxidative and glycolytic metabolism of hypothalamus. *Experientia*, **25**, 196–197.

Liew, C. C. and Korner, A. (1969) Growth hormone and the binding of aminoacyl-tRNA to liver ribosomes. *Biochem. J.*, **114**, 63P–64P.

Machlus, B. J. (1971) Phosphorylation of nuclear proteins during behavior of rats. *Thesis, University of North Carolina, Chapel Hill.*

Machlus, B. and Gaito, J. (1969) Successive competition hybridization to detect RNA species in a shock avoidance task. *Nature (Lond.)*, **222**, 573–574.

Machlus, B. J., Wilson, J. E. and Glassman, E. (1973a) Acid-extractable nuclear proteins in brain, I. The effect of short experiences on the incorporation of radioactive phosphate into nuclear proteins of rat brain. In preparation.

Machlus, B. J., Wilson, J. E. and Glassman, E. (1973b) Nuclear proteins in brain, II. The effect of various behaviors and reminding experiences on the incorporation of radioactive phosphate. In preparation.

McDonald, R. I. and Korner, A. (1971) Growth hormone stimulation of protein synthetic activity of membrane-bound ribosomes. *FEBS Letters*, **13**, 62–64.

Moguilevsky, J. A., Libertun, C. and Foglia, V. G. (1970) Oxidative metabolism of the hypothalamus in hypophysectomized, castrated rats. *Experientia*, **26**, 421.

Motta, M., Mangili, G. and Martini, L. (1965) A "short" feedback loop in the control of ACTH secretion. *Endocrinology*, **77**, 392–395.

Nasello, A. G. and Izquierdo, I. (1969) Effect of learning and of drugs on the ribonucleic acid concentration of brain structures of the rat. *Exp. Neurol.*, **23**, 521–528.

O'Malley, B. W. (1968) Hormonal regulation of nucleic acid and protein synthesis. *Trans. N.Y. Acad. Sci.*, 478–503.

Pohle, W. and Matthies, H. (1971) The incorporation of [^{3}H]-uridine monophosphate into the rat brain during the training period. A microautoradiographic study. *Brain Res.*, **29**, 123–128.

Reading, H. W. and Dewar, A. J. (1971) Effects of $ACTH_{4-10}$ on cerebral RNA and protein metabolism in the rat. *3rd Meeting International Society for Neurochemistry, Budapest*, J. Domonkos, A. Fonyó, I. Huszák and J. Szentágothai (Eds.), Akadémiai Kaidó, Budapest, p. 199.

Reiss, M. (1961) Hormones and mental disease. In *Proceedings International Neurochemistry Symposium, Strasbourg, 1958*, J. Folch-Pi (Ed.), Pergamon, New York, pp. 436–455.

Reith, M. E. A., Gispen, W. H., Schotman, P. (1973) Hypophysectomy and brain protein metabolism. In *Int. Symp. on Metabolic Regulation and Functional Activity in the Central Nervous System, Saint-Vincent (Aosta), Italy, September 16–17, 1972*, Springer, Berlin, in press.

Rodbell, M. (1967) Metabolism of isolated fat cells, V. Preparation of "ghosts" and their properties; adenyl cyclase and other enzymes. *J. biol. Chem.*, **242**, 5744–5750.

Rose, S. P. R., Bateson, P. P. G., Horn, A. L. D. and Horn, G. (1970) Effects of an imprinting procedure on reginal incorporation of tritiated uracil into chick brain RNA. *Nature (Lond.)*, **225**, 650–651.

Sawyer, C. H., Kawakami, M., Meyerson, B., Whitmoyer, D. I. and Lilley, J. I. (1968) Effects of ACTH, dexamethasone and asphyxia on electrical activity of the rat hypothalamus. *Brain Res.*, **10**, 213–226.

Schotman, P. (1971) Macromolecular metabolism in the brain stem of the hypophysectomized rat in relation to the conditioned avoidance behaviour. *Thesis, University of Utrecht.*

Schotman, P., Gispen, W. H., Jansz, H. S. and De Wied, D. (1972) Effects of ACTH analogues on macromolecule metabolism in the brain stem of hypophysectomized rats. *Brain Res.*, **46**, 349–362.

Schotman, P., Reith, M. E. A., Visser, J. H. and Gispen, W. H. (1973) RNA and protein metabolism in the brain stem of hypophysectomized rats. (in preparation)

Shashoua, V. E. (1968) RNA changes in goldfish brain during learning. *Nature (Lond.)*, **217**, 238–240.

Shashoua, V. E. (1970) RNA metabolism in goldfish brain during acquisition of new behavioral patterns. *Proc. natl. Acad. Sci. (U.S.)*, **65**, 160–167.

Shashoua, V. E. (1971) RNA metabolism in goldfish during acquisition of new behavioral patterns. (Abstr.) *1st National Meeting of the Society for Neuroscience, Washington D.C.*, p. 61.

Staehelin, M. (1965) Effect of hypophysectomy on rat liver polyribosomes. *Biochem. Z.*, **342**, 459–468.

Steiner, F. A. (1970) Effects of ACTH and corticosteroids on single neurons in the hypothalamus. In *Pituitary, Adrenal and the Brain* (Progress in Brain Research, Vol. 32), D. de Wied and J. A. W. M. Weijnen (Eds.), Elsevier, Amsterdam, pp. 102–107.

Sutherland, E. W., Øye, I. and Butcher, R. W. (1965) The action of epinephrine and the role of the adenyl cyclase system in hormone action. *Recent Progr. Hormone Res.*, **21**, 623–646.

Takahashi, S., Penn, M. V., Lajtha, A. and Reiss, M. (1970) Influence of growth hormone on phenylalanine incorporation into rat brain protein. In *Protein Metabolism of the Nervous System*, A. Lajtha (Ed.), Plenum, New York, pp. 355–366.

Tata, J. R. (1968) Hormonal regulation of growth and protein synthesis. *Nature (Lond.)*, **219**, 331–337.

Tata, J. R. and Williams-Ashman, H. G. (1967) Effects of growth hormone and tri-iodothyronine on amino acid incorporation by microsomal subfractions from rat. *Europ. J. Biochem.*, **2**, 366–374.

Tepperman, J. (1962) *Metabolic and Endocrine Physiology.* Year Book Medical Publisher, Chicago.

Uphouse, L. (1971) Effects of short-term training on macromolecules in mouse brain. *Thesis*, University of Colorado, Boulder, Colo.

UPHOUSE, L. L., MACINNES, J. W. AND SCHLESINGER, K. (1972) Effects of conditioned avoidance training on polyribosomes of mouse brain. *Physiol. Behav.*, **8**, 1013–1018.

VAN DELFT, A. M. L. AND KITAY, J. I. (1972) Effect of ACTH on single unit activity in the diencephalon of intact and hypophysectomized rats. *Neuroendocrinology*, **9**, 188–196.

VAN WIMERSMA GREIDANUS, TJ. B. AND DE WIED, D. (1971) Effects of systemic and intracerebral administration of two opposite acting ACTH-related peptides on extinction of conditioned avoidance behavior. *Neuroendocrinology*, **7**, 291–301.

VERSTEEG, D. H. G., GISPEN, W. H., SCHOTMAN, P., WITTER, A. AND DE WIED, D. (1972) Hypophysectomy and rat brain metabolism: effects of synthetic ACTH analogs. In *Studies of Neurotransmitters at the Synaptic Level.* (Advanc. Biochem. Psychopharmacol., Vol. 6), E. COSTA, L. L. IVERSEN AND R. PAOLETTI (Eds.), Raven, New York, pp. 219–239.

VON HUNGEN, K. (1971) Competitive hybridization with brain RNA fails to confirm new RNA induced by learning. *Nature (Lond.)*, **229**, 114–115.

WURFBAIN-MOOLENBURGH, M. C. W. (1968) De invloed van hypophysectomie en partiële hepatectomie op het aminozuur incorporerend systeem uit de rattenlever. *Thesis, University of Leiden, The Netherlands.*

YATES, F. E., RUSSELL, S. M. AND MARAN, J. W. (1971) Brain-adenohypophysial communications in mammals. *Ann. Rev. Physiol.*, **33**, 393–444.

ZEMP, J. W., WILSON, J. E., SCHLESINGER, K., BOGGAN, W. O. AND GLASSMAN, E. (1966) Incorporation of uridine into RNA of mouse brain during short-term training experience. *Proc. natl. Acad. Sci. (U.S.)*, **55**, 1423–1431.

ZEMP, J. W., WILSON, J. E. AND GLASSMAN, E. (1967) Brain function and macromolecules, II. Site of increased labeling of RNA in brains of mice during a short-term training experience. *Proc. natl. Acad. Sci. (U.S.)*, **58**, 1120–1125.

DISCUSSION

CIARANELLO: Hypophysectomy markedly alters the content of catecholamine-synthesizing enzymes in the adrenal. However, in work done with Drs. Danellis and Deguchi, we were unable to find any effects of the hypophysectomy on the activity of tryptophan hydroxylase or tyrosine hydroxylase in the brain stem.

GISPEN: It has been shown by several authors that hypophysectomy reduces the turnover rate of neurotransmittors in brain (Fuxe and Hökfelt, Progr. in Brain Res., Vol. 32, 42, 1970, Weiss *et al.*, Amer. J. Physiol., 218, 864, 1970). Also Dr. Versteeg in our laboratory showed a decrease in turnover of noradrenaline, dopamine and serotonin in rat brain after hypophysectomy (Versteeg *et al.*, Advanc. Biochem. Psychopharmacol., 6, 219, 1972). Maybe Dr. Hyyppä could elaborate on this.

HYYPPÄ. My data (Hyyppä and Valavaara, 1970) are relevant to their content; really we found a marked increase in noradrenaline concentration of rat diencephalon. No changes were found in cerebral cortex. Hypophysectomy was performed in 3-week-old rats and amine analyses were made 2 months later.

SHASKAN: In studies in collaboration with Dr. Snyder at Johns Hopkins (J. Neurochem., in press) we showed that the turnover of spermidine after intraventricular injection of [^{3}H]putresine had a high turnover rate in brain stem areas (*i.e.* hypothalamus, midbrain, pons and medulla oblongata). Other areas showed markedly lower turnover rates. Since the turnover rate of spermidine has been shown to be closely related to synthesis of ribosomal RNA I feel that our results substantiate your findings.

GISPEN: Our data on uridine and leucine incorporation do indeed suggest that the rate of macromolecule metabolism is relatively high in brain stem areas as compared to the cortex.

WEISS: I am sure you are aware that there are far more differences between an animal that can avoid or escape a shock, and a yoked animal that is helpless than just a difference in learning. I wonder how you feel other differences influenced the data you spoke about and how adequate you feel this design is for studying biochemical changes in learning.

GISPEN: At present I think the quiet control is the best one to use in comparing a trained animal to another animal. For, as you also indicated, the yoked control apparently goes through quite a different type of stress and experience. Therefore, a yoked animal should not be used as the only control for training specific stimuli. On the other hand I would say that the fact that in our studies on phosphorylation of synaptosomal proteins (Glassman *et al.*, 1972) the trained mouse differed in this respect from the quiet animal and that no difference in phosphorylation between yoked and quiet could be detected, might imply that the experimental design used (*i.e.* short-term jump-box conditioning) is indeed adequate to pick up biochemical changes related to a training experience involving learning.

Behavioral Aspects of Melanocyte-Stimulating Hormone (MSH)*

ABBA J. KASTIN, LYLE H. MILLER, RANSOM NOCKTON, CURT A. SANDMAN**, ANDREW V. SCHALLY AND LOIS O. STRATTON

VA Hospital, Tulane University School of Medicine and Louisiana State University at New Orleans and Medical Center, New Orleans, La. (U.S.A.)

Although melanocyte-stimulating hormone (MSH) is known to play a vital role in amphibians such as the frog, an important function for MSH in mammals such as the rat is not well recognized. The frog better adapts to the environment by changing the color of its skin, an effect mediated by MSH. Such rapid alterations in pigmentation do not occur in the rat. Nevertheless, by affecting behavior in mammals, MSH could be said to have retained its role in mediating responses to the environment. This review summarizes the evidence which established an effect of MSH upon the behavior of rats.

Extra-pigmentary effects of MSH upon bodily processes other than the central nervous system (CNS) have been described by several investigators, including ourselves, but will not be mentioned in this review. Work on the behavioral aspects of MSH has been confined primarily to two groups studying similar problems from different points of view. De Wied and his collaborators, who have done the pioneering work in this area, seem to have focused their interest upon corticotrophin (ACTH), considering MSH to be "an ACTH-like peptide" (De Wied and Bohus, 1966), whereas our primary interest has been directed toward MSH itself. Although much work on ACTH and its analogues probably applies to our understanding of the actions of MSH, this review has been restricted primarily to a discussion of MSH.

It was shown many years ago (Murphy and Miller, 1955; Miller and Ogawa, 1962) that administration of ACTH results in resistance to extinction of a conditioned avoidance response. De Wied (1965, 1966) demonstrated that MSH can have the same effect. A rat conditioned to leave its chamber at the sound of a buzzer, thus avoiding electrical shock, ceases this escape type of behavior faster (facilitated extinction) than a control if its pituitary gland has been previously removed. Treatment of hypophysectomized rats with certain peptides like MSH causes the rats to continue their escape behavior even when the shock has been discontinued (De Wied, 1965). Thus, MSH is considered to result in increased resistance to extinction of the con-

* The work reported here was supported in part by grants from the Veterans Administration and NIH (NS 07664 and AM 07467).

** Present address: Ohio State University, Columbus, O. (U.S.A.).

References p. 468–469

ditioned avoidance response. It was shown that the effect of ACTH peptides on extinction of a conditioned avoidance response was independent of the thyroid (De Wied and Pirie, 1968) and the adrenals. Actually, corticosterone had the opposite effect of ACTH, since it facilitated extinction of the avoidance response (De Wied, 1967, 1968).

Initially it was uncertain whether this extra-pigmentary effect of MSH and related peptides was restricted to conditioned avoidance responses, or whether it applied to other types of behavior as well. Accordingly, we studied the effect of MSH on animals tested in an appetitive task. Hungry rats were trained to run to the arm of a T-maze which contained food. After removal of the food, the rats which received MSH continued to run more times, and faster, to the goal box which had previously contained the food than did the rats injected with control solutions (Sandman *et al.*, 1969). MSH was shown, therefore, to affect behavior in appetitive as well as active avoidance conditions.

One of the possibilities explaining the results of these experiments was that MSH caused a rat to continue to make the same response. This perseveration, or lack of inhibition of a response tendency, was tested in a passive avoidance situation. Rats placed in one chamber of a two-chamber apparatus took about 10 sec to enter the second chamber. Electrical shock was then administered as soon as the rat entered the second chamber. After 2 days, the rats were placed in the first chamber again. If the main effect of MSH was to cause perseveration of behavior, it would be expected that the rats injected with MSH would not take any longer than the control rats to enter the chamber in which they had been previously shocked. It was found, however, that under certain lighting conditions rats injected with MSH took about three times longer ($p < 0.01$) to enter the second chamber than the rats injected with control solutions (Sandman *et al.*, 1971a). The study showed, therefore, that rats receiving MSH are capable of inhibiting a response and can avoid an aversive stimulus even better than controls. This finding made it unlikely that the results obtained after administration of MSH in a single conditioned avoidance task (De Wied, 1965) or appetitive task (Sandman *et al.*, 1969) were caused only by perseveration or increase of activity. One should be cautious, nevertheless, in comparing the conclusions obtained from one type of experiment with those obtained under different conditions.

Since a two-chambered apparatus had been used in the passive avoidance study mentioned above, it was possible that rats receiving MSH might have been "active" only in the safe chamber and yet still be considered "passive" because they did not enter the second chamber. This possibility was eliminated by the use of a small platform instead of one of the chambers. After being shocked when stepping down from the platform, rats injected with MSH took significantly ($p < 0.001$) longer to leave the platform than did the controls. This occurred regardless of whether MSH was administered during acquisition, extinction, or both (Dempsey *et al.*, 1972).

Another situation in which the effects of MSH on perseveration could be tested is in performance of a reversal discrimination task. Rats were trained to escape shock in a Y-maze by running to the door which was illuminated. After reaching the criterion of five out of six trials for 2 successive days, the task was reversed so that escape from shock was possible only by running to the arm of the Y-maze in which the door was not illuminated. When tested under conditions of constant illumination, which presumably decreases endogenous release of MSH (Kastin *et al.*, 1967a), rats injected with MSH reversed faster than the animals injected with the control solution (Sandman *et al.*, 1972a). This would not be expected if MSH only caused perseveration of activity in this relatively simple task.

It would seem that once a rat treated with exogenous MSH has learned a simple task, such as avoiding shock (De Wied, 1965) and obtaining food when hungry by running (Sandman *et al.*, 1969), it continues to make that response even when it is no longer rewarded. One might speculate that this behavior is analogous to the darkening of a frog by camouflage, but the darkening may be unrelated to the continued presence of danger since it can persist unrewarded even in the absence of a predator. This behavior can be construed as being adaptive in a simple situation even if it may not always be purposeful. The facilitated reversal learning (Sandman *et al.*, 1972a) in rats receiving MSH also seems adaptive, but the adaptive value of MSH in more complex discrimination tasks (Stratton and Kastin, 1973) may not be so obvious. Of course, all these experiments require replication, and methodological considerations such as the choice of light or dark for the reversal task (Sandman *et al.*, 1971a), may be important. Nevertheless, as an oversimplified construct for consideration of the various behavioral experiments considered so far, we can tentatively think of MSH as having some sort of "adaptive" value in certain simple situations for the rat just as it does for the frog.

Although perseveration does not seem fully to explain the effects of MSH upon behavior, can memory be considered as an explanatory construct? This depends upon how memory is defined. In our present state of knowledge, memory should be discussed only for the specific task being tested. One might infer that rats receiving MSH "remember" to continue to escape from shock, to continue running toward an area which previously contained food, and to avoid entering or stepping onto a chamber where they were previously shocked. Such speculations, however, must be substantiated.

One study specifically designed to test short-term memory utilized a variation of the delayed response paradigm developed by Hunter (1913). In the visual forms of this paradigm, the rat is presented with a response cue which is subsequently withdrawn or blocked from view. After a delay of several seconds, the animal is allowed to respond in the continued absence of the cue. In our study (L. H. Miller and A. J. Kastin, unpublished), hungry rats were trained to run for food to one of four identical goal boxes, the correct goal box being indicated by a light over the door. After the rats had learned this response to criterion, they were injected with either MSH or diluent and run under conditions of delayed response. That is, the rats were placed in a start box, presented with the cue indicating which goal box contained food, had the cue denied them, and then, after a delay of 1, 3, 5, 7, or 10 sec were given the opportunity to respond in the absence of the cue. Rats injected with MSH performed more poorly than did controls injected with saline. They made fewer correct runs than controls at all levels of delay. The animals receiving MSH, however, were much more agitated in

References p. 468–469

the start box and during the delay period it was not unusual for them to jump over the start box door (60 cm high) into the runway. It is possible that the agitation or hunger of the rats interfered with attention, resulting in a decrement in performance. Perhaps motivational variables interact with MSH in a complex way so that more sophisticated designs will be necessary to tease out the effects of MSH on memory. The rather bizarre type of behavior characterized by sporadic hyperactivity observed in the delayed experiment had been observed by us previously (Sandman *et al.*, 1969). It corresponds in some respects to the hyperexcitability seen by Sakamoto (1966) in mice, even though he claimed that MSH caused rats to become drowsy. The results of several experiments involving behavioral effects of MSH could be explained, at least in part, by increased activity.

Accordingly, we measured general activity with a special meter after injection of MSH (Kastin *et al.*, 1973a) in intact and hypophysectomized rats under conditions of rest and mild stimulation when they were either fed or hungry. No significant effects of MSH were found in any of the conditions. Individual variation, however, was very great. In goldfish, preliminary results indicate that intracranial injection of MSH does not cause hyperactivity (Bryant *et al.*, 1972).

The results of the delayed response experiment described above indicate that an effect of MSH on short-term memory cannot yet provide a comprehensive explanation for the various studies in which MSH changed the behavior of rats. Among the alternatives, careful consideration must be given to the possibility that MSH increases the general emotional state of arousal of the animal, at least under certain circumstances.

An increased arousal state may explain the results obtained after administration of MSH to rats tested in a complex brightness discrimination problem. After being trained to avoid electrical shock by running to the arm of a T-maze which was illuminated, rats had to learn to avoid shock by going to one goal box if the entire maze was illuminated, and to the other goal box if the maze was dark. Rats receiving MSH failed to learn the new task as fast as the controls. There was resistance to extinction of the first task and hence slower learning of the second task in the animals injected with MSH (Stratton and Kastin, 1973). It would seem as if MSH might have caused overlearning of a simple task. Since several investigators have shown that high levels of arousal reduce the range of stimulus cues to which an animal attends, it is possible that administration of MSH was associated with increased arousal and hence greater attention to the first problem. One can only conjecture whether the "increased feelings of nervousness, anxiety, and restlessness" which were observed in three women receiving i.v. infusions of MSH (Kastin *et al.*, 1968) reflected an increased state of arousal.

The interaction of emotional state with learning and activity after administration of MSH was investigated in a dual-chamber shuttle box. Both active and passive avoidance responses were tested with different visual cues in the same rats which received either 0.4 or 0.8 mA of electrical shock. No statistically significant differences in acquisition or extinction were found between the rats injected daily with synthetic α-MSH and those injected with diluent (Nockton *et al.*, 1972). The failure of MSH to affect acquisition has been noted many times previously. The lack of an effect of MSH on extinction may have been influenced by the fact that after 75 days of training, only some of the rats had learned the combination task. No differences between these groups of rats were found when tested with a general activity meter or in an open-field maze. This emphasizes again that increased activity does not explain the effects of MSH upon behavior. Body and adrenal weights were also the same in the two groups. To what extent the complexity of the experimental design affected the lack of distinguishable interactions among MSH, activity, emotional arousal, and attention cannot be ascertained at this time.

An effect of MSH upon attention however, was found to occur in some human beings. Tests of visual and verbal retention were performed in five subjects who received synthetic α-MSH and the effects compared with infusion of saline in these same subjects as well as four other controls. A significant improvement in the Benton Visual Retention Test occurred after the infusion of MSH, but no improvement in verbal retention was noted (Kastin *et al.*, 1971a). Perhaps MSH affects the registration of some sensory input in the brain.

A further indication of the effects of MSH upon the attentive process was suggested by measurements of the amplitude of electrical responses evoked in the human brain by threshold electrical stimulation of the median nerve. Administration of MSH caused a significant increase in the averaged somatosensory evoked responses when the subjects were relaxed; this increase became strikingly greater when the subjects paid particular attention to the sensory stimulation. Since the increased averaged somatosensory evoked response completely disappeared when the subjects were distracted, a non-specific arousal effect of MSH upon the CNS was unlikely (Kastin *et al.*, 1971a).

The first effects of MSH upon electrical activity of the human brain were shown several years ago (Kastin *et al.*, 1968). Similar high voltage, intermediate frequency activity and disintegration of alpha activity has been reported in rabbits (Dyster-Aas and Krakau, 1965), rats (Sandman *et al.*, 1971b), and frogs (Denman *et al.*, 1972). The pattern of the electroencephalogram (EEG) in the rat after injection of MSH resembled limbic system electrical activity (Sandman *et al.*, 1971b). In the frog, this type of activity has been found in the preoptic hypothalamic area, but not in the ventral forebrain or posterior hypothalamus (Denman *et al.*, 1972).

About the only other direct effects of MSH upon the CNS which have been reported involve potentiation of spinal reflexes (Krivoy and Guillemin, 1961), stretching activity after intracisternal injection (Ferrari *et al.*, 1961), and decreased amplitude of spontaneous electric discharge of the knife fish (Krivoy *et al.*, 1962). It is safe to predict that the next few years will see increasing investigation of the CNS effects of MSH and the hypothalamic hormone(s) which control its release.

If one were inclined to reason from a teleological point of view, one might interpret the many mechanisms which control the release of MSH as being evidence for its importance. These have been reviewed elsewhere (Kastin and Schally, 1971), and include the pineal, light and dark, stress, various drugs like phenothiazines and morphine, and most importantly, a hypothalamic inhibitor of MSH, named melanocyte-

References p. 468–469

stimulating hormone-release inhibiting factor (MIF). Since that review was published, a "mini-feedback" whereby MSH controls its own release at the pituitary level and complex interactions between the pineal hypothalamus, and pituitary have been shown (Kastin *et al.*, 1971b, 1972a). If the behavioral effects of MSH do have importance in the mammal, many interacting mechanisms are available to control its release.

The recent isolation, identification, and synthesis of two peptides from bovine hypothalamic tissue which inhibit MSH release (Nair *et al.*, 1971, 1972) now permit investigation of their behavioral effects. Recently, MIF has been shown to potentiate the behavior induced by 3,4-dihydroxyphenylalanine (DOPA) in mice (Plotnikoff *et al.*, 1971), reduce the tremor caused by oxotremorine (Plotnikoff *et al.*, 1972a), and reverse the sedative effects of deserpidine in mice and monkeys treated with pargyline and DOPA (Plotnikoff *et al.*, 1972b). The effects of MIF in these animal models of parkinsonism and depression, may involve dopamine metabolism, but do not require the presence of the pituitary gland (Plotnikoff *et al.*, 1971, 1972a, b).

Definite behavioral effects, therefore, have been observed after administration of exogenous MSH and MIF, even though they are not well understood. Does this necessarily mean, however, that endogenous MSH mediates some aspects of behavior in mammals? We have been more concerned, until now, in establishing whether exogenous MSH exerts any behavioral effects whatsoever and then determining the behavioral processes involved. That endogenous MSH is released by stress, such as exposure to ether vapors, was reported several years ago (Kastin *et al.*, 1967b, 1969). More recently, we showed that electrical shock releases MSH and that MSH release can be "conditioned" (Sandman *et al.*, 1972b). In this experiment, rats were shocked in a particular box. The levels of MSH released into the blood in response to this stress were elevated for only a few minutes. When the rat was replaced in the same box without shock 1 or 2 days later, the MSH levels in its plasma again increased, as compared with controls. These findings suggest that endogenous MSH may, indeed, modify or reflect the behavior of rats.

Plasma MSH levels were also measured in more than 500 hospitalized patients. Although the variation among patients was tremendous, the highest values were found in the group who had suffered brain trauma (Kastin *et al.*, 1973). Whether this reflects a non-specific stress or implicates MSH in some CNS processes remains completely unknown.

MSH is a hormone(s) whose presence has persisted in the pituitary gland of vertebrates from very low forms to man. The primary function of MSH in higher mammals no longer seems to be pigmentary, but this is not sufficient reason to assume that MSH has no role in mammals or that the effects of MSH can be ascribed to ACTH. Although the information cannot yet be definitely synthesized into a single, unifying hypothesis, the data presented in this report (Table I) seem to have relevance to such psychological constructs as attention, memory, emotional arousal, learning and perhaps others. The evidence discussed in this review strongly indicates that MSH, by itself, has distinct behavioral effects in mammals.

TABLE I

SUMMARY OF BEHAVIORAL EFFECTS OF MSH

Experiment	*Species*	*Principal effect of MSH*	*Reference*
Conditioned avoidance response			
shuttle box	rat	increased resistance to extinction	De Wied, 1965
pole jumping	rat	increased resistance to extinction	De Wied, 1966
Appetitive task (T-maze)	rat	increased resistance to extinction	Sandman *et al.*, 1969
Passive avoidance task (shuttle box)	rat	increased resistance to extinction	Sandman *et al.*, 1971a
(platform)	rat	increased resistance to extinction	Dempsey *et al.*, 1972
Simple reversal task (Y-maze)	rat	faster reversal	Sandman *et. al.*, 1972a
Complex brightness discrimination task (T-maze)	rat	increased resistance to extinction of first task	Stratton and Kastin, 1973
General activity	rat	no increase	Kastin *et al.*, 1973
	rat	no increase (drowsy)	Sakamoto, 1966
	mice	increased	Sakamoto, 1966
	goldfish	no increase	Bryant *et al.*, 1972
Infusion, i.v.	man	anxiety and restlessness	Kastin *et al.*, 1968
Delayed response for memory	rat	no improvement; agitation	L. H. Miller and A. J. Kastin (this review)
Active and passive avoidance with different visual cues and different shock levels	rat	none	Nockton *et al.*, 1972
Verbal retention test (Wechsler)	man	none	Kastin *et al.*, 1971a
Visual retention test (Benton)	man	increased	Kastin *et al.*, 1971a

References p. 468–469

SUMMARY

The pituitary hormone MSH has been tested in several different behavioral systems. It was found to increase resistance to extinction of a conditioned active avoidance response, a passive avoidance response, and an appetitive response. Perseveration, general activity levels, and memory could not be shown to fully explain the actions of MSH in the tasks studied, but subtle interactions may have been involved. Some studies in rats and human beings indicated an effect of MSH upon the attentive process, particularly visual attention. It is possible that MSH increases emotional arousal which leads to increased attention to some environmental cues. Electrical correlates of MSH activity have been found in animal and man, and endogenous MSH appears to respond to several types of stress. It is speculated that during the course of evolution, MSH has maintained its "adaptive" value for the organism, but that this may apply only to simple tasks. The conclusion is reached that in mammals MSH exhibits definite extra-pigmentary actions upon behavior.

REFERENCES

Bryant, R. C., Petty, F. and Kastin, A. J. (1972) Opposite effects on behavior in the goldfish of β-MSH and MSH-inhibiting factor. In *Proc. 2nd Annual Meeting of the Society for Neuroscience*, p. 118.

Dempsey, G. L., Kastin, A. J. and Schally, A. V. (1972) The effects of MSH on a restricted passive avoidance response. *Horm. Behav.*, **3**, 333–338.

Denman, P. M., Miller, L. H., Sandman, C. A., Schally, A. V. and Kastin, A. J. (1972) Electrophysiological correlates of melanocyte-stimulating hormone activity in the frog. *J. comp. physiol. Psychol.*, **80**, 59–65.

De Wied, D. (1965) The influence of the posterior and intermediate lobe of the pituitary and pituitary peptides on the maintenance of a conditioned avoidance response in rats. *Int. J. Neuropharmacol.*, **4**, 157–167.

De Wied, D. (1966) Inhibitory effect of ACTH and related peptides on extinction of conditioned avoidance behavior in rats. *Proc. Soc. exp. biol. Med.*, **122**, 28–32.

De Wied, D. (1967) Opposite effects of ACTH and glucocorticoids on extinction of conditioned avoidance behavior. In *Proc. 2nd Int. Congr. on Hormonal Steroids, Milan, May, 1966* (Congr. Series, No. 132), Excerpta Medica, Amsterdam, pp. 945–951.

De Wied, D. and Bohus, B. (1966) Long term and short term effects on retention of a conditioned avoidance response in rats by treatment with long acting pitressin and α-MSH. *Nature (Lond.)*, **212**, 1484–1486.

De Wied, D. and Pirie, G. (1968) The inhibitory effect of ACTH 1–10 on extinction of a conditioned avoidance response; its independence of thyroid function. *Physiol. Behav.*, **3**, 355–358.

De Wied, D., Bohus, B. and Greven, H. M. (1968) Influence of pituitary and adrenocortical hormones on conditioned avoidance behaviour in rats. In *Endocrinology and Human Behaviour*, R. P. Michael (Ed.), Oxford University Press, London, pp. 188–199.

Dyster-Aas, H. K. and Krakau, C. E. T. (1965) General effects of α-melanocyte stimulating hormone in the rabbit. *Acta endocrinol.*, **48**, 609–618.

Ferrari, W., Gessa, G. L. and Vargiu, L. (1961) Stretching activity in dogs intracisternally injected with a synthetic melanocyte-stimulating hexapeptide. *Experientia*, **17**, 90.

Hawley, W. D., Schally, A. V. and Lancaster, C. (1973b) Plasma MSH levels in 567 hospitalized patients. Submitted.

Hunter, W. S. (1913) The delayed reaction in animals and children. In *Behavior Monographs*, J. B. Watson (Ed.), Holt, New York, pp. 1–86.

Kastin, A. J., Schally, A. V., Viosca, S., Barrett, L. and Redding, T. W. (1967a) MSH activity in the pituitaries of rats exposed to constant illumination. *Neuroendocrinology*, **2**, 257–262.

KASTIN, A. J., ARIMURA, A., VIOSCA, S., BARRETT, L. AND SCHALLY, A. V. (1967b) MSH activity in pituitaries of rats exposed to stress. *Neuroendocrinology*, **2**, 200–208.

KASTIN, A. J., KULLANDER, S., BORGLIN, N. E., DAHLBERG, B., DYSTER-AAS, K., KRAKAU, C. E. T., INGVAR, D. H., MILLER, M. C., BOWERS, C. Y. AND SCHALLY, A. V. (1968) Extrapigmentary effects of MSH in amenorrheic women. *Lancet*, **1**, 1007–1010.

KASTIN, A. J., SCHALLY, A. V., VIOSCA, S. AND MILLER, M. C. (1969) MSH activity in plasma and pituitaries of rats after various treatments. *Endocrinology*, **84**, 20–27.

KASTIN, A. J. AND SCHALLY, A. V. (1971) Control of MSH release in mammals. In *Proc. VIIth Pan-American Congr. Endocrinol., Sao Paulo, August, 1970.* (Int. Congr. Series No. 238) Excerpta Medica, Amsterdam, pp. 311–317.

KASTIN, A. J., MILLER, L. H., GONZALEZ-BARCENA, D., HAWLEY, W. D., DYSTER-AAS, K., SCHALLY, A. V., PARRA, M. L. V. AND VELASCO, M. (1971a) Psychophysiologic correlates of MSH activity in man. *Physiol. Behav.*, **7**, 893–896.

KASTIN, A. J., ARIMURA, A., SCHALLY, A. V. AND MILLER, M. C. (1971b) Mass action type direct feedback control of pituitary release. *Nature (Lond.)*, **231**, 29–30.

KASTIN, A. J., VIOSCA, S., NAIR, R. M. G., SCHALLY, A. V. AND MILLER, M. C. (1972a) Interactions between pineal, hypothalamus and pituitary involving melatonin, MSH-release inhibiting factor, and MSH. *Endocrinology*, **91**, 1323–1328.

KASTIN, A. J., MILLER, M. C., FERRELL, L. AND SCHALLY, A. V. (1973) General activity in intact and hypophysectomized rats after administration of melanocyte-stimulating hormone (MSH), melatonin, and Pro-Leu-Gly-NH_2. *Physiol. Behav.* (February).

KRIVOY, W. A. AND GUILLEMIN, R. (1961) On a possible role of β-melanocyte stimulating hormone (β-MSH) in the central nervous system of mammalia: an effect of β-MSH in the spinal cord of the cat. *Endocrinology*, **69**, 170–175.

KRIVOY, W. A., LANE, M., CHILDERS, H. E. AND GUILLEMIN, R. (1962) On the action of β-melanocyte stimulating hormone (β-MSH) on spontaneous electric discharge of the transparent knife fish, *G. eigenmannia. Experientia*, **18**, 521.

MILLER, R. E. AND OGAWA, N. (1962) The effect of adrenocorticotrophic hormone (ACTH) on avoidance conditioning in the adrenalectomized rat. *J. comp. physiol. Psychol.*, **55**, 211–213.

MURPHY, A. V. AND MILLER, R. E. (1955) The effect of adrenocorticotrophic hormone (ACTH) on avoidance conditioning in the rat. *J. comp. physiol. Psychol.*, **48**, 47–49.

NAIR, R. M. G., KASTIN, A. J. AND SCHALLY, A. V. (1971) Isolation and structure of hypothalamic MSH release-inhibiting hormone. *Biochem. biophys. res. Commun.*, **43**, 1376–1381.

NAIR, R. M. G., KASTIN, A. J. AND SCHALLY, A. V. (1972) Isolation and structure of another hypothalamic peptide possessing MSH-release inhibiting activity. *Biochem. biophys. res. Commun.*, **47**, 1420–1425.

NOCKTON, R., KASTIN, A. J., SCHALLY, A. V. AND ELDER, T. (1972) Passive and active avoidance responses at two levels of shock after administration of MSH, *Horm. Behav.*, **3**, 339–344.

PLOTNIKOFF, N. P., KASTIN, A. J., ANDERSON, M. S. AND SCHALLY, A. V. (1971) DOPA potentiation; by a hypothalamic factor, MSH release-inhibiting hormone (MIF). *Life Sci.*, **10**, 1279–1283.

PLOTNIKOFF, N. P., KASTIN, A. J., ANDERSON, M. S. AND SCHALLY, A. V. (1972a) Oxotremorine antagonism by a hypothalamic hormone, MSH release-inhibiting factor (MIF). *Proc. soc. exp. biol. Med.*, **140**, 811.

PLOTNIKOFF, N. P., KASTIN, A. J., ANDERSON, M. S. AND SCHALLY, A. V. (1972b) Deserpidine antagonism by a tripeptide, L-Prolyl-L-Leucylglycinamide. *Neuroendocrinology*, submitted.

SAKAMOTO, A. (1966) Hypersensitivity induced in albino mice by melanocyte-stimulating hormone. *Nature (Lond.)*, **211**, 1370–1371.

SANDMAN, C. A., KASTIN, A. J. AND SCHALLY, A. V. (1969) Melanocyte-stimulating hormone and learned appetitive behavior. *Experientia*, **25**, 1001–1002.

SANDMAN, C. A., KASTIN, A. J. AND SCHALLY, A. V. (1971a) Behavioral inhibition as modified by melanocyte-stimulating hormone (MSH) and light-dark conditions. *Physiol. Behav.*, **6**, 45–48.

SANDMAN, C. A., DENMAN, P. M., MILLER, L. H., KNOTT, J. R., SCHALLY, A. V. AND KASTIN, A. J. (1971b) Electroencephalographic measures of melanocyte-stimulating hormone activity. *J. comp. physiol. Psychol.*, **76**, 103–109.

SANDMAN, C. A., MILLER, L. H., KASTIN, A. J. AND SCHALLY, A. V. (1972a) A neuroendocrine influence on attention and memory. *J. comp. physiol. Psychol.*, in press.

SANDMAN, C. A., KASTIN, A. J., SCHALLY, A. V., KENDALL, J. W. AND MILLER, L. H. (1972b) Neuroendocrine responses to physical and psychological stress. *J. comp. physiol. Psychol.*, in press.

STRATTON, L. AND KASTIN, A. J. (1973) Melanocyte-stimulating hormone (MSH) in learning and extinction of two problems. *Physiol. Behav.*, in press.

DISCUSSION

McCAULEY: May I inquire as to what type of mental disorder is associated with high levels of MSH?

KASTIN: In collaboration with Drs. Hawley, Miller and Schally, we have recently measured plasma MSH levels in 567 hospitalized patients who were classified by disease system and process. Patients with brain trauma were found to have the highest levels of plasma MSH. In these hospitalized patients, as in some other conditions in man and animals, no correlation was found between MSH and ACTH release even though they frequently are secreted together.

KRIVOY: I would like to call your attention to studies by Dr. Guillemin and by Drs. Lane and Kroeger in which they showed that β-MSH increased the Sherringtonian type of central excitatory state. I would also like to ask Dr. Kastin if he thinks that MSH might be synthesized by several tissues.

KASTIN: We have no evidence to support the possibility that tissues other than the pituitary produce MSH. However, those, including Dr. Schally, who have extracted hypothalamic tissues for other purposes have consistently found MSH in the hypothalamus. The question remains, is this MSH due to contamination or does this reflect some sort of feedback such as the short feedback we've shown to exist for MSH from the pituitary to the hypothalamus. A third possibility is the one that Dr. Krivoy just indicated, namely synthesis of MSH by the hypothalamus.

BOHUS: Do you have any explanation for the difference in the effect of MSH on two types of reversal learning.

KASTIN: We feel that the complexity of the task accounts for the differences. It is well known that, in a highly attentive animal, reversal learning is potentiated whereas tasks in which extradimensional shifts are involved are more difficult.

SACHS: We know that some of the pituitary peptide hormones can act in a short feedback loop mechanism on specific hypothalamic neurons. Is it possible that effects reported here reflect the non-specific influence of these specific feedback sensitive hypothalamic neurons on many other neurons of the CNS?

KASTIN: Of course this is a possibility, but it is not supported by our study in the human being where the effects of MSH were obtained only under conditions when the subjects were paying particular attention to the task; they were not present when the subject was distracted. This seems to mitigate against a non-specific effect of MSH on the CNS, but we can't rule it out.

Hormones and Avoidance Behavior: A Different Approach Points to a Role for Mineralocorticoids

JAY M. WEISS AND PETER GRAY

Rockefeller University, New York, N.Y. (U.S.A.)

INTRODUCTION

To date, investigators who have attempted to show that hormones can affect behavior have done so either by injecting hormones or by surgically removing glands to alter hormone secretion. While these methods clearly alter the hormonal composition of the organism, such approaches do not reproduce normal, physiological, hormonal changes. Consequently, we do not yet know whether the intriguing effects of hormones that have been discerned by various experimental procedures are actually important, or even valid, influences upon behavior when the hormones in question are secreted through physiologically normal pathways in physiological amounts. As a first step toward answering this question, the series of studies described in this paper was carried out. The investigation comprised the doctoral dissertation of one of the authors of this paper (Peter Gray), for which the other author (Jay Weiss) was the advisor.

The investigation was divided into three parts. First, normal animals were exposed to a stressful event that would presumably cause the endogenous secretion of various stress-induced hormones, thereby insuring that the hormonal secretion would occur through normal pathways in physiological amounts. Following exposure to the stressful event, the animals were tested in a behavioral task to observe any effects that these normally secreted hormones might have on behavioral performance. This paradigm constituted the first phase of the project; its purpose was simply to determine whether a "pre-stress", presumably causing endogenous release of hormones, could alter behavior. If the animals showed some consistent behavioral change following exposure to the stressor, this would clearly raise the possibility that hormones, secreted endogenously, do influence behavior.

The initial experiments showed that exposure to a pre-stress did, in fact, affect avoidance behavior. The second phase of the project was then initiated. In this phase, a series of experiments were carried out to describe the nature of this effect. Did the change in avoidance responding occur because a particular kind of pre-stress stimulus was used or would a wide variety of stressor stimuli also produce this effect? Could the effect of the pre-stress stimulus best be described as changing the motivational level of the animal? Questions such as these were asked in this section.

After a number of salient questions about the nature of the effect had been answered,

Reference p. 480

the investigation entered the third phase. This section was perhaps the most important from the point of view of hormonal study, for the experiments undertaken in it were designed to determine whether the behavioral change after pre-stress did, in fact, depend upon hormones secreted in response to the pre-stress, and to determine precisely which hormones were responsible.

GENERAL PROCEDURES USED IN ALL EXPERIMENTS

Subjects

All subjects were Sprague-Dawley albino rats, 250 to 500 g in weight. With only one exception, different subjects were used in each experiment; a total of 209 rats were used in the investigation. All animals were housed individually within sound-attenuated chambers that were kept in a quiet room used only for this study, so that the animals would not be aroused or disturbed by any extraneous stimuli.

Form of experiments

The general form of all experiments was the same. Principally, these experiments consisted of measuring the avoidance behavior of rats in a standard avoidance procedure. The basic experimental manipulation, also present in all experiments, was to expose an animal to a pre-stress stimulus at some time before the avoidance test or to omit this pre-stress experience. It is important to note that each individual animal was alternately tested in both conditions; on one day, it received the pre-stress stimulus before the test, on the next day it did not receive the pre-stress experience before the test, and so on, alternating between the two treatments. In this way, the avoidance behavior of each animal established the individual behavioral baseline for that animal, so that the effect of the pre-stress could be assessed by comparing each animal's avoidance behavior after the pre-stress with that same animal's base-rate of avoidance behavior when the pre-stress had not been given.

Avoidance test

The choice of avoidance procedure was governed by the fact that we were exploring for the first time the question of whether endogenous release of hormones could affect avoidance behavior. Therefore, an avoidance schedule was selected which seemed to us to offer the maximum opportunity to detect any behavioral change that might occur. The schedule used is called "free-operant" avoidance. The particular conditions employed demanded continual responding from the animal throughout the test session so that the test could detect changes in behavior that began at any time, and lasted for any period of time, during the test session.

The avoidance test was begun by placing the animal into a small compartment with plexiglas walls and a grid floor. Through this floor, the rat could receive an electric shock which consisted of shock pulses 0.5 sec in duration with 0.05 sec between pulses. However, the rat could control this shock by rotating a wheel mounted on one of the walls of the compartment. Whenever the shock occurred, the rat could turn the shock off by rotating the wheel, and the shock would not occur again for 5 sec. Also, if the rat turned the wheel when the shock was not on, this postponed the onset of shock for 5 sec. In short, every response the rat made produced 5 sec of shock-free time, with responses also terminating the shock if it had begun. To summarize the key aspects of this condition, responses in this situation were effective in avoiding and/or escaping shock, but the brief time between any response and onset of the next shock meant that animals were necessarily responding quite often, providing a continual baseline of behavior against which to measure change. In all experiments, animals were given at least five initial training sessions to acquire the response and stabilize their baseline of responding before the experiment was begun.

For the purpose of analyzing the results, those responses that turned off the shock, called escape responses, were separated from those responses made in the absence of the shock to postpone the onset of the shock, which are called avoidance responses. Any wheel-turn that occurred within the first 2-sec period after the shock was scored as an escape response, while any response that occurred after this 2-sec period was scored as an avoidance response.

I. DETERMINATION OF WHETHER A "PRE-STRESS" STIMULUS WOULD AFFECT SUBSEQUENT "FREE-OPERANT" AVOIDANCE BEHAVIOR

In the initial experiment, the pre-stress stimulus that each animal received consisted of two shocks (0.5 mA, 1.0 sec duration) given 1 min apart in a small Plexiglas cage (not the test apparatus). The total time for the pre-stress experience was 2 min. The

TABLE I

AVOIDANCE RESPONSE DATA FOR INDIVIDUAL SUBJECTS IN EXPERIMENT 1

Subject	*Mean avoidance responses*					*Percent of total*			
	1st 15 min		*2nd 15 min*		*Total of means*	*1st 15 min*		*2nd 15 min*	
	No pre-stress	*Pre-stress*	*No pre-stress*	*Pre-stress*		*No pre-stress*	*Pre-stress*	*No pre-stress*	*Pre-stress*
N1	59	45	92	166	362	16.3	12.4	25.4	45.9
N2	78	74	214	263	629	12.4	11.8	34.0	41.8
N3	67	162	247	462	938	7.1	17.3	26.3	49.3
N4	797	1047	1354	1522	4720	16.9	22.2	28.7	32.2
N5	770	774	1660	1920	5094	15.1	14.6	32.6	37.7
N6	69	52	197	185	503	13.7	10.3	39.2	36.8
N7	37	79	190	267	573	6.5	13.8	33.2	46.6
						12.6[a]	14.6	31.3	41.5
						1.6[b]	1.5	1.8	2.3

[a]mean; [b]S.E.M.

Reference p. 480

animal was then returned to its home cage. 30 min after the completion of the pre-stress, the animal was placed into the avoidance apparatus and the avoidance test was begun, which lasted 30 min in this particular experiment. On alternate days, no pre-stress experience was given; the animal simply remained undisturbed in its home cage until it was removed for the avoidance test session.

The results of this experiment will be explained in detail so that the method of data presentation can be understood. The "raw score" results are shown in Table I. First, it should be noted that only avoidance behavior is considered; escape behavior did not show consistent effects. Second, it should be noted that the 30-min test session is, for purposes of analysis, divided into periods of 15 min each. Third, it should be noted that the avoidance data are expressed in two ways in Table I: actual avoidance scores (on the left), which have been converted to percentages (on the right).

Looking at the columns on the left side of Table I, one can see that the individual animals varied greatly in their tendency to perform avoidance responses; for instance,

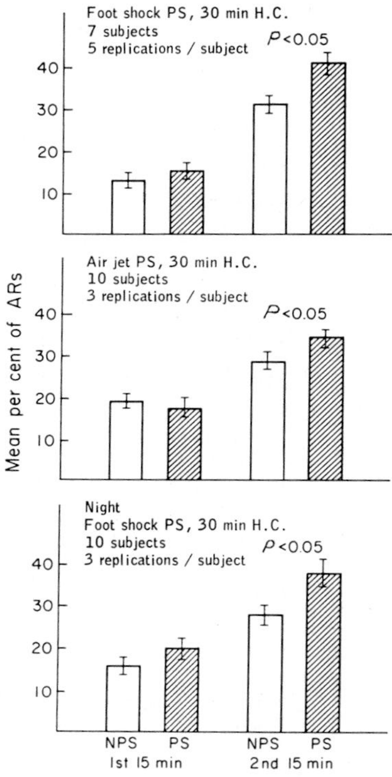

Fig. 1. Mean percentage of avoidance responses (AR) which occurred in each 15-min portion of avoidance test sessions that were preceded either by pre-stress (PS) or no pre-stress (NPS). At top are shown the results using foot shock as the pre-stress stimulus; at center are shown the results using an air jet; and at bottom are shown the results with the procedure conducted at night. A significant difference between two means is indicated by a "p" value above them. "30 min H.C." refers to the time that the animal spent in the home cage between pre-stress and avoidance test. The number of replications refers to the number of pairs of sessions (one PS, one NPS) that were carried out in the experiment.

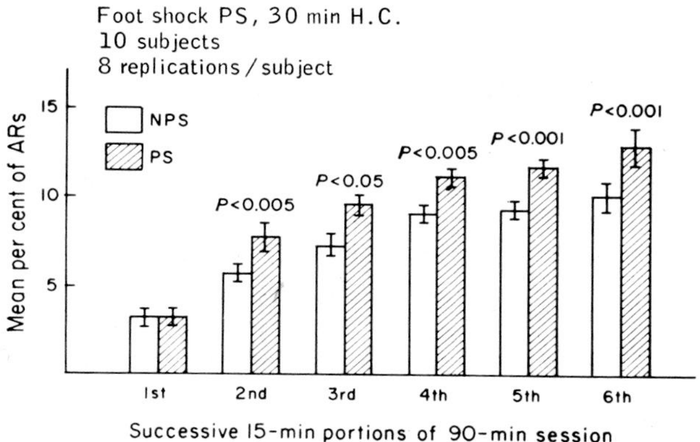

Fig. 2. Mean percentage of avoidance responses which occurred in each 15-min portion of 90-min avoidance test sessions that were preceded either by pre-stress or no pre-stress. Notations in the legend are explained in Fig. 1.

during the initial 15 min of sessions without pre-stress, one animal averaged 797 avoidance responses while another averaged only 37 such responses. But despite this variability, a rather consistent effect of the pre-stress stimulus can be seen. If one compares the avoidance responding made during the second half of the sessions, it is clear that six of the seven animals in the experiment performed more avoidance responses when the pre-stress stimulus was given than they did when it was not given. This effect is significant ($p < .05$ by a dependent "t" test). Although it seemed unusual that the pre-stress did not enhance avoidance behavior in the early part of the avoidance session but only did so in the latter part of the session, this particular effect appeared consistently in each experiment and is hereafter referred to as "the pre-stress effect".

It is much easier to see this pre-stress effect if the large amount of individual variation in overall responding is eliminated. This is done easily by converting raw avoidance scores to percentages, which are shown on the right side of Table I. The center column ("Total of Means") shows, for each animal, the overall measure of its avoidance responding under all conditions; this measure is the sum of the first four data columns on the left. With such a total, each individual column on the left then can be expressed as a percentage of this total, which appears in the four columns on the right. Since these percentages ignore the absolute size of the total, this statistical procedure simply does away with the differences that individual animals showed in their overall amount of avoidance behavior. Looking at the last two columns on the right, one can again see the pre-stress effect—animals made a larger percentage of avoidance responses in the second half of the session following the pre-stress stimulus than they did when no pre-stress was present. The percentage scores are shown in the top section of Fig. 1. Hereafter, the results of all experiments will be shown in this form.

Fig. 2 shows the results of a similar experiment except that the animals were given an avoidance test which lasted 90 min. Again, the pre-stress effect is evident after the first 15 min of the session, and remains throughout the session.

In summary, the initial experiments showed that a stimulus consisting of two shocks

Reference p. 480

would affect avoidance behavior in a test that began 30 min later. Further experiments were then carried out to characterize this effect.

II. FURTHER STUDIES TO CHARACTERIZE THE PRE-STRESS EFFECT

If the pre-stress stimulus affected avoidance behavior *via* hormonal secretion, then any stressful stimulus that would cause the release of "stress" hormones should produce the same result. On the other hand, the augmentation of avoidance behavior might be due to some special characteristic of the shock stimulus that was unrelated to hormones—for instance, receiving two shocks before the test might "alert" the animal to prepare for more shocks coming later. Were this the case, a pre-stress stimulus that was not a shock should fail to augment shock-motivated avoidance behavior. Therefore, an air blast stimulus lasting 1 min, directed into the animal's cage 30 min before the avoidance session, was tested as a pre-stress stimulus. The results using the air blast are shown in the center section of Fig. 1. It can be seen that the air blast was as effective in augmenting avoidance behavior as was the shock stimulus, demonstrating that the pre-stress effect did not depend upon using a shock.

Did these pre-stress stimuli augment avoidance simply because they "woke up" an otherwise lethargic, sleepy animal? Since albino rats sleep during the light portion of the day and the experiments were carried out in the morning, this might be the reason that a pre-stress augmented avoidance responding. However, this proved not to be the case. When the entire experimental procedure was carried out shortly after the onset of the animals' dark portion of the day, when the animals were quite active, the effect was also observed, as shown in the bottom section of Fig. 1.

The investigation now turned to the question of how the pre-stress might be affecting the animal so as to increase its avoidance behavior in the test. Historically, the most common way to explain an increase in avoidance behavior has been to postulate an increase in the subject's motivation; *i.e.*, an increase in fear. Was the pre-stress, perhaps *via* hormonal release, causing an increase in the animal's fear? An experiment was carried out to test this possibility. If the pre-stress added some amount of fear to the test situation, then the pre-stress effect should be virtually lost if the animal were made extremely afraid by the avoidance test itself; in this case, pre-stress could hardly add any substantial motivational increment to a fear level that was near, or at, a maximum. Also, if pre-stress adds fear, the pre-stress effect conversely should be very large if the animal were generally unafraid in the avoidance test; in this case, pre-stress would add a very large motivational increment to the otherwise low baseline of fear. To test these predictions, different shock levels were used in the avoidance test condition; some animals received 0.5 mA as in previous experiments, others were given 0.15 mA, found to be the lowest level that would still motivate responding, and others were given 1.7 mA, found to be the highest level that animals could safely be exposed to. These three shock intensities were also used for the pre-stress shocks, making a total of nine groups (three different pre-stress intensities for each of the three different avoidance intensities).

The results showed that altering shock intensity had no consistent influence on the pre-stress effect. The effect was found regardless of the shock intensity used in the avoidance test, occurring even at 1.7 mA with the same consistency seen at the other shock levels. Also, the effect was present regardless of the intensity used for the pre-stress stimulus, being produced even by pre-stress shocks of 0.15 mA. These findings make clear that the observed effect of a pre-stress on avoidance behavior is not readily explained by saying that pre-stress increases fear.

The final experiment in this section amplified this conclusion. This experiment used a pre-stress which consisted of simply removing the rat from its home cage and allowing it 2 min of exploration in a cage that it was accustomed to. The procedure was designed to elicit little, if any, fear and the animals did, in fact, show considerable exploration and no overt signs of fear (rearing behavior and defecation was counted). This kind of experience given 30 min before the avoidance test produced an increase in avoidance behavior that was just as large as these showed when given the usual shock pre-stress (two 0.5 mA shocks).

III. INVESTIGATION OF THE HORMONAL BASIS FOR THE "PRE-STRESS EFFECT"

The behavioral effects of a pre-stress experience, as defined by the experiments presented above, were quite consistent with the idea that the pre-stress stimulus stimulated hormonal release which, in turn, affected avoidance behavior. Experiments were therefore undertaken to determine whether this was, in fact, the case.

The first possibility explored was that the pre-stress effect depended upon secretion of adrenal hormones. Adrenalectomized animals were therefore tested just as were normal subjects in the first experiment. The results showed that unlike normal animals, adrenalectomized rats failed to show an augmentation in avoidance behavior as a result of the shock pre-stress. Thus, the pre-stress effect clearly depended upon the presence of adrenal hormones since it was eliminated by adrenalectomy. To test whether the effect was lost after the adrenalectomy because the animals no longer secreted adrenal corticoids, hypophysectomized rats were then tested. These animals, of course, can secrete other adrenal hormones but not the corticoids, since corticotrophin (ACTH) has been eliminated. Surprisingly, hypophysectomized rats showed a pre-stress effect, which meant that the effect did not depend upon secretion of hormones from the pituitary-adrenal axis.

The next possibility considered was that the effect depended upon the adrenal medullary hormones, adrenaline or noradrenaline. However, when demedullated animals were tested, they also showed the pre-stress effect. This left the adrenal mineralocorticoids, which seemed quite an unusual candidate for the role of mediator of an effect on avoidance responding. Nevertheless, when adrenalectomized rats, which otherwise did not show the pre-stress effect, were injected with desoxycorticosterone, the pre-stress effect reappeared. Fig. 3 shows the results of a further experiment in which adrenalectomized rats were run under four hormone injection conditions: (*a*) vehicle (sesame oil), and the acetate esters of (*b*) corticosterone (3.0 mg

Reference p. 480

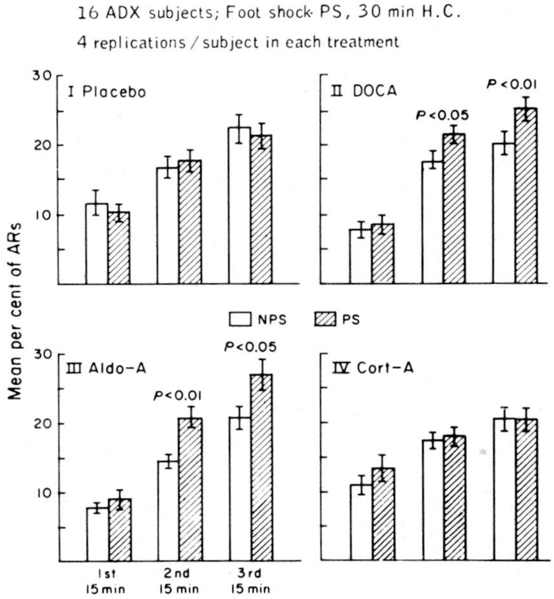

Fig. 3. Mean percentage of avoidance responses which occurred in each 15-min portion of avoidance test sessions that were preceded either by pre-stress or no pre-stress. Each subject was tested under four hormone-replacement conditions. The avoidance test sessions in this experiment were 45 min in length. Notations in the legend are explained in Fig. 1.

per day), (*c*) desoxycorticosterone (0.3 mg per day), and (*d*) aldosterone (0.03 mg per day), which is the natural mineralocorticoid of the rat. It can be seen that the pre-stress effect was absent in the first two conditions but returned when the animal was given either mineralocorticoid.

It was now apparent that the pre-stress effect was indeed dependent upon hormones, but that it was dependent upon mineralocorticoids and not upon any of the hormones classically associated with stress responses, such as ACTH, corticosteroids, or the adrenal catecholamines. Moreover, the pre-stress effect did not depend upon the secretion of such hormones to any stressful stimulus but, rather, simply depended upon the presence of the hormone. This was evident from the following: when adrenalectomized rats were given a single injection of long-acting mineralocorticoid, they showed the pre-stress effect thereafter throughout the course of the experiment. Clearly, these animals could not secrete the hormone since their adrenal gland was removed; their only supply of the hormone came from the circulating level resulting from the injection, and still they showed the pre-stress effect. Thus, the pre-stress effect depended upon the *presence* of some amount of mineralocorticoid in the body. This type of hormonal effect has been called a "permissive" action.

The next experiment showed that the pre-stress effect also could be manipulated in a normal animal that had not undergone adrenalectomy. Normal rats were maintained on 1.5% saline solution, which will greatly reduce, and possibly abolish, aldosterone secretion. Such animals did not show the pre-stress effect, but the effect was restored when they were given mineralocorticoid injection. This finding is important for two reasons. First, it indicates that mineralocorticoid did not restore the pre-stress effect because it restored body sodium and potassium distribution to normal. While desoxycortisone probably had this effect in the adrenalectomized animals because they could drink tap water, the normal animals in this experiment that were treated with desoxycorticosterone and maintained on 1.5% saline were very likely to have been high in sodium and low in potassium. Thus, the behavioral effect of mineralocorticoid described in these experiments represents an aspect of this hormone's action which is independent of its restoring overall electrolyte balance throughout the body. Second, the fact that normal rats lost the pre-stress effect because of a dietary change raises the possibility that the effect discussed above operates in the natural behavior of these animals.

In the final section of the investigation, the time interval between pre-stress and the avoidance test was varied; in all previous experiments this interval had been 30 min. When the interval was reduced to 5 min or less, surprisingly it was found that adrenalectomized rats showed a pre-stress effect. Fig. 4 shows the results for both normal rats and adrenalectomized animals under conditions of (*a*) no pre-stress, (*b*) pre-stress with a 1-min delay before the avoidance test, and (*c*) pre-stress with the usual 30-min delay. The results seen in the third 15-min portion of the test clearly shows how the adrenalectomized rats, unlike the normals, made more avoidance responses following the pre-stress *only* if the interval between the pre-stress and the test was brief (1 min in this case). This suggests that what the adrenalectomized animals lack, and the normal animals possess because of the presence of mineralocorticoid, is the ability to retain some aspect of the pre-stress experience. The nature of what is retained, however, and the role of mineralocorticoids in promoting this retention, is unknown at the present time.

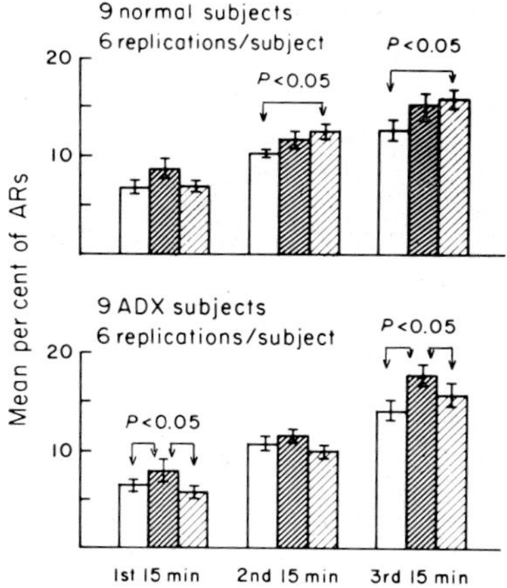

Fig. 4. Mean percentage of avoidance responses which occurred in each 15-min portion of avoidance test sessions that were preceded either by pre-stress or no pre-stress. The avoidance test sessions in this experiment were 45 min in length. Notations in the legend are explained in Fig. 1. □, NPS; ▨, PS_1 (1 min delay H.C.); ▨, PS_{30} (30 min delay H.C.).

Reference p. 480

In summary, it has been shown that a pre-stress stimulus administered to a normal rat 30 min before a free-operant avoidance test will augment its avoidance responding. This augmentation depends upon the presence of mineralocorticoids; without such hormones, this effect will not be seen. While it is not clear how mineralocorticoids permit this effect to occur, results suggest that they enable the animal to retain some aspect of the pre-stress experience which is lost if such hormones are not present.

In closing, we would like to emphasize that this is an initial series of studies which utilized only one avoidance test situation. Our failure to find a behavioral effect of pre-stress that is dependent upon the pituitary-adrenal axis therefore should not be interpreted to mean that ACTH and corticosterone do not affect behavior when secreted endogenously. Indeed, we have previously emphasized that hormonal effects on behavior are likely to be subtle (Weiss *et al.*, 1969), and the particular conditions used may have simply failed to detect the effects of these hormones. Nevertheless, the effects of mineralocorticoids observed in this investigation have led us to reexamine some of our earlier findings. We have reported that adrenalectomized rats show more pronounced passive avoidance behavior than do normal animals (Weiss *et al.*, 1969) and have attributed this effect to high circulating levels of ACTH in these animals. Recent experiments in our laboratory have now shown that the enhanced passive avoidance behavior of adrenalectomized rats is returned to a normal level if adrenalectomized rats are given a single injection of a long-acting mineralocorticoid. Whether the enhanced avoidance behavior that we observed in adrenalectomized subjects was due to ACTH is now open to question.

ACKNOWLEDGEMENTS

The authors wish to thank Dr. George Wolf for his helpful advice. The work described here was supported by grants MH 13189, MH 19991, and GM 01789 from the National Institutes of Health.

REFERENCE

WEISS, J. M., MCEWEN, B. S., SILVA, M. T. AND KALKUT, M. (1969) Pituitary-adrenal influences on fear-responding. *Science*, **163**, 197–199.

The Implication of Noradrenaline in Avoidance Learning in the Rat

K. D. CAIRNCROSS, SUE SCHOFIELD AND H. G. KING

School of Biological Sciences, Macquarie University, North Ryde, N.S.W. 2113 (Australia)

It has been reported that rats rendered anosmic following bilateral section of their olfactory tracts show a performance deficit in aversive learning (Marks *et al.*, 1971; Cairncross and King, 1971). The anatomical and physiological consequences of olfactory deafferentation are profound, and may be enumerated as follows:

(*i*) Degeneration occurs in primary olfactory neurones passing to the allocortex (in the terminology of Pigache, 1970).

(*ii*) Following primary neurone degeneration, transneuronal degeneration occurs involving the pyramidal cells of the allocortex, which is characterised in the rat by a lack of dendritic proliferation (Jones and Thomas, 1962; White and Westrum, 1964).

(*iii*) Following unilateral section of an olfactory tract, a reduction in telencephalic noradrenaline (NA) occurs in the side ipsilateral to the lesion, with no concomitant significant reduction in hypothalamic NA (Pohorecky *et al.*, 1969).

On the basis of the facts presented it appeared that the performance deficit in learning in aversive situations might be related to a reduction in NA availability in the telencephalon. Accordingly, male rats (Carworth CSF strain) 90 days old at the start of the experiment, were placed on a reverse 12-h night–day schedule, and housed in conditions of constant temperature and humidity. Following 14 days' equilibration, the experimental group were subjected to surgery, consisting of section of the lateral olfactory tracts. Control animals underwent the same surgical procedure without olfactory tract section.

The animals were sacrificed in groups of 6, 1–5 weeks after the surgical procedure. The brains were removed, and the cortex and hypothalamus assayed for endogenous NA after the spectrofluorimetric method of Haggendal (1963). The results of this experiment are illustrated in Fig. 1.

It can be seen that the procedure produced a reduction in cortical NA 14 days after the completion of surgery, and that there was no recovery in cortical NA levels during the ensuing 3 weeks. In accord with the findings of Pohorecky *et al.* (1969) there was no significant change in hypothalamic NA. It appeared, therefore, that bilateral olfactory tract section produced a reduction in endogenous NA specific to the cortical region.

Once the specificity of the surgical procedure on cortical endogenous NA levels was established, animals rendered anosmic were subjected to behavioural testing 14–21 days following surgery. The behavioural method consisted of one-way avoidance

References p. 484–485

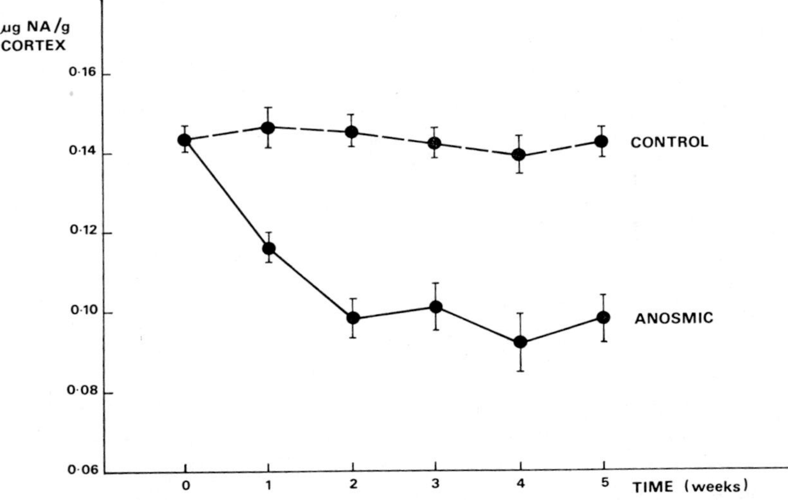

Fig. 1. Reduction in cortical noradrenaline following bilateral olfactory tract section.

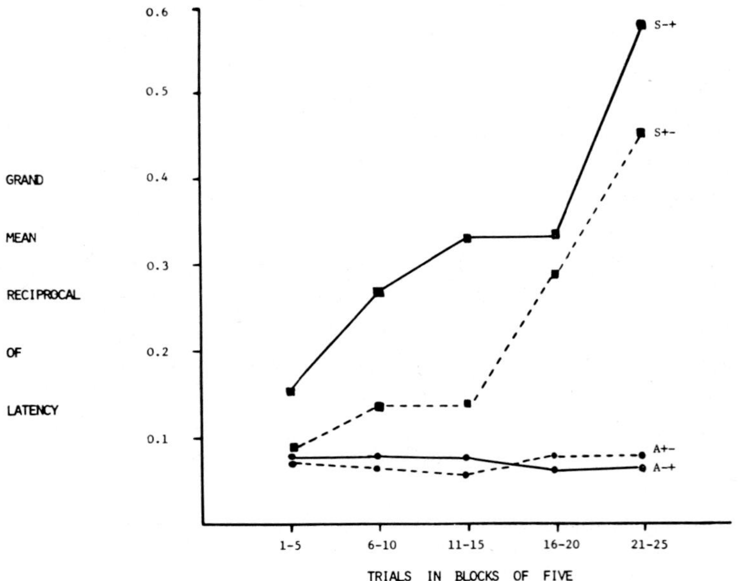

Fig. 2. Avoidance responding on a 1-way task in anosmic and sham operated rats. A, anosmic; S, sham.

learning. The performance of the anosmic animals was compared with sham-operated controls. The results of this experiment are illustrated in Fig. 2.

It can be seen that sham-operated animals quickly learned to escape the aversive stimulus, whereas the anosmic animals showed no such learning ability. It appeared, therefore, that a correlation existed between the physiological and behavioural parameters examined.

To test this hypothesis further, anosmic animals subjected to fear conditioning prior to the aversive avoidance task were examined. It was found that the anosmic group performed poorly when compared with the control group in such a situation. These observations further substantiated the hypothesis that a reduction in cortical NA availability reduced learning capacity. It was argued, therefore, that a pharmacological treatment aimed at increasing cortical NA availability should overcome the

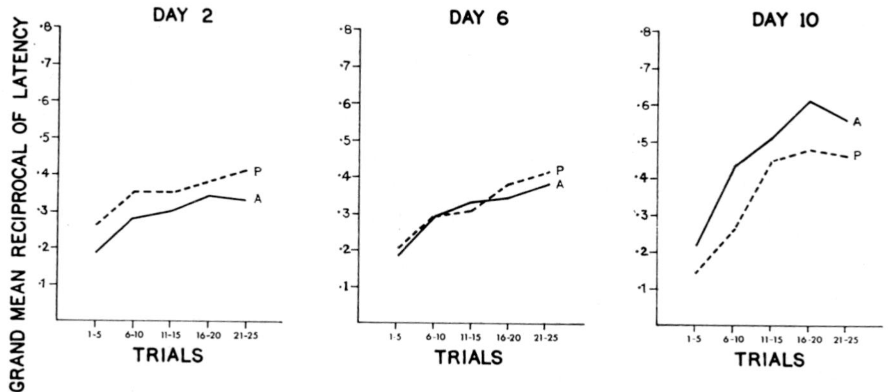

Fig. 3. Avoidance responding on a 1-way task following fear conditioning in anosmic rats. Group A received amitriptyline (1.5 mg/kg i.p., b.d.), group P received no drug, but a similar volume of isotonic saline i.p.

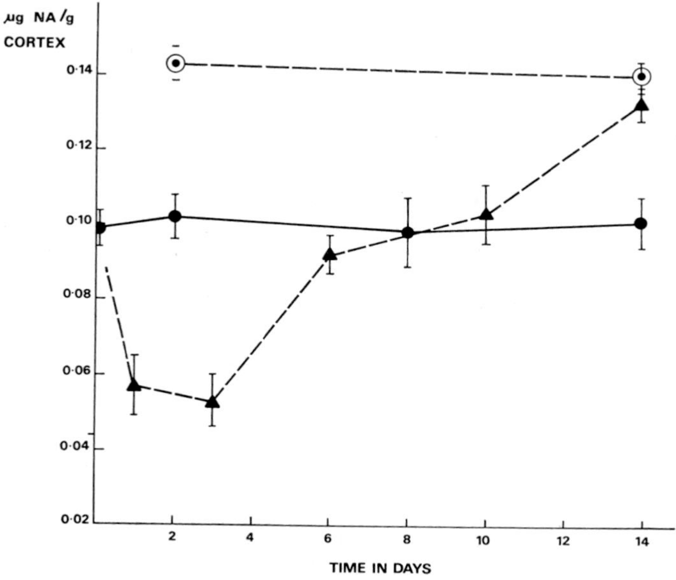

Fig. 4. Recovery of cortical noradrenaline following amitriptyline treatment in anosmic rats. ▲, amitriptyline (1.5 mg/kg i.p., b.d.); ●, saline (i.p., b.d.); ⊙, non-operated controls.

References p. 484–485

learning decrement exhibited by the anosmic animals. In this regard, the cortical and peripheral actions of the tricyclic anti-depressant drug amitriptyline were considered. This drug has been widely used in the treatment of depressive illness for many years, although its precise mode of action remains obscure. It is known, however, that amitriptyline and its metabolic derivatives enhance the peripheral actions of NA (Cairncross, 1965; Cairncross *et al.*, 1967), and that this action relates to the ability of the drug to inhibit the re-uptake of NA into the nerve ending. (Story and Story, 1968). Similar activity has been demonstrated for amitriptyline in the central nervous system (Schubert *et al.*, 1970; Cairncross and Martensz, 1972).

Accordingly amitriptyline was administered to anosmic rats for a 14-day period. A control group of anosmic animals received a similar volume of isotonic saline. The animals were then tested in one-way avoidance learning, following prior fear conditioning. Immediately following behavioural testing, the animals were killed, their brains removed, and the cortex assayed for endogenous NA. The behavioural results obtained are presented in Fig. 3.

Perusal of this figure illustrates that amitriptyline has a biphasic effect on behavioural performance. There is an initial reduction in performance in the amitriptyline-treated group apparent on day 2. By day 6 the amitriptyline-treated animals equate in performance with the placebo-treated anosmic animals, and by day 10 are statistically superior in performance to the placebo group, a situation remarkably similar to that described for the clinical situation (Hordern, 1965).

The effects of amitriptyline on endogenous NA levels in the cortex are illustrated in Fig. 4.

Again, a biphasic effect is evident. The initial response is a reduction in cortical NA, maximal at day 3, recovery to pre-drug anosmic levels by days 6–8, and thereafter an elevation of cortical endogenous NA levels to those found in non-operated control animals. The correlation between the improvement in behavioural performance and the recovery of endogenous NA to control values suggests that the supposition implicating NA in the development of avoidance learning is a phenomenon worthy of further investigation. It is suggested, also, that the results as presented offer a tentative explanation for the mode of action of amitriptyline in the clinical situation.

ACKNOWLEDGMENTS

The work was supported by Grant No. A65/15506 from the Australian Research Grants Committee.

REFERENCES

CAIRNCROSS, K. D. (1965) On the peripheral pharmacology of amitriptyline. *Arch. int. Pharmacodyn.*, **154**, 438–448.

CAIRNCROSS, K. D. AND KING, M. G. (1971) Facilitation of avoidance learning in anosmic rats by amitriptyline. *Proc. Aust. physiol. pharmacol. Soc.*, **2**, 25.

CAIRNCROSS, K. D. AND MARTENSZ, N. D. (1972) Unpublished results.

CAIRNCROSS, K. D., MCCULLOCH, MARION W., STORY, D. F. AND TRINKER, F. (1967) Modification of synaptic transmission in the superior cervical ganglion by epinephrine, norepinephrine and nortriptyline. *Int. J. Neuropharmacol.*, **6**, 293–300.

HAGGENDALL, J. (1963) An improved method for fluorimetric determination of small amounts of adrenaline and noradrenaline in plasma and tissues. *Acta physiol. scand.*, **59**, 242–254.

HORDERN, A. (1965) The antidepressant drugs. *New Engl. J. Med.*, **272**, 1159–1169.

JONES, W. H. AND THOMAS, D. B. (1962) Changes in the dendritic organisation of neurones in the cerebral cortex following deafferentiation. *J. Anat. (Lond.)*, **96**, 359–374.

MARKS, H. E., REMLEY, W. R., SEAGO, J. D. AND HASTINGS, D. W. (1971) The effects of bilateral lesion of olfactory bulbs of rats on measures of learning and motivation. *Physiol. Behav.*, **7**, 1–6.

PIGACHE, R. M. (1970) The anatomy of the "paleocortex", a critical review. In *Reviews of Anatomy, Embryology and Cell Biology*, Springer, Berlin, pp. 1–61.

POHORECKY, L. A., ZIGMUND, M. J., REIMER, L. AND WURTMAN, R. G. (1969) Olfactory bulb removal —effects on brain norepinephrine. *Proc. natl. Acad. Sci. (U.S.)*, **62**, 1052–1055.

SCHUBERT, J., NYBACH, H. AND SEDVALL, G. C. (1970) Effect of antidepressant drugs on accumulation and disappearance of monoamines formed *in vivo* from labelled precursors in mouse brain. *J. Pharm. Pharmacol.*, **22**, 136–139.

STORY, D. F. AND STORY, M. (1968) Studies on the uptake of H^3-noradrenaline by isolated guinea-pig atrial tissue. *Communication presented to Aust. Soc. clin. exp. Pharmacol.*, p. 38.

WHITE, L. E. AND WESTRUM, L. E. (1964) Dendritic spine changes in prepyriform cortex following olfactory bulb lesions—rat, Golgi method. *Anat. Rec.*, **148**, 410–411.

We thank the publishers, authors and editors of the following books and journals for their permission to reproduce material already published by them.

Mem. Soc. Endocrinol. (1971) **119**, 353 (for Fig. 3, p. 26 and Fig. 5, p. 29)
Mechanism of Release of Biogenic Amines, Pergamon Press, New York, 1966 (for Fig. 1, p. 23)
Nature (1971) **232**, 340; (1971) **232**, 341 (for Fig. 7, p. 30; Fig. 8, p. 31)
Structure and Function of the Nervous System, Vol. 5, G. H. BOURNE (Ed.), Academic Press, New York, 1972 (for Fig. 1, p. 89)
Amer. J. Anat. (1970) **129**, 219 (for Fig. 1, p. 50)
Steroid Hormones and Brain Function, C. H. SAWYER AND R. A. GORSKI (Eds.), Univ. of California Press, Los Angeles (for Fig. 2, p. 151)
Endocrinology (1968) **82**, 1010 (for Fig. 4, p. 154)
Neuroendocrinology (1972) **10**, 109 (for Fig. 5, p. 155)
The Neuroendocrinology of Human Reproduction, H. C. MACK (Ed.), Thomas, Springfield, Ill. (for Fig. 7, p. 157)
Frontiers in Neuroendocrinology, L. MARTINI AND F. W. GANONG (Eds.), Oxford Univ. Press, New York (for Fig. 8, p. 158)
Endocrinology (1970) **90**, 867 (for Fig. 1, p. 166; Fig. 2, p. 167)
Eur. J. Pharmacol. (1970) **11**, 266 (for Fig. 1, p. 173)
Neuropharmacology (1973) **12**, 57 (for Figs. 5 and 6, p. 177)
Neuroendocrinology (1972) **10**, 155; (1971) **8**, 257 (for Fig. 4, p. 176; Fig. 2, p. 174; Fig. 3, p. 175; Table I, p. 172)
Endocrinology (1971) **89**, 1464 (for Table II, p. 174)
J. Neurochem. (1970) **17**, 261 (for Fig. 1, p. 262; Figs. 2 and 3, p. 263)
Endocrinology (1970) **86**, 278 (for Fig. 5, p. 266)
Endocrinology (1969) **85**, 815; (1970) **87**, 1; (1971) **88**, 1003; (1972) **88**, 1012; (1971) **88**, 1288; (1971) **88**, 1294; (1971) **89**, 1042 (for data in Figs. 4, p. 265; 6 and 7, p. 267; 8, p. 268; 9 and 10, p. 269; 11, p. 270; 12, p. 271; 13, p. 272)
J. Endocrinol. (1971) **50**, 679 (for Table I, p. 290)
Experientia (1971) **27**, 844 (for Table II, p. 291)
Endocrinology (1972) **90**, 1231 (for Figs. 2 and 3, p. 293; Fig. 4, p. 294; Table III, p. 295)
Recent Progr. in Hormone Res., (1972) **28**, 527 (for Figs. 1 and 2, p. 312; Fig. 3, p. 313; Fig. 9, p. 319)
Endocrinology (1955) **57**, 205 (for Figs. 1 and 2, p. 362; Figs. 3, 4 and 5, p. 363, Fig. 10, p. 367)
J. Pharmacol. exp. Therap. (1959) **125**, 241; (1961) **132**, 323; (for Fig. 7, p. 364; Fig. 8, p. 365; Fig. 9, p. 366)
J. biol. Chem. (1971) **246**, 2058 (for Fig. 3, p. 422)

Author Index

Subject Index

International Symposium on Drug Effects on Neuroendocrine Regulation, Aspen, Colo., 1972.

Drug effects on neuroendocrine regulation, edited by E. Zimmermann [and others]. Amsterdam, New York, Elsevier Scientific Pub. Co., 1973.

vii, 502 p. illus. 27 cm. (Progress in brain research, v. 39)

Ne***

"Proceedings of an International Symposium ... sponsored by the National Institute of Mental Health and National Aeronautics and Space Administration, held at Snowmass-at-Aspen, Colorado, U. S. A., 17–19 July 1972."

Includes bibliographies.

1. Drugs — Physiological effect — Congresses. 2. Neuroendocrinology—Congresses. I. Zimmermann, Emery, ed. II. Series.

QP376.P7 vol. 39 612'.82'08 s 73-77069
[RM301] [615'.74] MARC
ISBN 0-444-41129-1
Library of Congress 74 [4]